Fitness Professional's Handbook

Fifth Edition

Edward T. Howley, PhD

University of Tennessee at Knoxville

B. Don Franks, PhD

University of Maryland at College Park

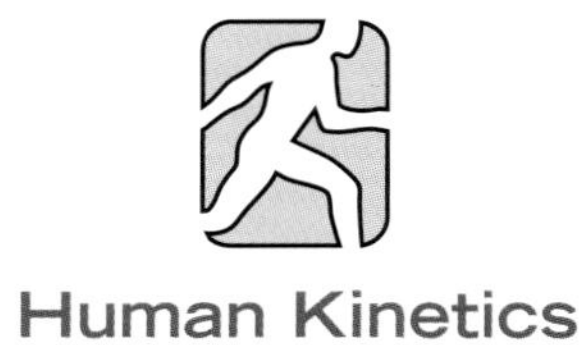

Human Kinetics

Library of Congress Cataloging-in-Publication Data

Howley, Edward T., 1943
Fitness professional's handbook / Edward T. Howley, B. Don Franks. -- 5th ed.
p. cm.
Rev. of: Health fitness instructor's handbook. 4th ed. c2003
Includes bibliographical references and index.
ISBN-13: 978-0-7360-6178-0 (hard cover)
ISBN-10: 0-7360-6178-9 (hard cover)
1. Physical fitness--Handbooks, manuals, etc. 2. Physical fitness--Testing--Handbooks, manuals, etc. 3. Exercise--Physiological aspects--Handbooks, manuals, etc. 4. Health. I. Franks, B. Don. II. Howley, Edward T., 1943- Health fitness instructor's handbook. III. Title.
GV481.H734 2007
613.7--dc22
2006025208

ISBN-10: 0-7360-6178-9
ISBN-13: 978-0-7360-6178-0

This book is a revised edition of *Health Fitness Instructor's Handbook, Fourth Edition*, published in 2003 by Human Kinetics.

The Web addresses cited in this text were current as of August 2006, unless otherwise noted.

Acquisitions Editor: Michael S. Bahrke, PhD; **Developmental Editor:** Amanda S. Ewing; **Assistant Editors:** Jillian Evans and Melissa McCasky; **Copyeditor:** Jocelyn Engman; **Proofreader:** Erin Cler; **Indexer:** Sharon Duffy; **Permission Manager:** Carly Breeding; **Graphic Designer:** Robert Reuther; **Graphic Artist:** Kathleen Boudreau-Fuoss; **Photo Manager:** Laura Fitch; **Cover Designer:** Keith Blomberg; **Photographer (cover):** Clockwise from top left photo: © Human Kinetics, © Human Kinetics, © Banana Stock, © Eyewire/PhotoDisc/Getty Images; **Photographers (interior):** Brenda Williams and Joe Jovanovich, unless otherwise noted. Photos on part openers from Left to Right: © Eyewire/PhotoDisc/Getty Images, © Human Kinetics, © Banana Stock/Gym, © Human Kinetics, © PhotoDisc, © Human Kinetics. Photos on chapter openers from top to bottom: © Eyewire/PhotoDisc/Getty Images, © Human Kinetics, © Human Kinetics, © PhotoDisc, © DigitalVision, © Banana Stock/Gym, © Human Kinetics, © Human Kinetics. Photos on pages 93, 135, and 137 © Human Kinetics; **Art Manager:** Kelly Hendren; **Illustrators:** Mic Greenberg and Al Wilborn

Printed in the United States of America 10 9 8 7

Human Kinetics
Web site: www.HumanKinetics.com

United States: Human Kinetics
P.O. Box 5076
Champaign, IL 61825-5076
800-747-4457
e-mail: humank@hkusa.com

Canada: Human Kinetics
475 Devonshire Road, Unit 100
Windsor, ON N8Y 2L5
800-465-7301 (in Canada only)
e-mail: info@hkcanada.com

Europe: Human Kinetics
107 Bradford Road
Stanningley
Leeds LS28 6AT, United Kingdom
+44 (0)113 255 5665
e-mail: hk@hkeurope.com

Australia: Human Kinetics
57A Price Avenue
Lower Mitcham, South Australia 5062
08 8372 0999
e-mail: info@hkaustralia.com

New Zealand: Human Kinetics
P.O. Box 80
Torrens Park, South Australia 5062
0800 222 062
e-mail: info@hknewzealand.com

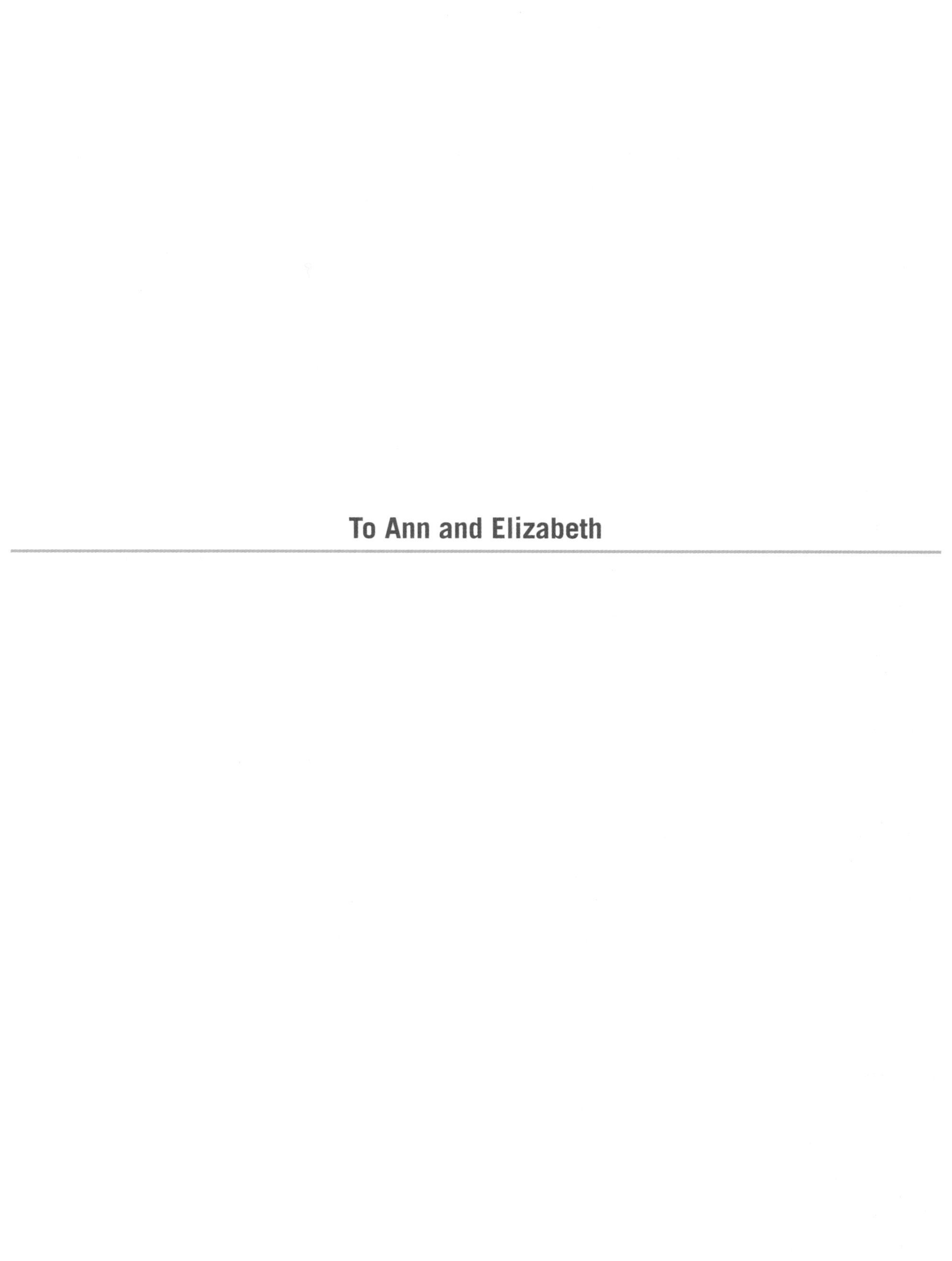

To Ann and Elizabeth

Contents

PART VI Scientific Foundations 415

Preface

You are different from most people. In all likelihood you are physically active, exercise each week, and are concerned about your fitness. In contrast, more than 60% of American adults do not engage in the recommended amounts of physical activity and are overweight. Further, the epidemic of obesity reaches right into the elementary classroom.

Your timing is perfect if you are interested in helping children, adults, or older citizens become more active and improve fitness, health, and quality of life. There is great support from all levels of government to do something about the problems of inactivity and obesity, and success stories already exist. This text will help you get on your way. You will learn how to screen participants for exercise programs, evaluate the various fitness components, and prescribe exercise to improve each fitness component. In addition, you will learn how to help people with chronic disease (e.g., hypertension) or a specific condition (e.g., pregnancy). Recent advances in how to approach these issues demanded a revision of the text, and we hope you enjoy the result.

Updates to the Fifth Edition

One of the first things you'll notice about the fifth edition of this book is the name change. We changed the title from *Health Fitness Instructor's Handbook* to *Fitness Professional's Handbook* for several reasons:

- The distinctions among the various types of fitness certifications have become blurred, with more similarities than differences given the common background that all fitness professionals must possess. The professionals performing the fitness testing must be able to communicate effectively with the personal fitness trainers and group exercise leaders who deliver the programming.
- The book has been used extensively as a reference text by those who are already certified and practicing as fitness professionals, not just by those pursuing the Health/Fitness Instructor® certification offered by the American College of Sports Medicine.
- This text has been used for the past two decades as a college textbook for fitness testing and prescription classes, even though many students in those classes plan to pursue careers in fields other than fitness (e.g., athletic training). For example, the majority of exercise science undergraduates at the University of Tennessee at Knoxville aim for a career in physical therapy (PT). However, with more PT facilities hiring fitness professionals to do fitness assessments and deliver structured exercise programs, it makes sense for them to be as informed about fitness testing and prescription as for those choosing career paths as fitness professionals. In essence, the content of this book has become a part of many exercise science programs, somewhat independent of students' career goals.

In addition to the title change, every chapter has been updated based on the latest standards, guidelines, and research, be they related to special populations or low-back pain and injury prevention. As you might expect, some chapters have required more updates than others; the chapters that received the most significant updates are the following:

- Chapter 3, Health Appraisal, has been completely rewritten to focus on the sequence of steps to follow in screening participants, such as completing health questionnaires and soliciting physician feedback, evaluating risk status, risk stratification, and making appropriate recommendations. The Health Status Questionnaire has been revised based on American College of Sports Medicine and American Heart Association questionnaires. Michael Shipe, a new author to this edition, has had extensive experience in both preventive and rehabilitative settings and brings this experience to the task.
- Chapter 7, Nutrition, has been updated based on the most recent *Dietary Guidelines of Americans* as well as on the current standards for nutritional intake.
- Chapter 12, Exercise Prescription for Resistance Training, has been modified extensively, with special attention to the most recent and relevant position stands from the American College of Sports Medicine and the National Strength and Conditioning Association. It provides a thorough explanation of how to develop exercise prescriptions for strength and endurance in a small space.
- Chapter 13, Exercise Prescription for Flexibility and Low-Back Function, has been thoroughly revised, with a special emphasis on core stability.
- Chapter 23, Mindful Exercise for Fitness Professionals, is new to the text and focuses on an approach to exercise that is getting more attention these days—yoga, Pilates, and other mind–body exercises. Ralph La Forge brings extensive background in this area to provide insights into the benefits of the different mind–body exercises.

• Chapter 26, Program Administration and Management, has been rewritten by Michael Shipe, taking advantage of his experiences in both fitness- and hospital-based programs, and provides additional detail on budget development.

Although many updates have been made, former users of the text will be comfortable with this new edition. The text continues to use *ACSM's Guidelines for Exercise Testing and Prescription* as a primary source of standards and expectations for fitness professionals. This has been and remains the standard-setting reference for professionals delivering fitness programs in any setting, whether club or hospital based. Consequently, the text is still helpful to those interested in taking appropriate ACSM certification exams, as well as those offered by other organizations.

In addition, this edition also retains many reproducible forms, interesting sidebars, useful key points, case study questions and answers, key terms and glossary, and extensive references, making it a useful textbook for students as well as a valuable reference for practitioners.

Intended Audience

This text continues to be written for the upper-level undergraduate or beginning graduate student with a general background in anatomy and physiology. The purpose of the text to is take someone with limited knowledge of what fitness testing and prescription is and enable them to screen participants, carry out standardized fitness tests to evaluate the major components of fitness, and write appropriate fitness prescriptions. Many academic programs incorporate lab experiences to drive the mastery of skills needed to accomplish these tasks. In that way, the class is not simply an academic experience, but is an experience that allows a person to move into practicum or internship experiences with the requisite skills and abilities. This text will work seamlessly with most lab experiences associated with fitness assessment because of its attention to detail regarding the most common fitness tests, from pretest concerns to posttest evaluation of results.

Text Organization

Part I, Activity, Fitness, and Health, contains three chapters and provides a general overview of the distinctions among the terms *activity, fitness,* and *health;* general information about each of those terms to set up the remainder of the text; and a step-by-step approach on how to screen potential participants for fitness programs.

Part II, Fitness Evaluation, provides extensive detail on how to assess cardiorespiratory fitness, body composition, flexibility, and muscular strength and endurance. In addition, chapters are also provided on nutrition assessment and how to evaluate the energy cost of activity, both of which are central to the issue of energy balance that is addressed in the next part.

Part III, Exercise Prescription for Health and Fitness, provides a separate chapter on how to deal with the test results for each of the fitness components assessed in part II and describes how to formulate an exercise prescription consistent with a client's goals and abilities. In addition, a chapter on exercise leadership provides general principles and specific examples of various modes of exercise programming.

Part IV, Special Populations, provides a separate chapter on exercise testing and prescription for each of the following: children and adolescents; older adults; women; and people with heart disease, obesity, diabetes, or pulmonary disease.

Part V, Exercise Programming, describes successful behavioral science approaches to changing behavior, a process that is central to helping people improve their lives; mind–body exercise programs and their benefits; exercise ECGs and medications; injury prevention and rehabilitation; and program administration and management.

Part VI, Scientific Foundations, covers basic anatomy and biomechanics and exercise physiology, useful for a quick review.

Instructor Resources

In addition to the thoroughly updated content, this edition also has several instructor resources available to aid in teaching a class with this textbook: a new instructor guide and revised test package and presentation package.

- The new instructor guide includes a syllabus; course outlines that detail lecture topics and lab and classroom activities; initial and final practical exams, including checklists for easy grading; and a laboratory notebook that students can use to track their completion of 12 fitness assessment and programming activities.
- The test package includes more than 400 questions, including true/false, multiple choice, and short answer/essay questions.
- The Microsoft PowerPoint® presentation package contains 580 slides that present the textbook material in a lecture-friendly format, including art, photos, and tables pulled from the text.

We hope that this book is helpful to you, whether you are using it as a textbook or a resource to help you stay up to date. Good luck in whatever career path you choose.

PART I

Activity, Fitness, and Health

Physical activity is an essential element in health and well-being. With that in mind, we wrote this book for current and future fitness professionals who help individuals, communities, and groups gain the benefits of regular physical activity in a positive and safe environment.

The chapters of part I explain the foundations underlying the study of physical activity and its relevance to fitness. In chapter 1, we summarize the current evidence regarding physical activity and health. Next, we describe the relationships among health, fitness, and performance in chapter 2. Finally, in chapter 3 we provide a process for screening potential fitness participants and recommend criteria for medical referrals and the development of supervised and unsupervised programs.

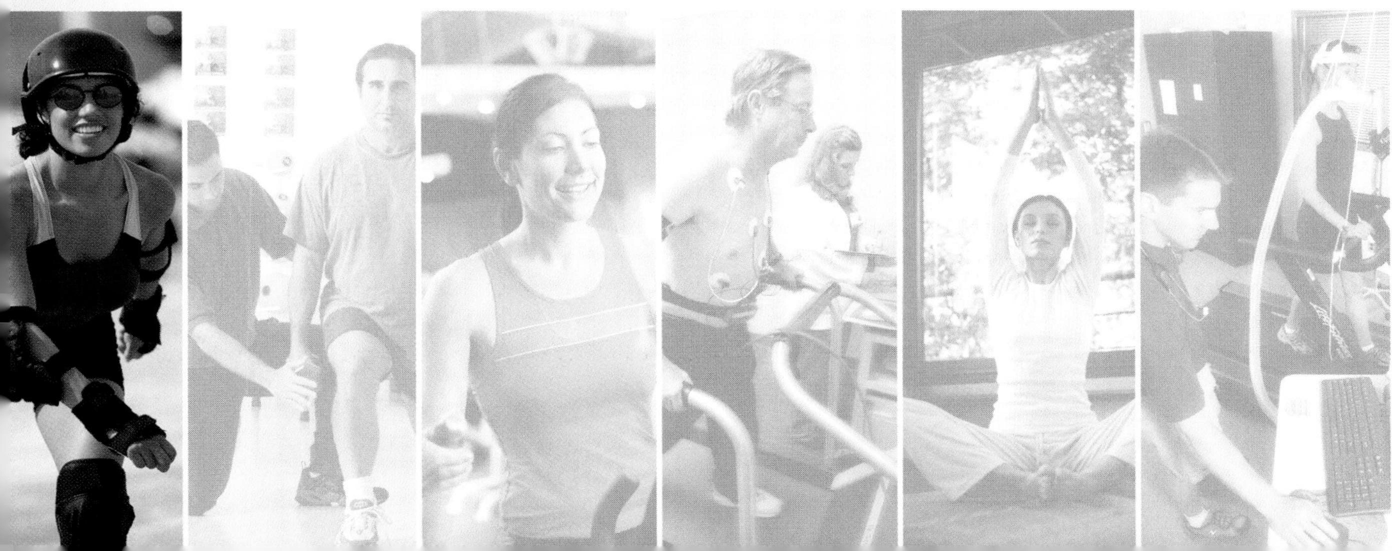

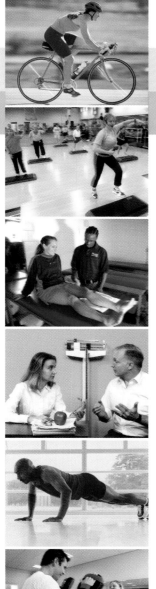

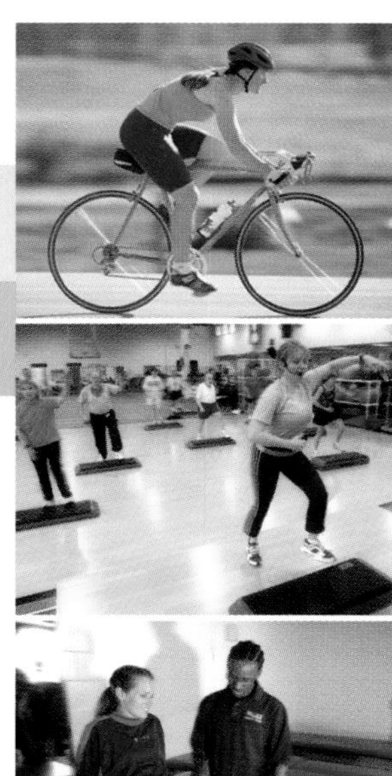

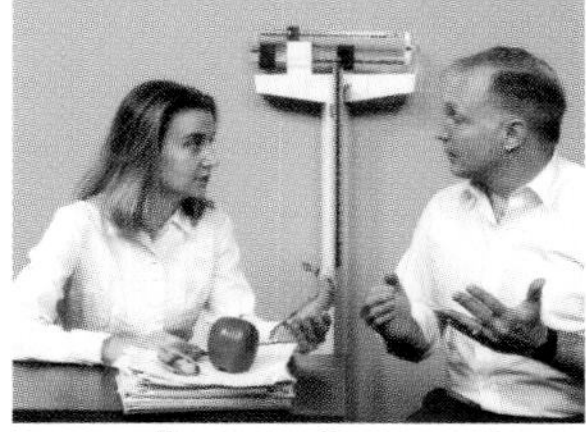

Physical Activity and Health

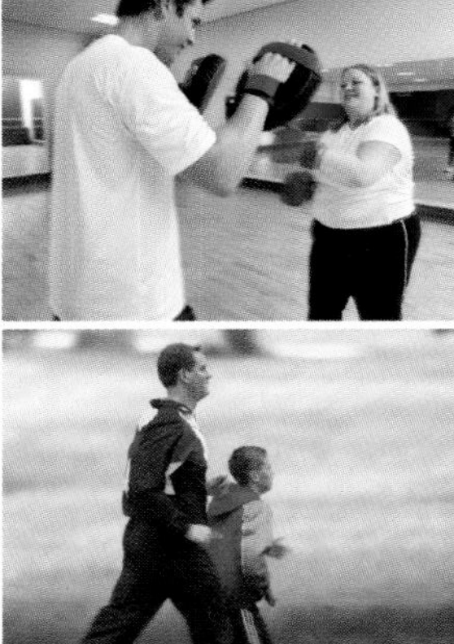

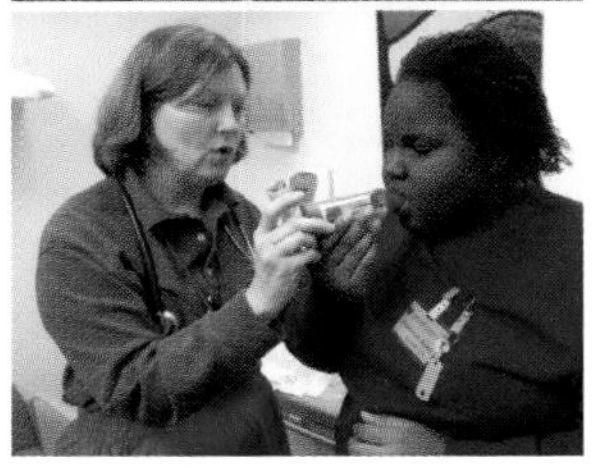

Objectives

The reader will be able to do the following:

1. Provide evidence that participation in regular physical activity has clear health benefits.
2. Describe some of the barriers that prevent individuals from participating in physical activity.
3. Describe how physical activity relates to health.

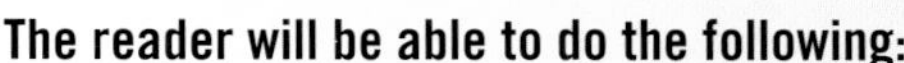

4. Describe the elements of total fitness.

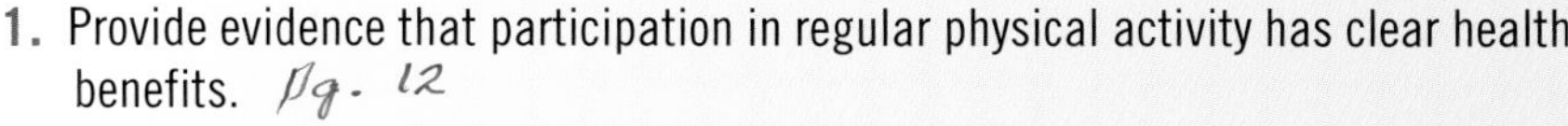

5. Understand the role of physical activity in quality of life.
6. Describe the goals and behaviors of a healthy life.
7. Describe the link between physical activity and lowered risk of premature health problems.
8. Understand the pathophysiology of atherosclerosis and other cardiovascular problems.
9. Identify risk factors for coronary heart disease and designate those that may be favorably modified by regular and appropriate physical activity habits.
10. Differentiate between the amount and type of exercise required for various health benefits and the amount and type required for fitness development.
11. Identify the short-term and long-term benefits of fitness.
12. Be aware of the risks associated with exercise participation or testing.
13. Describe three key elements of promoting physical activity.

From the beginning of recorded history, philosophers and health professionals have observed that regular physical activity is an essential part of a healthy life. Hippocrates wrote the following in *Regimen,* about 400 BC:

> *Eating alone will not keep a man [woman] well; he [she] must also take exercise. For food and exercise, while possessing opposite qualities, yet work together to produce health. . . . And it is necessary, as it appears, to discern the power of various exercises, both natural exercises and artificial, to know which of them tends to increase flesh and which to lessen it; and not only this, but also to proportion exercise to bulk of food, to the constitution of the patient, to the age of the individual . . . (20)*

Best of Times and Worst of Times for Fitness Professionals

In the past three decades, the public, professional groups (e.g., health-related scholarly societies), and medical community have accepted the importance of being physically active. It seems that almost everyone recognizes the overwhelming evidence, accumulated by exercise scientists over the past five decades, that points to the importance of regular physical activity for quality of life, health, and prevention and rehabilitation of many health problems. The information in the first half of the sidebar on page 5 (Good News and Bad News for Fitness Professionals) illustrates this widespread acceptance.

Public recognition of the need for physical activity for good health is a major accomplishment for fitness scholars and professionals who have conducted research and disseminated their findings on physical activity and health. To have so many statements promoting physical activity appear within the space of a few years indicates the excitement felt by all those involved with physical activity; however, there are many challenges left for fitness professionals who wish to promote the health benefits of physical activity for everyone (see the second half of Good News and Bad News for Fitness Professionals on page 5).

Key Point

Professional groups, such as the American College of Sports Medicine (ACSM) and the American Heart Association (AHA), and U.S. governmental agencies, such as the Centers for Disease Control and Prevention (CDC), the National Institutes of Health (NIH), the President's Council on Physical Fitness and Sports (PCPFS), and the Office of the Surgeon General, have released reports emphasizing the importance of physical activity to good health.

Key Point

Resources allocated for safe and supervised physical activities do not back up the position statements on the need for physical activity. The public is confused regarding what type and amount of physical activity are recommended for health, fitness, and weight control.

Physical Activity and Health

Starting in the 1940s with fitness pioneers such as T.K. Cureton, Bruno Balke, and Peter Karpovich, numerous experimental studies explored the effects of regular physical activity on fitness, especially cardiorespiratory fitness and body composition. These studies led to the 1978 ACSM position statement, with Michael Pollock as senior author, concerning the amount and type of physical activity needed to improve fitness (1). It appeared from these studies that doing small amounts of activity had little effect on cardiorespiratory fitness; in fact, results for groups assigned to perform less than the ACSM recommendations did not often differ from those for the sedentary control groups.

Epidemiological studies explore risk factors for various health problems, especially heart disease. The major findings of these epidemiological studies showed that smoking, high total cholesterol, and high blood pressure strongly related to the development of heart disease. It is now recognized that physical inactivity is also a major risk factor for heart disease (4, 29).

The 1978 ACSM statement summarized the experimental studies on what was needed for individuals to make fitness changes over a few months, but the large population studies spanning several years appeared to show that individuals with activity levels below the ACSM recommendations had reduced risk of heart disease and other health problems. Haskell (16) was one of the first scholars to observe the apparent contradiction of the relationship of physical activity to fitness and health. Two of the major population studies had sufficient data for analyzing different levels of physical activity (30) and different levels of cardiorespiratory fitness (7) to determine the relative risks of heart disease and all-cause mortality. Both the behavior (physical activity) and the outcome (cardiorespiratory fitness) appear to help reduce the risk of heart disease. Figures 1.1 and 1.2 (18) show the relationship between activity level or fitness level and risk of coronary heart disease (CHD). Risk is substantially

Good News and Bad News for Fitness Professionals

The Good News

People know that physical activity is necessary for good health: Surveys indicate that women and men of all ages, races, and socioeconomic backgrounds believe that regular physical activity is vital for health.

- The *Healthy People 2010* objectives (42) list physical activity and fitness as a priority. In addition, physical activity is listed as one of the 10 top health indicators.
- The AHA (4) includes physical inactivity and low fitness levels as primary risk factors for cardiovascular disease along with smoking, hypertension, and high cholesterol.
- The NIH (29) released a consensus statement on the importance of physical activity for cardiovascular health.
- The CDC and the ACSM (31) released a public health physical activity recommendation (accumulate 30 min of moderate-intensity physical activity on most, preferably all, days of the week) aimed to improve the health of the most sedentary Americans.
- The U.S. Department of Agriculture and U.S. Department of Health and Human Services published the seventh edition of the *Dietary Guidelines for the Nation* (39), which includes a statement on the vital role of physical activity.
- The Office of the Surgeon General released its report on physical activity and health, which strongly supports the role of physical activity for good health and prevention of major health problems (41).

The Bad News

More than 50% of adults in the United States do not meet the physical activity recommendation of 30 min of moderate-intensity daily exercise (10).

- The public is confused about the amount (30, 60, or 90 min) and type (moderate or vigorous) of physical activity recommended for health, fitness, and weight control (19, 39).
- The resources allocated for physical activity have lagged far behind money spent for other aspects of health: The resources for physical education and community physical activity programs are inadequate to provide safe and quality programs.
- Safe, attractive, and well-supervised facilities for participation in activity are not available for many individuals: Bike and walking trails are an exception rather than a rule in U.S. communities.
- Low-cost recreation programs for the masses are simply not sufficient to accommodate all who could benefit.
- In schools, health and physical education are low priorities and are often among the first curricular components cut during budget crises (12, 37).

reduced when an individual moves from the lowest activity or fitness level to a slightly increased level of activity or fitness. These studies also show additional benefit from higher levels of activity and fitness.

Drawing on these and other studies, the ACSM, the CDC, and the PCPFS (31) issued a position statement that supplemented the earlier ACSM recommendation and proclaimed that sedentary individuals could greatly reduce their risk of developing heart disease, type 2 diabetes, and other health problems simply by participating in 30 min of moderate-intensity physical activity most, but preferably all, days of the week. Additional fitness benefits can result from going beyond that to the 3 to 5 days per wk of vigorous aerobic activity specified in the original ACSM position statement, but the greatest boost in the health of the United States would come from sedentary individuals beginning a little bit of exercise every day. This view is reflected in the revised ACSM position statements (2, 3), which continue to be the gold standard for fitness improvement (see part III). *Healthy*

Key Point

An active lifestyle enhances quality of life. Regular participation in moderate-intensity physical activity decreases risk of heart disease and other diseases. Regular vigorous exercise reduces disease risk and also increases cardiorespiratory fitness.

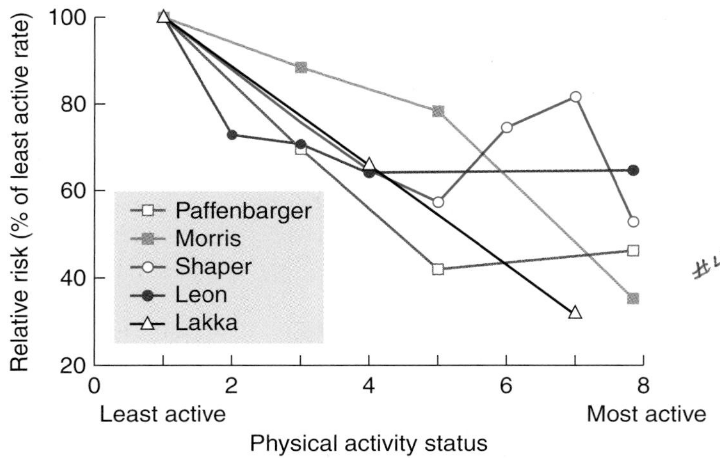

Figure 1.1 Physical activity and risk of coronary heart disease.

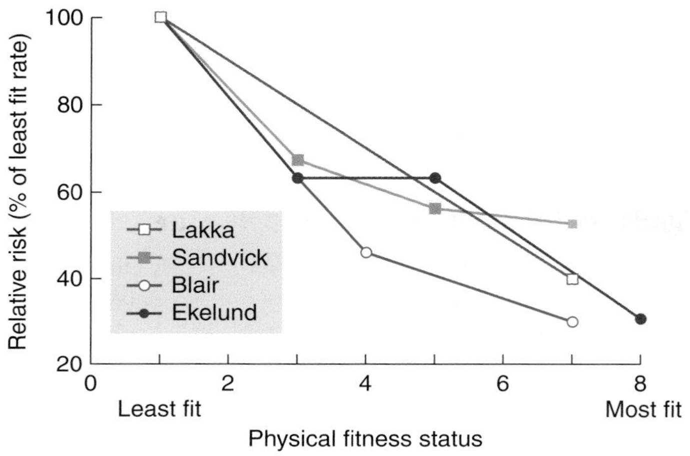

Figure 1.2 Physical fitness and risk of coronary heart disease.

People 2000 and *2010* (40, 42) include objectives for both daily moderate and regular vigorous activity. The NIH Consensus Conference on Physical Activity and Cardiovascular Health (29) drew the same conclusions.

What We Know About Physical Activity, Fitness, and Health

Many people would find it impossible to describe the highest level of positive, dynamic health without including physical activity. Physical activity is essential to optimal physical and mental health. Consistent with the link between activity and positive health, a sedentary lifestyle contributes to poor health for many people. Just adding regular physical activity to the lifestyle of sedentary individuals substantially increases their overall health.

Elements of Total Fitness

Although it is easy to recognize individuals enjoying an optimal quality of life, it is difficult to precisely describe this life. Many people have used the term **wellness** to emphasize that positive health is much more than simply being free from illness and that there is an added quality to being well. We use the term *total fitness* to capture this same concept. **Total fitness** is a condition reached through striving to optimize life in all aspects—social, mental, psychological, spiritual, and physical. This dynamic, multidimensional state has a positive health base and includes individual performance goals. The highest quality of life includes mental alertness and curiosity, positive emotional feelings, meaningful relationships with others, awareness and involvement in societal strivings, recognition of the broader forces of life, and the physical capacity to accomplish personal goals with vigor. These aspects of total fitness are interrelated; high fitness in one area enhances the other areas, and, conversely, lower fitness in any area restricts the accomplishments possible in other areas. Although physical activity plays a major role in the physical dimension, it also contributes to learning, relationships, and a sense of our human limitations within the broader perspective. An optimal quality of life requires individuals to strive, grow, and develop, though they may never achieve the highest level of fitness. The totally fit person nevertheless continually strives for the highest quality of life possible.

Heredity

People can achieve fitness goals up to their genetic potential, but it is not possible to establish the relative portion of a person's health or performance that is determined by heredity. Although heredity influences physical activity, fitness, and health (8), most people can lead healthy or unhealthy lives regardless of their genetic makeup. Thus, genetic background neither dooms a person to poor health nor guarantees good health.

Environment

We are born not only with fixed genetic potentials but also into environments that affect our development. An environment includes physical factors (e.g., climate, altitude, pollution) and social factors (e.g., friends, parental values, workplace characteristics) that affect activity, fitness, and health. Some elements, such as our nutrition or the air we breathe and water we drink, affect us directly. Other elements, such as the values and behaviors of people we admire, influence our lifestyles indirectly.

We can control certain aspects of our environments—we choose many of the mental and physical activities we undertake. However, our past and current environments affect us all in various ways. For example, some children have inadequate food because of their environment and cannot think about other aspects of fitness until that basic need is fulfilled.

Individual Interests

A major ingredient in total fitness is discretionary use of time. Selected activities are important to an individual in two ways: the nature of the activity and preparation for enjoyable participation. One of the purposes of education related to physical activity is to positively expose people to a wide variety of activities that enrich life. Thus, a well-educated person has many mentally and physically healthy activities from which to choose.

The long-term interests that a person develops may require additional preparation for their enjoyment. For example, someone may enjoy reading and tennis as a result of early positive involvement in both. In addition to becoming involved in groups interested in literature, the individual will need to pay attention to proper posture, lighting, and so on while reading. The person will need to develop underlying physical fitness and specific skills to enjoy playing tennis.

Key Point

Total fitness is striving for the highest level of existence, including mental, psychological, social, spiritual, and physical components. It is dynamic and multidimensional and is related to heredity, environment, and individual interests.

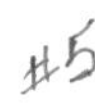

Quality of Life

The opening section of the chapter dealt with global notions of health to emphasize that there is more to physical activity than whether it can prolong life or prevent heart disease. Later in this chapter we explore the evidence that activity increases longevity and reduces risk of heart disease; however, the point here is that regular physical activity will improve quality of life even if it does not prolong life or ward off premature disease. Several studies have explored the relationship between physical activity and overall quality of life, including such variables as mental, psychological, and social well-being. Although the type and amount of physical activity essential for global quality of life are not as easily described, evidence that physical activity plays a role in quality of life is increasing (35) (see Research Insight).

Research Insight

In a comprehensive review of the research on quality of life and independent living in older adults, Spirduso and Cronin (36) found that physical activity postponed disability and enhanced independent living. Regular physical activity enhances physical function in people with chronic disease; however, there was insufficient evidence to differentiate the positive effects of aerobic and resistance training. In addition, there was no evidence for a dose–response relationship between exercise intensity and enhanced quality of life.

The energy and physical, mental, psychological, and social well-being that result from appropriate physical activity are reasons enough to promote activity. The reduced risk of developing premature health problems and the potential of a longer life are additional benefits.

Key Point

Physical activity influences quality of life because it increases energy and promotes physical, mental, and psychological well-being in addition to benefiting physical health.

Goals and Behaviors for a Healthy Life

Health is defined as being alive with no major health problem. The two primary health goals are to delay death and avoid disease. Although these goals provide a minimum basis for health and are desirable first steps, they fall far short of being goals for reaching optimal fitness.

Delaying Death

The death rate for humans is 100%! Death cannot be avoided, but, beyond inherited characteristics, it can be postponed. In general, you can practice a healthy lifestyle in a healthy and safe environment.

Avoiding Disease

Along with delaying death, the other minimum health goal is to be free from disease (i.e., to be apparently healthy). We try to prevent known illnesses through awareness, health checks, and healthy habits. You probably have assisted at or attended health fairs that help people identify signs, symptoms, and test scores that might indicate medical problems.

Positive activities and habits relate to total fitness and low risk of developing major health problems. These behaviors include exercising regularly, maintaining healthy nutrition, getting adequate sleep, relaxing and coping with stressors, practicing safety habits, and abstaining from using tobacco, excess alcohol, and nonessential drugs (table 1.1).

Table 1.1 Health Goals, Components, and Behaviors

Goal	Component	Behavior
Delay death	Heredity	Nutrition
	Healthy habits	Physical activity
		No smoking/drug use
		Limited alcohol consumption
	Safe habits	Relaxation
	Environment	Sleep
		Coping with stressors
		Wearing seat belts
		Avoiding high risks
		Clean air and water
Avoid disease	Heredity	Medical/dental exams
	Prevention	Immunization
	Awareness of symptoms	Check with health provider
	Lower CHD risk	Daily moderate physical activity
	Nutrition	Balance different foods
		Low fat, cholesterol, salt intake
		Balanced caloric intake and expenditure
		High complex carbohydrates

CHD = coronary heart disease

Key Point

The primary health goals are to avoid premature death and to prevent disease. Components related to these goals include heredity, environment, habits, and health status. Behaviors that contribute to a healthy life are regular exercise; proper nutrition; adequate sleep; relaxation; and abstinence from tobacco, excess alcohol, and nonessential drugs.

Physical Activity and Preventing Premature Health Problems

If a person lives long enough, health problems will develop, leading to an inability to function independently and eventually to death. One aspect influencing quality of life is delaying the development of these health problems, prolonging the healthy and independent living portions of life. Evidence shows that physical activity lowers the risk of prematurely developing many health problems, including atherosclerosis (26), back pain (32), some cancers (25), chronic lung disease (44), coronary heart disease (17), diabetes (23), hypertension (13), mental health problems (24), obesity (43), osteoporosis (34), and stroke (22). An active lifestyle also relates to estimates of prolonged quality of life (35) and independent living in the elderly (11, 36) and individuals with disabilities (33). In 1996, the *Surgeon General's Report on Physical Activity and Health* (41) reviewed the evidence relating physical activity to risks of health problems and concluded that physical activity reduces the risks of colon cancer, coronary heart disease, non-insulin-dependent diabetes, hypertension, obesity, osteoporosis, and all-cause mortality as well as enhances mental health. A later consensus conference dealing with dose–response issues of physical activity and health supported these findings (21).

Key Point

Regular physical activity helps prevent premature development of a variety of major health problems.

Pathophysiology of Arteriosclerosis and Other Cardiovascular Problems

Cardiovascular problems cause the majority of premature deaths in the United States, with heart disease being the number one killer (5). In addition, many who survive with these problems experience severely limited lives. Cardiovascular health problems take many different forms:

Arteriosclerosis
Atherosclerosis
Coronary artery thrombosis
Coronary heart disease (CHD)
Embolism
Hypertension
Myocardial infarction (MI)
Stroke
Thrombosis
Elevated serum **cholesterol**

Injury to the endothelial (innermost) lining of an artery caused by factors such as hypertension and smoking can generate an inflammation response, leading to a buildup of plaque (fatty fibrous deposits). Serum cholesterol contributes to the plaque buildup, which can clog arteries. As the coronary arteries narrow and harden, they may not be able to supply the oxygen needed by the heart muscle (myocardium). This inability to supply oxygen is likely to occur when more oxygen is needed (e.g., during stress or strenuous activity). The resulting imbalance between the need for and the supply of oxygen may cause pain in the chest (angina), neck, jaw, or left shoulder and arm. The narrowed artery may close or become totally occluded, which leads to an MI. (See chapter 3 for standards that define abnormal levels of cholesterol and blood pressure.)

High blood pressure (hypertension) is the most common cardiovascular disease (42). Hypertension relates to CHD and stroke. Stroke results from obstructions in or hemorrhages of blood vessels in the brain. It usually causes an abrupt disruption of bodily function and loss of consciousness and may cause partial paralysis. See Research Insight for more information on the leading versus actual causes of death.

Key Point

Cardiovascular problems cause the majority of premature deaths in the United States. Coronary heart disease is linked to the buildup of fatty deposits in the coronary arteries and to limited oxygen delivery to the myocardium.

Research Insight

As mentioned earlier, the leading cause of death is heart disease. CHD is followed by cancer, stroke (cerebrovascular disease), chronic lung disease, unintentional injuries, and diabetes (5). However, such a list does not provide information about the underlying causes of death. It is not surprising that the leading actual cause of death is tobacco use, accounting for 18% of all deaths. This is followed by poor diet and physical inactivity, alcohol consumption, infection (microbial agents), toxic agents, motor vehicles, and firearms (27). Although these investigators later corrected their estimate of the number of deaths due to poor diet and physical inactivity (28), this correction did not affect the order of actual causes and only slightly lowered the percent contribution (from 16.6% to 15.2%) to the death rate. In contrast to smoking and poor diet and physical inactivity, the next leading cause of death, alcohol consumption, was responsible for only 3.5% of deaths. This information underscores the theme in this book: Our ability to modify poor health behaviors (smoking, physical inactivity, and poor diet) can dramatically affect our health and well-being. This is an important message for the fitness professional.

Risk Factors for Cardiovascular Disease

Large-population epidemiological studies of cardiovascular problems have found that several characteristics (risk factors) highly relate to the premature development of cardiovascular disease. One way to classify risk factors is to distinguish between inherited factors that cannot be altered and unhealthy lifestyle behaviors that can be modified. Risk factors that cannot be altered include the family history of premature cardiovascular disease (3), sex (15) (men are at greater risk), race (42) (e.g., African Americans are at greater risk), and age (3) (risk increases with age).

Part of the risk associated with family history and age cannot be changed. The good news, however, is that some of the risks of family history can be changed. These include an unhealthy diet, a sedentary lifestyle, smoking, and poor coping behaviors that tend to be transmitted from parents to children. These behaviors can be corrected with proper attention throughout life, especially in early childhood.

In terms of aging, many fitness characteristics (e.g., maximum cardiovascular function and amount of body fat) worsen with age; that is, if the fitness characteristics of people from 20 to 80 yr are plotted against age, fitness steadily deteriorates (i.e., cardiovascular function decreases, fat increases) with each decade. This decline, starting in the mid-20s, has been called the *aging curve.* However, lack of optimal participation in physical activity contributes to a portion of the deterioration seen in aging curves. People who maintain active lifestyles slow the decline in fitness seen in typical aging curves (see chapter 16).

Modifiable characteristics that increase CHD risk include smoking (3), high levels of serum cholesterol (3), high blood pressure (3), low levels of physical activity (3) and cardiorespiratory fitness (7), glucose intolerance (3), high fibrinogen (29), obesity (3), psychosocial factors (15), and low socioeconomic status (15). Fortunately, many of these characteristics can be favorably altered with healthy habits. (See chapter 3 for use of risk factors in screening for fitness programs.)

Numerous studies have shown that active people have a lower risk of heart disease than sedentary individuals have; however, in the past, physical inactivity was viewed as less important than controlling serum cholesterol, blood pressure, and smoking. Studies indicate that both physical activity, such as expending 2000 kcal $\cdot$ wk^{-1} in various activities (30), and high cardiorespiratory fitness, such as being able to last longer on a treadmill test (7), are major factors that reduce the relative risk of heart disease and all-cause mortality. Physical inactivity and poor fitness deserve the same emphasis that the traditional primary risk factors deserve. Regular exercise also affects many of the CHD risk factors, improving serum cholesterol levels, blood pressure, glucose tolerance, fibrinogen, and body fat (29). Activity also helps people learn to cope with stressors. Table 1.2 summarizes how physical activity affects disease risk factors.

Although these risk factors have normally been linked with cardiovascular disease, many of them are also related to pulmonary (e.g., chronic obstructive pulmonary disease) and metabolic (e.g., type 2 diabetes) health problems.

Low-Back Problems

Clinical evidence indicates that several risk factors are associated with low-back problems (see chapters 9 and 13):

- Lack of abdominal muscle endurance
- Lack of flexibility in the midtrunk and hamstrings
- Poor posture while lying, sitting, standing, and moving
- Poor lifting habits
- Injury of low back
- Overuse of low-back muscles
- Inability to cope with stressors

Key Point

Some inherited characteristics and behaviors place certain people at higher risk of premature health problems (such as cardiovascular disease and low-back problems) and death. Physical activity can reduce or eliminate risk factors of high serum cholesterol levels, high blood pressure, glucose intolerance, high fibrinogen, obesity, and high stress.

Regular activities that strengthen the abdominal muscles and increase flexibility in the low back and hamstrings are highly recommended to prevent low-back problems (see chapter 13).

Implications for Fitness Professionals

Fitness professionals need to keep up with the constantly evolving recommendations for health and physical fitness that directly apply to fitness program and exercise recommendations. Because the media use brief headlines and

Table 1.2 Effect of Physical Activity on Risk Factors

	Effect of regular physical activity		
Risk factor	**Improve**	**May improve**	**No effect**
Older age			X
Smoking		X	
High total cholesterol	X		
High low-density cholesterol	X		
African American			X
Low HDL-cholesterol	X		
High fibrinogen	X		
Male			X
High very low-density cholesterol	X		
Family history			X
High blood pressure	X		
Physical inactivity	X		
Low cardiorespiratory fitness	X		
High-fat diet		X	
Obesity	X		
Insulin needs, glucose tolerance	X		
Inability to cope with stress		X	

HDL-cholesterol = high-density lipoprotein cholesterol

TV sound bites that provide only limited and confusing information about the latest fitness recommendations, many people may need more in-depth explanations to help put each new report into perspective in terms of overall recommendations for a healthy life.

Exercise Prescription

One of the most controversial and confusing areas for the public is how much and what type of physical activity benefit health and fitness. One reason for this confusion is that recommendations differ for individuals depending on their current activity levels and their fitness, health, and performance goals (14). It is not surprising that headlines and 20 sec sound bites send conflicting messages when one recommendation is aimed at the most sedentary people, another is for improving cardiorespiratory fitness in active adults, and yet another involves how to train for a marathon. Any set of exercise guidelines that does not address activity status and health and fitness goals will add to the confusion. It is possible to have clear and consistent recommendations for physical activity (see the activity pyramid in figure 1.3).

This section provides an overview of how fitness professionals can deal with questions about exercise prescription. Refer to part III for a more comprehensive treatment of exercise prescription. As the past few years have illustrated, providing exercise recommendations is a dynamic process that should stay in tune with new research findings. Thus, although we are confident that the recommendations in this book are appropriate for the beginning of the 21st century, they will need periodic updating as research findings are continually reviewed.

Physical activity includes any muscular activity that expends energy, whereas exercise is a subset of physical activity that is structured and planned to improve or maintain physical fitness (9). Everyone is encouraged to include physical activity in daily life, by using stairs instead of elevators, walking or cycling for visits or errands, and participating in active leisure-time pursuits with family and friends. Sedentary individuals should accumulate at least 30 min of moderate-intensity physical activity every day. Everything counts, from housework to gardening to the activities mentioned previously. Additional 10 to 15 min exercise breaks during the day are a good way to meet the 30 min goal (31).

Persons who are already active for 30 min daily can enhance their fitness and health by including 20 min of

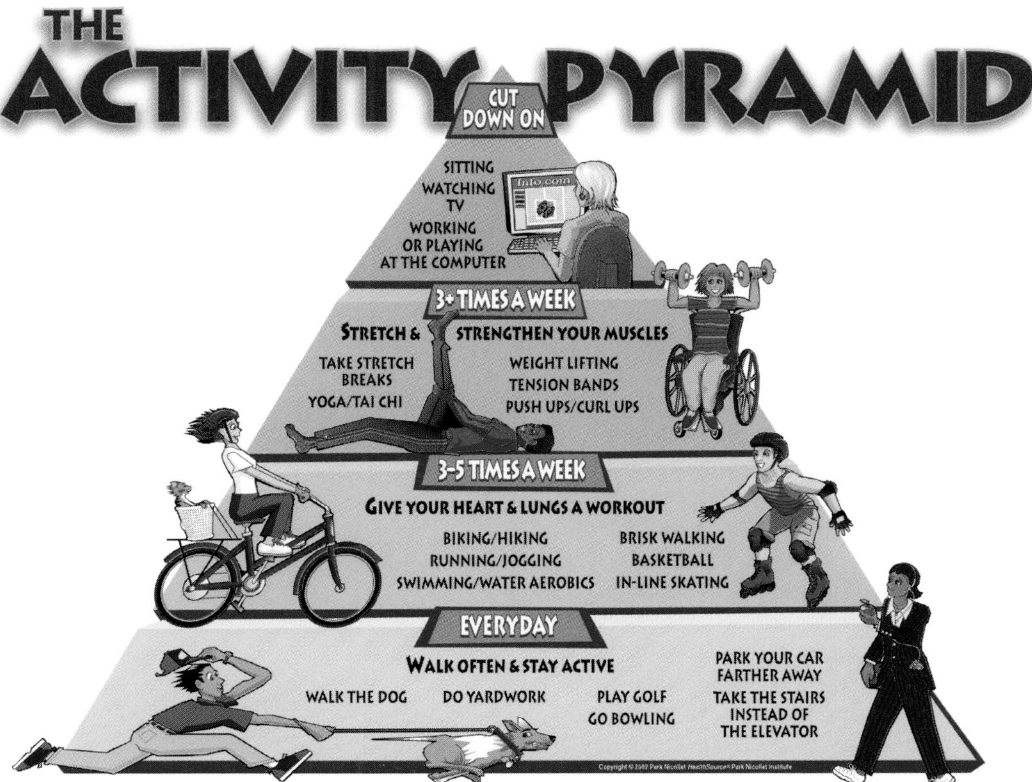

Figure 1.3 Activity pyramid.

The Activity Pyramid © 2003 Park Nicollet Health*Source*®, Minneapolis, U.S.A. 1-888-637-2675. Reprinted with permission.

> **Key Point**
>
> Exercise prescription must consider the individual's current activity status and desired outcomes. By making some simple changes, everyone can include more physical activity in daily life. Sedentary individuals should include at least 30 min of daily moderate-intensity activity. Moderately active individuals can improve their overall health and fitness by incorporating regular aerobic, resistance, and flexibility activities in an enjoyable atmosphere.

vigorous physical activity 3 to 5 days each week (cardiovascular fitness and health) or engaging in daily activities that use large amounts of energy (body composition and obesity). The activities should include weight-bearing activities (bone health), resistance training 2 to 3 days each week (muscular strength and endurance and bone health), regular stretching (flexibility and low-back health), and activities with an enjoyable atmosphere (enhanced adherence and psychological health).

Persons with high levels of fitness can increase their exercise levels and work on skills for a variety of performance goals (see chapter 2).

Intensity

One of the major differences in recommendations based on current activity status is the intensity of exercise. Table 10.1 on page 159 describes intensity levels, but usually the daily activities for the general population and for sedentary people require light-to-moderate intensity. Fitness activities fall into the category of hard (vigorous) intensity, and performance-related activities demand even greater intensities.

Benefits of Physical Activity

The long-term health and fitness benefits of regular activity are well known, including reduced risk of major health problems and improved cardiorespiratory function, muscular strength and endurance, flexibility, and body composition (fat content). Although we normally focus on the long-term (chronic) effects of regular physical activity, part of the benefit of physical activity is derived from repeated short-term (acute) activity. For example, chronic activity reduces resting blood pressure, but blood pressure is additionally lowered after each acute bout of exercise. A single bout of activity has positive psychological effects for many people, such as a positive mood after exercise. Finally, the time spent on physical activity is time not spent on unhealthy behaviors, such as smoking or eating unhealthy snacks. Table 1.3 summarizes some of the acute and chronic effects of physical activity.

Exercise-Related Risks

Exercise and fitness tests involve risk of injury, cardiovascular problems, or death. High-intensity exercise and competition in many sports place extreme demands on the cardiovascular system and increase the risk of musculoskeletal injury. In addition, some fitness participants become obsessed with exercise and train too much (overtrain), which decreases fitness and leads to frequent injuries.

Moderate-intensity physical activity is very low risk. There is an increased risk of MI or sudden death with vigorous exercise, but these risks are still quite low. For the general population, it is estimated that during vigorous exercise only one sudden cardiac death occurs per year for every 15,000 to 18,000 people (3, 38). The risk of a cardiac event occurring when cardiac patients engage in vigorous exercise is considerably greater but is still low (3). Because of the lower risk of heart disease in active or fit persons, the overall risk of a cardiovascular problem is greater for those who maintain sedentary habits (41).

• Table 1.3 Short- and Long-Term Benefits of Physical Activity •

Variable	Short-term benefits	Long-term benefits
Heart rate	+, then –	– (except max)
Stroke volume		+
Ejection fraction		+
Lactate threshold		+
Fibrinogen	–	–
Fibrinolysis	+	+
Blood pressure	+, then –	–
Oxygen uptake, max		+
Muscle mass		+
Strength/endurance		+
Fat		–
Cholesterol, HDL		+
LDL, VLDL		–
Flexibility		+
Appetite	–	+
Use of leisure time	+	+
Positive mood	+	
Anxiety	–	–
Depression	–	–
Self-esteem		+
Stress	+, then –	–
Overreaction to stress		–

+ = increases; – = decreases; HDL = high-density lipoprotein; LDL = low-density lipoprotein; VLDL = very low-density lipoprotein.

The risk of cardiac events occurring during exercise testing is low in previously healthy individuals, but it increases as the number of CHD risk factors increases. In a mixed population, the overall risk of severe cardiovascular complications or death is about 6 out of 10,000 tests (3).

Exertion-related deaths are uncommon and generally relate to congenital heart defects (e.g., hypertrophic cardiomyopathy, Marfan syndrome, severe aortic-valve stenosis, prolonged QT syndromes, cardiac conduction abnormalities) or to acquired myocarditis. The NIH consensus statement on physical activity and cardiovascular health (29) recommends that individuals with these conditions remain active but not participate in vigorous or competitive athletics.

We deal with the question of risk by identifying classes of individuals for whom a certain type of medical examination is recommended before initiation of an exercise program (see chapter 3). Per-Olof Åstrand, a well-known Swedish physiologist, has offered another view. He stated that consulting a physician is advisable if there are any doubts about health but that there is less risk in being active than in continuous inactivity; it is more advisable to pass a careful medical examination if one intends to be sedentary to determine whether one's state of health is good enough to stand the inactivity (6)! This view is consistent with the evidence that regular physical activity and good cardiorespiratory fitness directly relate to a lower risk of heart disease and death (42).

Key Point

Exercise carries some risk of injury, cardiovascular problems, and death. The health risk of an inactive lifestyle is greater than the risk associated with the fitness activities and tests recommended in this book.

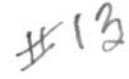

Promoting Physical Activity

The obvious need is for communities, schools, states, and countries to endorse regular physical activity for improving a nation's health by working with fitness professionals and allocating resources to encourage everyone to choose activity as part of a healthy lifestyle. Three elements of a strategy to enhance Americans' health through physical activity are clarity, access, and safety.

- **Clarity.** Fitness scholars and professionals must interpret and explain the evidence about physical activity as it relates to health, fitness, and performance variables. New evidence must be viewed within a clearly articulated model that indicates what type of physical activity relates to which outcomes for particular groups of individuals. In addition, fitness professionals must become more adept at providing short and simple explanations for the media's use.
- **Access.** Access to physical activity is largely outside fitness professionals' direct control. Fitness professionals must nonetheless work with public and private partners to provide an environment that makes regular physical activity available and attractive to people of all ages and socioeconomic backgrounds. This environment includes good health and physical education programs in the schools for all children and youth; community activity programs that are convenient and open to everyone; and programs at work sites, in preschools, and in facilities serving older adults. Qualified fitness professionals are an essential part of these programs.
- **Safety.** Fitness professionals must advocate that participation in all physical activities take place in a positive and safe environment. Safe equipment, activities appropriate to age and fitness level, and careful monitoring of signs and symptoms of participants are all part of a quality program. For example, helmets should be worn for cycling, skating, and other activities; pregnant women should avoid intense activity in hot environments; and older adults should be monitored carefully for any signs of cardiovascular problems.

Key Point

Fitness professionals must provide clear physical activity recommendations combined with adequate resources so that everyone can participate in quality physical activity in an enjoyable and safe atmosphere.

Case Studies

You can check your answers by referring to page 469 in appendix A.

1. You have just presented a speech on physical fitness to a local service club. One of the members says that he knows of two men who died in incidents related to exercise during the past few years and that he has read of other exercise-related deaths. He has decided that it will be safer to lead a quiet life and not take the risk of exercising. How would you respond?
2. A client complains that she has been deceived by all the exercise recommendations you have given her over the past several years. She just read a report from the CDC indicating that a person has to only do moderate-intensity physical activity (walking) to achieve health benefits. She wants to know if she should continue her vigorous exercise program in which she exercises at her target heart rate for 30 min 3 to 4 times each week or whether she should switch to a walking program. How would you respond?

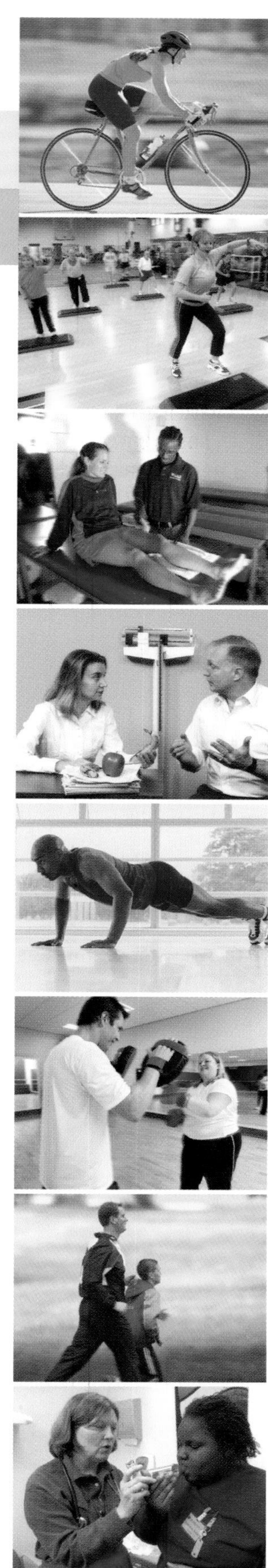

CHAPTER 2

Physical Fitness and Performance

Objectives

The reader will be able to do the following:

1. Describe the goals of fitness and performance.
2. Demonstrate an understanding of the components of fitness.
3. Define terms related to fitness and performance.
4. Define the major components of performance.
5. Describe healthy behaviors related to fitness.
6. Describe factors related to setting individual fitness goals.
7. Explain the role of fitness professionals in encouraging healthy behavior.

Chapter 1 dealt with the importance of physical activity for total fitness, health, and prevention of premature health problems. It presented the two-prong recommendation for moderate- and vigorous-intensity activity. The first part emphasizes that sedentary individuals should perform regular moderate-intensity activity to achieve health goals. The second part of the recommendation is to use vigorous activity (exercise) to enhance fitness benefits and build the basis for participation in performance activities that also enrich life. Using recommended definitions (1, 2) the first chapter dealt with physical activity and health, whereas this chapter explores exercise, physical fitness, and performance. We continue the discussion of activity, fitness, and health by comparing the goals, components, and behaviors related to **physical fitness** and **performance.**

Physical Fitness Goals

The physical fitness goals include lowering the risks of developing health problems and maintaining positive physical health. You are undoubtedly familiar with the components of these goals.

Lowering Health Risks

This goal is an extension of the health goal to avoid disease (chapter 1). Many of the health problems responsible for premature deaths can be prevented with careful screening and preventive action (e.g., immunization). There are still many people in the world who need this basic health care, and medical science can provide this service. The solution to this aspect of health care is finding the resources and political will to make it available to everyone.

In more affluent societies, where preventive health care is routine, another set of health problems has emerged (e.g., cardiovascular and metabolic diseases) that cause premature death or disability. As discussed in chapter 1, physical activity plays a major role in preventing premature health problems.

Maintaining Physical Well-Being

Many of the characteristics that lower the risk for developing serious health problems also provide a higher quality of life. In other words, optimizing cardiorespiratory fitness and body composition helps us feel good and gives us the energy to do the activities that enrich our lives. In addition, muscular endurance and flexibility in the midtrunk relate to a healthy low back. Weight-bearing activities enhance bone density, helping prevent osteoporosis. As people increase their physical fitness, they move toward a better life, whereas decreases in physical fitness lead to health problems and poorer quality of life.

Performance Goals

The primary performance goals are to complete daily tasks efficiently and to achieve desired levels in selected sports. These goals also involve a number of components.

Completing Daily Tasks

To get through the day efficiently, we must have fundamental motor skills that allow us to accomplish various tasks. We must be able to move from place to place and push, pull, pick up, carry, and perform other tasks requiring the hands and arms. Moderate levels of muscular strength and endurance, flexibility, and cardiorespiratory function are essential for these routine tasks. In addition, we need special abilities to perform the unique activities related to work or home.

This goal also relates to the positive health goal of independent functional living. It is an extension of the physical fitness goal of having healthy cardiorespiratory function, relative leanness, muscular strength and endurance, and flexibility.

Achieving Desired Sport Performance

Many individuals also engage in selected games, sports, and high-level physical performances. In addition to requiring good physical fitness, these activities require specific motor abilities (such as agility, balance, coordination, power, and speed) as well as the particular skills of the sport.

Key Point

The goals of physical fitness are achieving a positive physical health base with a low risk of health problems. Performance goals include the ability to engage in daily tasks with adequate energy and to participate successfully in selected sports.

Components of Physical Fitness and Performance

The components of physical fitness and performance derive directly from their goals. The physical fitness goals are achieved through exercise that improves and maintains cardiorespiratory function, healthy body composition, muscular strength and endurance, and flexibility. The performance goals are enhanced by specific conditioning to achieve and maintain high levels of aerobic and anaerobic energy; muscular strength, endurance, and power; speed; agility; coordination; balance; and sport skills.

Physical Fitness Components

The components of physical fitness are **cardiorespiratory function, relative leanness, muscular strength, muscular endurance,** and **flexibility.**

Cardiorespiratory function is essential not only for preventing premature cardiovascular problems but also for providing the energy to accomplish other elements related to quality of life. Chapter 28 explains the physiology underlying cardiorespiratory function, chapter 5 describes ways to test it, and chapter 10 deals with exercise prescription for improving it.

Unhealthy levels of body fat relate to numerous health and psychological problems. Obesity has become a problem of epidemic proportions, affecting both adults and children, and it is unlikely that the United States will be able to achieve the standards for body composition stipulated in the *Healthy People 2010* objectives (3). This is a complex area involving nutrition, physical activity, and behavior modification, which are covered in chapters 6, 7, 11, and 22.

The activities that improve and maintain muscular strength and endurance appear to benefit bone density, thus helping prevent osteoporosis, a problem of decreasing bone mass that particularly affects older women. Chapter 27 discusses basic human anatomy, chapter 8 describes ways to assess strength and endurance, and chapter 12 deals with exercise prescription for increasing strength and endurance.

Midtrunk strength, endurance, and flexibility are essential to maintaining a healthy low back. Flexibility and low-back function are covered in chapters 9 and 13.

Key Point

Physical fitness components are cardiorespiratory function, relative leanness, muscular strength and endurance, and flexibility. These fitness elements relate to a higher quality of life and prevention of major health problems.

Performance Components

Appropriate cardiorespiratory function, body composition, muscular strength and endurance, and flexibility allow people to achieve performance goals. In the first place, modest levels of these fitness components increase the efficiency with which we can do daily tasks around the home, in the yard, and at work. Although successful daily living is important at all ages, it is a top priority for elderly individuals because it allows them to continue to live independently.

Second, higher levels of these fitness components also support successful participation in sport and performance activities. Although an individual can attain health and fitness goals through other activities, sports and games provide enjoyable health and fitness supplements. In addition to requiring basic fitness, each sport places unique demands on energy, body composition, strength, endurance, and flexibility, and each requires specific skills. Many sports demand high **agility, balance, coordination, power,** and **speed.**

Because most of this book deals with health and fitness, the following example illustrates the differing needs for meeting the two performance goals. The first goal is to complete daily tasks efficiently. Most people move around during the day, doing some bending, lifting, carrying, pushing, and pulling, all of which require appropriate cardiorespiratory function, muscular strength and endurance, flexibility, and body leanness. In addition, a person's lifestyle adds other needs. Contrast, for example, a computer programmer, a firefighter, and a parent staying at home with an infant. The computer programmer needs stretching and relaxation activities to prevent low-back and postural problems and can benefit from short activity breaks. The firefighter is sedentary for most of the time but must be able to respond quickly with near-maximal levels of anaerobic energy and muscular strength and endurance, all within an adverse environment with heavy equipment. This person must engage in regular vigorous aerobic, anaerobic, and resistance exercise to maintain the conditioning necessary to respond to emergencies. The parent needs flexibility, strength, and endurance to lift and carry the infant and other items through an obstacle course of toys, clothes, and so on, in addition to learning to perform under sleep deprivation.

The second performance goal is to achieve desired levels in selected sports, games, and competitions. Although high fitness levels are desirable as an athletic base, individuals here also have very different needs. Compare, for example, 10K runners, basketball players, and golfers. The runners rely on great aerobic power that comes from lots of distance running, with careful stretching before and after. Basketball players depend on aerobic and anaerobic energy, coordination, and specific passing, shooting, and defensive skills. Golfers require a moderate cardiorespiratory base, some muscular power, and coordination of a complex skill used in a variety of settings (e.g., fairway, bunker, woods).

Physical activity recommendations for performing sports or work tasks are shown on page 18 and extend to vigorously active individuals who want to engage in sports and endurance performances. These individuals should enhance fitness components related to their selected sports and increase the skills directly related to the sports.

Recommendations for Vigorously Active Individuals Performing Specific Sports or Work Tasks

A vigorously active individual is able to jog 3 mi (4.8 km) at moderate to vigorous intensities (e.g., 60%-80% maximal oxygen uptake or heart rate reserve) 3 to 5 times each week without discomfort or undue fatigue.

Activity Goal

- To engage successfully in selected work or sport performance activities

Fitness Goal

- To have the underlying fitness and the specific skills needed to perform the tasks at the desired level with minimum risks of health problems or injury

Preactivity Screening

- If the training involves maximal exertion, a medical examination including a maximal exercise test is recommended (see chapter 3).

Recommended Activities

- Perform fitness activities as a base (see part III).
- Add additional training related to specific requirements of sport or activity. You may need to exceed total work, intensity, duration, or frequency of fitness workouts.
- Develop and maintain skills related to the sport or work task. Be aware of safety concerns during performance.
- Incorporate a warm-up, including moderate-intensity activities directly related to performance of the sport or work task.

Key Point

Performance components include a general fitness base. Specific levels of fitness components and unique skills related to the sport or game are needed for performance.

Behaviors That Support Fitness and Performance Components

The first two sections of this chapter discussed definitions, goals, and components related to physical fitness and performance. To achieve physical fitness, a person must adopt healthy behaviors.

Behaviors that contribute to fitness goals include eating healthily; exercising regularly; avoiding smoking, illegal drug use, and excessive alcohol use; getting adequate sleep and managing stress; and performing regular stretching and resistance training. Performance goals can be achieved by adopting healthy behaviors such as developing a resistance training program, using static stretching exercises, participating in regular vigorous exercise, practicing specific sport-related movements, using interval training, and practicing skills in game-like conditions. Figure 2.1 summarizes the goals, components, and behaviors for physical fitness and performance.

Common Behaviors for Fitness and Health

Although behaviors for promoting fitness or health can be differentiated, they are interrelated. People who exercise and exhibit other healthy behaviors are more likely to be fit. Achieving fitness standards leads to a healthy, longer life. On the other hand, sedentary existence relates to low fitness and major health problems that shorten life.

In these first two chapters, we have tried to show both the common and the unique elements of health, fitness, and performance. You have probably noticed some repetition in the behaviors recommended for delaying death, avoiding disease, preventing major health problems, and developing positive health. Although individuals need to be educated about signs, symptoms, and risk factors related to major health problems, a fitness program should emphasize the behaviors on the Health and Fitness Behaviors list on page 20.

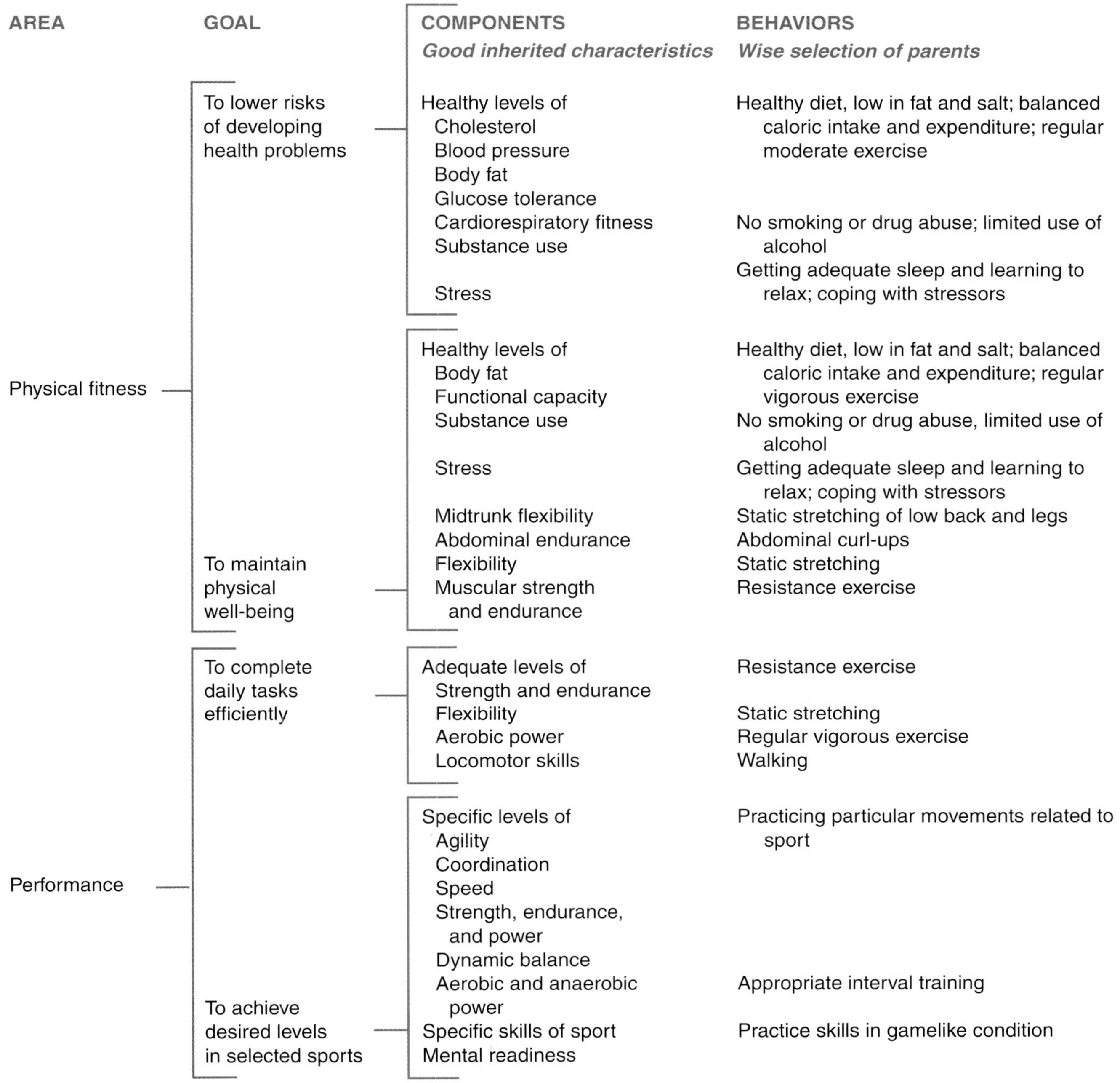

Figure 2.1 Physical fitness and performance goals, components, and behaviors.

Key Point

Although health and fitness goals differ somewhat, many of the recommended behaviors are common to both goals. Health and fitness are enhanced with regular exercise and sleep, nutritious diet, no smoking or drug abuse, limited alcohol intake, ability to cope with stressors, ability to relax, preventive checkups, and safe habits.

Setting Fitness Goals

People entering your fitness class or asking you to be their fitness professional have taken a first step toward improving their fitness. It is your responsibility to help them

- understand the components of fitness,
- analyze their current fitness status and begin or continue appropriate exercise habits,

Health and Fitness Behaviors

Regular Physical Activity

- Moderate-intensity activity
- Vigorous-intensity exercise
- Abdominal curl-ups
- Static stretching for low-back flexibility
- Whole-body flexibility and strength and endurance exercise

Healthy Diet

- Proper proportions of fat, carbohydrate, and protein
- Balance between energy expenditure and energy intake
- Balance among food groups
- High levels of complex carbohydrates
- Low levels of saturated and total fat
- Low levels of saltO

Substance Use

- No smoking
- No drugs (except as prescribed by physician)
- Limited alcohol use

Stress

- Coping with stressors
- Relaxation
- Regular sleep

Regular Tests for Fitness and Health

- Health risk appraisal
- Healthy habits
- Fitness status

- determine other health behaviors that need change, and
- take appropriate steps to change unhealthy behavior.

Information in chapters 1 and 2 will help fitness professionals assist individuals in setting appropriate health, fitness, and performance goals. Chapter 22 suggests ways to help participants start changing unhealthy behaviors. Chapter 14 provides tips for leading fitness programs and suggests specific activities that can be used.

Taking Control of Personal Health

One of the most frustrating and exciting aspects of dealing with current health problems is that individuals can modify their health status and control major health risks. The frustrating side is that many people find it difficult to change an unhealthy lifestyle. The exciting element is that they can gain control of their health. Fitness professionals are at the cutting edge of health, in much the same way the scientists discovering vaccines for major health problems were at the turn of the 20th century. The opportunity to help people alter their unhealthy lifestyles carries the responsibility of making recommendations based on the best scientific evidence available. Fitness professionals can help people gain control of their lives through evaluating their health-related risk factors and behaviors. Chapter 3 examines this type of health appraisal.

#1

Key Point

Fitness professionals live in an exciting time because of the increasing evidence and recognition that regular physical activity is essential to the good life. It is a worthwhile challenge to motivate people to begin and continue an active lifestyle, especially when there is so much competition for everyone's time.

Fred - Health related - moderate intensity to begin with. May add fitness goals later.

Susan - performance goals. Has already reached health & fitness goals.

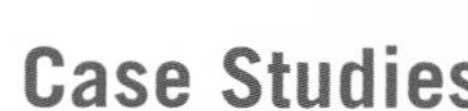

Case Studies

You can check your answers by referring to page 469 in appendix A.

1. Two people come to you and say they want to get in shape. After talking with them, you discover that Fred seems free of major health problems, but he hasn't done any regular activity for 20 yr. Susan, also apparently healthy, has been jogging and exercising to music 2 to 4 times each week for the past 5 yr. She has just joined an adult soccer league and wants to compete at a higher level. How would you help Fred and Susan formulate and achieve their goals?

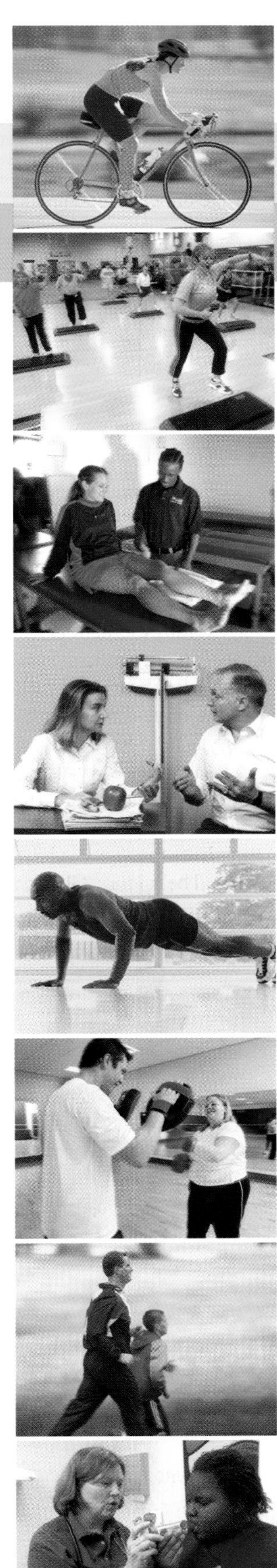

3 CHAPTER

Health Appraisal

Michael Shipe

Objectives

The reader will be able to do the following:

1. Understand the purpose of evaluating the health status of potential participants in fitness programs and identify appropriate instruments for health appraisal.
2. Describe the screening protocol for moderate- and vigorous-intensity exercise.
3. Learn how to identify risk factors for heart disease and risk-stratify patients.
4. Describe the categories of participants who should receive physician consent before undergoing an exercise test or participating in an exercise program.
5. Recommend an appropriate fitness program for participants based on their health screening and fitness test results.
6. List the conditions and test scores that indicate the need for a supervised program or for special attention during exercise.
7. Identify conditions requiring a change in exercise recommendations and describe the signs and symptoms of participants (including special populations) who should defer, delay, or terminate an exercise session.

After an individual has joined an exercise facility, the fitness professional is responsible for properly screening prospective exercise participants to determine their current health status, their readiness to undergo fitness testing and begin regular physical activity. To properly screen an exercise participant, the fitness professional should begin with a preparticipation health screening questionnaire, such as the Physical Activity Readiness Questionnaire (PAR-Q) or the Health Status Questionnaire (HSQ). The choice of the questionnaire should be appropriate to the fitness facility's target population. (These two questionnaires are discussed in detail later in this chapter.)

In some instances, physician consent or referral of the participant to initially participate in a clinic-based supervised exercise program may be necessary before the participant begins a moderate- or vigorous-intensity exercise program. There are no universal guidelines for determining when physician consent is necessary before exercise participation or when a supervised exercise program is warranted. To help the fitness professional make these decisions, this chapter provides the recommendations of the American Heart Association (AHA) and American College of Sports Medicine (ACSM) guidelines for both situations. In situations where a definitive answer is uncertain, the participant's primary care physician or the medical counsel of the facility should make the final decision regarding exercise participation.

When deciding to obtain physician consent or recommend a supervised program, the fitness professional should consider the participant's preparticipation health screening questionnaire answers, risk stratification category, physician recommendations, and fitness test results. Next, the participant undergoes a fitness test in which the results are evaluated relative to age and gender norms. Now the fitness professional has the necessary information to prescribe an appropriate exercise prescription for improving the participant's health and fitness in relation to their present health status and personal exercise goals. To update records of the participant's health status, the preparticipation health screening questionnaire and fitness test should be readministered periodically.

Evaluating Health Status

The ACSM and AHA recommend that exercise facilities provide their adult members with a preparticipation health screening that is consistent with the exercise programs they plan to pursue. These organizations support "all facilities offering exercise equipment or services should conduct a cardiovascular screening of all new members and/or prospective users" (1, 2, 4). Although an exercise facility may not have an expressed legal responsibility to conduct a preparticipation health screening, the aforementioned published standards of care serve the best health and safety considerations of exercise participants. Further, the health screening results should be interpreted by qualified staff and documented (3).

Preparticipation Health Screening

A well-designed preparticipation health screening questionnaire serves as the initial step in the fitness professional's health appraisal of exercise participants and includes the following categories:

Medical history review
Risk factor assessment and stratification
Prescribed medications
Level of physical activity
Establishing whether physician consent is necessary
Administration of fitness tests and evaluation of results
Setup of exercise prescription
Evaluation of progress with follow-up tests

It may help the fitness professional to remember the recommended health appraisal categories and order in which they are performed by using the acronym MR. PLEASE, which could represent the individual asking, "Mr., may I please exercise?" This protocol expands on previous recommendations for working with new clients in fitness settings (12).

Two standard preparticipation health screening questionnaires commonly used in the fitness industry are the PAR-Q and the Health Status Questionnaire. Both of these questionnaires address the categories in the acronym MR. PLEASE. Each level of MR. PLEASE is discussed in detail following the Health Status Questionnaire, and additional categories of screening are discussed after that.

Physical Activity Readiness Questionnaire

The Physical Activity Readiness Questionnaire (PAR-Q; see form 3.1) has been recommended as a simple, concise, and safe preexercise screening tool when individuals want to engage exclusively in light to moderate exercise activities (e.g., 20-60% $\dot{V}O_2R$ or HRR). Therefore, when individuals want to pursue only a moderate-intensity walking program, the PAR-Q might be considered appropriate for screening participants.

If a participant answers yes to any of the seven questions in this self-administered questionnaire, he or she is directed to contact a physician before undergoing a fitness test or pursuing regular physical activity (7). The PAR-Q produces an inordinate number of false-positives with older individuals (e.g., >60 yr), especially those

FORM 3.1 Physical Activity Readiness Questionnaire

Physical Activity Readiness
Questionnaire - PAR-Q
(revised 2002)

PAR-Q & YOU

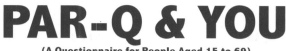

(A Questionnaire for People Aged 15 to 69)

Regular physical activity is fun and healthy, and increasingly more people are starting to become more active every day. Being more active is very safe for most people. However, some people should check with their doctor before they start becoming much more physically active.

If you are planning to become much more physically active than you are now, start by answering the seven questions in the box below. If you are between the ages of 15 and 69, the PAR-Q will tell you if you should check with your doctor before you start. If you are over 69 years of age, and you are not used to being very active, check with your doctor.

Common sense is your best guide when you answer these questions. Please read the questions carefully and answer each one honestly: check YES or NO.

YES	NO		
☐	☐	1.	**Has your doctor ever said that you have a heart condition and that you should only do physical activity recommended by a doctor?**
☐	☐	2.	**Do you feel pain in your chest when you do physical activity?**
☐	☐	3.	**In the past month, have you had chest pain when you were not doing physical activity?**
☐	☐	4.	**Do you lose your balance because of dizziness or do you ever lose consciousness?**
☐	☐	5.	**Do you have a bone or joint problem (for example, back, knee or hip) that could be made worse by a change in your physical activity?**
☐	☐	6.	**Is your doctor currently prescribing drugs (for example, water pills) for your blood pressure or heart condition?**
☐	☐	7.	**Do you know of any other reason why you should not do physical activity?**

If you answered

YES to one or more questions

Talk with your doctor by phone or in person BEFORE you start becoming much more physically active or BEFORE you have a fitness appraisal. Tell your doctor about the PAR-Q and which questions you answered YES.

- You may be able to do any activity you want — as long as you start slowly and build up gradually. Or, you may need to restrict your activities to those which are safe for you. Talk with your doctor about the kinds of activities you wish to participate in and follow his/her advice.
- Find out which community programs are safe and helpful for you.

NO to all questions

If you answered NO honestly to all PAR-Q questions, you can be reasonably sure that you can:

- start becoming much more physically active – begin slowly and build up gradually. This is the safest and easiest way to go.
- take part in a fitness appraisal – this is an excellent way to determine your basic fitness so that you can plan the best way for you to live actively. It is also highly recommended that you have your blood pressure evaluated. If your reading is over 144/94, talk with your doctor before you start becoming much more physically active.

DELAY BECOMING MUCH MORE ACTIVE:

- if you are not feeling well because of a temporary illness such as a cold or a fever – wait until you feel better; or
- if you are or may be pregnant – talk to your doctor before you start becoming more active.

PLEASE NOTE: If your health changes so that you then answer YES to any of the above questions, tell your fitness or health professional. Ask whether you should change your physical activity plan.

Informed Use of the PAR-Q: The Canadian Society for Exercise Physiology, Health Canada, and their agents assume no liability for persons who undertake physical activity, and if in doubt after completing this questionnaire, consult your doctor prior to physical activity.

No changes permitted. You are encouraged to photocopy the PAR-Q but only if you use the entire form.

NOTE: If the PAR-Q is being given to a person before he or she participates in a physical activity program or a fitness appraisal, this section may be used for legal or administrative purposes.

"I have read, understood and completed this questionnaire. Any questions I had were answered to my full satisfaction."

NAME ______________________________

SIGNATURE ______________________________ DATE ______________________

SIGNATURE OF PARENT ______________________________ WITNESS ______________________
or GUARDIAN (for participants under the age of majority)

Note: This physical activity clearance is valid for a maximum of 12 months from the date it is completed and becomes invalid if your condition changes so that you would answer YES to any of the seven questions.

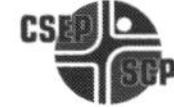

Supported by: 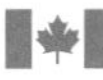 Health Canada Santé Canada

continued on other side...

(continued)

FORM 3.1 Physical Activity Readiness Questionnaire *(continued)*

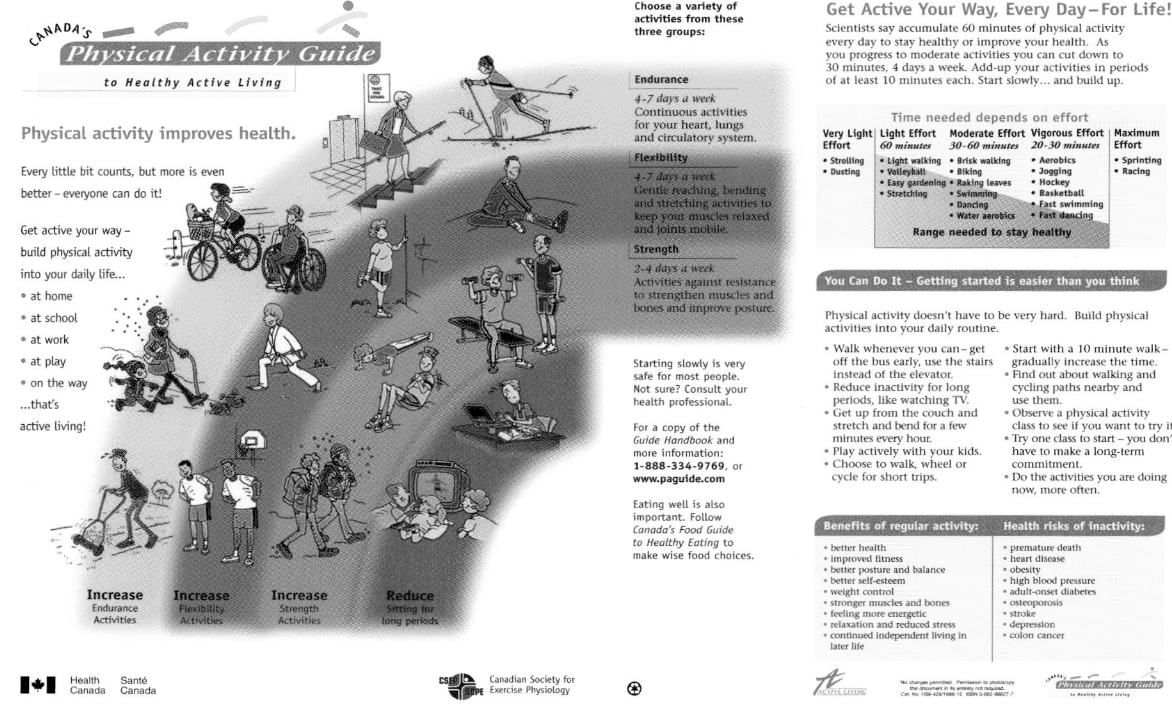

...continued from other side

PAR-Q & YOU

Physical Activity Readiness
Questionnaire - PAR-Q
(revised 2002)

Canada's **Physical Activity Guide** to Healthy Active Living

Physical activity improves health.

Every little bit counts, but more is even better – everyone can do it!

Get active your way – build physical activity into your daily life...

- at home
- at school
- at work
- at play
- on the way

...that's active living!

Choose a variety of activities from these three groups:

Endurance
4-7 days a week
Continuous activities for your heart, lungs and circulatory system.

Flexibility
4-7 days a week
Gentle reaching, bending and stretching activities to keep your muscles relaxed and joints mobile.

Strength
2-4 days a week
Activities against resistance to strengthen muscles and bones and improve posture.

Increase Endurance Activities | **Increase** Flexibility Activities | **Increase** Strength Activities | **Reduce** Sitting for long periods

Starting slowly is very safe for most people. Not sure? Consult your health professional.

For a copy of the *Guide Handbook* and more information: **1-888-334-9769**, or **www.paguide.com**

Eating well is also important. Follow *Canada's Food Guide to Healthy Eating* to make wise food choices.

Get Active Your Way, Every Day – For Life!

Scientists say accumulate 60 minutes of physical activity every day to stay healthy or improve your health. As you progress to moderate activities you can cut down to 30 minutes, 4 days a week. Add-up your activities in periods of at least 10 minutes each. Start slowly... and build up.

Time needed depends on effort

Very Light Effort	Light Effort *60 minutes*	Moderate Effort *30-60 minutes*	Vigorous Effort *20-30 minutes*	Maximum Effort
• Strolling • Dusting	• Light walking • Volleyball • Easy gardening • Stretching	• Brisk walking • Biking • Raking leaves • Swimming • Dancing • Water aerobics	• Aerobics • Jogging • Hockey • Basketball • Fast swimming • Fast dancing	• Sprinting • Racing

Range needed to stay healthy

You Can Do It – Getting started is easier than you think

Physical activity doesn't have to be very hard. Build physical activities into your daily routine.

- Walk whenever you can – get off the bus early, use the stairs instead of the elevator.
- Reduce inactivity for long periods, like watching TV.
- Get up from the couch and stretch and bend for a few minutes every hour.
- Play actively with your kids.
- Choose to walk, wheel or cycle for short trips.
- Start with a 10 minute walk – gradually increase the time.
- Find out about walking and cycling paths nearby and use them.
- Observe a physical activity class to see if you want to try it.
- Try one class to start – you don't have to make a long-term commitment.
- Do the activities you are doing now, more often.

Benefits of regular activity:	Health risks of inactivity:
• better health • improved fitness • better posture and balance • better self-esteem • weight control • stronger muscles and bones • feeling more energetic • relaxation and reduced stress • continued independent living in later life	• premature death • heart disease • obesity • high blood pressure • adult-onset diabetes • osteoporosis • stroke • depression • colon cancer

Health Canada Santé Canada

Canadian Society for Exercise Physiology

Active Living

Cat. No. H39-429/1998-1E ISBN 0-662-86627-7

Canada's Physical Activity Guide to Healthy Active Living

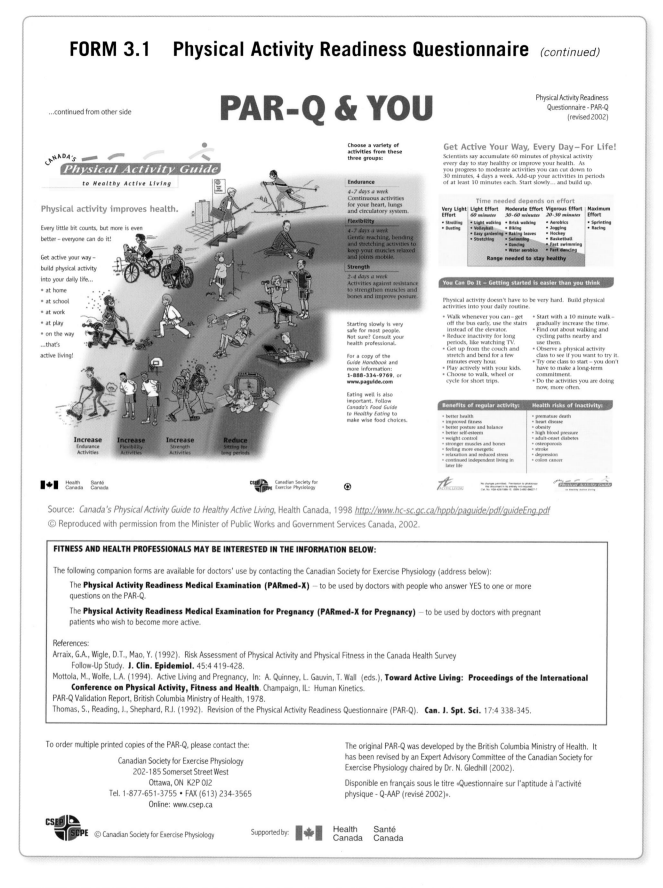

Source: *Canada's Physical Activity Guide to Healthy Active Living*, Health Canada, 1998 http://www.hc-sc.gc.ca/hppb/paguide/pdf/guideEng.pdf

FITNESS AND HEALTH PROFESSIONALS MAY BE INTERESTED IN THE INFORMATION BELOW:

The following companion forms are available for doctors' use by contacting the Canadian Society for Exercise Physiology (address below):

The **Physical Activity Readiness Medical Examination (PARmed-X)** – to be used by doctors with people who answer YES to one or more questions on the PAR-Q.

The **Physical Activity Readiness Medical Examination for Pregnancy (PARmed-X for Pregnancy)** – to be used by doctors with pregnant patients who wish to become more active.

References:

Arraix, G.A., Wigle, D.T., Mao, Y. (1992). Risk Assessment of Physical Activity and Physical Fitness in the Canada Health Survey Follow-Up Study. **J. Clin. Epidemiol.** 45:4 419-428.

Mottola, M., Wolfe, L.A. (1994). Active Living and Pregnancy, In: A. Quinney, L. Gauvin, T. Wall (eds.), **Toward Active Living: Proceedings of the International Conference on Physical Activity, Fitness and Health**. Champaign, IL: Human Kinetics.

PAR-Q Validation Report, British Columbia Ministry of Health, 1978.

Thomas, S., Reading, J., Shephard, R.J. (1992). Revision of the Physical Activity Readiness Questionnaire (PAR-Q). **Can. J. Spt. Sci.** 17:4 338-345.

To order multiple printed copies of the PAR-Q, please contact the:

Canadian Society for Exercise Physiology
202-185 Somerset Street West
Ottawa, ON K2P 0J2
Tel. 1-877-651-3755 • FAX (613) 234-3565
Online: www.csep.ca

The original PAR-Q was developed by the British Columbia Ministry of Health. It has been revised by an Expert Advisory Committee of the Canadian Society for Exercise Physiology chaired by Dr. N. Gledhill (2002).

Disponible en français sous le titre «Questionnaire sur l'aptitude à l'activité physique - Q-AAP (revisé 2002)».

Supported by:  Health Canada Santé Canada

with orthopedic problems (8). The fitness professional should ask additional questions to those individuals who check yes to a given question to determine whether they have legitimate medical reasons to seek physician consent before exercising. Given that most facilities offer vigorous-intensity exercise, the remainder of this chapter addresses how to screen individuals for this level of activity.

Health Status Questionnaire

A more thorough preparticipation screening tool, the Health Status Questionnaire (HSQ; see form 3.2), provides the fitness professional with enough information to quickly and accurately identify medical contraindications to exercise, **risk factors** for coronary heart disease (CHD), and lifestyle behaviors that may affect the individual's ability to begin exercising safely. The HSQ provided in this text has been expanded from the AHA and ACSM health and fitness facility preparticipation screening questionnaire to include sections on specific physical activity patterns, current medications, and a patient information release form (1). This information will help the fitness professional determine whether a physician's consent is required before proceeding with the fitness test. Fitness professionals who administer an HSQ should also consider its legal and personal content.

A completed HSQ will contain a significant amount of personal health information, which is protected under the Health Insurance Portability and Accountability Act (HIPAA) of 1996 (17). Thus, a completed HSQ should be kept in a secure location and accessible only by designated staff. A participant's medical history and fitness test results constitute personal health information. This information should be shared only with other health professionals who will be working with the participant and should be discussed, if necessary, in a private setting in which fellow staff or participants cannot overhear. For instance, a violation of HIPAA regulations would occur if a participant's body composition results were discussed with another participant or fellow staff member where other individuals could listen to the conversation.

Fitness professionals should note the patient information release form at the end of the HSQ. Participants must sign this section so that their respective physician(s) may release their pertinent medical information to the fitness professional, if warranted, in accordance with the HIPAA of 1996 (17).

Aside from legal rights that protect personal health information, the fitness professional should consider that many participants may feel uncomfortable sharing their detailed medical history with a person they have just met. To make them feel more at ease, ask additional questions concerning medical diagnoses. For instance, when a participant has checked the box for heart disease, you might ask, "Are your heart disease symptoms stable (if present)?" "How has your heart attack affected your activities of daily life?" "Has your physician given you any restrictions regarding your physical activity levels?" "Have you been able to return to the activities you were doing before the event?" "Did you participate in cardiac rehabilitation?" Relevant responses should be documented on the HSQ. Reviewing the HSQ conversationally allows the fitness professional to learn more about the participant's health status and to convey empathy. Then participants are more likely to consider the fitness professional as being genuinely concerned with helping them improve their health.

It is important to understand that no HSQ can address all possible medical conditions that might warrant physician consent. Thus, the fitness professional is encouraged to ask additional questions relevant to the participant's medical history while reviewing the HSQ. By doing so, all probable medical diagnoses or symptoms that may possibly place the participant at additional CHD risk during exercise are addressed. A fitness facility may want to make minor alterations to the HSQ presented so that it may be more applicable to their participant population.

If a prospective exercise participant refuses to complete a HSQ, then they cannot be properly screened according to the standards of care for fitness facilities advocated by the AHA and ACSM. In this case, the participant should be informed that the HSQ is a safety-oriented screening tool and the information will be shared only with proper health care professionals. If the prospective participant still refuses, the fitness supervisor or director of the facility should be consulted for further direction.

Medical History Review

The first step of evaluating health status—the medical history review—is addressed in section 2 of the HSQ. The history is assessed with a series of questions covering the participant's heart history, symptoms, and additional health

> **Key Point**
>
> Evaluation of a preparticipation health screening questionnaire helps the fitness professional determine a participant's current health status and whether it is appropriate for the participant to undergo fitness testing or begin regular physical activity. In addition, fitness professionals can assess the presence of relevant medical conditions, risk factors for CHD, lifestyle behaviors, and medications that will assist in the determination of the necessity of a physician's consent before beginning an exercise program. This information is protected by the Health Insurance Portability and Accountability Act (HIPAA) of 1996.

FORM 3.2 Health Status Questionnaire

This questionnaire identifies adults for whom physical activity might be inappropriate or adults who should seek physician consultation before beginning a regular physical activity program.

Section 1 Personal and Emergency Contact Information

Name: ______________________________ Date of birth: ____________

Address: ________________________________ Phone: ____________

Physician's name: ____

Height: ____________ Weight: ____________

Person to contact in case of emergency

Name: ________________________________ Phone: ____________

Section 2 General Medical History

Please check the following conditions you have experienced.

Heart History

____ Heart attack

____ Heart surgery

____ Cardiac catheterization

____ Coronary angioplasty (PTCA)

____ Cardiac pacemaker

____ Cardiac rhythm disturbance

____ Heart valve disease

____ Heart failure

____ Heart transplantation

____ Congenital heart disease

Symptoms

____ You experience chest discomfort with exertion.

____ You experience unreasonable shortness of breath at any time.

____ You experience dizziness, fainting, or blackouts.

____ You take heart medications.

Additional Health Issues

____ You have diabetes (type 1 or type 2).

____ You have asthma or other lung disease (e.g., emphysema).

____ You have burning or cramping sensations in your lower legs with minimal physical activity.

____ You have joint problems (e.g., arthritis) that limit your physical activity.

____ You have concerns about the safety of exercise.

____ You take prescription medications.

____ You are pregnant.

Section 3 Risk Factor Assessment

Risk Factors for Coronary Heart Disease

_____ You are a man older than 45 yr.

_____ You are a woman older than 55 yr, have had a hysterectomy, or are postmenopausal.

_____ You smoke or you quit smoking within the previous 6 mo.

_____ Your blood pressure is >140/90 mmHg.

_____ Your blood cholesterol is >200 mg · dl^{-1}.

_____ You have a close male blood relative (father or brother) who had a heart attack or heart surgery before the age of 55 or a close female blood relative (mother or sister) who had a heart attack or heart surgery before the age of 65.

_____ You are physically inactive (you get <30 min of physical activity at least 3 days per wk).

_____ Your waist circumference is >40 in. (101.6 cm in men) or >35 in. (88.9 cm in women).

Section 4 Medications

Are you currently taking any medication? ❏ Yes ❏ No

If yes, please list all of your prescribed medications and how often you take them, whether daily (D) or as needed (PRN). ______________________________

____

Of the medications you have listed, are there any you do not take as prescribed?

____

Section 5 Physical Activity Patterns and Objectives

List the type, frequency, intensity (e.g., low, moderate, strenuous), and duration of your weekly exercise. ______________________________

____

List your specific goals for your exercise program. ______________________________

____

Please inform the fitness professional immediately of any changes that occur in your health status.

Patient Information Release Form

If you have answered yes to questions indicating that you have significant cardiac, pulmonary, metabolic, or orthopedic problems that may be exacerbated with exercise, you agree it is permissible for us to contact your physician regarding your health status.

Signature: ______________________________ Date: ____________

Fitness staff signature: ______________________________ Date: ____________

To be completed by fitness professional (circle one):

AHA/ACSM risk stratification: ❏ Low ❏ Moderate ❏ High

Physician consent: ❏ Yes ❏ No

issues. This information helps the fitness professional determine whether physician consent is warranted before the participant engages in a regular exercise program. The AHA and ACSM recommend that individuals who mark any of the statements in this section should consult a physician or an appropriate health care provider before pursuing a regular exercise program. Participants diagnosed with CHD, symptoms suggestive of a chronic pulmonary disease, or type 1 or 2 diabetes require physician consent before they undergo fitness testing or regular exercise participation (1, 2).

The decision-making processes in the following sections are based on the premise that the fitness professional works in a structured fitness facility. Personal trainers who work with individuals on their own are encouraged to use the same guidelines.

It is important to note the AHA and ACSM recommendations for seeking physician consent are guidelines, and the fitness professional must rely on his or her professional experience and academic knowledge when making decisions on physician consent. For example, a prospective participant indicates she is taking a prescription medication. Does this medical history automatically warrant physician consent? Not necessarily, because many people take medications for a variety of health reasons. The fitness professional could use the answer as a cue to indicate the participant may take medications for CHD or other diseases that may be aggravated with exercise. The fitness professional will review the participant's prescribed medications (i.e., section 4) to help make a more definitive decision regarding physician consent. This instance should encourage the fitness professional to analyze the results of the entire HSQ before making a final decision regarding physician consent.

The fitness professional should be able to identify specific medical conditions which significantly increase the risks of a coronary event occurring during exercise testing (2). The risks of exercise testing exceed its benefits for individuals with certain conditions. A list of the absolute and relative contraindications to exercise testing identified by the ACSM for nonhospital settings is provided on page 29 (13). The fitness professional should be aware that a contraindication indicates the most health professionals would not recommend that participant undergo fitness testing or participate in regular physical activity without physician consent.

Additional clarification and suggestions on when the fitness professional should seek physician consent or when clinic-based supervised exercise program is necessary for a participant is provided in the following sections. In the event that the fitness professional is still uncertain whether a medical history requires physician consent before performing a fitness test, the professional should consult a supervisor or medically qualified personnel for further clarification.

Risk Factor Assessment and Stratification

Risk factor assessment and stratification take place by reviewing section 3 of the HSQ, which contains specific information concerning the individual's risk factors for CHD. For the remainder of this chapter, the term *risk factor* refers to a primary risk factor for CHD. The AHA and ACSM recommend obtaining consent from a physician or an appropriate health care provider before exercise participation if two or more statements are marked in section 3 (1, 2, 4).

The fitness professional should establish and quantify the participant's specific CHD risk factors using the thresholds listed in table 3.1. The scope of this table is not exhaustive, because emerging risk factors such as elevated triglycerides, which have been highly correlated with the progression of CHD, are not included. The conditions and values listed in the table were chosen to help fitness professionals identify individuals who likely have CHD but have not been clinically diagnosed. Also, the information in table 3.1 should be cross-referenced with sections 2 and 3 of the HSQ to ensure that each risk factor is acknowledged. These results will help the fitness professional establish whether physician consent is necessary, which is the case if an individual has two or more risk factors for CHD (1, 2).

When analyzing the HSQ, it is imperative to acknowledge that the risk status of individuals with and without CHD varies significantly. Regular physical activity reduces the cardiovascular morbidity and mortality for persons with established CHD (10). Yet the incidence of a coronary event during exercise for these individuals is estimated to be 10 times greater than that of healthy adults (11). Further, each risk factor does not cause an equal increase in an individual's risk for a coronary event. For example, a diagnosis of diabetes is considered a CHD equivalent. A person who has diabetes but not CHD is as likely to have a coronary event as is a person who has CHD or who has already experienced a coronary event (9). These facts underline the necessity of fitness professionals to understand a participant's medical history before administering fitness tests or administering exercise prescriptions.

Fitness professionals should educate participants about their risk factors for CHD and their significance. Initially, they should explain the meaning of a risk factor (i.e., a clinical diagnosis or lifestyle behavior that has been proven to increase a person's chances of developing heart disease). Some fitness professionals may want to quantify the severity of a participant's individual risk factors and overall relative risk for developing CHD by using the Framingham algorithm (14).

Next, fitness professionals should address which risk factors can be modified and inform participants that

Contraindications to Exercise Testing

Absolute contraindications

- Recent significant change in the resting ECG suggesting significant ischemia, recent myocardial infarction (within 2 days), or other acute event
- Unstable angina
- Uncontrolled cardiac dysrhythmias causing symptoms or hemodynamic compromise
- Symptomatic severe aortic stenosis
- Uncontrolled symptomatic heart failure
- Acute pulmonary embolus or pulmonary infarction
- Acute myocarditis or pericarditis
- Suspected or known dissecting aneurysm
- Acute systemic infection, accompanied by fever, body aches, or swollen lymph glands

Relative contraindications†

- Left main coronary stenosis
- Moderate stenotic valvular heart disease
- Electrolyte abnormalities (i.e., hypokalemia, hypomagnesemia)
- Severe arterial hypertension (i.e., systolic blood pressure >200 mmHg or diastolic blood pressure >100 mmHg at rest)
- Tachydysrhythmia or bradydysrhythmia
- Hypertrophic cardiomyopathy and other forms of outflow tract obstruction
- Neuromuscular, musculoskeletal, or rheumatoid disorders that are exacerbated by exercise
- High-degree atrioventricular block
- Ventricular aneurysm
- Uncontrolled metabolic disease (i.e., diabetes, thyrotoxicosis, or myxedema)
- Chronic infectious disease (i.e., mononucleosis, hepatitis, AIDS)
- Mental or physical impairment leading to inability to exercise adequately

†Relative contraindications can be superseded if the benefits of exercise testing outweigh the risks of exercise. In some instances, individuals with relative contraindications can exercise with caution and with using low-level end points, especially if they are asymptomatic at rest.

Reprinted, by permission, from American College of Sports Medicine (ACSM), 2006, *ACSM's guidelines for exercise testing and prescription*, 7th ed. (Philadelphia, PA: Lippincott, Williams & Wilkins), 50. Modified from R.J. Gibbons, G.J. Balady, J. Bricker et al., 2002, ACC/AHA 2002 guideline update for exercise testing: a report of the American College of Cardiology/American Heart Association Task Force on Practice Guidelines (Committee on Exercise Testing), American College of Cardiology web site. Available: www.acc.org/clinical/guidelines/exercise/dirIndex.htm.

adequate amounts of regular physical activity can modify most risk factors for CHD and prevent additional ones from developing (1, 2, 5). The possibility that regular physical activity may help manage and prevent these risk factors can serve as powerful motivation for long-term exercise adherence.

Fitness professionals should next consider participants' health status, symptoms, and risk factors and classify them into one of the following three risk strata (adapted from table 2.4 in the *ACSM's Guidelines for Exercise Testing and Prescription* [1]):

- **Low risk.** Men <45 yr and women <55 yr who are asymptomatic and meet no more than one risk factor threshold from table 3.1
- **Moderate risk.** Men >45 yr and women >55 yr *or* people who meet the threshold for two or more risk factors from table 3.1
- **High risk.** Individuals who have known cardiovascular (e.g., cardiac, peripheral vascular, or cerebrovascular), pulmonary (e.g., chronic obstructive pulmonary diseases), or metabolic disease (e.g., type 1 and type 2 diabetes) or who show signs or symptoms suggestive of these diseases. Major signs and symptoms are angina, shortness of breath at rest or with mild exertion, dizziness, loss of consciousness, ankle swelling, palpitations, tachycardia, heart murmurs, and intermittent claudication.

Table 3.1 Coronary Artery Disease Risk Factor Thresholds for ACSM Risk Stratification

Positive risk factors	Defining criteria
1. Family history	Myocardial infarction, coronary revascularization, or sudden death before age 55 in father or other male first-degree relative or before age 65 in mother or other female first-degree relative
2. Cigarette smoking	Current cigarette smoker *or* Smoker who quit within the previous 6 mo
3. Hypertension	Systolic blood pressure ≥ 140 mmHg or diastolic blood pressure ≥ 90 mmHg, confirmed by measurements on at least two separate occasions *or* On antihypertensive medications
4. Dyslipidemia	Low-density lipoprotein (LDL) cholesterol > 130 mg · dl^{-1} (3.4 mmol · L^{-1}), high-density lipoprotein (HDL) cholesterol < 40 mg · dl^{-1} (1.03 mmol · L^{-1}), or total serum cholesterol (if only measurement available) > 200 mg · dl^{-1} (5.2 mmol · L^{-1}) *or* On lipid-lowering medication
5. Impaired fasting	Fasting blood glucose > 100 mg · dl^{-1} (5.6 mmol · L^{-1}), confirmed by glucose measurements on at least two separate occasions
6. Obesity*	Body mass index > 30 kg · m^{-2} *or* Waist girth > 102 cm for men and > 88 cm for women *or* Waist–hip ratio ≥ 0.95 for men and ≥ 0.86 for women
7. Sedentary lifestyle	Individuals not participating in a regular exercise program or not accumulating 30 min or more of moderate physical activity on most days or week
Negative risk factor	**Defining criteria**
1. High serum cholesterol±	HDL > 60 mg · dl^{-1} (1.6 mmol · L^{-1})

* Professional opinions vary regarding the most appropriate thresholds for obesity; thus allied health professionals should use clinical judgment when evaluating this risk factor.

± It is common to sum risk factors in making clinical judgments. If HDL is high, subtract one risk factor from the sum of positive risk factors, since high HDL decreases CAD risk.

Reprinted, by permission, from American College of Sports Medicine (ACSM), 2006, *ACSM's guidelines for exercise testing and prescription*, 7th ed. (Philadelphia, PA: Lippincott, Williams & Wilkins), 22.

To ensure that each participant is stratified, the last notation of the HSQ prompts the fitness professional to document whether the participant is considered low, moderate, or high risk. Proper stratification is critical in determining a participant's current health status and whether physician consent is warranted before beginning fitness testing or regular exercise participation. Proper stratification also should be used to prescribe an appropriate exercise program.

Key Point

Analyzing the first three sections of the HSQ allows the fitness professional to identify risk factors and medical conditions that will be aggravated with exercise testing as well as categorize the health risks of exercise participants. This information coupled with the participant's desired activity level will determine whether a participant requires physician consent to begin exercising.

Prescribed Medications

Identifying prescribed medications is the next step in the health evaluation process. Section 4 of the HSQ requires the individual to document prescribed medications. The fitness professional should study appendix D of this book to be aware of common medications and their effects. An individual's medication regimen can provide additional insight into their medical history and diagnosed risk factors. In addition, the fitness professional should be able to determine whether a prescribed medication will alter the typical physiological responses to physical activity. For example, if a participant is taking a medication from the class of drugs known as beta blockers, the fitness professional should be aware that the participant's heart rate is unlikely to exceed 120 beats/min even though the participant is exercising strenuously. This response should not be considered abnormal; instead, it indicates the efficacy of the medication.

As mentioned previously, section 2 of the HSQ asks whether the participant takes heart medications or any prescribed medications. When these questions are checked, it should prompt the fitness professional to review the participant's medication list to determine whether he or she takes medications commonly prescribed for chronic diseases such as high blood pressure, elevated cholesterol, or diabetes. In this manner, risk factors can be more readily identified, which expedites the participant's risk stratification and the determination of whether physician consent is warranted. This instance underlines the importance of evaluating the overall HSQ rather than simply relying on one section to determine whether physician consent is necessary.

Level of Physical Activity

Section 5 indicates the individual's present level of physical activity as well as specific goals regarding the exercise program. As indicated in table 3.1, if an individual does not accumulate 30 min of physical activity at least three days a week, then the individual has the risk factor of physical inactivity (1, 2). Further, the ACSM recommends that the physical activity should be at least moderate intensity (2). Section 5 asks the participant to note the intensity of exercise he or she performs as low, moderate, or strenuous. Because exercise intensity is subjective, the fitness professional should discuss an example of each one of these intensity designations. Thus, the fitness professional will have further insight regarding the participant's actual physical activity level. Further, the fitness professional should ask if exercising causes any physiological responses the participant considers unusual (e.g., exceptional shortness of breath, significant joint or muscle pain or soreness). If so, the participant's remarks should be documented and taken into consideration regarding whether or not physician consent is warranted.

Establishing Necessity of Physician Consent

The information obtained in the prior sections of the HSQ should be used by the fitness professional to determine if the participant needs physician consent before they begin a moderate- or vigorous-intensity exercise program.

Individuals in the low-risk category may begin a regular program of vigorous exercise (1, 2, 4). For instance, a 43-yr-old female with only hypertension who walks for 30 min four times a week is considered a low-risk participant. Further, the ACSM does not recommend physician consent for individuals in the moderate-risk category if they plan to engage in no greater than moderate-intensity exercise (e.g., <60% $\dot{V}O_2R$ or HRR) (1). Therefore, an apparently healthy person who has two or more risk factors for CHD (see table 3.1) can safely initiate a walking program without physician consent. Fitness professionals should provide individuals in this category with specific examples of recommended exercise (e.g., walking briskly at 3-4 mi $\cdot$ hr^{-1}, or 4.8-6.4 km $\cdot$ hr^{-1}) as well as adequate supervision to ensure they are exercising in the correct intensity range.

Most health or fitness facilities offer vigorous-intensity physical activity, and staff at the facilities cannot reasonably supervise each participant at moderate risk during each visit. Thus, they might consider developing a standard protocol in which all individuals classified as moderate risk or greater receive physician consent before pursuing a regular exercise program. This protocol helps ensure the greatest safety for exercise participants.

Individuals classified as moderate or high risk should obtain physician consent before they begin a vigorous-intensity exercise program (e.g., >60% $\dot{V}O_2R$ or HRR) (1). For example, a 48-yr-old physically inactive male with high cholesterol and hypertension who wants to pursue a new jogging program has three risk factors. This individual would be classified as moderate risk and wants to begin a vigorous exercise program, thus physician consent is required before the person can participate in the program. The fitness professional should be aware that participants with diabetes (type 1 or type 2) are classified as high risk regardless of additional risk factors for CHD and thus warrant physician consent before exercising (1, 2). Although the AHA and ACSM offer specific recommendations regarding medical clearance before exercise participation, it is in the best interest of each fitness facility director to determine the facility's preparticipation screening policy in consideration of the qualifications of personnel, emergency preparedness, and the target population they serve (1, 2, 4, 6).

Administration of Fitness Tests and Evaluation of Results

The next step of the health appraisal involves administering and evaluating fitness tests. When combined with the HSQ, the test results provide greater insight into an individual's current level of physical fitness. Although a participant's HSQ may not warrant physician consent, the participant's fitness test results may indicate that it is necessary. Further, the fitness test results may necessitate the referral of the participant to a medically supervised exercise program (see table 3.2). A common instance the fitness professional will encounter is individuals with low fitness levels or test scores since they do not exercise regularly. These individuals will likely have one or more additional risk factors. These risk factors, combined with the results of the fitness test, will guide the decision of whether physician consent is necessary.

Common measurements obtained before a cardiovascular fitness test are resting heart rate (HR) and blood pressure (BP), percent body fat, waist circumference, and low-back flexibility. Next, a submaximal graded exercise

Table 3.2 Criteria for Decisions on Physical Activity

Basis for physician consent		
Conditions		
Breathless with slight exertion	Heart disease, operation, or problem	
Cirrhosis	Pain in the abdomen, leg, arm, shoulder, or chest	
Concussion	Phlebitis	
Current medication for diabetes	Pregnancy	
Faintness or dizziness	Stroke	
Test scores[a]		
Resting HR > 100 beats · min^{-1}	LDL > 130 mg · dl^{-1}	
Resting SBP > 160 mmHg	Fasting glucose > 126 mg · dl^{-1}	
Resting DBP > 100 mmHg	Vital capacity < 75% predicted	
% fat > 40 female; > 30 male	Vital capacity < 75% predicted	
Cholesterol > 240 mg · dl^{-1}	FEV_1 < 75%	
Basis for a supervised program		
Conditions (currently under control)[b]		
Alcoholism	Bronchitis	Epilepsy
Anemia	Cancer	Hypoglycemia
Anorexia	Colitis	Mental illness
Asthma	Diabetes	Peptic ulcer
Bleeding trait	Emphysema	Thyroid problem
Test scores[c]		
Hypertension ≥ 140 or ≥ 90 mmHg	Waist circumference > 100 cm	
High cholesterol > 240 mg · dl^{-1}	Smoking > 20 cigarettes a day	
LDL > 130 mg · dl^{-1}	Obesity 32%-38% females; 25%-28% males	
Basis for special attention		
Conditions		
Arthritis	Hearing loss	
Back, eye, joint, lung, or neck operations	Hernia	
Eye problems	Low-back pain	
Gout		
Test scores		
Values of risk factors approaching those in supervised programs		
% fat < 15% or > 30% female; < 6% or > 25% male[d]		
Curl-ups < 10		
Any of the reasons for stopping a maximal that occur at light to moderate work		
Sit and reach < 15 cm		
Modified pull-ups < 5		
Max METs < 8		
Push-ups < 10		
Max $\dot{V}O_2$ < 30		

Any condition or test value that causes the person or the fitness professional to be concerned for the person's health or safety forms the basis for physician consent. HR = heart rate; LDL = low-density lipoprotein; SBP = systolic blood pressure; DBP = diastolic blood pressure; FEV_1 = forced expiratory volume in 1 sec; RPE = rating of perceived exertion.

[a]Any of these individual scores would be the basis for physician consent. A person might also require consent if more than one test score approached these values.

[b]Severe or uncontrolled levels should be referred for medical attention.

[c]Persons with higher scores should be referred for medical attention.

[d]Participants who have either too little fat or too much fat may have health problems that need special attention. If there is any question, refer them to the program director.

From American College of Sports Medicine (ACSM), 2006, *ACSM's guidelines for exercise testing and prescription*, 7th ed. (Philadelphia, PA: Lippincott, Williams, & Wilkins).

Key Point

The last two sections of the HSQ enable the fitness professional to learn what medications the participant takes to address medical conditions and their specific level of physical activity. These results should be considered along with the participant's risk factors so that the participant can be readily risk stratified and the fitness professional can determine whether physician consent is necessary before undergoing fitness testing. In addition, certain fitness test results or changes in health status may also necessitate physician consent.

Health Appraisal Overview

Medical history review. Use a pre-participation health screening questionnaire to determine if any medical conditions indicate the participant should seek physician consent before undergoing fitness testing and regular physical activity participation.

Risk factor assessment and risk stratification. Identify risk factors and stratify participant (e.g., low, moderate, high) based on their number of risk factors for CHD and if they have known cardiovascular, pulmonary, and metabolic disease.

Prescribed medications. Identify medications that will alter the typical physiological responses to exercise and make certain diagnosed risk factors are being treated pharmacologically.

Level of physical activity. How frequently, intensely, and for what duration do they perform specific physical activities.

Establishing whether physician consent is necessary. The participant's medical history, risk stratification, and current level of physical activity should be used to determine if physician consent is necessary prior to fitness test administration and/or regular physical activity participation according to the AHA/ACSM standards of practice.

Administration of fitness tests and evaluation of results. Determine what fitness tests are appropriate given the participant's health status.

Setup of exercise prescription. Consider the participant's medical history, past physical activity patterns, fitness results, and personal goals to prescribe an appropriate exercise program.

Evaluation of progress with follow-up tests. Determine if the participant's fitness level and risk stratification have changed.

test is conducted to determine how the participant's HR, BP, and rating of perceived exertion (RPE) respond to gradually increasing exercise workloads. Further, fitness tests may determine muscular strength and endurance. Fitness testing procedures are included in chapters 5, 6, 8, and 9. The participant's values for these tests, combined with their medical history and exercise goals, should serve as the framework for their exercise prescription.

Setup of Exercise Prescription

At this point, the fitness professional should be prepared to address the next step in the health appraisal process: setting up the individual's exercise prescription. An appropriate exercise prescription considers a person's health status, personal goals, and fitness test results. Chapters 10, 11, 12, and 13 address exercise prescriptions for aerobic fitness, weight management, muscular strength and endurance, flexibility, and low-back function for generally healthy adults. In addition, chapters 15 through 21 suggest exercise prescriptions for special populations.

Evaluation of Progress With Follow-Up Tests

The participant's exercise goals and health status are certain to change, which necessitates the last step in the health appraisal: Evaluate progress with follow-up tests. Fitness tests should be periodically repeated and a HSQ should be periodically readministered. Follow-ups involving fitness tests and updates to the participant's health status serve several purposes: documenting the participant's health and fitness progress, identifying any changes in health status or response to activity, and indicating whether changes are necessary in the exercise prescription or level of supervision should change. A follow-up fitness test may be conducted 3 mo after the participant has been exercising regularly, with biannual testing thereafter. An overview of the health appraisal process is provided above.

Fitness Program Decisions

This chapter has addressed the guidelines supported by the AHA and ACSM concerning when physician consent is necessary before a participant begins an exercise program. The following section discusses additional criteria to consider as the fitness professional decides which of the following actions to pursue:

- Immediate referral for physician consent or proper medical consultation
- Admission to one of the following fitness programs:
  - Clinic-based supervised exercise program
  - Carefully prescribed exercise under the supervision of a fitness professional
  - Vigorous-intensity exercise
  - Any unsupervised physical activity
- Educational information, seminars, or referral to other health professionals

Fitness professionals will encounter individuals who don't specifically meet the criteria for moderate or high risk but are on the verge of meeting these criteria. Do they require physician consent? Should they exercise in a supervised capacity? The following section helps resolve these dilemmas.

Determining Necessary Supervision

Altogether, the fitness professional should consider the participant's health status, fitness test results, and desired activity level to determine whether physician consent or referral to a supervised exercise program is necessary. Table 3.2 lists additional criteria for evaluating medical conditions and fitness test scores, which should provide further guidance on whether physician referral or a supervised program is warranted. A supervised program entails professionally qualified staff that have academic training in and clinical knowledge of monitoring special populations classified as high risk (e.g., individuals diagnosed with CHD, pulmonary, or metabolic disease) (1, 2).

The AHA and ACSM risk stratification classifications (i.e., low, moderate, and high risk) are not all inclusive, and not every person fits precisely into one of these categories (1). In kind, the AHA and ACSM recommendations for seeking physician consent do not always apply. Therefore, fitness professionals must rely on their professional experience and academic knowledge to decide on physician referrals. For example, a review of the HSQ for a 52-yr-old female includes an acknowledgment that she checked yes to having a musculoskeletal problem that limits her physical activity. Upon further questioning, she states she has consistent pain in her right knee when she takes her daily morning walk, which limits her walking speed. She has been diagnosed with arthritis. She did not check yes for any other condition in section 2 or 3 of the HSQ. According to the AHA and ACSM guidelines, since she acknowledged having a condition listed in section 2 of the HSQ, her physician should be consulted before she begins exercising. Given that she exercises regularly and cites no risk factors, she could undergo a fitness test without her physician's consent, although her exercise prescription should be modified to account for her arthritis. If the fitness professional is uncertain whether a medical condition requires physician consent before performing a fitness test, he should consult a supervisor or medically qualified personnel for further clarification. Similar instances may occur when assessing additional metabolic and fitness tests.

Numerous conditions and fitness test scores warrant additional supervision and special attention (see table 3.2). Using physical conditions to indicate low, moderate, and high risk is somewhat arbitrary. Consider each variable as residing on a continuum that begins with low risk and progresses to high risk. For instance, when a person has a fasting blood glucose level of 118 $mg \cdot dl^{-1}$ (clinically considered as impaired glucose tolerance), is he necessarily at less cardiovascular risk than a person with a fasting value of 128 $mg \cdot dl^{-1}$ (clinically diagnosed as having type 2 diabetes)? Both individuals have significant cardiovascular risks and should pursue lifestyle changes to lower their blood glucose levels. Do they both warrant physician consent for exercise participation? Again, the knowledge and experience of the fitness professional will help make this decision. Type 2 diabetes typically requires 2 to 5 yr to become clinically discernable (13). Thus, the participant's cardiovascular system has been exposed to elevated blood sugars for a prolonged time. Since type 2 diabetes is a CHD equivalent, fasting blood glucose levels on the borderline of the clinical diagnosis for type 2 diabetes indicate physician consent is necessary (1, 2).

The decision to seek physician consent or refer to a supervised exercise program can be solidified by considering additional medical history and fitness test values. For instance, individuals with elevated blood sugar commonly have high blood pressure, have elevated cholesterol, and are overweight. Also, they are likely to have exceptionally poor cardiovascular fitness levels (a maximum $\dot{V}O_2$ of $<25\ ml \cdot kg^{-1} \cdot min^{-1}$). Such individuals are on the borderline for several primary risk factors for CHD and are likely to have a fitness test score indicating that they require special attention (see table 3.2). Together, the participants' health status and fitness test results indicate that physician consent is necessary for exercise participation.

Borderline fitness test and resting values, such as resting BP and HR measurements, should be replicated before seeking physician consent. Either value could be temporarily elevated if the participant ate, smoked, or performed physical activity shortly before being measured. Also, apprehension about BP measurements or the presence of excessive noise may elevate the test results. In this case, permit the participant to relax for a couple of minutes, reassure the participant about the safety of the test, and perform the measurements again. After several measurements have confirmed a borderline or questionable test result, the fitness professional may decide to obtain physician consent before conducting further fitness tests (6).

Referral to Supervised Programs

The values that serve as the basis for a recommendation to a supervised exercise program are listed in table 3.2. As when making other decisions, fitness professionals should combine these guidelines with their professional experience and training with similar populations, the qualifications of other personnel in the facility, and the facility's emergency preparedness (6, 12). A participant who has exercise-induced asthma but controls it readily with an inhaler is likely to be safe during unsupervised exercise. In contrast, a participant with emphysema who is prone to low oxygen levels (i.e., O_2 saturation <88%) would benefit by initially exercising in a clinic-based supervised exercise program, such as pulmonary rehabilitation. Again, the fitness professional must decide when to refer a participant to a supervised exercise program by considering the participant's health status, fitness test results, and desired intensity of physical activity.

Structured exercise programs that offer immediate access to medical and emergency personnel (versus exercise facilities without these resources) may want to use higher values than those listed in table 3.2 (4). Each exercise facility, in conjunction with its medical advisors, should establish its own standards for physician consent and supervised exercise referrals that will ensure the greatest safety for participants.

Obtaining Physician Consent

After determining that a person requires physician consent, the fitness professional should promptly inform the participant of this requirement. The appropriate medical personnel, typically the participant's primary care physician, should provide the consent. A sample physician form is presented in form 3.3 (6). The form provides the physician with the option to refer the patient to a clinic-based supervised exercise facility. When a physician makes this recommendation, the fitness professional should contact the participant promptly and place him or her in contact with the nearest supervised exercise facility. In accordance with HIPAA regulations, the physician consent request must be accompanied by a medical release form (17).

Physician consent can be sought in one of two ways. First, the participant can be given the paperwork to be signed by a physician. After consulting with a physician, the participant can return the paperwork to the fitness professional for verification. Second, fitness professionals can contact the appropriate physician directly (e.g., fax the consent form to the physician's administrative office). Taking the initiative to contact a physician has both benefits and challenges. The following are benefits of taking the initiative:

- Demonstrates proper recognition of conditions requiring physician consent
- Permits a relatively prompt reply from the physician
- Acquires additional medical information so that the participant receives appropriate exercise testing and prescription
- Develops a rapport with local physicians conducive to obtaining future exercise referrals from those physicians

The workload of general practitioners does not allow them to quickly respond to each medical request they receive. Therefore, it is recommended to wait 3 business days before sending a second physician consent request. Thereafter, participants should be encouraged to contact the physician personally to expedite the return of the consent form. Participants requiring physician consent should be informed of the facility's protocol for contacting physicians so that they understand their clearance to begin exercising may take time. Although they may have to wait to exercise, participants should be assured that the steps taken in accordance with established protocols are based on serving their best health interest.

Key Point

The conditions and test scores listed in table 3.2 for physician consent or supervised programs are guidelines to be used with additional information about the participant in making a decision concerning safe and appropriate physical activity. Altogether, the exercise professional's academic knowledge and professional experience, coupled with the facility's preparticipation health screening standards and emergency preparedness, should be considered when making the decision concerning the level of necessary supervision for each participant.

Key Point

The participant's physician or appropriate medical personnel should be contacted immediately when physician consent is required for exercise participation.

FORM 3.3 Sample Physician Consent Form*

Dear Dr.: ____

Your patient ______________________________ would like to begin an exercise program at ______________________________ (name of health or fitness facility).

After reviewing ______________________________'s (patient's name) responses to our health status questionnaire, we would appreciate your medical opinion and recommendations concerning participation in regular exercise. Please provide the following information and return this form to

____ (Name)

____ (Address)

____ (Phone/fax)

1. Are there specific concerns or conditions our staff should be aware of before this individual engages in regular exercise at our facility? Yes/No. If yes, please specify.

   ____

   ____

2. If this individual has completed a graded exercise test, please provide the following:

   a. Date of test ____

   b. A copy of the final exercise test report and interpretation

   c. Your specific recommendations for exercise training, including heart rate limits

      during exercise: ____

3. Please provide the following information so that we may contact you if we have any further questions:

   ____ I AGREE to the participation of this individual in regular exercise activity at your fitness facility.

   ____ I DO NOT AGREE that this individual is a candidate for exercise at your fitness facility, and this individual should be referred to a supervised exercise facility because ____.

Physician's signature ____

Physician's name ____

Address____

Thank you for your consideration.

(Insert signature of fitness staff member) ______________________________

* Must be accompanied by a medical release form in accordance with HIPAA regulations.

From Edward T. Howley and B. Don Franks, 2007, *Fitness Professional's Handbook,* 5th ed. (Champaign, IL: Human Kinetics). Adapted, by permission, from American College of Sports Medicine and American Heart Association, 1998, "Recommendations for cardiovascular screening, staffing, and emergency policies at health/fitness facilities." *Medicine and Science in Sports and Exercise* 30: 1009-1018.

To prevent the delay of fitness tests for individuals requiring physician clearance, the HSQ should be completed and furnished to the appropriate fitness professional for review 2 to 3 business days before the fitness test is scheduled. Therefore, the appropriate paperwork is obtained before the fitness test and the participant can readily begin an exercise program.

Education

All participants with documented primary risk factors or borderline clinical values for CHD should be educated about their increased risk for heart disease. In addition, the fitness professional should discuss sensible lifestyle changes that the participants can pursue to more readily control their risk factors. However, information alone is unlikely to lead participants to make significant changes. Chapter 22 provides several approaches to changing behavior that fitness professionals can use to help the participant. In addition, the fitness professional can inform the participant of support groups, upcoming educational seminars, and other health professionals (e.g., dietitians) who can assist with proper lifestyle choices.

Changing Health or Fitness Status

People who regularly participate in physical activity are likely to experience significant positive changes in their fitness and in their risk factors for CHD. In most cases, these changes can be readily observed by an increase in the participant's exercise duration or intensity or a decrease in body weight.

In contrast, some new medical conditions may develop and not be readily apparent after a participant completes a fitness test. For instance, a participant may have chest pain consistently during exercise but may keep this information to himself. The HSQ directs participants to contact the fitness director when they experience significant changes in their health status. Although some people will notify staff members when health changes occur, many will not. Therefore, periodic fitness retesting and readministration of the HSQ are advisable to determine whether or not participants experiencing changes in health status should seek physician consent or be assigned to a supervised program.

If someone develops symptoms such as significant chest pain during exercise, the person should be referred to a physician. In addition, any participant initially classified as low to moderate risk who develops a medical condition that reclassifies him as high risk should be referred to a physician (1, 2, 4). Additional situations in which moderate- and vigorous-intensity exercise should be discontinued are musculoskeletal problems exacerbated with activity and severe psychological, medical, or drug or alcohol problems that are not responding to therapy (15). In addition, exercise should be deferred with major changes in resting blood pressure (1). It is the responsibility of the fitness professional to determine the length of time between follow-up fitness tests or HSQ administrations to ensure participants are properly risk stratified and pursuing the appropriate exercise program.

Key Point

Fitness professionals should be aware of temporary or chronic conditions that alter a participant's health status and warrant medical clearance, additional supervision, or changes in exercise recommendations. These conditions can de identified with periodic readministration of the HSQ and follow-up fitness tests.

Case Studies

You can check your answers by referring to page 469 in appendix A.

1. Tom, a 47-yr-old marketing agent who has been physically inactive for several years, visits your fitness facility to begin his fitness assessment. He has seen his physician recently and brings his recent lab results with him. Reviewing his HSQ, you note that he does not have a family history of heart disease. He is 5 ft 9 in. (1.75 m), weighs 185 lb (83.9 kg), and has a 39 in. (99.1 cm) waist. His HSQ states that he does have high blood pressure and high cholesterol, for which he is taking medication. His resting blood pressure is 124/82 and his resting pulse rate is 76. His blood chemistry values include a total cholesterol of 195 mg · dl^{-1}, an LDL cholesterol of 114 mg · dl^{-1}, an HDL cholesterol of 52 mg · dl^{-1}, and a fasting glucose of 130 mg · dl^{-1}. (Consult table 3.1 for the defining criteria for CHD risk factors.)
   a. List Tom's risk factors for CHD.
   b. Does he warrant physician consent before exercise testing and participation?
2. You are the instructor for a chair-based arthritis class that involves moderate calisthenics, stretching, and weightlifting and is open to the public. Everyone in the class completes a PAR-Q and answers no to all of the questions on the checklist. One of the participants is a woman of normal weight who mentions that she is 65 yr old when you speak with her. Upon further questioning, you find out she does not have any additional risk factors. Further, she walks 4 times a week for 45 min at a brisk pace. She has seen her physician recently for her annual physical and was given a clean bill of health. She recently read that resistance training would be good for her and therefore wants to attend your class. Would you permit her to participate in the class? Why or why not? What advice would you give her?
3. Barbara is a 48-yr-old female who has recently signed up at your fitness facility. She appears to be somewhat apprehensive as she taps her foot while you review her HSQ. You conclude she can engage in unsupervised exercise and take her resting measurements. Her resting HR is 104 beats · min^{-1} and BP is 158/90 mmHg. What would you do?

PART II

Fitness Evaluation

Fitness professionals must know how to answer the question "What does it mean?" This question is often raised regarding fitness test scores. In the chapters in part II, we examine the evaluation of energy cost (chapter 4), cardiorespiratory fitness (chapter 5), body composition (chapter 6), nutrition (chapter 7), muscular strength and endurance (chapter 8), and flexibility and low-back function (chapter 9).

Before you begin, you may want to review the general principles supporting fitness testing. How do you select appropriate tests? How can you obtain more accurate results? For a more complete introduction to the topic of fitness evaluation, please see appendix E.

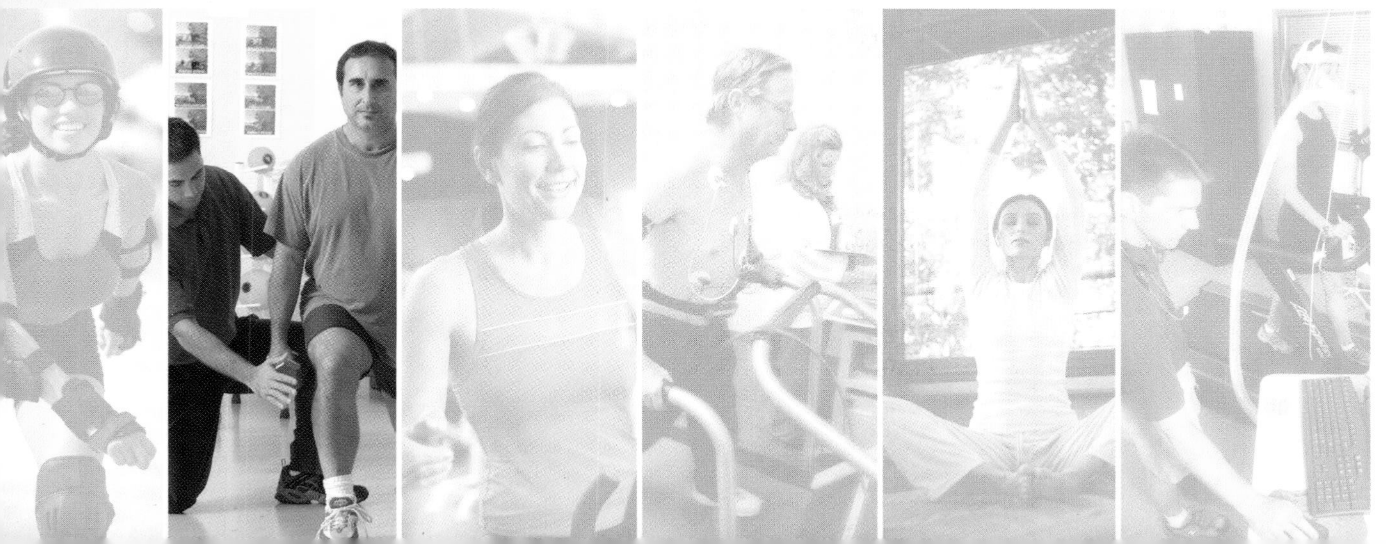

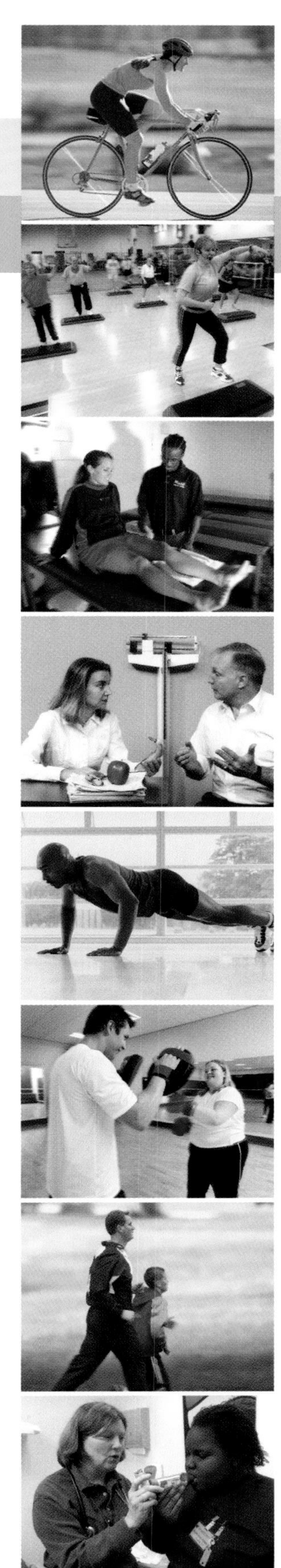

4 CHAPTER

Energy Costs of Physical Activity

Objectives

The reader will be able to do the following:

1. Describe how measurements of oxygen consumption can be used to estimate energy production, and list the number of calories derived per liter of oxygen and per gram of carbohydrate, fat, and protein.
2. Express energy expenditure as $L \cdot min^{-1}$, $kcal \cdot min^{-1}$, $ml \cdot kg^{-1} \cdot min^{-1}$, metabolic equivalents (METs), and $kcal \cdot kg^{-1} \cdot hr^{-1}$.
3. Estimate the oxygen cost of walking, jogging, and running, including the cost of walking and running 1 mi (1.6 km).
4. Estimate the oxygen cost of cycle ergometry exercise for both arm and leg work.
5. Estimate the oxygen cost of bench stepping.
6. Identify the approximate energy cost of recreational activities, sport, and other activities, and describe the effect of environmental factors on the HR response to a fixed work rate.

Fitness professionals usually ask the following two questions when they recommend specific physical activities to participants:

1. Are the activities of the appropriate exercise intensity to achieve the target HR (see chapter 10)?
2. Is the combination of intensity and duration appropriate for achieving an energy expenditure that balances or exceeds caloric intake (see chapter 11)?

To answer these questions, the fitness professional should become familiar with the energy costs of activities. This chapter offers basic information about how to estimate the energy requirement of physical activities and summarizes the values associated with common recreational activities.

Measuring Energy Expenditure

Energy expenditure can be measured by direct and indirect calorimetry. **Direct calorimetry** requires that the person perform an activity within a specially constructed chamber that is insulated and has water flowing through its walls. The water is warmed by the heat given off by the subject, and heat production can be calculated by knowing the volume of water flowing through the chamber per minute and the change in the water temperature from entry to exit. For example, a person in the chamber does bench stepping at the rate of 30 steps · min^{-1} using a 20 cm bench. The water flows through the walls of the chamber at 20 L · min^{-1}, and the increase in the temperature of the water from entry to exit is 0.5 °C. Because it takes approximately 1 kcal to raise the temperature of 1 L of water 1 °C, the following calculation yields the approximate energy expenditure.

$$\frac{20\text{ L}}{\text{min}} \cdot \frac{1\text{ kcal}}{°\text{C}} \cdot 0.5\ °\text{C} = \frac{10\text{ kcal}}{\text{min}}$$

The subject loses additional heat through evaporation of water from the skin and respiratory passages. This heat loss can be measured and added to that picked up by the water in the chamber walls to yield the rate of energy the individual produced for that task.

Indirect calorimetry estimates energy production by measuring oxygen consumption; the procedures for these estimates are described in chapter 28. These calculations use certain constants for converting liters of oxygen consumption to calories expended. The constants are derived from measurements made in a bomb calorimeter, a heavy metal chamber into which carbohydrate, fat, or protein can be placed with 100% oxygen under pressure. The chamber is immersed in a water bath, and the foodstuff is oxidized to CO_2 and H_2O when an electric spark sets this combustion reaction in motion. The heat given off by the combustion warms the water, and it has been determined that carbohydrate, fat, and protein give off approximately 4.0, 9.0, and 5.6 kcal of heat per gram, respectively. Because the nitrogen in protein cannot be completely oxidized in the body and is excreted as urea, the physiological value for protein is actually 4.0 kcal · g^{-1}.

Knowing how much oxygen is required to oxidize 1 g of carbohydrate, fat, and protein allows you to calculate the number of calories of energy produced when 1 L of oxygen is consumed. This is called the **caloric equivalent of oxygen.** Values for carbohydrate, fat, and protein are listed in table 4.1. The table shows that carbohydrate gives about 6% more energy per liter of oxygen than fat gives (5.0 versus 4.7 kcal · L^{-1}), whereas fat gives more than twice as much energy per gram than carbohydrate gives (9 versus 4 kcal · g^{-1}). If a person is deriving energy from a 50/50 mixture of carbohydrate and fat during exercise, the caloric equivalent is approximately 4.85 kcal · L^{-1}, halfway between the value of 4.7 for fat and 5.0 for carbohydrate (18). The ratio of carbon dioxide produced to oxygen consumed at the cell is called the respiratory quotient (RQ). The same ratio, when measured by conventional gas exchange procedures, is called the respiratory exchange ratio (R) and is used to indicate fuel use (carbohydrate versus fat) during exercise (see chapter 28).

Indirect calorimetry employs two techniques to measure oxygen consumption: **closed-circuit** and **open-circuit spirometry.** In the closed-circuit technique, the subject breathes 100% oxygen from a spirometer, and the exhaled air passes through a chemical that absorbs the carbon dioxide. Over time, the volume of oxygen contained in the spirometer decreases, giving a measure of the

• Table 4.1 Caloric Density, Caloric Equivalent, and Respiratory Quotient Associated With Oxidation of Carbohydrate, Fat, and Protein •

Measurement	Carbohydrate	Fat	Protein[a]
Caloric density (kcal · g^{-1})	4.0	9.0	4.0
Caloric equivalent of 1 L of O_2 (kcal · L^{-1})	5.0	4.7	4.5
Respiratory quotient	1.0	0.7	0.8

[a]Does not include the energy derived from the oxidation of nitrogen in the amino acids because the body excretes this as urea.
Adapted, by permission, from L.K. Koebel, 1984, Energy metabolism. In *Physiology*, 5th ed., edited by E. Selkurt (Boston, MA: Little, Brown & Co.), 635-650.

Research Insight

Carbohydrate yields about 6% more energy (5 kcal) per liter of oxygen than fat (4.7 kcal), making carbohydrate a better fuel for high-intensity exercise, when oxygen delivery to the working muscles is limited. However, with rare exceptions, carbohydrate makes up at least 50% of the fuel used during a workout in the intensity range of 60% to 80% of maximal oxygen uptake, a typical intensity range for individuals with average levels of cardiorespiratory fitness (see chapter 10). Consequently, the range of values that might be used to convert oxygen uptake to kilocalories is reduced to 4.85 to 5.0 kcal · L^{-1} (with about a 3% difference between the low and high ends of the range). Therefore, using a constant value of 5 kcal · L^{-1} to convert oxygen uptake to kilocalories involves little error.

Key Point

Oxygen consumption ($\dot{V}O_2$) is a measure of how much energy (calories) is produced by the body. When we know how many calories are generated per gram of carbohydrate and fat and how much oxygen is used to burn these calories, liters of oxygen consumed can be converted to calories of energy produced. The following values are the number of calories gained per gram of food when the food is metabolized in the body: 4 kcal · g^{-1} for carbohydrate, 9 kcal · g^{-1} for fat, and 4 kcal · g^{-1} for protein. Knowing how much oxygen is used to metabolize food, we know that we obtain 4.7 kcal · L^{-1} when fat is oxidized and 5.0 kcal · L^{-1} when carbohydrate is oxidized. When a 50/50 mixture of carbohydrate and fat is used for energy, we obtain 4.85 kcal · L^{-1}.

oxygen consumption in milliliters per minute (ml · min^{-1}). Because the carbon dioxide is absorbed, R cannot be calculated, so a caloric equivalent of 4.82 kcal · L^{-1} is used to indicate that a mixture of carbohydrate, fat, and protein is used to produce the energy. This closed-circuit technique was used extensively to measure basal metabolic rate but has been replaced with modern open-circuit methods (18).

The open-circuit technique for measuring oxygen consumption and carbon dioxide production is the most common indirect calorimetry technique. In this procedure, oxygen consumption is calculated by simply subtracting the volume of oxygen exhaled from the volume of oxygen inhaled. The difference is taken as the oxygen uptake, or oxygen consumption (see chapter 28). Carbon dioxide production is calculated in the same manner. Knowing carbon dioxide production makes it possible to calculate R. Knowing R allows you to determine which substrate, fat or carbohydrate, provided the most energy during work and also what value to use for the caloric equivalent of 1 L of oxygen in the calculation of energy expenditure (i.e., 5.0 kcal · L^{-1} for carbohydrate and 4.7 kcal · L^{-1} for fat). However, as described in the Research Insight, an average value of 5.0 kcal · L^{-1} is typically used to convert oxygen uptake to kilocalories.

Expressing Energy Expenditure

The energy requirement for an activity is calculated from the subject's steady-state oxygen uptake ($\dot{V}O_2$) measured during an activity. Once the subject reaches steady-state (level) oxygen uptake, the energy (adenosine triphosphate, or ATP) supplied to the muscles is derived from aerobic metabolism. The measured oxygen uptake then can be used to express energy expenditure in different ways. The five most common expressions follow.

1. **$\dot{V}O_2$ ($L \cdot min^{-1}$).** The calculation of oxygen uptake (see chapter 28) yields a value expressed in liters of oxygen used per minute. For example, the following data were collected for an 80 kg man performing a submaximal run on a treadmill: ventilation (STPD) = 60 $L \cdot min^{-1}$; inspired O_2 = 20.93%; expired O_2 = 16.93%.

$$\dot{V}O_2\ (L \cdot min^{-1}) = 60\ L \cdot min^{-1}\ (20.93\%\ O_2 - 16.93\%\ O_2) = 2.4\ L \cdot min^{-1}$$

2. **$kcal \cdot min^{-1}$.** Oxygen uptake can be expressed in kilocalories used per minute. The caloric equivalent of 1 L of O_2 ranges from 4.7 $kcal \cdot L^{-1}$ for fat to 5.0 $kcal \cdot L^{-1}$ for carbohydrate. For practical reasons, and with little loss in precision, 5 kcal per liter of O_2 is used to convert the oxygen uptake to kilocalories per minute. Energy expenditure is calculated by multiplying the kilocalories expended per minute ($kcal \cdot min^{-1}$) by the duration of the activity in minutes. For example, if the 80 kg man mentioned previously runs on the treadmill for 30 min at a $\dot{V}O_2$ of 2.4 $L \cdot min^{-1}$, the total energy expenditure can be calculated as follows.

$$\frac{2.4\ L\ O_2}{min} \cdot \frac{5\ kcal}{L\ O_2} = \frac{12\ kcal}{min}$$

$$\frac{12\ kcal}{min} \cdot 30\ min = 360\ kcal$$

3. **$\dot{V}O_2$ ($ml \cdot kg^{-1} \cdot min^{-1}$).** If the measured oxygen uptake, expressed in liters per minute, is multiplied by 1,000 to yield milliliters per minute and then divided by the subject's body weight in kilograms, the value is expressed in milliliters of O_2 per kilogram of body weight per minute, or $ml \cdot kg^{-1} \cdot min^{-1}$. This expression helps you compare values for people of different body sizes. For example, for the 80 kg man with a $\dot{V}O_2$ of 2.4 $L \cdot min^{-1}$,

$$\frac{2.4\ L}{min} \cdot \frac{1000\ ml}{L} \div 80\ kg = 30\ ml \cdot kg^{-1} \cdot min^{-1}$$

4. **METs.** *MET (metabolic equivalent)* is a term used to describe resting metabolism. Resting metabolic rate (oxygen uptake) is measured with the individual at quiet, supine rest, after a time of fasting and no exercise. The resting metabolic rate varies with age and gender, being smaller in females than in males, and decreases with age (18). The MET is taken, by convention, to be 3.5 $ml \cdot kg^{-1} \cdot min^{-1}$. This is called *1 MET.* Activities are expressed in terms of multiples of the MET unit. For example, using the $\dot{V}O_2$ values presented previously in number 3,

$$30\ ml \cdot kg^{-1} \cdot min^{-1} \div 3.5\ ml \cdot kg^{-1} \cdot min^{-1} = 8.6\ METs$$

5. **$kcal \cdot kg^{-1} \cdot hr^{-1}$.** The MET expression of energy expenditure carries a special bonus; the value also indicates the number of calories the subject uses per kilogram of body weight per hour. In the example mentioned previously, the subject is working at 8.6 METs, or about 30 $ml \cdot kg^{-1} \cdot min^{-1}$. When this value is multiplied by 60 $min \cdot hr^{-1}$, it equals 1,800 $ml \cdot kg^{-1} \cdot hr^{-1}$, or 1.8 $L \cdot kg^{-1} \cdot hr^{-1}$. If the person is using a mixture of carbohydrate and fat as fuel, then this oxygen consumption is multiplied by 4.85 kcal per liter of O_2 to give 8.7 $kcal \cdot kg^{-1} \cdot hr^{-1}$. The following steps show the details of this calculation.

$$8.6\ METs \cdot \frac{3.5\ ml \cdot kg^{-1} \cdot min^{-1}}{MET} = 30\ ml \cdot kg^{-1} \cdot min^{-1}$$

$$30\ ml \cdot kg^{-1} \cdot min^{-1} \cdot 60\ min \cdot hr^{-1} = 1{,}800\ ml \cdot kg^{-1} \cdot hr^{-1} = 1.8\ L \cdot kg^{-1} \cdot hr^{-1}$$

$$1.8\ L \cdot kg^{-1} \cdot hr^{-1} \cdot 4.85\ kcal \cdot L\ O_2^{-1} = 8.7\ kcal \cdot kg^{-1} \cdot hr^{-1}$$

Key Point

Energy expenditure can be expressed in $L \cdot min^{-1}$, $kcal \cdot min^{-1}$, $ml \cdot kg^{-1} \cdot min^{-1}$, METs, and $kcal \cdot kg^{-1} \cdot hr^{-1}$. To convert $L \cdot min^{-1}$ to $kcal \cdot min^{-1}$, multiply by $5.0\ kcal \cdot L^{-1}$. To convert $L \cdot min^{-1}$ to $ml \cdot kg^{-1} \cdot min^{-1}$, multiply by 1,000 and divide by body weight in kilograms. To convert $ml \cdot kg^{-1} \cdot min^{-1}$ to METs or $kcal \cdot kg^{-1} \cdot hr^{-1}$, divide by $3.5\ ml \cdot kg^{-1} \cdot min^{-1}$.

Equations for Estimating the Energy Cost of Activities

In the mid-1970s, the ACSM identified some simple equations to estimate the steady-state energy requirement associated with common modes of activities used in graded exercise tests (GXTs), including walking, stepping, running, and cycle ergometry (2). Over the years the equations have been modified to reflect the best information available and this chapter discusses the current thinking in estimating energy costs (3). The oxygen uptake calculated from these equations is an estimate, and a typical **standard deviation** associated with the actual measured average value is about 7% to 9% (3, 10). Remember this normal variation in the energy costs of activities when you use these equations in prescribing exercise.

The ACSM equations have been applied to GXTs to estimate maximal aerobic power. This application has been shown to give reasonable estimates when the subjects are healthy and the rate at which the GXT progresses is slow enough to allow the subject to achieve steady-state oxygen uptake at each stage (20, 21). When the increments between the stages of the GXT are large or the person is somewhat unfit, oxygen uptake will not keep pace with each stage of the test. In these cases, the equations overestimate the actual measured oxygen uptake (14), because the equations are designed to estimate steady-state energy requirements. This overestimation is more likely to happen in populations with disease (e.g., cardiac patients), suggesting that the GXTs used to test these populations may be too aggressive. A test that progresses at a slower rate and allows the subject to reach the steady-state VO_2 at each stage reduces the chance of overestimating functional capacity and still requires the subject to work at an appropriate metabolic rate to overload the system (see chapter 10).

When the ACSM equations were developed, an attempt was made to use a true physiological oxygen cost for each type of work. Each activity is broken down into the energy components. That is, in estimating the total oxygen cost of walking up a grade, you add the net oxygen cost of the horizontal walk (one component) to the net oxygen cost of the vertical (grade) walk (one component) to the resting metabolic rate (one component), which is taken to be 1 MET ($3.5\ ml \cdot kg^{-1} \cdot min^{-1}$).

$$\text{Total } O_2 \text{ cost} = \text{net oxygen cost of activity} + 3.5\ ml \cdot kg^{-1} \cdot min^{-1}$$

For the equations to properly estimate the oxygen cost of the activity, the subject must follow instructions carefully (e.g., not hold on to the treadmill railing, maintain the pedal cadence) and the work instruments (treadmill, cycle ergometer) must be calibrated so the settings are correct (see chapter 5).

Energy Requirements of Walking, Running, Cycle Ergometry, and Stepping

The following sections provide equations to estimate the energy cost of walking, running, cycle ergometry, and stepping. These activities are common to cardiac rehabilitation and adult fitness programs. Examples are provided to show how the equations are used in designing exercise programs.

Oxygen Cost of Walking

Equations to determine the oxygen cost of walking differ depending on the walking speed and whether the walker is on a horizontal or a graded surface.

Horizontal Surface

One of the most common activities used in exercise programs and GXTs is walking. The following equation can be used to estimate the energy requirement between the walking speeds of 50 and 100 $m \cdot min^{-1}$, or 1.9 and 3.7 $mi \cdot hr^{-1}$. (Multiply miles per hour by 26.8 to obtain meters per minute. Divide meters per minute by 26.8 to obtain miles per hour.) Dill (12) showed that the net cost of walking 1 $m \cdot min^{-1}$ on a horizontal surface is 0.100 to 0.106 $ml \cdot kg^{-1} \cdot min^{-1}$. A value of 0.1 $ml \cdot kg^{-1} \cdot min^{-1}$ is used in the ACSM equations to simplify calculations without losing too much precision. The equation for calculating the oxygen cost ($ml \cdot kg^{-1} \cdot min^{-1}$) of walking on a flat surface is as follows:

$$\dot{V}O_2 = 0.1\ ml \cdot kg^{-1} \cdot min^{-1}\ (\text{horizontal velocity}) + 3.5\ ml \cdot kg^{-1} \cdot min^{-1}$$

QUESTION: What are the estimated steady-state $\dot{V}O_2$ and METs for a walking speed of 90 $m \cdot min^{-1}$ (3.4 $mi \cdot hr^{-1}$)?

Answer:

$$\dot{V}O_2 = 90\ m \cdot min^{-1} \cdot \frac{0.1\ ml \cdot kg^{-1} \cdot min^{-1}}{m \cdot min^{-1}} + 3.5\ ml \cdot kg^{-1} \cdot min^{-1}$$

$$\dot{V}O_2 = 9.0\ ml \cdot kg^{-1} \cdot min^{-1} + 3.5\ ml \cdot kg^{-1} \cdot min^{-1} = 12.5\ ml \cdot kg^{-1} \cdot min^{-1}$$

$$\text{METs} = 12.5\ ml \cdot kg^{-1} \cdot min^{-1} \div 3.5\ ml \cdot kg^{-1} \cdot min^{-1} = 3.6$$

The equations also can be used to predict the level of activity required to elicit a specific energy expenditure.

QUESTION: An unfit participant is told to exercise at 11.5 $ml \cdot kg^{-1} \cdot min^{-1}$ to achieve the proper exercise intensity. What walking speed would you recommend?

Answer:

$$11.5\ ml \cdot kg^{-1} \cdot min^{-1} = ?\ m \cdot min^{-1} \cdot \frac{0.1\ ml \cdot kg^{-1} \cdot min^{-1}}{m \cdot min^{-1}} + 3.5\ ml \cdot kg^{-1} \cdot min^{-1}$$

Subtract the resting metabolic rate of 3.5 $ml \cdot kg^{-1} \cdot min^{-1}$ from both sides of the equation. Subtracting 3.5 $ml \cdot kg^{-1} \cdot min^{-1}$ from 11.5 $ml \cdot kg^{-1} \cdot min^{-1}$ gives you the net oxygen cost of the activity (8.0 $ml \cdot kg^{-1} \cdot min^{-1}$):

$$8\ ml \cdot kg^{-1} \cdot min^{-1} = ?\ m \cdot min^{-1} \cdot \frac{0.1\ ml \cdot kg^{-1} \cdot min^{-1}}{m \cdot min^{-1}}$$

The net cost (8 $ml \cdot kg^{-1} \cdot min^{-1}$) is divided by 0.1 $ml \cdot kg^{-1} \cdot min^{-1}$ per $m \cdot min^{-1}$ to yield 80 $m \cdot min^{-1}$. To obtain miles per hour, divide meters per minute by 26.8 to get 3 $mi \cdot hr^{-1}$:

$$80\ m \cdot min^{-1} = 8\ ml \cdot kg^{-1} \cdot min^{-1} \div \frac{0.1\ ml \cdot kg^{-1} \cdot min^{-1}}{m \cdot min^{-1}}$$

$$3.0\ mi \cdot hr^{-1} = 80\ m \cdot min^{-1} \div \frac{26.8\ m \cdot min^{-1}}{mi \cdot hr^{-1}}$$

Walking Up a Grade

The oxygen cost of walking up a grade is the sum of the oxygen cost of horizontal walking, the oxygen cost of the vertical component of walking on a grade, and the resting metabolic rate of 3.5 $ml \cdot kg^{-1} \cdot min^{-1}$. Studies have shown that the oxygen cost of moving (walking or stepping) 1 $m \cdot min^{-1}$ vertically is 1.8 $ml \cdot kg^{-1} \cdot min^{-1}$ (7, 22). The vertical component (vertical velocity) is calculated by multiplying the grade (expressed as a fraction) times the speed in meters per minute. A person walking at 80 $m \cdot min^{-1}$ on a 10% grade is walking 8 $m \cdot min^{-1}$ vertically ($0.10 \cdot 80\ m \cdot min^{-1}$). The equation for calculating the oxygen cost ($ml \cdot kg^{-1} \cdot min^{-1}$) of walking on a grade is as follows:

$$\dot{V}O_2 = 0.1 \text{ ml} \cdot \text{kg}^{-1} \cdot \text{min}^{-1} \text{ (horiz. velocity)} + 1.8 \text{ ml} \cdot \text{kg}^{-1} \cdot \text{min}^{-1} \text{ (vert. velocity)} + 3.5 \text{ ml} \cdot \text{kg}^{-1} \cdot \text{min}^{-1}$$

QUESTION: What is the total oxygen cost of walking 90 m · min^{-1} up a 12% grade?

Answer:
The horizontal component is calculated as in the preceding equation for walking on a horizontal surface and equals 9 ml · kg^{-1} · min^{-1}. The following equations show how to calculate the vertical component and finally the total oxygen cost for walking 90 m · min^{-1} up a 12% grade:

$$\dot{V}O_2 = 0.12 \text{ (grade)} \cdot 90 \text{ m} \cdot \text{min}^{-1} \cdot \frac{1.8 \text{ ml} \cdot \text{kg}^{-1} \cdot \text{min}^{-1}}{\text{m} \cdot \text{min}^{-1}} = 19.4 \text{ ml} \cdot \text{kg}^{-1} \cdot \text{min}^{-1}$$

$$\dot{V}O_2 \text{ (ml} \cdot \text{kg}^{-1} \cdot \text{min}^{-1}) = 9.0 \text{ (horizontal)} + 19.4 \text{ (vertical)} + 3.5 \text{ (rest)} = 31.9 \text{ ml} \cdot \text{kg}^{-1} \cdot \text{min}^{-1}, \text{ or } 9.1 \text{ METs}$$

As indicated earlier, the equations can be used to estimate the treadmill settings needed to elicit a specific oxygen uptake.

QUESTION: How would you set the treadmill grade to achieve an energy requirement of 6 METs (21.0 ml · kg^{-1} · min^{-1}) when walking at 60 m · min^{-1}?

Answer:
The net oxygen cost of the activity is 21 – 3.5, or 17.5, ml · kg^{-1} · min^{-1}. Now we must calculate the vertical and horizontal energy components to reach the final answer:

$$\text{Horizontal component} = 60 \text{ m} \cdot \text{min}^{-1} \cdot \frac{0.1 \text{ ml} \cdot \text{kg}^{-1} \cdot \text{min}^{-1}}{\text{m} \cdot \text{min}^{-1}} = 6.0 \text{ ml} \cdot \text{kg}^{-1} \cdot \text{min}^{-1}$$

$$\text{Vertical component} = 17.5 - 6.0 = 11.5 \text{ ml} \cdot \text{kg}^{-1} \cdot \text{min}^{-1}$$

$$11.5 \text{ ml} \cdot \text{kg}^{-1} \cdot \text{min}^{-1} = \text{fractional grade} \cdot 60 \text{ m} \cdot \text{min}^{-1} \cdot \frac{1.8 \text{ ml} \cdot \text{kg}^{-1} \cdot \text{min}^{-1}}{\text{m} \cdot \text{min}^{-1}}$$

$$11.5 \text{ m} \cdot \text{kg}^{-1} \cdot \text{min}^{-1} = \text{fractional grade} \cdot 108 \text{ ml} \cdot \text{kg}^{-1} \cdot \text{min}^{-1}$$

$$\text{Fractional grade} = 11.5 \div 108 = 0.106 \cdot 100\% = 10.6\% \text{ grade}$$

Walking at Different Speeds

The preceding equations are useful for walking speeds of 50 to 100 m · min^{-1} (1.9-3.7 mi · hr^{-1}); beyond that, the oxygen requirement for walking increases curvilinearly (10). Because many people choose to walk quickly rather than jog, knowing the energy requirements for walking at these higher speeds is useful in prescribing exercise. Values for the energy requirements for walking horizontally and at various grades at these faster speeds (4.0-5.0 mi · hr^{-1}, or 107-134 m · min^{-1}) are included in table 4.2.

One of the most common and useful ways to express the energy cost of walking is in kilocalories per minute. In this way, the fitness professional can simply locate the walking speed in a table, identify the number of calories used per minute, and calculate the total energy expenditure, depending on the duration of the walk. Table 4.3 presents the energy cost (in kcal · min^{-1}) for walking at speeds of 2 to 5 mi · hr^{-1} (54-134 m · min^{-1}) and includes values for people of different body weights. The energy cost of walking increases with the speed of the walk; however, the rate of increase is larger at the higher speeds. For example, when a 170 lb (77.3 kg) participant increases his walking speed from 2 to 3 mi · hr^{-1} (from 54 to 80 m · min^{-1}), the energy cost increases from 3.2 to 4.2 kcal · min^{-1}. But going from 4 to 5 mi · hr^{-1} (from 107 to 134 m · min^{-1}) increases energy cost from 6.3 to 10.2 kcal · min^{-1}. The very sedentary individual can walk at slow speeds and achieve the desired exercise intensity, and the relatively fit individual can walk at higher speeds at which the elevated energy requirement provides the necessary stimulus for a training effect. As a participant loses weight, the energy cost of walking at a certain speed decreases because the energy cost of walking depends on body weight. The participant can compensate for the lower energy cost by walking for a longer duration or for a greater distance.

• Table 4.2 Energy Requirement in METs for Walking at Various Speeds and Grades •

Grade (%)	Speed ($mi \cdot hr^{-1}/m \cdot min^{-1}$) 2.0/54	2.5/67	3.0/80	3.5/94	4.0/107	4.5/121	5.0/134
0	2.5	2.9	3.3	3.7	4.9	6.2	7.9
2	3.1	3.6	4.1	4.7	5.9	7.4	9.3
4	3.6	4.3	4.9	5.6	7.1	8.7	10.6
6	4.2	5.0	5.8	6.6	8.1	9.9	12.0
8	4.7	5.7	6.6	7.5	9.3	11.1	13.4
10	5.3	6.3	7.4	8.5	10.4	12.4	14.8
12	5.8	7.1	8.3	9.5	11.4	13.6	16.6
14	6.4	7.7	9.1	10.4	12.6	14.9	17.5
16	6.9	8.4	9.9	11.4	13.6	16.1	18.9
18	7.5	9.1	10.7	12.4	14.8	17.4	20.3
20	8.1	9.8	11.6	13.3	15.9	18.6	21.7
22	8.6	10.3	12.4	14.3	17.0	19.9	23.1
24	9.1	11.1	13.2	15.3	18.1	21.1	
26	9.7	11.9	14.0	16.2	19.2	22.3	
28	10.3	12.5	14.9	17.2	20.3	23.6	
30	10.8	13.2	15.7	18.2	21.4		

Based on data found in ACSM's *Guidelines for exercise testing and prescription* (3) and Bubb et al (10).

Oxygen Cost of Jogging and Running

Jogging and running are common in fitness programs for apparently healthy individuals. It is possible to use the ACSM equations to estimate the oxygen cost of these activities for a broad range of speeds, generally from 130 to 350 $m \cdot min^{-1}$. The equations are also useful at speeds below 130 $m \cdot min^{-1}$ as long as the person is really jogging. The fact that a person can walk or jog at speeds below 130 $m \cdot min^{-1}$ complicates the issue. The oxygen cost of walking is less than that of jogging at slow speeds; however, at approximately 140 $m \cdot min^{-1}$ (5.2 mph), the oxygen costs of jogging and walking are about the same. Above this speed, the oxygen cost of walking exceeds that of jogging (5).

Jogging and Running on a Horizontal Surface

The net oxygen cost of jogging or running 1 $m \cdot min^{-1}$ on a horizontal surface is about twice that of walking, 0.2 $ml \cdot kg^{-1} \cdot min^{-1}$ per $m \cdot min^{-1}$ (6, 9, 19). Remember that the equation will, in general, reasonably estimate the oxygen cost of running for average individuals. However, it is well known that trained runners are more economical (in terms of energy expenditure) than the average person is and also that running economy varies within any specific group, trained or untrained (9, 11, 21). The equation for estimating the oxygen cost ($ml \cdot kg^{-1} \cdot min^{-1}$) of running on a flat surface is as follows:

$$\dot{V}O_2 = 0.2\ ml \cdot kg^{-1} \cdot min^{-1}\ (\text{horizontal velocity}) + 3.5\ ml \cdot kg^{-1} \cdot min^{-1}$$

QUESTION: What is the oxygen requirement for running a 10K race on a track in 60 min?

Answer:

$$10{,}000\ m \div 60\ min = 167\ m \cdot min^{-1}$$

$$\dot{V}O_2 = 167\ m \cdot min^{-1} \cdot \frac{0.2\ ml \cdot kg^{-1} \cdot min^{-1}}{m \cdot min^{-1}} + 3.5\ ml \cdot kg^{-1} \cdot min^{-1}$$

$$= 36.9\ ml \cdot kg^{-1} \cdot min^{-1}, \text{ or } 10.5\ \text{METs}$$

• Table 4.3 Energy Costs of Walking ($kcal \cdot min^{-1}$) •

Body weight		Speed ($mi \cdot hr^{-1}/m \cdot min^{-1}$)						
kg	lb	2.0/54	2.5/67	3.0/80	3.5/94	4.0/107	4.5/121	5.0/134
50.0	110	2.1	2.4	2.8	3.1	4.1	5.2	6.6
54.5	120	2.3	2.6	3.0	3.4	4.4	5.6	7.2
59.1	130	2.5	2.9	3.2	3.6	4.8	6.1	7.8
63.6	140	2.7	3.1	3.5	3.9	5.2	6.6	8.4
68.2	150	2.8	3.3	3.7	4.2	5.6	7.0	9.0
72.7	160	3.0	3.5	4.0	4.5	5.9	7.5	9.6
77.3	170	3.2	3.7	4.2	4.8	6.3	8.0	10.2
81.8	180	3.4	4.0	4.5	5.0	6.7	8.4	10.8
86.4	190	3.6	4.2	4.7	5.3	7.0	8.9	11.4
90.9	200	3.8	4.4	5.0	5.6	7.4	9.4	12.0
95.4	210	4.0	4.6	5.2	5.9	7.8	9.9	12.6
100.0	220	4.2	4.8	5.5	6.2	8.2	10.3	13.2

Multiply value by the duration of the activity to obtain total calories expended.
Based on *ACSM's Guidelines for Exercise Testing and Prescription* (3) and Bubb et al. (10).

QUESTION: A 20-yr-old female distance runner with a $\dot{V}O_2max$ of 50 $ml \cdot kg^{-1} \cdot min^{-1}$ wants to run intervals at 90% of $\dot{V}O_2max$. At what speed should she run on a track given that 1 mi equals 1,610 m?

Answer:
90% of 50 = 45 $ml \cdot kg^{-1} \cdot min^{-1}$, and the net cost of the run equals 45 $ml \cdot kg^{-1} \cdot min^{-1}$ – 3.5 $ml \cdot kg^{-1} \cdot min^{-1}$, or 41.5 $ml \cdot kg^{-1} \cdot min^{-1}$.

$$41.5\ ml \cdot kg^{-1} \cdot min^{-1} \div \frac{0.2\ ml \cdot kg^{-1} \cdot min^{-1}}{m \cdot min^{-1}} = 207\ m \cdot min^{-1}$$

$$1610\ m \cdot min^{-1} \div 207\ m \cdot min^{-1} = 7.78\ \text{min, or 7:47 (min:s) mile pace}$$

Jogging and Running Up a Grade

There is not as much information about the oxygen cost of running up a grade as there is about the cost of walking up a grade or running on a flat track. But one thing is clear—the oxygen cost of running up a grade is about one half that of walking up a grade (8, 19). Some of the vertical lift associated with running on a flat surface is used to accomplish some of the grade work during inclined running, lowering the net oxygen requirement for the vertical work. The oxygen cost of running 1 $m \cdot min^{-1}$ vertically is about 0.9 $ml \cdot kg^{-1} \cdot min^{-1}$. As in the calculations for uphill walking, the vertical velocity is calculated by multiplying the fractional grade times the horizontal velocity. The following equation is used for calculating the oxygen cost of running up a grade.

$$\dot{V}O_2 = 0.2\ ml \cdot kg^{-1} \cdot min^{-1}\ \text{(horiz. velocity)} + 0.9\ ml \cdot kg^{-1} \cdot min^{-1}\ \text{(vert. velocity)} + 3.5\ ml \cdot kg^{-1} \cdot min^{-1}$$

QUESTION: What is the oxygen cost of running 150 $m \cdot min^{-1}$ up a 10% grade?

Answer:
Horizontal component:

$$\dot{V}O_2 = 150\ m \cdot min^{-1} \cdot \frac{0.2\ ml \cdot kg^{-1} \cdot min^{-1}}{m \cdot min^{-1}} = 30\ ml \cdot kg^{-1} \cdot min^{-1}$$

Vertical component:

$$\dot{V}O_2 = 0.10\ \text{(fractional grade)} \cdot 150\ m \cdot min^{-1} \cdot \frac{0.9\ ml \cdot kg^{-1} \cdot min^{-1}}{m \cdot min^{-1}}$$

$$= 13.5\ ml \cdot kg^{-1} \cdot min^{-1}$$

$$\dot{V}O_2 = 30.0\ \text{(horizontal)} + 13.5\ \text{(vertical)} + 3.5\ \text{(rest)} = 47\ ml \cdot kg^{-1} \cdot min^{-1}$$

QUESTION: The oxygen cost of running 350 m · min^{-1} on a flat surface is about 73.5 ml · kg^{-1} · min^{-1}. What grade should be set on a treadmill for a speed of 300 m · min^{-1} to achieve the same $\dot{V}O_2$?

Answer:
Horizontal component:

$$\dot{V}O_2 = 300 \text{ m} \cdot \text{min}^{-1} \cdot \frac{0.2 \text{ ml} \cdot \text{kg}^{-1} \cdot \text{min}^{-1}}{\text{m} \cdot \text{min}^{-1}} = 60 \text{ ml} \cdot \text{kg}^{-1} \cdot \text{min}^{-1}$$

Vertical component:

$$\text{Net } \dot{V}O_2 = 73.5 \text{ (total)} - 60 \text{ (horizontal)} - 3.5 \text{ (rest)} = 10.0 \text{ ml} \cdot \text{kg}^{-1} \cdot \text{min}^{-}$$

$$10.0 \text{ ml} \cdot \text{kg}^{-1} \cdot \text{min}^{-1} = \text{fractional grade} \cdot 300 \text{ m} \cdot \text{min}^{-1} \cdot \frac{0.9 \text{ ml} \cdot \text{kg}^{-1} \cdot \text{min}^{-1}}{\text{m} \cdot \text{min}^{-1}}$$

$$\text{Fractional grade} = 10 \text{ ml} \cdot \text{kg}^{-1} \cdot \text{min}^{-1} \div 270 \text{ ml} \cdot \text{kg}^{-1} \cdot \text{min}^{-1}$$

$$= .037, \text{ or } 3.7\% \text{ grade}$$

Table 4.4 summarizes oxygen costs of running on a level surface and up a grade.

Jogging and Running at Different Speeds

In contrast to the energy cost of walking, the energy cost of jogging and running increases linearly with increasing speed. Table 4.5 shows the caloric cost of running, in kilocalories per minute, for runners of different body weights. For the 170 lb (77.3 kg) participant, the energy cost increases from 7.2 to 11.2 kcal · min^{-1} when speed jumps from 3 to 5 mi · hr^{-1} (from 80 to 134 m · min^{-1}); the increase is also 4 kcal · min^{-1} when speed increases from 7 to 9 mi · hr^{-1} (from 188 to 241 m · min^{-1}). As with walking, the energy cost is higher for heavier individuals.

Oxygen Cost of Walking and Running 1 Mi (1.6 km)

Despite the vast amount of information regarding the costs of walking and running, a good deal of misunderstanding still exists. We hear claims that the energy cost of walking 1 mi (1.6 km) is equal to that of running the same distance. In general, this is not the case (16). The equations for estimating the energy cost of walking and running can be used to estimate the caloric cost of walking and running 1 mi (1.6 km), information that is useful in achieving energy expenditure goals.

• Table 4.4 Energy Requirement in METs for Jogging or Running at Various Speeds and Grades •

	Speed (mi · hr^{-1}/m · min^{-1})							
Grade (%)	**3/80**	**4/107**	**5/134**	**6/161**	**7/188**	**8/215**	**9/241**	**10/268**
0	5.6	7.1	8.7	10.2	11.7	13.3	14.8	16.3
1	5.8	7.4	9.0	10.6	12.2	13.8	15.4	17.0
2	6.0	7.7	9.3	11.0	12.7	14.4	16.0	17.7
3	6.2	7.9	9.7	11.4	13.2	14.9	16.6	18.4
4	6.4	8.2	10.0	11.9	13.7	15.5	17.3	19.1
5	6.6	8.5	10.4	12.3	14.2	16.1	17.9	19.8
6	6.8	8.8	10.7	12.7	14.6	16.6	18.5	20.4
7	7.0	9.0	11.0	13.1	15.1	17.1	19.1	21.1
8	7.2	9.3	11.4	13.5	15.6	17.7	19.7	21.8
9	7.4	9.6	11.7	13.9	16.1	18.3	20.3	22.5
10	7.6	9.9	12.1	14.3	16.6	18.8	21.0	23.2

Based on data found in ACSM's *Guidelines for exercise testing and prescription* (3).

• Table 4.5 Energy Costs of Jogging and Running (kcal · min^{-1}) •

Body weight		Speed (mi · hr^{-1}/m · min^{-1})							
kg	lb	3.0/80	4.0/107	5.0/134	6.0/161	7.0/188	8.0/215	9.0/241	10.0/268
50.0	110	4.7	5.9	7.2	8.5	9.8	11.1	12.3	13.6
54.5	120	5.1	6.4	7.9	9.3	10.6	12.1	13.4	14.8
59.1	130	5.5	7.0	8.6	10.0	11.5	13.1	14.6	16.1
63.6	140	5.9	7.5	9.2	10.8	12.4	14.1	15.7	17.3
68.2	150	6.4	8.1	9.9	11.6	13.3	15.1	16.8	18.5
72.7	160	6.8	8.6	10.5	12.4	14.2	16.1	17.9	19.8
77.3	170	7.2	9.1	11.2	13.1	15.1	17.1	19.1	21.0
81.8	180	7.6	9.7	11.8	13.9	15.9	18.1	20.2	22.2
86.4	190	8.1	10.2	12.5	14.7	16.8	19.1	21.3	23.5
90.9	200	8.5	10.8	13.2	15.4	17.7	20.1	22.4	24.7
95.4	210	8.9	11.3	13.8	16.2	18.6	21.1	23.5	25.9
100.0	220	9.3	11.8	14.5	17.0	19.5	22.2	24.7	27.2

Multiply value by the duration of the activity to obtain total calories expended.

If a person walks at 3 mi · hr^{-1} (80 m · min^{-1}), he completes 1 mi (1.6 km) in 20 min. The caloric cost for walking 1 mi (1.6 km) for a 70 kg person is calculated as follows:

$$\dot{V}O_2 = 80 \text{ m} \cdot \text{min}^{-1} (0.1 \text{ ml} \cdot \text{kg}^{-1} \cdot \text{min}^{-1}) + 3.5 \text{ ml} \cdot \text{kg}^{-1} \cdot \text{min}^{-1}$$
$$= 11.5 \text{ ml} \cdot \text{kg}^{-1} \cdot \text{min}^{-1}$$
$$\dot{V}O_2 \text{ (ml} \cdot \text{mile}^{-1}) = 11.5 \text{ ml} \cdot \text{kg}^{-1} \cdot \text{min}^{-1} \cdot 70 \text{ kg} \cdot 20 \text{ min} \cdot \text{mi}^{-1} = 16{,}100 \text{ ml} \cdot \text{mi}^{-1}, \text{ and so}$$
$$\dot{V}O_2 \text{ (L} \cdot \text{min}^{-1}) = 16{,}100 \text{ ml} \cdot \text{mi}^{-1} \div 1{,}000 \text{ ml} \cdot \text{L}^{-1} = 16.1 \text{ L} \cdot \text{mi}^{-1}.$$

At about 5.0 kcal per liter of O_2, the gross caloric cost per mile of walking is 80.5 kcal (5 kcal · L^{-1} · 16.1 L · mi^{-1}). The net caloric cost for the mile walk can be calculated by subtracting the oxygen cost of 20 min of rest from the gross cost of the 3 mi · hr^{-1} walk. For example, 20 min of rest · 70 kg (3.5 ml · kg^{-1} · min^{-1}) = 4,900 ml, or 4.9 L. At 5 kcal · L^{-1}, this equals 24.5 kcal for 20 min of rest. The net cost of the mile walk is 80.5 kcal – 24.5 kcal, or 56 kcal for each mile.

If the same 70 kg individual ran the mile at 6 mi · hr^{-1} (161 m · min^{-1}), his oxygen cost could be calculated by the following method.

$$\dot{V}O_2 = 161 \text{ m} \cdot \text{min}^{-1} (0.2 \text{ ml} \cdot \text{kg}^{-1} \cdot \text{min}^{-1}) + 3.5 \text{ ml} \cdot \text{kg}^{-1} \cdot \text{min}^{-1}$$
$$= 35.7 \text{ ml} \cdot \text{kg}^{-1} \cdot \text{min}^{-1}$$
$$\dot{V}O_2 \text{ (ml} \cdot \text{mile}^{-1}) = 35.7 \text{ ml} \cdot \text{kg}^{-1} \cdot \text{min}^{-1} \cdot 70 \text{ kg} \cdot 10 \text{ min} \cdot \text{mi}^{-1} = 25{,}000 \text{ ml} \cdot \text{mi}^{-1}, \text{ and so}$$
$$\dot{V}O_2 \text{ (L} \cdot \text{min}^{-1}) = 25{,}000 \text{ ml} \cdot \text{mi}^{-1} \div 1{,}000 \text{ ml} \cdot \text{L}^{-1} = 25 \text{ L} \cdot \text{mi}^{-1}.$$

At about 5 kcal per liter of O_2, 125 kcal are used to jog or run 1 mi (5 kcal · L^{-1} · 25 L · mi^{-1}). The gross caloric cost per mile (or per 1.6 km) is about 50% higher for jogging than for walking (125 versus 80 kcal). The net caloric cost of jogging or running 1 mi or 1.6 km (calories used above resting), however, is relatively independent of speed and is about twice that of walking. For example, when we subtract the caloric cost for 10 min of rest (12 kcal) from the gross caloric cost of the run (125 kcal), the net cost is 113 kcal, or twice that for the walk (56 kcal). Table 4.6 lists values for the net and gross caloric costs of walking and running 1 mi (1.6 km) for a variety of body weights, with the values expressed in kilocalories per mile.

For weight control it is important to use the net cost of the activity, because it measures the energy used above that used for sitting. When a person moves at slow to moderate speeds (2-3.5 mi · hr^{-1}, or 54-94 m · min^{-1}), the net cost of walking a mile is about half that of jogging or running the mile. This means that a person who jogs a mile at 3 mi · hr^{-1} (80 m · min^{-1}) works at a higher metabolic rate than someone who walks at the same speed, and the HR response is greater as well. Because many people walk at these slower speeds, it is important to remember that the

Key Point

The oxygen cost of walking increases linearly between the speeds of 50 and 100 m · min^{-1}; it increases faster at higher walking speeds. The oxygen cost of jogging or running increases linearly with speed from slow jogging (3 mi · hr^{-1}, or 80 m · min^{-1}) to fast running. The net caloric cost of jogging or running a mile is twice that of walking a mile at a moderate pace.

net energy cost of the mile is half that of running. If we look at very high walking speeds such as 5 mi · hr^{-1}(134 m · min^{-1}), or 1 mi in 12 min, however, we see that the net energy cost of walking 1 mi is only slightly less than that of running.

Table 4.6 shows that the net cost of running a mile is independent of speed. It does not matter whether participants jog at 3 mi · hr^{-1} (80 m · min^{-1}) or run at 6 mi · hr^{-1} (161 m · min^{-1})—the net

Table 4.6 Gross and Net (Gross/Net) Cost for Walking and Running (kcal · mi^{-1})

Walking								
Body weight		Speed (mi · hr^{-1})						
kg	lb	2.0	2.5	3.0	3.5	4.0	4.5	5.0
50.0	110	64/39	58/39	54/39	53/39	60/48	68/57	79/67
54.5	120	69/42	63/42	59/42	57/42	66/52	75/63	86/81
59.1	130	75/45	68/45	64/45	62/45	71/57	81/68	93/81
63.6	140	80/49	73/49	69/49	67/49	77/61	87/73	100/88
68.2	150	87/52	79/52	74/52	72/52	82/65	93/78	108/94
72.7	160	92/56	84/56	79/56	76/56	88/70	100/84	115/100
77.3	170	98/59	90/59	84/59	81/59	93/74	106/89	122/107
81.8	180	104/63	95/63	89/63	86/63	99/78	112/94	139/113
86.4	190	110/66	100/66	94/66	91/66	104/83	118/99	136/119
90.9	200	115/70	105/70	99/70	95/70	110/87	124/104	144/125
95.4	210	121/73	111/73	104/73	100/73	115/92	131/110	151/132
100.0	220	127/77	116/77	109/77	105/77	121/96	137/115	158/138

Running									
Body weight		Speed (mi · hr^{-1})							
kg	lb	3.0	4.0	5.0	6.0	7.0	8.0	9.0	10.0
50.0	110	93/77	89/77	86/77	84/77	84/77	82/77	82/77	81/77
54.5	120	101/83	97/83	94/83	92/83	92/83	89/83	89/83	89/83
59.1	130	110/90	105/90	102/90	100/90	99/90	97/90	97/90	96/90
63.6	140	118/97	113/97	110/97	108/97	107/97	104/97	104/97	104/97
68.2	150	127/104	121/104	118/104	115/104	114/104	112/104	112/104	111/104
72.7	160	135/111	129/111	125/111	123/111	122/111	119/111	119/111	119/111
77.3	170	144/118	137/118	133/118	131/118	130/118	127/118	127/118	126/118
81.8	180	152/125	146/125	141/125	138/125	137/125	134/125	134/125	133/125
86.4	190	161/132	154/132	149/132	146/132	145/132	141/132	141/132	141/132
90.9	200	169/139	162/139	157/139	154/139	153/139	149/139	149/139	148/139
95.4	210	177/146	170/146	165/146	161/146	160/146	156/146	156/146	155/146
100.0	220	186/153	178/153	173/153	169/153	168/153	164/153	164/153	163/153

Multiply value by the number of miles walked or run to obtain the total (gross/net) calories expended.

caloric cost is the same. At 6 mi · hr^{-1} the individual expends energy at about twice the rate measured at 3 mi · hr^{-1} (161 m · min^{-1}), but because the mile is finished in half the time, the net energy expenditure is about the same. HR will, of course, be higher in the 6 mi · hr^{-1} (161 m · min^{-1}) run in order to deliver the oxygen to the muscles at the higher rate.

Oxygen Cost of Cycle Ergometry

Cycle ergometry is a popular exercise done at a sport club, at home, or as part of a rehabilitation program. Generally, cycle ergometry expends energy while causing less trauma to the ankle, knee, and hip joints than jogging. Cycle ergometers are used for conventional leg-exercise programs, but they are also adapted for arm exercise (by placing the ergometer on a table). The following sections describe how to estimate the energy costs of leg and arm cycle ergometry.

Leg Ergometry

In the previous activities the individuals were carrying their body weight, and the oxygen requirement was therefore proportional to body weight (ml · kg^{-1} · min^{-1}). This is not the case in cycle ergometry, in which an individual's body weight is supported by the cycle seat and the work rate is determined primarily by the pedal rate and the resistance on the wheel. The oxygen requirement, in liters per minute, is approximately the same for people of different sizes for the same work rate. Thus, when a light person is doing the same work rate as a heavy person, the relative $\dot{V}O_2$ (ml · kg^{-1} · min^{-1}), or MET level, is higher for the lighter person.

The work rate is set on the simple, mechanically braked cycle ergometers by varying the force (weight, or load) on the wheel and the number of pedal revolutions per minute (rev · min^{-1}). On the Monark cycle ergometer, the wheel travels 6 m per pedal revolution; on the Tunturi ergometer, the wheel travels only 3 m per revolution. If we use the Monark ergometer as an example, a pedal rate of 50 rev · min^{-1} causes the wheel to travel a distance of 300 m (6 m · 50 rev · min^{-1}). If a 1 kg force (1 kg weight) is applied to the wheel, the work rate is 300 kgm · min^{-1} (kilogram-meters per minute). Work rates also are expressed in watts (W), where 6.1 kgm · min^{-1} equals 1 W; the 300 kgm · min^{-1} work rate would be expressed as 50 W. The work rate can be doubled by changing the force from 1 to 2 kg or by changing the pedal rate from 50 to 100 rev · min $^{-1}$. In contrast, some cycle ergometers are electronically controlled to deliver a specific work rate somewhat independent of pedal rate; as the pedal rate decreases, the load on the wheel is increased proportionally to maintain the work rate (4).

The total oxygen cost of leg cycle ergometry exercise is the sum of the resting oxygen uptake, the cost of unloaded cycling (movement of the legs against no resistance), and the cost of the work itself. The oxygen cost of doing 1 kgm of work is 1.8 ml. The energy required to move the pedals against no resistance has been estimated to be 1 MET, or 3.5 ml · kg^{-1} · min^{-1}, and as with the other equations, resting oxygen uptake is 3.5 ml · kg^{-1} · min^{-1} (3). The latter two terms are combined in the equation to yield 7 ml · kg^{-1} · min $^{-1}$. The estimates from the following equations are reasonable for work rates between approximately 150 and 1,200 kgm · min^{-1} (see table 4.7). The equations for work rates expressed in kgm · min^{-1} and watts follow.

$$\dot{V}O_2\ (\text{ml} \cdot \text{kg}^{-1} \cdot \text{min}^{-1}) = (\text{kgm} \cdot \text{min}^{-1} \cdot 1.8\ \text{ml}\ O_2 \cdot \text{kgm}^{-1}) \div \text{body weight (kg)} + 7\ \text{ml} \cdot \text{kg}^{-1} \cdot \text{min}^{-1}$$

$$\dot{V}O_2\ (\text{ml} \cdot \text{kg}^{-1} \cdot \text{min}^{-1}) = (\text{W} \cdot 10.8\ \text{ml}\ O_2 \cdot \text{W}^{-1}) \div \text{body weight (kg)} + 7\ \text{ml} \cdot \text{kg}^{-1} \cdot \text{min}^{-1}$$

QUESTION: What is the oxygen cost of doing 600 kgm · min^{-1} (100 W) on a cycle ergometer for 50 kg and 100 kg subjects?

Answer:

For the 50 kg subject:

$$\dot{V}O_2\ (\text{ml} \cdot \text{kg}^{-1} \cdot \text{min}^{-1}) = (600\ \text{kgm} \cdot \text{min}^{-1} \cdot 1.8\ \text{ml}\ O_2 \cdot \text{kgm}^{-1}) \div 50\ \text{kg} + 7\ \text{ml} \cdot \text{kg}^{-1} \cdot \text{min}^{-1}$$
$$= 28.6\ \text{ml} \cdot \text{kg}^{-1} \cdot \text{min}^{-1}, \text{ or } 8.2\ \text{METs}$$

For the 100 kg subject:

$$\dot{V}O_2\ (\text{ml} \cdot \text{kg}^{-1} \cdot \text{min}^{-1}) = (600\ \text{kgm} \cdot \text{min}^{-1} \cdot 1.8\ \text{ml}\ O_2 \cdot \text{kgm}^{-1}) \div 100\ \text{kg} + 7\ \text{ml} \cdot \text{kg}^{-1} \cdot \text{min}^{-1}$$
$$= 17.8\ \text{ml} \cdot \text{kg}^{-1} \cdot \text{min}^{-1}, \text{ or } 5.1\ \text{METs}$$

• Table 4.7 Energy Expenditure in METs for Cycle Ergometry for Legs and Arms •

Body weight		Work rate ($kgm \cdot min^{-1}$/W)						
kg	lb	300/50	450/75	600/100	750/125	900/150	1,050/175	1,200/200
50	110	5.1(6.1)	6.6(8.7)	8.2(11.3)	9.7(13.9)	11.3(–)	12.8(–)	14.3(–)
60	132	4.6(5.3)	5.9(7.4)	7.1(9.6)	8.4(11.7)	9.7(–)	11.0(–)	12.3(–)
70	154	4.2(4.7)	5.3(6.5)	6.4(8.3)	7.5(10.2)	8.6(12.0)	9.7(–)	10.8(–)
80	176	3.9(4.2)	4.9(5.8)	5.9(7.4)	6.8(9.0)	7.8(10.6)	8.8(12.3)	9.7(–)
90	198	3.7(3.9)	4.6(5.3)	5.4(6.7)	6.3(8.1)	7.1(9.6)	8.0(11.0)	8.9(12.4)
100	220	3.5(3.6)	4.3(4.9)	5.1(6.1)	5.9(7.4)	6.6(8.7)	7.4(10.0)	8.2(11.3)

Values in ( ) are for arm work.

Based on data found in ACSM's *Guidelines for exercise testing and prescription*, 7th ed., 2006.

In some exercise programs, a participant might use a variety of exercise equipment to achieve a training effect and might like to be able to set about the same intensity on each machine. In this regard, the equation for the cycle ergometer can be used to set the load to achieve a particular MET value on the cycle ergometer and bring it in balance with what is done during walking or jogging.

QUESTION: A 70 kg participant must work at 6 METs ($21\ ml \cdot kg^{-1} \cdot min^{-1}$) to match the intensity of his walking program. What force (load) should be set on a Monark cycle ergometer at a pedal rate of $50\ rev \cdot min^{-1}$?

Answer:

$$21\ ml \cdot kg^{-1} \cdot min^{-1} = (?\ kgm \cdot min^{-1} \cdot 1.8\ ml\ O_2 \cdot kgm^{-1}) \div 70\ kg + 7\ ml \cdot kg^{-1} \cdot min^{-1}$$

$$\text{Net cost of cycling} = 21 - 7\ ml \cdot kg^{-1} \cdot min^{-1} = 14\ ml \cdot kg^{-1} \cdot min^{-1}$$

$$14\ ml \cdot kg^{-1} \cdot min^{-1} = (?\ kgm \cdot min^{-1} \cdot 1.8\ ml\ O_2 \cdot kgm^{-1}) \div 70\ kg$$

Multiply each side by 70 kg.

$$980\ ml \cdot min^{-1} = ?\ kgm \cdot min^{-1} \cdot 1.8\ ml\ O_2 \cdot kgm^{-1}$$

Divide each side by $1.8\ ml\ O_2 \cdot kgm^{-1}$ to obtain the work rate

$$\text{Work rate} = 544\ kgm \cdot min^{-1}$$

Because the Monark wheel travels $300\ m \cdot min^{-1}$ at $50\ rev \cdot min^{-1}$, the load on the wheel should be $544\ kgm \cdot min^{-1} \div 300\ m \cdot min^{-1}$, or 1.8 kg.

Arm Ergometry

A cycle ergometer can be used to exercise the muscles of the arms and shoulder girdle by modifying the pedals and placing the cycle on a table. Arm ergometry is used on a limited basis as a GXT to evaluate cardiovascular function. It is used more generally as a routine exercise in rehabilitation programs (13). There are a variety of factors to keep in mind when considering arm ergometry:

- $\dot{V}O_2max$ for the arms is only 70% of that measured with the legs in a normal healthy population and is less in an unfit, elderly, or diseased population.
- The natural endurance of the muscles used in this work is less than that of the legs.
- The HR and BP responses are higher for arm work compared with leg work at the same $\dot{V}O_2$.
- There is no need to account for unloaded arm cycling, but the oxygen cost of doing 1 kgm is about $3\ ml\ O_2 \cdot kgm^{-1}$ for arm work because of the action's inefficiency (3).

The equations for estimating the oxygen cost of arm work for work rates expressed in $kgm \cdot min^{-1}$ or W are as follows:

$$\dot{V}O_2\,(ml \cdot kg^{-1} \cdot min^{-1}) = (kgm \cdot min^{-1} \cdot 3\ ml\ O_2 \cdot kgm^{-1}) \div \text{body weight (kg)} + 3.5\ ml \cdot kg^{-1} \cdot min^{-1}$$
$$\dot{V}O_2\,(ml \cdot kg^{-1} \cdot min^{-1}) = (W \cdot 18\ ml\ O_2 \cdot W^{-1}) \div \text{body weight (kg)} + 3.5\ ml \cdot kg^{-1} \cdot min^{-1}$$

See table 4.7 for estimates of the oxygen cost of arm work on a cycle ergometer.

QUESTION: What is the oxygen requirement for a 70 kg man doing 150 kgm · min^{-1} on an arm ergometer?

Answer:

$$\dot{V}O_2\,(ml \cdot kg^{-1} \cdot min^{-1}) = (150\ kgm \cdot min^{-1} \cdot 3\ ml\ O_2 \cdot kgm^{-1}) \div 70\ kg + 3.5\ ml \cdot kg^{-1} \cdot min^{-1} = 9.9\ ml \cdot kg^{-1} \cdot min^{-1}, \text{ or } 2.8\ METs$$

Key Point

The oxygen cost of cycle ergometry primarily depends on the work rate because body weight is supported. The net oxygen cost of leg ergometry is 1.8 ml · kgm^{-1} versus 3 ml · kgm^{-1} for arm ergometry. Physiological responses (HR, BP) are exaggerated for arm work compared with leg work at the same work rate because the oxygen cost is higher and represents a higher percentage of the arm $\dot{V}O_2$max.

Oxygen Cost of Bench Stepping

One of the most useful and inexpensive forms of exercise is bench stepping. The activity can be done at home and requires little or no equipment. The work rate is adjusted easily by simply increasing step height or cadence (number of lifts per minute).

The total oxygen cost of this exercise is the sum of the costs of (a) stepping up, (b) stepping down, (c) moving back and forth on a level surface at the specified cadence, and (d) resting oxygen uptake (3.5 ml · kg^{-1} · min^{-1}). The oxygen cost of stepping up is 1.8 ml · kg^{-1} · min^{-1} per m · min^{-1}, as in walking (22). The oxygen cost of stepping down is a third of the cost of stepping up; therefore, the oxygen cost of stepping up and down is 1.33 times the cost of stepping up. The oxygen cost of stepping back and forth on a flat surface is equal to 0.2 ml O_2 per kilogram of body mass for the four-cycle step (3). The number of meters moved up or down per minute is calculated by multiplying the number of lifts per minute by the height of the step; for example, if the step height is 0.2 m (20 cm) and the cadence is 30 steps · min^{-1}, then the total lift or descent per minute is 30 times 0.2 m, or 6 m · min^{-1}. To determine step height, multiply inches by 2.54 to obtain centimeters, and divide centimeters by 100 to obtain meters. The equation for estimating the energy requirement for stepping follows:

$$\dot{V}O_2\,(ml \cdot kg^{-1} \cdot min^{-1}) = (0.2 \cdot \text{step rate}) + (1.8 \cdot 1.33 \cdot \text{step rate} \cdot \text{step height in meters}) + 3.5\ ml \cdot kg^{-1} \cdot min^{-1}$$

QUESTION: What is the oxygen requirement for stepping at a rate of 20 steps · min^{-1} on a 20 cm bench?

Answer:

$$\begin{aligned}\dot{V}O_2 &= \left(\frac{0.2\ ml \cdot kg^{-1} \cdot min^{-1}}{steps \cdot min^{-1}} \cdot 20\ steps \cdot min^{-1}\right) + \\ &\left(\frac{1.8\ ml}{kgm} \cdot 1.33 \cdot \frac{0.2\ m}{step} \cdot \frac{20\ steps}{min}\right) + 3.5\ ml \cdot kg^{-1} \cdot min^{-1} \\ &= 4.0\ ml \cdot kg^{-1} \cdot min^{-1} + 9.6\ ml \cdot kg^{-1} \cdot min^{-1} + 3.5\ ml \cdot kg^{-1} \cdot min^{-1} \\ &= 17.1\ ml \cdot kg^{-1} \cdot min^{-1}, \text{ or } 4.9\ METs\end{aligned}$$

Table 4.8 summarizes the energy requirement of stepping at different rates.

• Table 4.8 Energy Expenditure in METs During Stepping at Different Rates on Steps of Different Heights •

Step height		Steps · min^{-1}			
cm	in.	12	18	24	30
0	0	1.7	2.0	2.4	2.7
4	1.6	2.0	2.5	3.0	3.5
8	3.2	2.3	3.0	3.7	4.4
12	4.7	2.7	3.5	4.3	5.2
16	6.3	3.0	4.0	5.0	6.0
20	7.9	3.3	4.5	5.7	6.8
24	9.4	3.7	5.0	6.3	7.6
28	11.0	4.0	5.5	7.0	8.5
32	12.6	4.3	6.0	7.6	9.3
36	14.2	4.6	6.5	8.3	10.1
40	15.8	5.0	7.0	8.9	10.9

Based on data found in ACSM's *Guidelines for exercise testing and prescription*, 6th ed., 2000.

Key Point

The oxygen cost of bench stepping includes the cost of stepping up and down, moving horizontally back and forth, and resting oxygen uptake. The oxygen cost of stepping up is the same as in walking. The oxygen cost of stepping up and down is 1.33 times the cost of stepping up. The oxygen cost of stepping back and forth is proportional to the cadence.

Energy Requirements of Other Activities

Many activities are available for designing a fitness program (see chapter 14). These include exercising to music, rope skipping, swimming, and playing games. Not surprisingly, the energy expenditure associated with these activities is difficult to predict compared with walking or running, in which the energy cost between people is similar because of the natural movements associated with those activities. In contrast, these other activities have variable energy costs depending on the skill level of the participants and the motivation they bring to the activity. This will be clear in the following examples. Estimates of the energy requirements of some common aerobic activities also are presented.

Exercising to Music

Exercising to music is a fun alternative to walking and running. The energy requirement depends on whether the session is high or low impact; done at a low, medium, or high intensity; and done with or without hand weights (24). A person who is starting out might simply walk through the movements, whereas an experienced person might go through the full range of motion with each step. Thus, the energy costs of this activity vary considerably, ranging from as low as 4 METs for someone walking through the routine to 10 METs for the experienced participant working at a high intensity in either a low- or a high-impact session (24). Remember that this activity often involves small muscle groups and includes some static (stabilizing) muscle contractions; as a result, HR response is higher for the same oxygen uptake measured in walking and running. Table 4.9 summarizes the caloric expenditure associated with exercise to music at low, moderate, and high intensities.

• Table 4.9 Gross Energy Cost of Exercise to Music (kcal · min^{-1}) •

Body weight (kg)	Body weight (lb)	Low intensity	Moderate intensity	High intensity
50.0	110	3.3	5.8	8.3
54.5	120	3.6	6.4	9.1
59.1	130	3.9	6.9	9.8
63.6	140	4.2	7.4	10.6
68.2	150	4.5	7.9	11.3
72.7	160	4.8	8.5	12.1
77.3	170	5.1	9.0	12.8
81.8	180	5.4	9.5	13.6
86.4	190	5.7	10.1	14.3
90.9	200	6.0	10.6	15.1
95.4	210	6.3	11.1	15.9
100.0	220	6.6	11.7	16.7

Multiply value by the duration of the aerobic phase to obtain total calories expended.

Rope Skipping

In walking and running, the energy requirement is proportional to the rate at which the person moves. But the energy requirement for rope skipping at only 60 to 80 turns · min^{-1} (about as slow as the rope can be turned) is about 9 METs. At 120 turns · min^{-1}, the energy cost increases to only 11 METs (17). Consequently, rope skipping is not a graded activity as are walking and running. Second, the HR response is higher than expected from the oxygen cost of the activity. This, again, may be because a small muscle mass (lower leg) is the primary muscle group involved in the activity. Despite this, rope skipping can be included in a fitness program when done intermittently using target heart rate (THR) as the guide (see chapter 14). Rope skipping should not be used, however, in the early phase of a fitness program because the energy cost and the loading on the ankle, knee, and hip joints are relatively high. Table 4.10 summarizes the energy costs of skipping rope at two speeds.

• Table 4.10 Gross Energy Cost of Rope Skipping (kcal · min^{-1}) •

Body weight (kg)	Body weight (lb)	Slow skipping	Fast skipping
50.0	110	3.3	5.8
54.5	120	3.6	6.4
59.1	130	8.9	10.9
63.6	140	9.5	11.7
68.2	150	10.2	12.5
72.7	160	10.9	13.4
77.3	170	11.6	14.2
81.8	180	12.3	15.0
86.4	190	13.0	15.9
90.9	200	13.6	16.7
95.4	210	14.3	17.5
100.0	220	15.0	18.4

Multiply value by the duration of the rope skipping to obtain total calories expended.

Swimming

Swimming is a preferred activity for many people because it is dynamic, uses large muscle groups, and causes little joint trauma. The limitation is in finding a convenient facility that allows lap swimming and, of course, in having enough skill to swim. The energy requirement depends on the swimming velocity and on the stroke being used, but it is also influenced by the skill of the swimmer. A skilled swimmer requires less energy to move through the water, so the skilled swimmer has to swim a greater distance to achieve the same caloric expenditure.

The energy cost of simply treading water can be as high as 1.5 $L \cdot min^{-1}$ (7.5 $kcal \cdot min^{-1}$). Elite swimmers use this same number of kilocalories per minute to swim at 36 $m \cdot min^{-1}$, whereas an unskilled swimmer might require twice that to maintain the same velocity. For elite swimmers, the front and back crawl are the most economical strokes and the butterfly is the least economical stroke. The net caloric cost per mile of swimming has been estimated to be more than 400 kcal, or about 4 times that of running the mile and about 8 times that of walking the mile. However, the actual caloric cost per mile of swimming varies greatly, depending on skill and gender. Table 4.11 summarizes the caloric costs presented by Holmer (15) for men and women.

The HR response measured during swimming at a specific $\dot{V}O_2$ is lower than that measured during running at the same $\dot{V}O_2$. In fact, the maximal HR response is about 14 $beats \cdot min^{-1}$ lower for swimming (see chapter 18). With this in mind, when you prescribe swimming activities you should instruct participants to decrease the THR range.

• Table 4.11 Caloric Cost per Mile ($kcal \cdot mi^{-1}$) of Swimming the Front Crawl •

Skill level	Women	Men
Competitive	180	280
Skilled	260	360
Average	300	440
Unskilled	360	560
Poor	440	720

Adapted from I. Holmer, 1979, "Physiology of swimming man," *Exercise and Sports Sciences Review* 7: 87-123.

Estimation of Energy Expenditure Without Equations

Appendix C contains a summary of the energy requirements for a wide variety of physical activities, including exercises, sports, occupations, and home-related tasks (1). These values are helpful in estimating the energy expenditure associated with an individual's structured physical activity program; however, there is considerable variability in many of these estimates. What follows is another approach for estimating the energy costs of an exercise session without using equations.

The fitness professional selects activities that cause participants to exercise in the range of 40% to 85% of their $\dot{V}O_2max$, the intensity needed to improve or maintain cardiorespiratory fitness (see chapter 10). It should be possible, therefore, to estimate the energy expenditure for each individual on the basis of the subject's $\dot{V}O_2max$ and the portion of the THR range at which the person is working. If a person has a $\dot{V}O_2max$ of 10 METs, energy expenditure can be estimated in the following way. Ten METs equals about 10 $kcal \cdot kg^{-1} \cdot hr^{-1}$. If a person exercises at the bottom of the THR range for young healthy persons, at about 60% $\dot{V}O_2max$, then the energy expenditure should be about 6 METs (60% of 10 METs). If the person weighs 70 kg, then 420 kcal are expended per hour (70 $kg \cdot 6\ kcal \cdot kg^{-1} \cdot hr^{-1}$). A 30 min workout expends half this, or about 210 kcal. These simple calculations assume that the person is performing an activity that uses large muscle groups. Table 4.12 shows the estimated calorie expenditure for a 30 min workout at 70% $\dot{V}O_2max$ for a variety of fitness levels ($\dot{V}O_2max$ expressed as METs) and body weights (23).

• **Table 4.12 Estimated Gross Energy Expenditure for a 30 Min Workout at 70% Functional Capacity for People of Various Fitness Levels ($\dot{V}O_2$max) and Body Weights** •

$\dot{V}O_2$max, in METs ($kcal \cdot kg^{-1} \cdot hr^{-1}$)	70% max, in METs ($kcal \cdot kg^{-1} \cdot hr^{-1}$)	50 kg/110 lb	70 kg/154 lb	90 kg/198 lb
20	14.0	350	490	630
18	12.6	315	441	567
16	11.2	280	392	504
14	9.8	245	343	441
12	8.4	210	294	378
10	7.0	175	245	315
8	5.6	140	196	252
6	4.2	105	147	189

MET = metabolic equivalent.

Environmental Concerns

Although changes in temperature, relative humidity, pollution, and altitude do not change the energy requirements for submaximal exercise, they do change the participant's response to the exercise. Remember that a person's HR response is the best indicator of the relative stress being experienced due to the interaction of exercise intensity, exercise duration, and environmental factors. The participant should cut back on the intensity of the activity when environmental factors increase the HR response. The duration of the activity can be increased to accommodate any energy expenditure goal.

Key Point

The energy cost of exercising to music varies from 4 to 10 METs, depending on effort and whether the exercise is high or low impact. Rope skipping requires about 10 METs, whereas the oxygen cost of swimming is inversely related to skill. Energy expenditure can be estimated without equations. If a person works at 60% of $\dot{V}O_2$max and has a $\dot{V}O_2$max of 10 METs, the person is expending energy at 6 METs, or 6 $kcal \cdot kg^{-1} \cdot hr^{-1}$. If the person weighs 80 kg, 480 kcal are expended per hour. Environmental factors such as heat, humidity, altitude, and pollution can increase the HR response to work while not really affecting the energy cost. HR should be monitored more frequently in these settings to adjust the intensity of the activity downward to keep the person in the appropriate HR range.

Case Studies

You can check your answers by referring to page 470 in appendix A.

1. A 75 kg man walks at 3.5 $mi \cdot hr^{-1}$ for 30 min. How many calories does he expend?
2. A 60 kg woman rides a cycle ergometer at a work rate of 100 W. What is her oxygen uptake?
3. A 70 kg college student runs 3 mi in 24 min. How many calories does he expend?
4. An 85 kg man with a functional capacity of 12 METs works at 70% of his capacity for 30 min. How many calories does he expend?
5. A client has read that he can expend the same number of calories per mile whether he walks it at 3 $mi \cdot hr^{-1}$ or jogs it at 6 $mi \cdot hr^{-1}$. How would you respond?

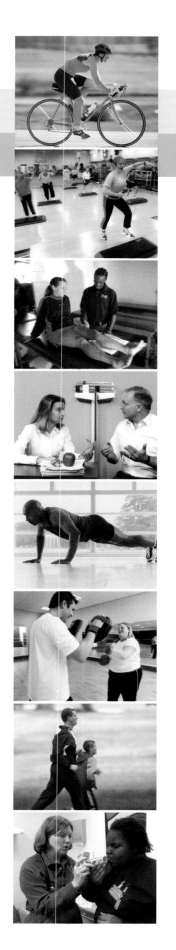

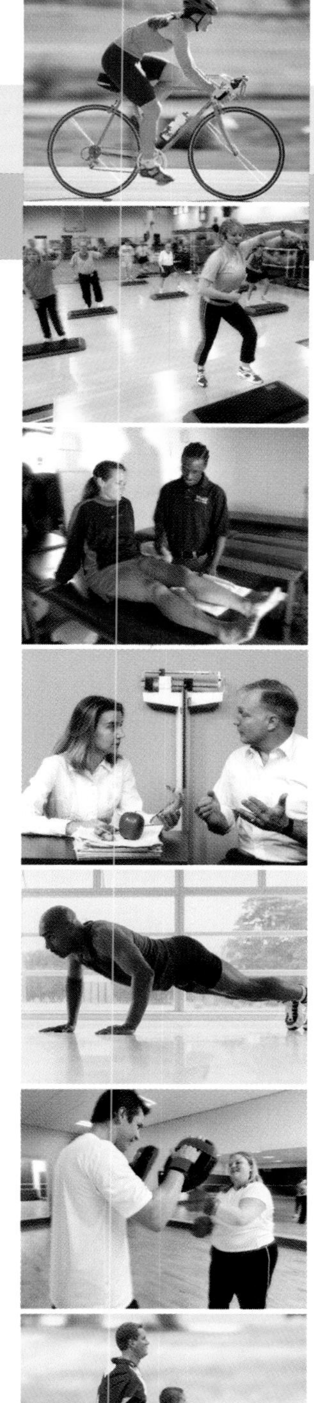

Cardiorespiratory Fitness

Objectives

The reader will be able to do the following:

1. Describe how cardiorespiratory fitness (CRF) relates to health and list reasons for testing CRF as well as risks associated with CRF testing.
2. Present a logical sequence of testing.
3. Describe procedures for walking and jogging or running field tests to estimate CRF.
4. Contrast the treadmill, cycle ergometer, and bench step as instruments for GXTs.
5. List variables measured during a GXT.
6. Describe procedures used before, during, and after testing.
7. Contrast submaximal and maximal GXTs.
8. Describe the HR extrapolation procedures to estimate $\dot{V}O_2$max using submaximal treadmill, cycle, and bench-step GXTs.
9. Calibrate a treadmill, a Monark cycle ergometer, and a sphygmomanometer.

The usual introduction to cardiorespiratory fitness (CRF) delineates heart disease as the major cause of death and proceeds to describe the role of exercise in prevention and rehabilitation programs. It is also important, however, to focus on good CRF as a normal, lifelong goal that makes life more enjoyable. That benefit alone merits including CRF in any discussion about positive health. Cardiorespiratory fitness, also called *cardiovascular* or *aerobic fitness,* is a good measure of the heart's ability to pump oxygen-rich blood to the muscles. Although the terms *cardio* (heart), *vascular* (blood vessels), *respiratory* (lungs and ventilation), and *aerobic* (working with oxygen) differ technically, they all reflect aspects of CRF. A person with a healthy heart that can pump great volumes of blood with each beat has a high level of CRF. CRF values are expressed in the following ways:

- Liters of oxygen used by the body per minute ($L \cdot min^{-1}$)
- Milliliters of oxygen used per kilogram of body weight per minute ($ml \cdot kg^{-1} \cdot min^{-1}$)
- METs, multiples of resting metabolic rate, where 1 MET = $3.5\ ml \cdot kg^{-1} \cdot min^{-1}$

A person with the ability to use $35\ ml \cdot kg^{-1} \cdot min^{-1}$ during maximal exercise is said to have a CRF equal to 10 METs ($35 \div 3.5 = 10$). Aerobic training programs increase the heart's ability to pump blood, so it is no surprise that such programs improve CRF.

Chapter 28 describes how CRF variables respond to acute or short-term exercise and how endurance training affects those responses. Chapter 10 explains how to recommend activities to clients to improve their CRF. This chapter emphasizes how to evaluate CRF. The reader is referred to other resources for additional details (1, 2).

Historically, measurements of HR, BP, and electrocardiogram (ECG) taken at rest were used to evaluate CRF. In addition, some static pulmonary function tests (e.g., vital capacity) were used to characterize respiratory function. It became clear, however, that measurements made at rest revealed little about the way a person's cardiorespiratory system responds to physical activity. We are now familiar with using graded exercise tests (GXTs) to evaluate HR, ECG, BP, ventilation, and oxygen uptake responses during work.

Why Test Cardiorespiratory Fitness?

Results from cardiorespiratory fitness tests are used to write exercise recommendations and allow the fitness professional or physician to evaluate positive or negative changes in CRF resulting from physical conditioning, aging, illness, or inactivity. Given the recent increase in obesity and inactivity in persons of all ages, it makes good sense to evaluate CRF throughout life, from early childhood to old age. This information can indicate where the individual stands on health-criterion tests, and it alerts the individual to subtle changes in lifestyle that may compromise positive health. The nature of the tests and the level of monitoring should vary across age groups to reflect the information that is needed.

CRF testing depends on the purposes of the test, the type of person to be evaluated, and the work tasks available. Reasons for testing include

- determining physiological responses at rest and during **submaximal** or maximal work,
- providing a basis for exercise programming,
- screening for CHD, and
- determining a person's ability to perform a specific work task.

Choosing an appropriate test depends on several factors. People differ in age, fitness level, known health problems, and risks of CHD. Also, financial considerations determine the amount of time that can be devoted to each individual (e.g., physician versus fitness professional administering test) and the work tasks available.

Risks of CRF Testing

As indicated in chapter 1, the risks associated with exercise testing are quite low. Health professionals should emphasize that the overall CHD risk is greater for those who remain sedentary than for those who take an exercise test and then embark on a regular exercise program (1). This is consistent with evidence showing that low cardiorespiratory fitness directly relates to a higher risk of heart disease and death (11).

Key Point

CRF is an important aspect of quality of life as well as a risk factor for CHD. The ability to use oxygen during exercise is the basis for CRF and can be expressed in $L \cdot min^{-1}$, $ml \cdot kg^{-1} \cdot min^{-1}$, and METs. CRF testing is used for exercise programming, screening for heart disease, and determining a person's ability to do a specific work task. The risk of death attributable to exercise testing is very low.

Testing Sequence

A logical sequence for fitness testing (and activities) can be followed when people attend the same fitness

Sequence of Testing and Activity Prescription

1. Informed consent
2. Health history
3. Screening
4. Resting CRF, body composition, and psychological tests
5. Submaximal CRF tests
6. Tests for low-back function
7. Beginning of light activity program
8. Tests for muscular strength and endurance
9. Maximal CRF tests
10. Activity program revision (include games and sports here)
11. Periodic retest (and activity revision)

center over time. This sequence progresses from the initial screening to fitness testing and programming, with opportunities for periodic retesting and revision of the program as fitness gains are made. The sequence of testing and activity prescription is shown on page 65. The rest of this section details the process. For people who request fitness testing but are not continually involved with the fitness center, the submaximal and maximal tests are usually part of the same GXT protocol.

Informed Consent

Fitness participants should be informed volunteers. The fitness program should clearly describe all of its procedures and potential risks and benefits. The participants should understand that their individual data are confidential and that they can terminate any test or activity at any time should they feel uncomfortable. They should sign a written informed consent form after reading a description of the program and having all questions answered. A sample consent form is included in chapter 26.

Health History

Chapter 3 describes procedures for determining current health status. The current health status can be used to determine appropriate testing protocols and activity recommendations. People with symptoms of health problems should undergo fitness testing. Referrals to other professionals might be warranted based on the person's history.

Screening

We recommended in chapter 3 that individuals undergo regular medical examinations and health screenings and engage in moderate-intensity exercise. Fitness programs need to determine whether a person needs medical permission to begin fitness programs involving vigorous activities. Older individuals and people with CHD or other known major health problems must have medical supervision or clearance before embarking on any fitness testing or program that goes beyond moderate-intensity exercise.

In chapter 3 (table 3.2 on page 32) we listed the conditions (absolute contraindications) that the ACSM has identified in which the risk of testing outweighs the possible benefits. Other conditions (relative contraindications) may increase the risk of exercise testing; people with these conditions should only be tested if a doctor determines that the need for the test outweighs the potential risk.

Apparently healthy people who have no known major health problems or symptoms can be tested or begin the type of fitness program recommended in this book with minimal risk. Chapter 3 identifies the people who need medical clearance for exercising, a carefully supervised program, and educational information about health problems and behaviors.

Resting Measurements

Typical resting tests may include CRF measures (e.g., 12-lead ECG, HR, BP, blood chemistry profile) as well as other fitness variables such as body composition and psychological traits. Evaluation of the ECG by a physician determines whether any abnormalities require further medical attention. People with extreme BP or blood chemistry values (see chapter 3) should also be referred to their personal physicians.

Submaximal Tests to Estimate CRF

If the resting tests reflect normal values, then a submaximal test is administered. The submaximal test usually provides the HR and BP responses to different intensities of work ranging from light intensity up to a predetermined point (usually 85% of predicted maximum HR). This test can use a bench step, cycle ergometer, or treadmill. Once again, if unusual responses to the submaximal test appear, the person is referred for further medical tests. If the results appear normal, then the person begins an activity program at intensities less than those reached on the test (e.g., a person goes to 85% of maximum HR on the test and starts the fitness program at 70%). After the person has become accustomed to regular exercise and appears to be adjusting to fitness activities, a maximal test can be administered.

Submaximal tests also can be used to estimate maximal functional capacity (maximal oxygen uptake) by extrapolating HR to a predicted maximum and then using the linear relationship between HR and oxygen uptake to estimate maximal oxygen uptake. Although this estimated maximum is useful for evaluating a person's current CRF status and prescribing or revising exercise, the estimation involves considerable error (15%). In addition to submaximal CRF, flexibility and muscular strength and endurance (especially for low-back function) are often measured at this stage (see chapters 8 and 9).

Maximal Tests to Estimate or Measure CRF

If no problems occur up to this point, a maximal test is administered. Two types of maximal tests are used to estimate CRF: laboratory tests that measure physiological responses (e.g., HR, BP) to increasing workloads and all-out endurance performance tests (e.g., time on a 1 mi, or 1.6 km run). The results of the maximal test can be used to revise the activity program (i.e., the person's maximal functional capacity provides a new basis for selecting fitness activities). The person's measured maximal HR (instead of estimated maximal HR) should now be used to determine THR.

Program Modification and Periodic Retests

After the program participant achieves a minimum level of fitness, a wider variety of activities (e.g., games and sports) can be included in the fitness program. All of the fitness tests should be readministered periodically to determine the progress being made and to revise the program in areas where the gains are not as great as desired.

Key Point

A logical sequence of steps to follow in fitness testing includes informed consent, health history, screening, resting CRF, submaximal CRF and other tests, light activity prescription, maximal CRF, program modification, and periodic retesting (see box on page 63).

Field Tests

A variety of field tests can be used to estimate CRF. These are called *field tests* because they require very little equipment, can be done just about anywhere, and use the simple activities of walking and running. Because these tests involve running or walking as fast as possible over a set distance, they are not recommended at the start of an exercise program. Instead, participants should complete the graduated walking program before taking the walking test and the graduated jogging program before taking the running test. The walking and jogging programs are found in chapter 14. The graduated nature of the fitness programs allows participants to start at a low and safe level of activity and gradually improve. It is then appropriate to administer an endurance run test to evaluate fitness status.

Field tests rely on the observation that for a person to walk or run at high speeds over long distances, the heart must pump great volumes of oxygen to the muscles. In this way, the average speed maintained in these walk or run tests gives an estimate of CRF. The higher the CRF score, the greater the heart's capacity to transport oxygen. An endurance run of a set distance for a given time or of a set time for a given distance provides information about a person's CR endurance as long as the run is 1 mi (1.6 km) or longer. The advantages of an endurance run test include its moderately high correlation to maximum oxygen uptake, the use of a natural activity, and the large numbers of participants who can be tested in a short time. The disadvantages of endurance running are that it is difficult to monitor physiological responses, other factors affect the outcome (e.g., motivation), endurance running cannot be used for graded or submaximal testing, and the *SEE* is about 5 ml · kg^{-1} · min^{-1} (32).

1 Mi (1.6 km) Walk Test

A 1 mi (1.6 km) walk test to predict CRF accommodates individuals of different ages and fitness levels. Follow the steps on page 65 to administer the 1 mi walk test.

In this test, the individual walks as fast as possible on a measured track, and HR is measured at the end of the mile. The following equation is used to calculate $\dot{V}O_2max$ (ml · kg^{-1} · min^{-1}):

$$\dot{V}O_2max = 132.853 - 0.0769\ (weight) - 0.3877\ (age) + 6.315\ (sex) - 3.2649\ (time) - 0.1565\ (HR),$$

where weight is body weight in pounds, age is in years, sex equals 0 for female and 1 for male, time is in minutes and hundredths of minutes, and HR is in beats per minute. The formula was developed and validated on men and women aged 30 to 69 yr (25), and the *SEE* is about 5 ml · kg^{-1} · min^{-1} (1, 25).

QUESTION: What is the CRF of a 25-yr-old, 170 lb (77.1 kg) man who walks the mile in 20 min and has an immediate postexercise HR of 140 beats · min^{-1}?

Answer:

$$\dot{V}O_2max = 132.853 - 0.0769\ (weight) - 0.3877\ (age) + 6.315\ (sex) - 3.2649\ (time) - 0.1565\ (HR) = 132.853 - 0.0769\ (170) - 0.3877\ (25) + 6.315\ (1) - 3.2649\ (20.0) - 0.1565\ (140) = 29.2\ ml \cdot kg^{-1} \cdot min^{-1}$$

Steps to Administer the 1 Mi (1.6 km) Walk Test

Before Test Day

1. Arrange to have the following elements at the test site:
    - A person to start and read the time from a stopwatch
    - A partner with a watch (with a second hand) for each walker (perhaps with a sheet to mark off laps)
    - A stopwatch for the timer (with a spare ready)
    - A score sheet or scorecard
2. Explain the purpose of the test (i.e., to determine how fast the participants can walk 1 mi (1.6 km), which reflects the endurance of their cardiovascular system).
3. Select and mark off (if needed) a level area for the walk.
4. Explain to people being tested that they are to walk the mile in the fastest time possible. Only walking is allowed, and the goal is to cover the distance as fast as possible.

Test Day

1. Participants warm up with stretching and slow walking.
2. Several people will walk at the same time.
3. Explain the procedure again. Remind the participants not to speed up at the end of the walk but to maintain a fast and steady pace throughout.
4. The timer says, "Ready, go," and starts the stopwatch.
5. Each individual has a partner standing at the start/finish line with a watch with a second hand.
6. The partner counts the laps and tells the individual at the end of each lap how many more laps to walk.
7. The timer calls out the minutes and seconds as each person finishes the mile walk.
8. The partner listens for the time when her walker finishes the mile and records it (to the nearest second) immediately on a scorecard.
9. The walker takes a 10 sec HR immediately after the end of the mile walk, with the partner timing it.

To simplify the calculations for this 1 mi walk test, table 5.1 was generated on the basis of the preceding formula for men weighing 170 lb (77.1 kg) and women weighing 125 lb (56.7 kg). For each 15 lb (6.8 kg) above (or below) these weights, subtract (or add) 1 ml · kg^{-1} · min^{-1}.

To use table 5.1, find the part of the table for the individual's sex and age, then go across the top until you find the time (to the nearest minute) that person took to walk a mile, and then go down that column until it intersects with the person's postexercise HR (listed on the left side). The number at which the mile time and postexercise HR meet is the CRF value in terms of ml · kg^{-1} · min^{-1}. For example, a 25-yr-old man who walked the mile in 20 min and had a postexercise HR of 140 has an estimated maximal oxygen uptake of 29.2 ml · kg^{-1} · min^{-1}. You can evaluate CRF by comparing that number with the standards presented in table 5.2. In the example of the 25-yr-old man, his maximal oxygen uptake is <30, indicating a need for improvement. The standards in table 5.2 represent the levels of oxygen uptake for females and males who wish to achieve health-related fitness. Those wishing to focus on performance should strive for higher values.

Jog or Run Test

One of the most common CRF field tests is the 12 min or 1.5 mi (2.4 km) run popularized by Cooper (15). This test is very much like the walk test mentioned previously: Participants jog or run as fast as possible for 12 min or for 1.5 mi (2.4 km). This test is based on work by Balke (8), who showed that 10 to 20 min running tests could be used to estimate $\dot{V}O_2max$. Balke found the optimal duration for the run test to be 15 min. The test relies on the relationship between a running velocity and the oxygen uptake required to run at that velocity (figure 5.1). The greater the running speed, the greater the oxygen uptake required. The reason for the duration of 12 to 15 min is that the running test has to be long enough to diminish the contribution of anaerobic energy (immediate and short-term energy) to the average velocity. In essence, the average velocity that can be maintained in a 5 or 6 min run overestimates

Table 5.1 Estimated Maximal Oxygen Uptake (ml · kg^{-1} · min^{-1}) for Men and Women, 20-69 Years Old

	Min · mile^{-1}										
HR	10	11	12	13	14	15	16	17	18	19	20
Men (20-29)											
120	65.0	61.7	58.4	55.2	51.9	48.6	45.4	42.1	38.9	35.6	32.3
130	63.4	60.1	56.9	53.6	50.3	47.1	43.8	40.6	37.3	34.0	30.8
140	61.8	58.6	55.3	52.0	48.8	45.5	42.2	39.0	35.7	32.5	29.2
150	60.3	57.0	53.7	50.5	47.2	43.9	40.7	37.4	34.2	30.9	27.6
160	58.7	55.4	52.2	48.9	45.6	42.4	39.1	35.9	32.6	29.3	26.1
170	57.1	53.9	50.6	47.3	44.1	40.8	37.6	34.3	31.0	27.8	24.5
180	55.6	52.3	49.0	45.8	42.5	39.3	36.0	32.7	29.5	26.2	22.9
190	54.0	50.7	47.5	44.2	41.0	37.7	34.4	31.2	27.9	24.6	21.4
200	52.4	49.2	45.9	42.7	39.4	36.1	32.9	29.6	26.3	23.1	19.8
Women (20-29)											
120	62.1	58.9	55.6	52.3	49.1	45.8	42.5	39.3	36.0	32.7	29.5
130	60.6	57.3	54.0	50.8	47.5	44.2	41.0	37.7	34.4	31.2	27.9
140	59.0	55.7	52.5	49.2	45.9	42.7	39.4	36.1	32.9	29.6	26.3
150	57.4	54.2	50.9	47.6	44.4	41.1	37.8	34.6	31.3	28.0	24.8
160	55.9	52.6	49.3	46.7	42.8	39.5	36.3	33.0	29.7	26.5	23.2
170	54.3	51.0	47.8	44.5	41.2	38.0	34.7	31.4	28.2	24.9	21.6
180	52.7	49.5	46.2	42.9	39.7	36.4	33.1	29.9	26.6	23.3	20.1
190	51.2	47.9	44.6	41.4	38.1	34.8	31.6	28.3	25.0	21.8	18.5
200	49.6	46.3	43.1	39.8	36.5	33.3	30.0	26.7	23.5	20.2	16.9
Men (30-39)											
120	61.1	57.8	54.6	51.3	48.0	44.8	41.5	38.2	35.0	31.7	28.4
130	59.5	56.3	53.0	49.7	46.5	43.2	39.9	36.7	33.4	30.1	26.9
140	58.0	54.7	51.4	48.2	44.9	41.6	38.4	35.1	31.8	28.6	25.3
150	56.4	53.1	49.9	46.6	43.3	40.1	36.8	33.5	30.3	27.0	23.8
160	54.8	51.6	48.3	45.0	41.8	38.5	35.2	32.0	28.7	25.5	22.2
170	53.3	50.0	46.7	43.5	40.2	36.9	33.7	30.4	27.1	23.9	20.6
180	51.7	48.4	45.2	41.9	38.6	35.4	32.1	28.8	25.6	22.3	19.1
190	50.1	46.9	43.6	40.3	37.1	33.8	30.5	27.3	24.0	20.8	17.5
Women (30-39)											
120	58.2	55.0	51.7	48.4	45.2	41.9	38.7	35.4	32.1	28.9	25.6
130	56.7	53.4	50.1	46.9	43.6	40.4	37.1	33.8	30.6	27.3	24.0
140	55.1	51.8	48.6	45.3	42.1	38.8	35.5	32.3	29.0	24.7	22.5
150	53.5	50.3	47.0	43.8	40.5	37.2	34.0	30.7	27.4	24.2	20.9
160	52.0	48.7	45.4	42.2	38.9	35.7	32.4	29.1	25.9	22.6	19.3
170	50.4	47.1	43.9	40.6	37.4	34.1	30.8	27.6	24.3	21.0	17.8
180	48.8	45.6	42.3	39.1	35.8	32.5	29.3	26.0	22.7	19.5	16.2
190	47.3	44.0	40.8	37.5	34.2	31.0	27.7	24.4	21.2	17.9	14.6

	Min · mile^{-1}										
HR	**10**	**11**	**12**	**13**	**14**	**15**	**16**	**17**	**18**	**19**	**20**
Men (40-49)											
120	57.2	54.0	50.7	47.4	44.2	40.9	37.6	34.4	31.1	27.8	24.6
130	55.7	52.4	49.1	45.9	42.6	39.3	36.1	32.8	29.5	26.3	23.0
140	54.1	50.8	47.6	44.3	41.0	37.8	34.5	31.2	28.0	24.7	21.4
150	52.5	49.3	46.0	42.7	39.5	36.2	32.9	29.7	26.4	23.1	19.9
160	51.0	47.7	44.4	41.2	37.9	34.6	31.4	28.1	24.8	21.6	18.3
170	49.4	46.1	42.9	39.6	36.3	33.1	29.8	26.5	23.3	20.0	16.7
180	47.8	44.6	41.3	38.0	34.8	31.5	28.2	25.0	21.7	18.4	15.2
Women (40-49)											
120	54.4	51.1	47.8	44.6	41.3	38.0	34.8	31.5	28.2	25.0	21.7
130	52.8	49.5	46.3	43.0	39.7	36.5	33.2	29.9	26.7	23.4	20.1
140	51.2	48.0	44.7	41.4	38.2	34.9	31.6	28.4	25.1	21.8	18.6
150	49.7	46.4	43.1	39.9	36.6	33.3	30.1	26.8	23.5	20.3	17.0
160	48.1	44.8	41.6	38.3	35.0	31.8	28.5	25.2	22.0	18.7	15.5
170	46.5	43.3	40.0	36.7	33.5	30.2	26.9	23.7	20.4	17.2	13.9
Men (50-59)											
120	53.3	50.0	46.8	43.5	40.3	37.0	33.7	30.5	27.2	23.9	20.7
130	51.7	48.5	45.2	42.0	38.7	35.4	32.2	28.9	25.6	22.4	19.1
140	50.2	46.9	43.7	40.4	37.1	33.9	30.6	27.3	24.1	20.8	17.5
150	48.6	45.4	42.1	38.8	35.6	32.3	29.0	25.8	22.5	19.2	16.0
160	47.1	43.8	40.5	37.3	34.0	30.7	27.5	24.2	20.9	17.7	14.4
170	45.5	42.2	39.0	35.7	32.4	29.2	25.9	22.6	19.4	16.1	12.8
Women (50-59)											
120	50.5	47.2	43.9	40.7	37.4	34.1	30.9	27.6	24.3	21.1	17.8
130	48.9	45.6	42.4	39.1	35.8	32.6	29.3	26.0	22.8	19.5	16.2
140	47.3	44.1	40.8	37.5	34.3	31.0	27.7	24.5	21.2	17.9	14.7
150	45.8	42.5	39.2	36.0	32.7	29.4	26.2	22.9	19.6	16.4	13.1
160	44.2	40.9	37.7	34.4	31.1	27.9	24.6	21.3	18.1	14.8	11.5
170	42.6	39.4	36.1	32.8	29.6	26.3	23.0	19.8	16.5	13.2	10.0
Men (60-69)											
120	49.4	46.2	42.9	39.6	36.4	33.1	29.8	26.6	23.3	20.0	16.8
130	47.9	44.6	41.3	38.1	34.8	31.5	28.3	25.0	21.7	18.5	15.2
140	46.3	43.0	39.8	36.5	33.2	30.0	26.7	23.4	20.2	16.9	13.6
150	44.7	41.5	38.2	34.9	31.7	28.4	25.1	21.9	18.6	15.3	12.1
160	43.2	39.9	36.6	33.4	30.1	26.8	23.6	20.3	17.0	13.8	10.5
Women (60-69)											
120	46.6	43.3	40.0	36.8	33.5	30.2	27.0	23.7	20.5	17.2	13.9
130	45.0	41.7	38.5	35.2	31.9	28.7	25.4	22.2	18.9	15.6	12.4
140	43.4	40.2	36.9	33.6	30.4	27.1	23.8	20.6	17.3	14.1	10.8
150	41.9	38.6	35.3	32.1	28.8	25.5	22.3	19.0	15.8	12.5	9.2
160	40.3	37.0	33.8	30.5	27.2	24.0	20.7	17.5	14.2	10.9	7.7

Note. Calculations assume 170 lb for men and 125 lb for women. For each 15 lb beyond these values, subtract 1 ml · kg^{-1} · min^{-1}. HR = heart rate.

Values generated from formula in G.M. Kline, J.P. Porcari, R. Hintermeister, P.S. Freedson, A. Ward, R.F. McCarron, J. Ross and J.M. Rippe, 1987, "Estimation of $\dot{V}O_2$max from a 1-mile track walk, gender, age, and bodyweight," *Medicine and Science in Sports and Exercise* 19: 253-259.

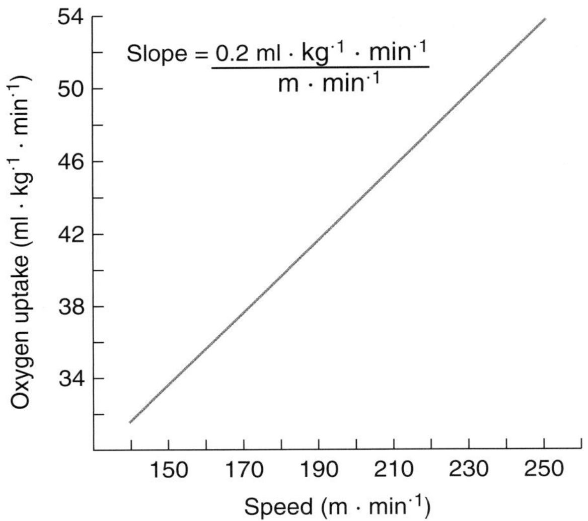

Figure 5.1 Relationship between steady-state oxygen uptake and running speed (13).

$\dot{V}O_2$max because anaerobic energy sources contribute substantially to total energy production in a 5 min run compared with a 12 to 15 min run. If the run lasts too long, the person is not able to run close to 100% of $\dot{V}O_2$max, and then the estimate is too low (figure 5.2).

The $\dot{V}O_2$ associated with a specific running speed can be calculated from the following formula (see chapter 4 for details):

$$\dot{V}O_2 = \text{horizontal velocity } (\text{m} \cdot \text{min}^{-1}) \cdot \frac{0.2 \text{ ml} \cdot \text{kg}^{-1} \cdot \text{min}^{-1}}{(\text{m} \cdot \text{min}^{-1})} + 3.5 \text{ ml} \cdot \text{kg}^{-1} \cdot \text{min}^{-1}$$

These estimates are reasonable for adults who jog or run the entire 12 min or 1.5 mi (2.4 km). The formula underestimates $\dot{V}O_2$max in children because they have a higher oxygen cost of running (18). In contrast, the formula overestimates $\dot{V}O_2$max in trained runners because of their better running economy (17) and in those who walk the test because the net oxygen cost of walking is half that of running (see chapter 4).

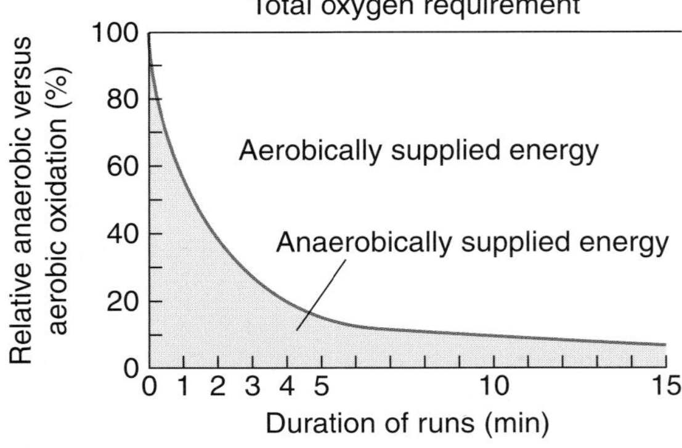

Figure 5.2 The relative role of aerobic and anaerobic energy sources in best-effort runs of various durations.
From B. Balke, 1963, "A simple field test for the assessment of physical fitness," *Federal Aviation Agency* 63: 7.

QUESTION: A 20-yr-old woman takes the Cooper 12 min run test following a 15 wk walk and jog program and completes 6 laps on a 440 yd (402.3 m) track. What is her $\dot{V}O_2$max?

Answer:

$$402.3 \text{ m} \cdot \text{lap}^{-1} \cdot 6 \text{ laps} = 2{,}414 \text{ m, and}$$

$$2{,}414 \text{ m} \div 12 \text{ min} = 201 \text{ m} \cdot \text{min}^{-1}$$

$$\dot{V}O_2 = 201 \text{ m} \cdot \text{min}^{-1} \cdot \frac{0.2 \text{ ml} \cdot \text{kg}^{-1} \cdot \text{min}^{-1}}{(\text{m} \cdot \text{min}^{-1})} + 3.5 \text{ ml} \cdot \text{kg}^{-1} \cdot \text{min}^{-1}$$

Applying the 12 Min Run Test

The advantage of the 12 min run is that it can be used to regularly evaluate CRF without expensive equipment. It is easily adapted to cyclists and swimmers, who can evaluate their CRF progress by determining how far they can ride or swim in 12 min. Although no equations exist that can relate cyclists' and swimmers' respective performances to $\dot{V}O_2$max, participants can personally judge their current CRF and improvement attributable to training by monitoring the distance they can cover in 12 min.

As Cooper (15) and others agree, an endurance run should not be used for testing CRF at the beginning of an exercise program. A person new to exercise should progress through the jogging program (at low exercise intensities) to make fitness improvements before taking an endurance run test.

Table 5.2 lists values to classify CRF as good, adequate, borderline, and needs extra work. The table takes age and sex into consideration. For example, a 40-yr-old woman who runs 1.5 mi (2.4 km) in 14 min and 15 sec (14:15) would rate between adequate and good. Her time of 14:15 corresponds to a CRF value of about 37 to 40 ml · kg^{-1} · min^{-1}. Encourage participants to achieve and maintain the good value for their age and sex. If people

> **Key Point**
>
> A 1 mi (1.6 km) walking test can be used to estimate CRF. The time of the walk and the HR measured at the end of the walk are used to calculate $\dot{V}O_2$max. A 1.5 mi (2.4 km) run test also can be used to estimate CRF. The time for the 1.5 mi (2.4 km) is used to determine average velocity, and a formula (see chapter 4) is used to calculate $\dot{V}O_2$max.

Table 5.2 Standards for Maximal Oxygen Uptake and Endurance Runs

$\dot{V}O_2max$ (ml · kg^{-1} · min^{-1})			1.5 mi (2.4 km) run (min:sec)		12 min run in mi (km)	
Age[a]	Female[b]	Male	Female	Male	Female	Male
			Good			
15-30	>40	>45	<12	<10	>1.5 (2.4)	>1.7 (2.7)
35-50	>35	>40	<13:30	<11:30	>1.4 (2.3)	>1.5 (2.4)
55-70	>30	>35	<16	<14	>1.2 (1.9)	>1.3 (2.1)
			Adequate for most activities			
15-30	35	40	13:30	11:50	1.4 (2.3)	1.5 (2.4)
35-50	30	35	15	13	1.3 (2.1)	1.4 (2.3)
55-70	25	30	17:30	15:30	1.1 (1.8)	1.3 (2.1)
			Borderline			
15-30	30	35	15	13	1.3 (2.1)	1.4 (2.3)
35-50	25	30	16:30	14:30	1.2 (1.9)	1.3 (2.1)
55-70	20	25	19	17	1.0 (1.6)	1.2 (1.9)
			Needs extra work on CRF			
15–30	<25	<30	>17	>15	<1.2 (1.9)	<1.3 (2.1)
35-50	<20	<25	>18:30	>16:30	<1.1 (1.8)	<1.2 (1.9)
55-70	<15	<20	>21	>19	<0.9 (1.4)	<1.0 (1.6)

These standards are for fitness programs. People wanting to do well in endurance performance need higher levels than those listed. People at the *good* level should emphasize maintaining this level the rest of their lives. Those in the lower levels should emphasize setting and reaching realistic goals for CRF.

[a]CRF declines with age.

[b]Women have lower standards because they have a larger amount of essential fat.

Reprinted from E.T. Howley and B.D. Franks, 1986, *Health fitness instructor's handbook* (Champaign, IL: Human Kinetics), 85.

are not at that level, help them make small and systematic progress toward that goal by using the walking and jogging programs in chapter 14.

Administrating an Endurance Run Test

The 1 mi (1.6 km) run is used in many youth fitness programs (16, 33). The steps to administering the 1 mi (1.6 km) run are listed on page 70. They can be used for other endurance runs (e.g., 1.5 mi or 12 min run); the 1 mi run is used as an example.

Graded Exercise Tests

Many fitness programs use a **graded exercise test (GXT)** to evaluate CRF. These multilevel tests can be administered with a bench, cycle ergometer, or treadmill.

Bench Step

Bench stepping is very economical. It can be used for both submaximal and maximal testing. The disadvantages include the limited number of stages that can be included for any one bench height and individual fitness level and the difficulty of taking certain measurements during the test (e.g., BP). The oxygen costs for stepping at different rates on steps of different heights were presented in chapter 4.

Cycle Ergometer

Cycle ergometers are portable, moderately priced work instruments that allow easy measurement of heart rate and blood pressure because the participant's upper body is essentially stationary. Their disadvantages, however, are that the exercise load is self-paced and that fatigued leg muscle may be a limiting factor. On mechanically braked cycle ergometers such as the Monark models, altering the pedal rate or the resistance on the flywheel changes the work rate. Generally, the pedal rate is maintained constant during a GXT at a rate appropriate to the individual being tested: 50 to 60 rev · min^{-1} for individuals of low to average fitness and 70 to 100 rev · min^{-1} for highly fit and competitive cyclists (23). A metronome or some other source of feedback such as a speedometer helps the individual

Steps to Administer the 1 Mi (1.6 km) Run

Before Test Day

1. Arrange to have the following elements at the test site:
   - A person to start and read the time from a stopwatch
   - A partner for each runner (perhaps with a sheet to mark off laps)
   - A stopwatch for the tester (with a spare ready)
   - A score sheet or scorecard
2. Explain the purpose of the test (i.e., to determine how fast participants can run 1 mi, or 1.6 km, which reflects the endurance of their cardiovascular system).
3. Do not administer the test until participants have had several fitness sessions, including some with running.
4. Have participants practice running at a set submaximal pace for 1 lap, then 2, and so on, several times before the test day.
5. Select and mark off (if needed) a level area for the run.
6. Explain to people being tested that they are to run the mile in the fastest time possible. Walking is allowed, but the goal is to cover the distance as quickly as possible.

Test Day

1. Participants warm up with stretching, walking, and slow jogging.
2. Several people will run at the same time.
3. The procedure is explained again.
4. The timer says, "Ready, go," and starts the stopwatch.
5. Each individual has a partner with a watch with a second hand.
6. The partner counts the laps and tells the individual at the end of each lap how many more laps to run.
7. The timer calls out the minutes and seconds as the runner finishes the mile run.
8. The partner listens for the time when the runner finishes the mile and records it (to the nearest second) immediately on a scorecard.
9. The runner continues to walk 1 lap after finishing the run.

maintain the pedal rate. The resistance (load) on the wheel is increased sequentially to systematically overload the cardiovascular system. The starting work rate and the increment from one stage to the next depend on the fitness of the person being tested and the purpose of the test. $\dot{V}O_2$ can be estimated from a formula (1) that gives reasonable estimates of $\dot{V}O_2$ up to work rates of about 1,200 kgm · min^{-1} or 200 W (see chapter 4 for details):

$$\dot{V}O_2\ (\text{ml} \cdot \text{kg}^{-1} \cdot \text{min}^{-1}) = (\text{work rate [kgm} \cdot \text{min}^{-1}] \cdot 1.8\ \text{ml O}_2 \cdot \text{kgm}^{-1}) \div \text{body weight (kg)} + 7\ \text{ml} \cdot \text{kg}^{-1} \cdot \text{min}^{-1}, \text{ or}$$

$$\dot{V}O_2\ (\text{ml} \cdot \text{kg}^{-1} \cdot \text{min}^{-1}) = (\text{work rate [W]} \cdot 10.8\ \text{ml O}_2 \cdot \text{W}^{-1}) \div \text{body weight (kg)} + 7\ \text{ml} \cdot \text{kg}^{-1} \cdot \text{min}^{-1}.$$

The cycle ergometer differs from the treadmill in that the seat supports the body weight and the work rate depends primarily on pedal rate and on the load on the wheel. This means that the relative $\dot{V}O_2$ at any work rate is higher for a smaller person than for a bigger person.

QUESTION: What is the relative difficulty of a work rate of 900 kgm · min^{-1} for two individuals, one weighing 60 kg and the other 90 kg?

Answer:

For the 60 kg subject,

$$\dot{V}O_2\ (\text{ml} \cdot \text{kg}^{-1} \cdot \text{min}^{-1}) = (900\ \text{kgm} \cdot \text{min}^{-1} \cdot 1.8\ \text{ml O}_2 \cdot \text{kgm}^{-1}) \div 60\ \text{kg} + 7\ \text{ml} \cdot \text{kg}^{-1} \cdot \text{min}^{-1}, \text{ and}$$

$$\dot{V}O_2\ (\text{ml} \cdot \text{kg}^{-1} \cdot \text{min}^{-1}) = 34\ \text{ml} \cdot \text{kg}^{-1} \cdot \text{min}^{-1}, \text{or } 9.7\ \text{METs}.$$

For the 90 kg subject,

$$\dot{V}O_2\ (\text{ml} \cdot \text{kg}^{-1} \cdot \text{min}^{-1}) = (900\ \text{kgm} \cdot \text{min}^{-1} \cdot 1.8\ \text{ml O}_2 \cdot \text{kgm}^{-1}) \div 90\ \text{kg} + 7\ \text{ml} \cdot \text{kg}^{-1} \cdot \text{min}^{-1}, \text{ and}$$

$$\dot{V}O_2\ (\text{ml} \cdot \text{kg}^{-1} \cdot \text{min}^{-1}) = 25\ \text{ml} \cdot \text{kg}^{-1} \cdot \text{min}^{-1}, \text{or } 7.1\ \text{METs}.$$

In addition, the increments in the work rate, by demanding a fixed increase in the $\dot{V}O_2$ (e.g., an increment

Table 5.3 Work Differences Based on Body Weight in Work Tasks

	$\dot{V}O_2max$			
Work task	**L · min^{-1}**	**ml · kg^{-1} · min^{-1}**	**Total work (kcal)**	**METs**
A heavier person will respond with the following differences when compared with a lighter person when both are doing the same task at the same rate:				
Bench	↑	=	↑	=
Walk	↑	=	↑	=
Jog	↑	=	↑	=
Body-weight supported cycle	=	↓	=	↓

MET = metabolic equivalent.

of 150 kgm · min^{-1} equals a $\dot{V}O_2$ change of 270 ml · min^{-1}), force the small or unfit subject to make cardiovascular adjustments greater than those of a large or highly fit subject. As we will see, these factors are considered in selecting work rates for a cycle ergometer test used to evaluate CRF. Table 5.3 summarizes how differences in body weight affect the metabolic responses to weight-supported (e.g., cycle ergometry) and weight-carrying (e.g., bench stepping, jogging) work tasks. Thus, for tasks in which the body weight provides the resistance (weight-carrying tasks), a larger person achieves a greater absolute $\dot{V}O_2$ (L · min^{-1}) than a smaller person achieves, but both work at the same MET level. In cycling (a weight-supported task), the two people achieve a similar absolute $\dot{V}O_2$, but the larger person has a lower MET level.

Treadmill

Treadmill protocols are very reproducible because they set the pace for the subject, whereas the subject may go too slow or too fast on either the bench step or the cycle ergometer. Treadmill tests can accommodate people of any fitness level and use the natural activities of walking and running, with the running tests placing the greatest potential load on the cardiovascular system. Treadmills, however, are expensive, are not portable, and make some measurements (BP and blood sampling) difficult. The type of treadmill test influences the measured $\dot{V}O_2$max, with the graded running test giving the highest value, the running test at 0% grade giving the next highest value, and the walking test giving the lowest value (7, 27).

To estimate $\dot{V}O_2$ by varying grade and speed, the grade and speed settings on the treadmill must be calibrated correctly (see details on how to calibrate a treadmill and other equipment later in this chapter). Further, the subject cannot hold on to the treadmill railing during the test if the estimated $\dot{V}O_2$ values are going to be reasonable. For example, it was observed that HR decreased 17 beats · min^{-1} when a subject who was walking on a treadmill at 3.4 mi · hr^{-1} (5.5 km · hr^{-1}) and at a 14% grade held onto the treadmill railing (5). Holding onto the railing results in an overestimation of the $\dot{V}O_2$max because the HR is lower at any stage of the test and so the test lasts longer. With the treadmill test, there is no need to adjust the $\dot{V}O_2$ calculation for differences in body weight because the person being tested carries his own weight; therefore, the $\dot{V}O_2$ (ml · kg^{-1} · min^{-1}) is independent of body weight (28).

Key Point

CRF response to exercise intensity can be determined with bench stepping, cycle ergometers, or a treadmill protocol. The oxygen uptake values (expressed in ml · kg^{-1} · min^{-1}) are similar for most adults at specific stages of a treadmill or step test because the energy cost is proportional to the body weight, which is carried by the test participant. In contrast, the absolute oxygen uptake (expressed in L · min^{-1}) is similar for most adults at each stage of a cycle ergometer test; however, the relative oxygen cost (ml · kg^{-1} · min^{-1}) is higher for the lighter participant.

Common Variables Measured During a GXT

The variables commonly measured for resting and submaximal tests include HR, BP, and rating of perceived exertion (RPE). For maximal testing, $\dot{V}O_2$ max and the final stage achieved on a GXT are often measured.

Heart Rate

Heart rate (HR) often is used as a fitness indicator at rest and during a standard submaximal work task. Maximal

HR is useful for determining the target heart rate (THR) for fitness workouts (see chapter 10), but it is not a good fitness indicator because it changes very little with training. Table 5.4 summarizes how aerobic exercise or conditioning affects HR in different situations.

When an ECG is recorded, the HR can be taken from the ECG strip (see chapter 24). Without an ECG, HR can be taken by an HR watch, a stethoscope, or manual palpation of an artery at the wrist or neck. HR watches have been found to be accurate and are the easiest way to measure HR. When palpating, fingers (not the thumb) should be used to take HR, preferably at the wrist (radial artery). Taking the HR at the neck (carotid artery) requires caution because applying too much pressure can trigger a reflex that slows the HR. Reliable measures are obtained, however, when people are trained in this procedure (31). The HR at rest or during steady-state exercise should be taken for 30 sec for higher reliability. When HR is taken after exercise, the measurement should begin soon after exercise ends (e.g., within 5 sec) and should be taken for 10 or 15 sec because the HR changes so rapidly. The 10 or 15 sec rate is multiplied by 6 or 4, respectively, to calculate beats per minute. For example, if a 10 sec postexercise HR is 20 beats · min $^{-1}$, the HR is 120 beats · min $^{-1}$ (6 · 20).

Blood Pressure

Systolic blood pressure (SBP) and diastolic blood pressure (DBP) are often determined at rest, during work, and after work. Proper cuff size (in which the bladder overlaps two thirds of the arm) and a sensitive stethoscope are required to get accurate values at rest and during work. At rest, the person should have both feet flat on the floor and be in a relaxed position with the arm supported. The cuff should be wrapped securely around the arm at heart level, usually with the tube on the inside of the arm. The stethoscope should be below (not under) the cuff—the placement will depend on where the sound can be most easily heard, often toward the inside of the arm (21). The first and fourth Korotkoff sounds (the first sound heard and the sound when the tone changes or becomes muffled) should be used for SBP and DBP, respectively, during exercise. The fifth Korotkoff sound (disappearance of sound) is used to classify BP at rest (1).

Table 5.4 Effects of Fitness Conditioning on HR

Condition	Effects of fitness on HR
Rest	↓
Standard submaximal work (same external work rate)	↓
Maximal work	No change
Set % of maximal	No change

HR = heart rate.

Rating of Perceived Exertion

Borg introduced the **rating of perceived exertion (RPE),** that is, how hard the participant perceives the workout is on a scale from 6 to 20 (roughly based on resting to maximal HR, i.e., 60-200 beats · min $^{-1}$). Table 5.5 presents this scale as well as Borg's revised 10-point RPE scale (12). Either can be used with a GXT to provide useful information during the test as the person approaches exhaustion and to serve as a reference for exercise prescription. When you administer the RPE scale, we recommend that you provide the following instructions (1, p. 78):

> During the exercise test we want you to pay close attention to how hard you feel the exercise work rate is. This feeling should reflect your total amount of exertion and fatigue, combining all sensations and feelings of physical stress, effort, and fatigue. Don't concern yourself with any one factor such as leg pain, shortness of breath, or exercise intensity, but try to concentrate on your total, inner feeling of exertion. Try not to underestimate or overestimate your feelings of exertion; be as accurate as you can.

Estimating Versus Measuring Functional Capacity

Functional capacity is defined as the highest work rate (oxygen uptake) reached in a GXT during which HR, BP, and ECG responses are within the normal range for heavy work. For cardiac patients, the highest work rate normally does not reflect the maximal capacity of their cardiorespiratory systems because the GXT might be stopped for ECG changes, angina, claudication pain, and so on. For the apparently healthy person, functional capacity can be called *maximal aerobic power* or *maximal oxygen uptake* ($\dot{V}O_2$max) (see chapter 28 for procedures for measuring oxygen uptake).

Oxygen uptake increases with each stage of the GXT until the CRF reaches its upper limit. At that point, $\dot{V}O_2$ does not increase when the test moves to the next stage; the person's $\dot{V}O_2$max has been reached. Given the complexity and cost of procedures for directly measuring $\dot{V}O_2$max, it is usually estimated with equations relating the stage of the GXT to a specific oxygen uptake.

As discussed in chapter 4, many formulas may be used to estimate oxygen uptake from the stage reached in a GXT. In general, these formulas reasonably estimate the $\dot{V}O_2$ if the GXT is suited to the individual. However, if the increments in the stages of the GXT are too large relative to the person's CRF, or if the time spent at each stage is too short, then the person might not reach the

Table 5.5 Category and Category-Ratio Scales for Ratings of Perceived Exertion (RPE)

Category scale		Category-ratio scale		
6		0	Nothing at all	No *I*
7	Very, very light	0.3		
8		0.5	Extremely weak	Just noticeable
9	Very light	0.7		
10		1	Very weak	
11	Fairly light	1.5		
12		2	Weak	
13	Somewhat hard	2.5		
14		3	Moderate	
15	Hard	4		
16		5	Strong	Heavy
17	Very hard	6		
18		7	Very strong	
19	Very, very hard	8		
20		9		
		10	Extremely strong	Strongest *I*
		11		
		•	Absolute maximum	Highest possible

On the category-ratio scale, *I* represents intensity.

To correctly use the Borg scales, follow the administration and instructions given in G. Borg's *Perceived Exertion and Pain Scales.* Champaign, IL: Human Kinetics, 1998.

steady-state oxygen requirement associated with that stage (29). Failure to achieve the oxygen requirement for a GXT stage results in overestimating $\dot{V}O_2$ at each stage of the test, with the overestimation growing larger with each stage. The inability to reach the oxygen requirement is a common problem with individuals who are less fit (e.g., cardiac patients). This inability suggests that more conservative (i.e., smaller increments between stages) GXT protocols should be used to allow these individuals to reach the oxygen demand at each stage. This problem is explained more completely in chapter 28.

Key Point

Common variables measured during a resting or submaximal GXT include HR, BP, and RPE. Oxygen uptake can be measured at each stage of a test and at maximal exertion; however, $\dot{V}O_2$max usually is estimated (using the formulas described in chapter 4) from the final stage achieved during the GXT.

In contrast, shorter stages and larger increments between stages in a GXT can be used if the purpose of the tests is to screen for ECG abnormalities (rather than to estimate $\dot{V}O_2$max). In addition, changes in CRF over time can be determined by periodically using the same GXT on an individual.

Procedures for GXTs

This section explains how to administer a GXT and uses examples of different testing protocols. Before administering any GXT, the tester should

- calibrate the equipment,
- check supplies and data forms,
- select the appropriate test protocol for the participant,
- obtain informed consent,
- instruct the participant about the task, including the cool-down,
- have the participant practice the task (if needed), and

- check to see that the participant followed pretest instructions.

Because HR, BP, and RPE responses to submaximal work are influenced by a variety of factors, variation in each factor from test to test should be carefully minimized. These factors include, but are not limited to,

- temperature and relative humidity of the room;
- number of hours of sleep before testing;
- emotional state;
- hydration state;
- medication;
- time of day;
- time since last meal, cigarette smoking, caffeine intake, and exercise; and
- psychological environment for the test (i.e., the participant's comfort level with the surroundings during testing).

Attention to these factors increases the likelihood that changes in HR, BP, or RPE from one test to the next actually reflect changes in physical fitness and physical activity habits. A form such as the Pretest Instructions for a Fitness Test (see form 5.1) helps ensure that the client is ready for testing.

Typical procedures to follow during GXTs are shown on page 75, in Steps to Administering a GXT. A series of end points should be used to stop a GXT (see page 75) (1). These guidelines are for nondiagnostic testing performed without direct physician involvement or electrocardiographic monitoring.

Key Point

Equipment for measuring and recording CRF variables should be checked for availability and calibration before testing. Carefully attending to procedures before and during a test enhances the safety and accuracy of the test. The tester should know when to stop a test, given certain signs, symptoms, or CRF measurements.

When to Use Submaximal and Maximal Tests

GXTs have been used to evaluate CRF in fitness programs for healthy populations and in the clinical assessment of ischemic heart disease—a condition in which an inadequate blood flow to the heart muscle can alter the ECG. Exercise is used to place a load on the heart to determine the cardiovascular response and to see if the ECG changes (19).

FORM 5.1 Pretest Instructions for a Fitness Test

Name ______________________ Test date ______________ Time ____________

Report to ______________________

Instruction

Please observe the following:

1. Wear running shoes, shorts, and a loose-fitting shirt.
2. No food, drink (except water), tobacco, or medication for 3 hr before test.
3. Minimal physical activity on day of test.

Cancellation

If you cannot keep this appointment, please call ______________ or ______________.

Steps to Administering a GXT

1. Greet the client.
2. Obtain consent (oral and written).
3. Record age and measure height and weight. Calculate and record estimated HRmax and 70% to 85% HRmax.
4. Obtain resting HR and BP.
5. Instruct participant on how to do a step test.
   - Instruct participant to step all the way up and all the way down.
   - Tell participant to keep pace with the metronome.

   OR

   Instruct participant in how to use the cycle ergometer.
   - Tell participant to adjust seat height so the knee is slightly flexed when the foot is at the bottom of the pedal swing and parallel to the floor.
   - Instruct participant to keep pace with the metronome.
   - Tell participant not to tightly hold on to the handlebars; tell participant to release hold when BP is taken.

   OR

   Instruct participant in how to walk on the treadmill.
   - Have the participant hold on to railing and get the feel of the belt speed by putting one foot on the belt, keeping up with belt speed.
   - Instruct participant to step on, keeping eyes ahead and back straight, and to walk relaxed with arms swinging.
   - Initially, the person can hold on for balance and then touch the railing lightly with just a finger or the back of the hand.
6. Follow test protocol.
   - Advise the person to talk about how he or she feels during the test.
   - Follow criteria for terminating the test.

For fitness evaluations HR, BP, and RPE are the usual variables measured.

Reprinted, by permission, from E.T. Howley, 1988, The exercise testing laboratory. In *Resource manual for guidelines for exercise testing and prescription*, edited by S.N. Blair et al. (Philadelphia, PA: Lea & Febiger), 406-413.

General Indications for Stopping an Exercise Test in Low-Risk Adults*

- Onset of angina or angina-like symptoms
- Drop in systolic blood pressure of >10 mmHg from baseline blood pressure despite an increase in workload
- Excessive rise in blood pressure: systolic pressure > 250 mmHg or diastolic pressure > 115 mmHg
- Shortness of breath, wheezing, leg cramps, or claudication
- Signs of poor perfusion: light-headedness, confusion, ataxia, pallor, cyanosis, nausea, or cold and clammy skin
- Failure of heart rate to increase with increased exercise intensity
- Noticeable change in heart rhythm
- Subject requests to stop
- Physical or verbal manifestations of severe fatigue
- Failure of the testing equipment

*Assumes that testing is nondiagnostic and is being performed without direct physician involvement or ECG monitoring.

Reprinted, by permission, from American College of Sports Medicine (ACSM), 2006, *ACSM's guidelines for exercise testing and prescription*, 7th ed. (Philadelphia, PA: Lippincott, Williams & Wilkins), 78.

Some controversy has arisen concerning whether to use submaximal or maximal GXTs. On the basis of thousands of exercise stress tests conducted since the mid-1950s, a maximal or sign and symptom limited exercise test is generally recommended for finding ischemic heart disease in asymptomatic individuals (1). Although submaximal exercise tests are not as effective in identifying disease, they are appropriate for evaluating CRF before and after exercise programs.

When a fitness center is responsible for both fitness testing and the fitness program, the sequence of testing and activity recommended earlier provides the advantages of each while minimizing their disadvantages. The main objection to using maximal tests is that they stress people who have been inactive. Although the health risk of a maximal GXT is very small with adequate screening and qualified testing personnel, the discomfort of reaching CRF maximum without previous conditioning may discourage some people from participating in a fitness program. Objections to the submaximal test include finding fewer abnormal responses to exercise and inaccurately estimating $\dot{V}O_2max$ from submaximal data. In a fitness program for apparently healthy people, the objections against giving either maximal or submaximal tests are overcome by administering the submaximal test early in the fitness program and the maximal test after the participant has been involved in regular exercise. Any of the GXT protocols can be used for submaximal or maximal testing—the only difference is the criteria for stopping the test. Either test is stopped if any of the abnormal responses listed in the box on page 75 occur. In the absence of abnormal responses, the submaximal test is usually terminated when the person reaches a certain HR (often 85% of maximum HR), and the maximal test is stopped when the person reaches voluntary exhaustion.

Maximal Exercise Test Protocols

No one GXT protocol is appropriate for all people. The durations, starting points, and increments between stages vary with the person. Young active people, normal sedentary people, and people with questionable health status should start at 6, 4, and 2 METs, respectively. The same three groups should increase by 2 to 3, 1 to 2, and 0.5 to 1 METs, respectively, for progressive stages of the test. If the test is for comparing CRF at different times, then 1 or 2 min per stage can be used. If it is for predicting $\dot{V}O_2max$, however, the time per stage should be 2 to 3 min. Table 5.6 illustrates how these criteria might be used for a bench, cycle, or treadmill test administered to different fitness levels.

The following testing protocols are examples of tests used for different populations. The first protocol, shown in table 5.7, could be used with deconditioned subjects, who would start at a very low MET level, walk slowly, and increase 1 MET per 3 min stage (30). The Balke standard protocol (9) could be used for typical inactive adults by having them start at a higher MET level and progress 1 MET per 2 min stage. More active or younger people could be tested on the Bruce protocol (14), which starts at a moderate MET level and goes up 2 or 3 METs per 3 min stage. Unfortunately, some testing centers use the same testing protocol for all people, with the result that the initial stage is often too high or too low and the

Key Point

GXT protocols can be used for submaximal tests (early in the testing sequence) or maximal tests (for active persons who have reached minimal fitness levels). Submaximal and maximal tests can use the same GXT protocol; however, their criteria for test termination differ. Maximal tests are more effective in identifying ischemic heart disease. Submaximal tests are useful in assessing fitness and are relatively inexpensive to administer. Although the $\dot{V}O_2max$ estimated from a submaximal test is not as accurate as that obtained from a maximal test, it is useful in evaluating changes in CRF due to an exercise program.

Research Insight

When introducing each test, we have provided the *SEE* associated with estimating $\dot{V}O_2max$ from that test. If the standard error is 4 $ml \cdot kg^{-1} \cdot min^{-1}$, 68% of the true $\dot{V}O_2max$ values are within 4 $ml \cdot kg^{-1} \cdot min^{-1}$ of the estimated $\dot{V}O_2max$ value, and 95% of the true values are within 8 $ml \cdot kg^{-1} \cdot min^{-1}$ of the estimated value. The problem is that you don't know where an individual is within that 8 $ml \cdot kg^{-1} \cdot min^{-1}$. Consequently, if you estimate that a person's $\dot{V}O_2max$ is 38 $ml \cdot kg^{-1} \cdot min^{-1}$, it is probably between 30 and 46 $ml \cdot kg^{-1} \cdot min^{-1}$. For that reason, fitness professionals must interpret the test results with caution, especially when comparing them with norms. On the other hand, given that endurance training easily alters the HR response to submaximal work, the submaximal tests are good educational and motivational devices to show gradual improvements in CRF.

• Table 5.6 Testing Protocol for Different Groups •

		Bench		Cycle		Treadmill	
Stage	METs	Height (cm)	Steps · min^{-1}	Work rate (kpm · min^{-1})	RPM	Speed (km · min^{-1})	Grade (%)
Individuals with questionable health							
1	2	0	24	0	50	3.2	0
2	3	16	12	150	50	4.8	0
3	4	16	18	300	50	4.8	2.5
4	5	16	24	450	50	4.8	5.0
5	6	16	30	600	50	4.8	7.5
Normal sedentary individuals							
1	4	16	18	360	60	4.8	2.5
2	6	16	30	540	60	4.8	7.5
3	7-8	36	18-24	720-900	60	4.8-5.5	10.0
4	9	36	27	900-1,080	60	5.5	12.0
5	10-11	36	30-33	1,080-1,260	60	9.7	0-1.75
Young active individuals							
1	6	16	30	630	70	4.8	7.5
2	9	36	27	1,060	70	5.5	12.0
3	12	36	36	1,270	70	9.7	3.5
4	15	50	33	1,900	70	11.3	7.0
5	17	50	39	2,110	70	11.3	11.0

MET = metabolic equivalent.

Reprinted, by permission, from B.D. Franks, 1979, Methodology of the exercise ECG test. In *Exercise electrocardiography: Practical approach*, edited by E.K. Chung (Baltimore, MD: Lippincott, Williams & Wilkins), 46-61.

work increments for each stage too small or too large for the individual being tested. Estimating $\dot{V}O_2max$ from the final stage of a maximal GXT has a *SEE* of about 3 ml · kg^{-1} · min^{-1} (32).

Submaximal Exercise Test Protocols

Any GXT protocol can be used for submaximal or maximal testing. The fitness professional typically uses a submaximal GXT to estimate $\dot{V}O_2max$ or to simply show how the exercise program changes selected variables. Predicting maximal oxygen uptake from any submaximal test involves substantial error (see Research Insight on page 76). However, it can provide useful information for estimating a person's functional capacity and for determining the person's fitness category and what exercise programming therefore is most appropriate. The only way to determine an individual's true functional capacity is to measure it during a maximal test. However, submaximal tests are very reliable, and changes in HR, BP, and RPE resulting from exercise conditioning make a submaximal test a good mechanism for showing improvements in CRF. Estimating $\dot{V}O_2max$ from submaximal exercise test protocols has a *SEE* of about 5 ml · kg^{-1} · min^{-1} (32).

Submaximal Treadmill Test Protocol

The initial stage and rate of progression of the GXT should be selected using the criteria mentioned earlier. In the following example, a Balke standard protocol (3 mi · hr^{-1}, or 4.8 km · hr^{-1}, 2.5% grade increase every 2 min) was used; HR was monitored in the last 30 sec of each stage. The test was terminated at 85% of the age-adjusted maximal HR (with the equation 220 – age). Maximal aerobic power was estimated by extrapolating the HR response to the person's estimated maximal HR. Figure 5.3 presents the results of this test with a graph showing the HR response at each work rate. The HR response is rather flat between the 0% and 5% grades. This is not uncommon (see the discussion that follows the YMCA test); perhaps the subject is too excited, or perhaps the stroke volume changes are accounting for the changes in cardiac output at these

• Table 5.7 Treadmill Protocols for Various Categories •

Stage	METs	Speed (km · hr⁻¹)	Grade (%)	Time (min)
Deconditioned individuals[a]				
1	2.5	3.2	0	3
2	3.5	3.2	3.5	3
3	4.5	3.2	7	3
4	5.4	3.2	10.5	3
5	6.4	3.2	14	3
6	7.3	3.2	17.5	3
7	8.5	4.8	12.5	3
8	9.5	4.8	15	3
9	10.5	4.8	17.5	3
Normal inactive individuals[b]				
1	4.3	4.8	2.5	2
2	5.4	4.8	5	2
3	6.4	4.8	7.5	2
4	7.4	4.8	10	2
5	8.5	4.8	12.5	2
6	9.5	4.8	15	2
7	10.5	4.8	17.5	2
8	11.6	4.8	20	2
9	12.6	4.8	22.5	2
10	13.6	4.8	25	2
Young active individuals[c]				
1	5	2.7	10	3
2	7	4	12	3
3	9.5	5.4	14	3
4	13	6.7	16	3
5	16	8	18	3

MET = metabolic equivalent.

[a]From J.P. Naughton and R. Haider, 1973, Methods of exercise testing. In *Exercise testing and exercise training in coronary heart disease*, edited by J.P. Naughton, H.R. Hellerstein and L.C. Mohler (New York, NY: Academic Press).

[b]From B. Balke, 1970, "Advanced Exercise Procedures for Evaluation of the Cardiovascular System," *Monograph* (Milton, WI: Burdick Corporation).

[c]From R.A. Bruce, 1972, Multi-stage treadmill test of maximal and submaximal exercise. In *Exercise testing and training of apparently healthy individuals: A handbook for physicians*, American Heart Association (New York, NY: American Heart Association), 32-34.

low work rates. The HR response is usually quite linear between 110 beats · min^{-1} and the subject's 85% HRmax.

To estimate $\dot{V}O_2$max, the procedures of Maritz and colleagues (26) are followed. A line is drawn through the HR points from the 7.5% grade to the final work rate. This line is extended (extrapolated) to the person's estimated maximal HR (183 beats · min^{-1}). A vertical line is dropped from the last point to the baseline to estimate the subject's maximal aerobic power, which in this example is 11.8 METs, or 41.3 ml · kg $^{-1}$ · min $^{-1}$. Any formula used to estimate maximal HR has a *SEE* of about 10 beats · min^{-1}. Consequently, this possible inaccuracy influences any estimate of maximal oxygen uptake derived from extrapolating HR to an estimated maximal HR. If this person's true (measured) maximal HR is 173 or 193 beats · min^{-1}, the estimated maximal MET level is 11.0 METs or 12.6 METs, respectively.

Submaximal Cycle Ergometer Test Protocol

The steps in administering submaximal cycle ergometer tests are provided on page 80. One of the most common submaximal cycle ergometer protocols (figure 5.4) comes from the *YMCA Fitness Testing and Assessment Manual* (22). This protocol relies on the linear relationship between HR and work rate ($\dot{V}O_2$) that occurs once an HR of approximately 110 beats · min^{-1} is reached. The test requires the person to complete one more stage beyond the one that induces an HR of 110 beats · min^{-1}. The line describing the HR–work rate relationship is extrapolated out to the person's age-adjusted maximal HR (as was done for the treadmill protocol) to estimate the person's $\dot{V}O_2$max. Each stage of the test lasts 3 min, unless a person's HR has not yet reached a steady state (there is >5 beats · min $^{-1}$ difference between 2nd and 3rd min HR). In that case, an extra minute is added to that stage. The pedal rate is maintained at 50 rev · min^{-1} so that, on a Monark cycle ergometer, a 0.5 kg increase in load equals 150 kgm · min^{-1} (25 W). Seat height is adjusted so that the knee is slightly bent (6) when the pedal is at the bottom of the swing through 1 revolution. The seat height is recorded for future reference. HR is monitored during the later half of the 2nd and 3rd min of each stage.

Selection of the initial work rate and the rate of progression on the cycle ergometer should consider body weight, sex, age, and level of fitness. In general, absolute $\dot{V}O_2$max (L · min^{-1}) is lower in smaller people, women have lower absolute $\dot{V}O_2$max values than men have, $\dot{V}O_2$max decreases with age, and inactivity is associated with low $\dot{V}O_2$max. The YMCA test addresses body weight, fitness, and so on by starting everyone at 150 kgm · min^{-1} and using the HR response to that specified work rate to set subsequent stages in the test (see figure 5.4). Large or fit individuals would have a low HR response to this work rate and would use the most strenuous sequence of work rates (far left boxes in the figure). A small or unfit individual would have a high HR response to the 150 kgm · min $^{-1}$ work rate and would follow the sequence with the smallest increments in the power output. People being tested should complete only one additional work rate beyond the one demanding an HR of 110 beats · min^{-1}.

The HR values for the 2nd and 3rd min of each work rate are recorded, and directions are followed to estimate

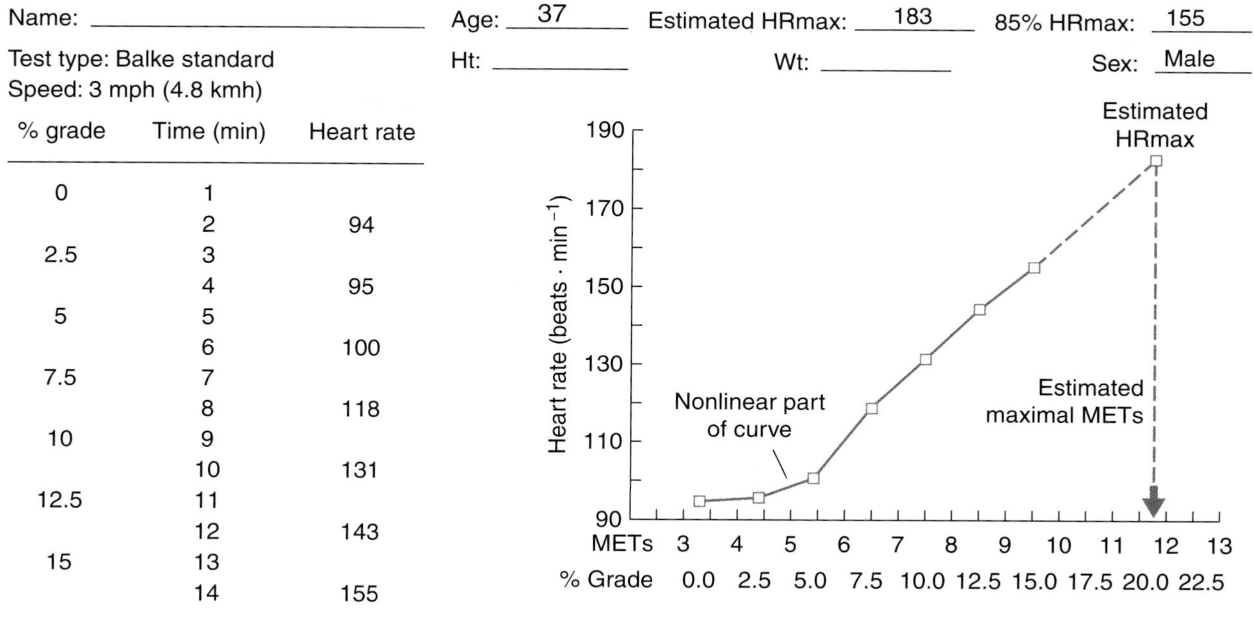

Figure 5.3 Maximal aerobic power estimated by measuring the HR response to a submaximal GXT on a treadmill.

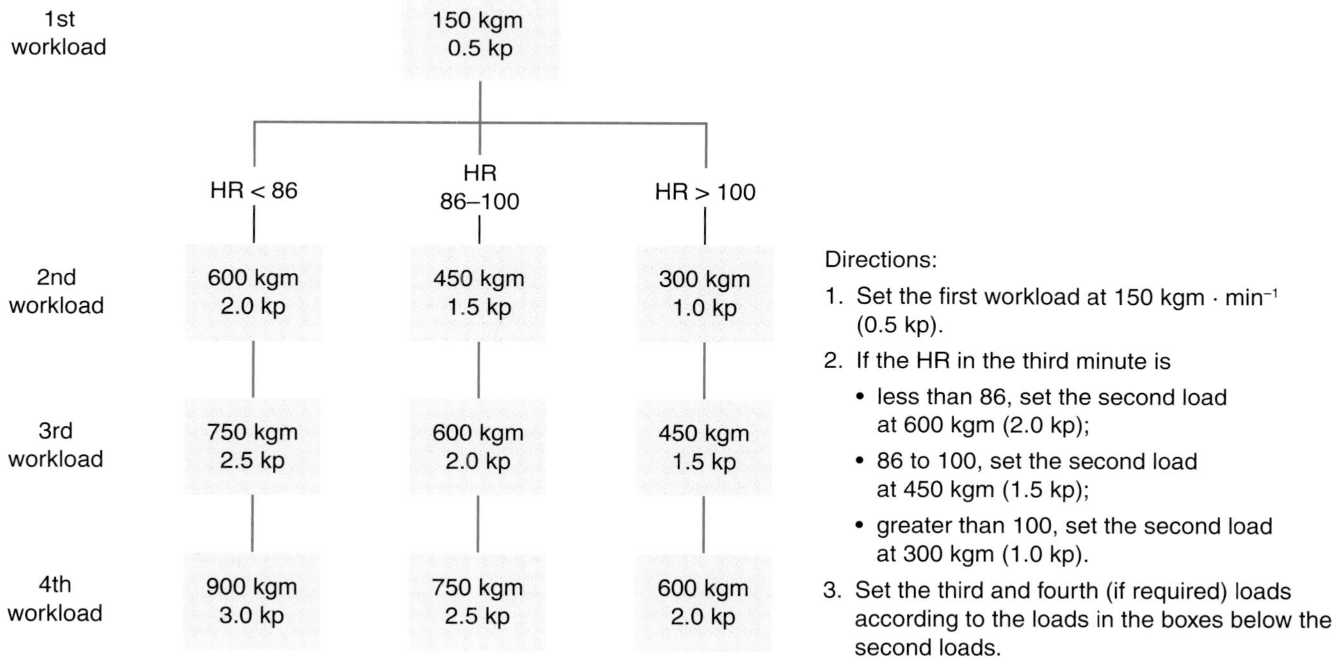

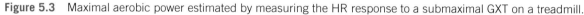

Figure 5.4 Guide for setting power outputs (workloads) on YMCA submaximal cycle ergometer test.
Reprinted from *YMCA fitness testing and assessment manual* with permission of the YMCA of the USA, 101 N. Wacker Drive, Chicago, IL 60606.

$\dot{V}O_2$max in liters per minute. Figure 5.5 presents the YMCA protocol directions and an example test for a 50-yr-old woman who weighs 59 kg. The stages followed the pattern dictated by the HR response to the initial work rate of 150 kgm · min^{-1}. A line was drawn through the last two HR values and extrapolated to the estimated maximal HR. A vertical line, dropped from the last point of the extrapolated line to the baseline, estimated the subject's maximal work rate to be 750 kgm · min^{-1}. With the formula described earlier (and in chapter 4) for the cycle

Steps to Administering a Submaximal Cycle Ergometer Test

1. Complete pretest items.
2. Select the test protocol.
3. Estimate the participant's HRmax (220 – age = HRmax in beats · min^{-1}).
4. Determine 85% of participant's HRmax (HRmax · 0.85 = 85% HRmax).
5. Review the procedure with participant.
6. Set and record the seat height (leg should be slightly bent at the knee when foot is at the bottom of the pedaling stroke).
7. Start the metronome (set at 100 beats · min^{-1} so that one foot is at the bottom of the pedaling stroke on each beat, resulting in 50 complete rev · min^{-1}).
8. Have the participant begin pedaling in rhythm with the metronome.
9. As soon as the correct pace is achieved, set the resistance according to the protocol chosen.
10. Start the timer for the beginning of the 3 min stage.
11. Check the resistance setting (it may drift) and observe the participant for signs or symptoms that require terminating the test.
12. At 1:30 into the stage, measure and record BP and HR.
13. At 2:30, measure and record HR.
14. At 2:50, ask for and record the participant's RPE.
15. At 2:55, ask the participant, "How are you doing?"
16. At 3:00, if HR is less than 85% of HRmax, BP is responding normally, and participant is all right, increase resistance to the next stage. If the two HR values (from minutes 2 and 3) are not within 5 beats · min^{-1}, the YMCA protocol calls for adding another minute to the stage to obtain a steady-state value.
17. Repeat steps 10 through 16 until the participant reaches 85% of HRmax or there is another reason to stop the test. Go back to stage 1 (for cool-down) and repeat steps 10 through 15, stopping at 3:00 in the cool-down stage.
18. Talk with the participant and check out any problems.

Reprinted from B.D. Franks and E.T. Howley, 1989, *Fitness leader's handbook* (Champaign, IL: Human Kinetics), 87.

ergometer, $\dot{V}O_2max$ for this woman was estimated to be ~30 ml · kg^{-1} · min^{-1}, or about 1.77 L · min^{-1}.

In contrast to the YMCA test, the Åstrand and Rhyming cycle ergometer test (6) requires the subject to complete only one 6 min work rate demanding an HR between 125 and 170 beats · min^{-1}. These investigators observed that for young (18-30 yr) subjects, the average HR was 128 beats · min^{-1} for males and 138 beats · min^{-1} for females at 50% $\dot{V}O_2max$, while at 70% $\dot{V}O_2max$ the average HRs were 154 and 164 beats · min^{-1}, respectively. So if you know from an HR response that a person is at 50% $\dot{V}O_2max$ at a work rate equal to 1.5 L · min^{-1}, then you know the estimated $\dot{V}O_2max$ is twice that, or 3.0 L · min^{-1}. Table 5.8 is used to estimate $\dot{V}O_2max$ from the subject's HR response to one 6 min work rate (4).

Using the data from the example of the woman taking the YMCA test (discussed earlier), we can see how $\dot{V}O_2max$ is estimated in the Åstrand and Rhyming protocol. The 50-yr-old woman had an HR of 140 beats · min^{-1} at a work rate of 450 kgm · min^{-1}. Using table 5.8, for women, look down the leftmost column to an HR of 140, and look across to the second column of values (for a work rate of 450 kgm · min^{-1}).

The estimated $\dot{V}O_2max$ is 2.4 L · min^{-1}. Because maximal HR decreases with increasing age, however, and the data in table 5.8 were collected on young subjects, I. and P.O. Åstrand (3, 4) established the following age correction factors to correct for the lower maximal HR:

Age	Factor	Age	Factor	Age	Factor
15	1.10	40	0.83	55	0.71
25	1.00	45	0.78	60	0.68
35	0.87	50	0.75	65	0.65

To calculate the corrected $\dot{V}O_2max$, the estimated $\dot{V}O_2max$ is multiplied by the appropriate correction factor. For our 50-yr-old subject, the correction factor is 0.75, and the corrected $\dot{V}O_2max$ is 0.75 · 2.4 L · min^{-1} = 1.8 L · min^{-1}. This value compares well with that estimated by the

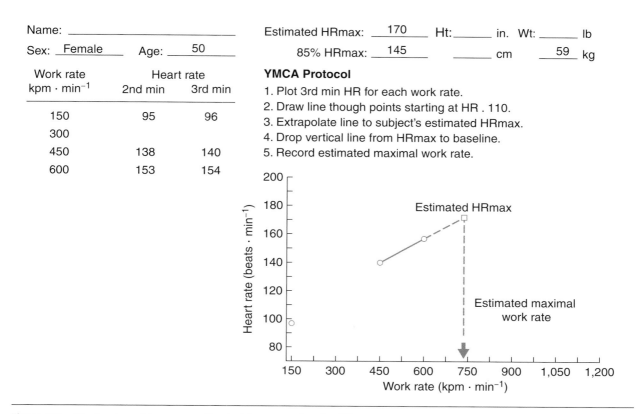

Name: ____________________ Estimated HRmax: 170 Ht: ______ in. Wt: ______ lb

Sex: Female Age: 50 85% HRmax: 145 ______ cm 59 kg

Work rate kpm · min^{-1}	Heart rate 2nd min	Heart rate 3rd min
150	95	96
300		
450	138	140
600	153	154

YMCA Protocol

1. Plot 3rd min HR for each work rate.
2. Draw line though points starting at HR . 110.
3. Extrapolate line to subject's estimated HRmax.
4. Drop vertical line from HRmax to baseline.
5. Record estimated maximal work rate.

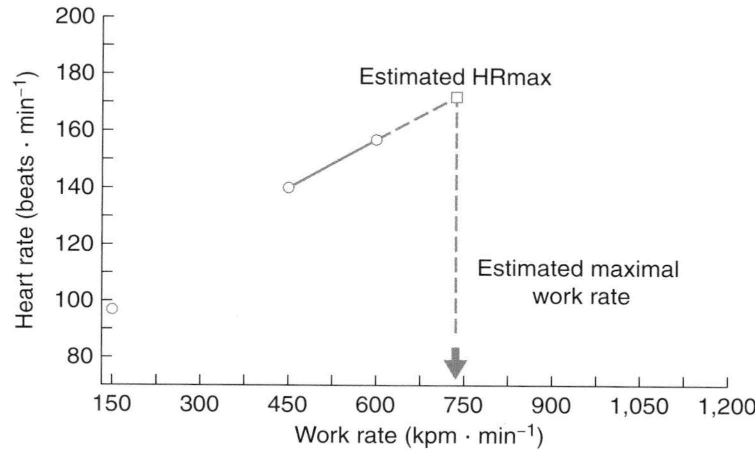

Figure 5.5 Maximal aerobic power estimated by measuring the HR response to a submaximal GXT on a cycle ergometer, using the protocol from the *YMCA Fitness Testing and Assessment Manual*

YMCA protocol. The Åstrand and Rhyming calculations can be simplified by using formulas developed by Shephard (34).

Submaximal Step Test Protocol

A multistage step test can be used to estimate $\dot{V}O_2$max and to show changes in CRF resulting from training or detraining. As always, the initial stage and rate of progression of the stages must be suited to the individual. Table 5.6 presented three examples of step test protocols (page 77). The subject must follow the metronome (4 counts per cycle, i.e., up-up-down-down) and step all the way up and all the way down. Each stage should last at least 2 min, with HR monitored in the last 30 sec of each 2 min.

HR is more difficult to monitor during a step test if the palpation technique is used. The HR watch simplifies the process, but when one is not available, a BP cuff can be used. When an HR measure is needed, pump the cuff up just above diastolic pressure (around 80-100 mmHg). With the stethoscope, count the pulse rate for 15 to 30 sec. Release the pressure after each measurement. An alternative is for the participant to stop stepping after each stage, taking the HR for a 10 sec count 5 sec after completing the stage.

As in most submaximal GXT protocols, HR is plotted against work rate or $\dot{V}O_2$ for each stage, and a line is drawn through the points to the estimated maximal HR. A vertical line is then drawn to the baseline to estimate the step rate that would have been achieved if the subject had completed a maximal test. Figure 5.6 shows the results of a step test for a sedentary 55-yr-old man. His estimated maximal step rate was 40 steps · min^{-1}. The $\dot{V}O_2$max, calculated with the formula for stepping given in chapter 4, was 7.7 METs, or about 27 ml · kg^{-1} · min^{-1}.

Posttest Procedures

When the test is over, the tester should conduct a cooldown, monitor test variables, and give posttest instructions. The tester should also organize the test data (see Posttest Protocol on page 83).

• Table 5.8 Predicting Maximal Oxygen Uptake From Heart Rate and Workload During a 6 Min Cycle Ergometer Test •

	Values for women for $\dot{V}O_2max$ ($L \cdot min^{-1}$)						Values for men for $\dot{V}O_2max$ ($L \cdot min^{-1}$)				
Heart rate	300 kgm · min⁻¹	450 kgm · min⁻¹	600 kgm · min⁻¹	750 kgm · min⁻¹	900 kgm · min⁻¹	Heart rate	300 kgm · min⁻¹	600 kgm · min⁻¹	900 kgm · min⁻¹	1,200 kgm · min⁻¹	1,500 kgm · min⁻¹
120	2.6	3.4	4.1	4.8		120	2.2	3.5	4.8		
121	2.5	3.3	4.0	4.8		121	2.2	3.4	4.7		
122	2.5	3.2	3.9	4.7		122	2.2	3.4	4.6		
123	2.4	3.1	3.9	4.6		123	2.1	3.4	4.6		
124	2.4	3.1	3.8	4.5		124	2.1	3.3	4.5	6.0	
125	2.3	3.0	3.7	4.4		125	2.0	3.2	4.4	5.9	
126	2.3	3.0	3.6	4.3		126	2.0	3.2	4.4	5.8	
127	2.2	2.9	3.5	4.2		127	2.0	3.1	4.3	5.7	
128	2.2	2.8	3.5	4.2	4.8	128	2.0	3.1	4.2	5.6	
129	2.2	2.8	3.4	4.1	4.8	129	1.9	3.0	4.2	5.6	
130	2.1	2.7	3.4	4.0	4.7	130	1.9	3.0	4.1	5.5	
131	2.1	2.7	3.4	4.0	4.6	131	1.9	2.9	4.0	5.4	
132	2.0	2.7	3.3	3.9	4.5	132	1.8	2.9	4.0	5.3	
133	2.0	2.6	3.2	3.8	4.4	133	1.8	2.8	3.9	5.3	
134	2.0	2.6	3.2	3.8	4.4	134	1.8	2.8	3.9	5.2	
135	2.0	2.6	3.1	3.7	4.3	135	1.7	2.8	3.8	5.1	
136	1.9	2.5	3.1	3.6	4.2	136	1.7	2.7	3.8	5.0	
137	1.9	2.5	3.0	3.6	4.2	137	1.7	2.7	3.7	5.0	
138	1.8	2.4	3.0	3.5	4.1	138	1.6	2.7	3.7	4.9	
139	1.8	2.4	2.9	3.5	4.0	139	1.6	2.6	3.6	4.8	
140	1.8	2.4	2.8	3.4	4.0	140	1.6	2.6	3.6	4.8	6.0
141	1.8	2.3	2.8	3.4	3.9	141		2.6	3.5	4.7	5.9
142	1.7	2.3	2.8	3.3	3.9	142		2.5	3.5	4.6	5.8
143	1.7	2.2	2.7	3.3	3.8	143		2.5	3.4	4.6	5.7
144	1.7	2.2	2.7	3.2	3.8	144		2.5	3.4	4.5	5.7
145	1.6	2.2	2.7	3.2	3.7	145		2.4	3.4	4.5	5.6
146	1.6	2.2	2.6	3.2	3.7	146		2.4	3.3	4.4	5.6
147	1.6	2.1	2.6	3.1	3.6	147		2.4	3.3	4.4	5.5
148	1.6	2.1	2.6	3.1	3.6	148		2.4	3.2	4.3	5.4
149		2.1	2.6	3.0	3.5	149		2.3	3.2	4.3	5.4
150		2.0	2.5	3.0	3.5	150		2.3	3.2	4.2	5.3
151		2.0	2.5	3.0	3.4	151		2.3	3.1	4.2	5.2
152		2.0	2.5	2.9	3.4	152		2.3	3.1	4.1	5.2
153		2.0	2.4	2.9	3.3	153		2.2	3.0	4.1	5.1
154		2.0	2.4	2.8	3.3	154		2.2	3.0	4.0	5.1
155		1.9	2.4	2.8	3.2	155		2.2	3.0	4.0	5.0
156		1.9	2.3	2.8	3.2	156		2.2	2.9	4.0	5.0
157		1.9	2.3	2.7	3.2	157		2.1	2.9	3.9	4.9
158		1.8	2.3	2.7	3.1	158		2.1	2.9	3.9	4.9
159		1.8	2.2	2.7	3.1	159		2.1	2.8	3.8	4.8
160		1.8	2.2	2.6	3.0	160		2.1	2.8	3.8	4.8
161		1.8	2.2	2.6	3.0	161		2.0	2.8	3.7	4.7
162		1.8	2.2	2.6	3.0	162		2.0	2.8	3.7	4.6
163		1.7	2.2	2.6	2.9	163		2.0	2.8	3.7	4.6
164		1.7	2.1	2.5	2.9	164		2.0	2.7	3.6	4.5
165		1.7	2.1	2.5	2.9	165		2.0	2.7	3.6	4.5
166		1.7	2.1	2.5	2.8	166		1.9	2.7	3.6	4.5
167		1.6	2.1	2.4	2.8	167		1.9	2.6	3.5	4.4
168		1.6	2.0	2.4	2.8	168		1.9	2.6	3.5	4.4
169		1.6	2.0	2.4	2.8	169		1.9	2.6	3.5	4.3
170		1.6	2.0	2.4	2.7	170		1.8	2.6	3.4	4.3

Reprinted, by permission, from P.-O. Astrand, 1979, *Work tests with the bicycle ergometer* (Varberg, Sweden: Monark Exercise AB), 24.

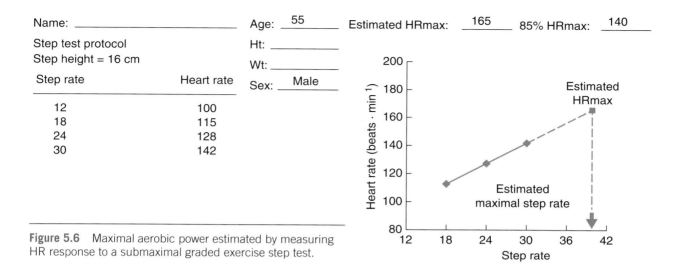

Name: ______ Age: 55 Estimated HRmax: 165 85% HRmax: 140

Step test protocol

Step height = 16 cm

Ht: ______

Wt: ______

Sex: Male

Step rate	Heart rate
12	100
18	115
24	128
30	142

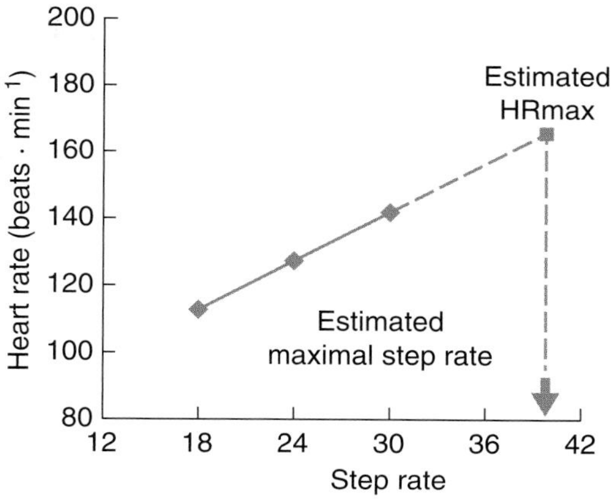

Heart rate (beats · min^{-1})

200

180

160

140

120

100

80

Estimated HRmax

Estimated maximal step rate

12 18 24 30 36 42

Step rate

Figure 5.6 Maximal aerobic power estimated by measuring HR response to a submaximal graded exercise step test.

Key Point

A plot of HR responses (>110 beats · min^{-1}) to a GXT on a treadmill, cycle ergometer, or bench step can be used to estimate $\dot{V}O_2max$. A line is drawn through the HR values and is extrapolated to the subject's age-adjusted estimate of maximal HR. A vertical line is drawn to the x-axis to estimate the work rate and $\dot{V}O_2$ the person would have achieved if the test had been a maximal test.

Posttest Protocol

1. Use a cool-down as programmed per physician or other guidelines:
   - Have the individual sit down or lie down depending on posttest (nuclear).
   - Monitor HR, BP, and ECG immediately and after 1, 2, 4, and 6 min.
   - Remove cuff and electrodes when double product (HR · SBP) is close to pretest value.
2. Provide instructions for showering:
   - Ask subject to wait about 30 min before showering.
   - Ask subject to move around in the shower and use warm (not hot) water. Check for return of person from the shower.
3. Organize test data and discuss test results with the participant.

Adapted, by permission, from E.T. Howley, 1988, The exercise testing laboratory. In *Resource manual for guidelines for exercise testing and prescription*, edited by S.N. Blair et al. (Philadelphia, PA: Lea & Febiger), 413.

Case Studies

You can check your answers by referring to page 470 in appendix A.

1. You are contacted by a fitness club to review the test it uses to evaluate CRF in middle-aged participants. The club requires the participants to perform the 1.5 mi (2.4 km) run test during their first exercise session. The club director says he uses this test because so many data exist for it—the test has been used for more than 10 yr. What is your reaction?
2. You conduct the 1 mi walk test with a 45-yr-old male client and record the following information: time = 15 min, HR = 140 beats · min $^{-1}$, weight = 170 lb (77.1 kg).

   Calculate and evaluate his estimated $\dot{V}O_2max$.
3. A 50-yr-old male, weighing 180 lb (81.7 kg), completes a submaximal GXT on a cycle ergometer, and the following data are obtained:

kgm · min^{-1}	HR	kgm · min^{-1}	HR
300	100	600	125
450	110	750	140

   Estimate the subject's $\dot{V}O_2max$ by the extrapolation procedure. Express the value in METs.
4. A 30-yr-old woman, weighing 120 lb (54.4 kg), completes four stages of a submaximal Balke treadmill test at 3 mi · hr^{-1} (4.8 km · hr^{-1}), and the following data are obtained:

% Grade	HR	% Grade	HR
2.5	96	7.5	135
5	120	10	150

   Estimate the subject's $\dot{V}O_2max$ by the extrapolation method and express it in ml · kg^{-1} · min^{-1}, L · min^{-1}, and METs.
5. A Monark cycle ergometer is calibrated with 0.5, 1.0, 1.5, and 2.0 kg weights, and each of the values is 0.25 kg too high on the scale. What could have caused this?

Calibrating Equipment

To calibrate is to check the accuracy of a measuring device by comparing it with a known standard and adjusting the device so that it provides an accurate reading. This section explains how to calibrate equipment used in exercise testing. These are suggestions only and should not be viewed as a substitute for the specific procedures recommended by the equipment manufacturers (24).

Treadmill Speed and Elevation Settings

The speed and grade settings on the treadmill must be calibrated because they determine physiological demand and are crucial in estimating cardiorespiratory fitness.

Calibrating Speed

An easy way to calibrate the speed on any treadmill is to measure the length of the belt and count the number of belt revolutions in a certain amount of time. To calibrate treadmill speed, follow these specific steps (24):

1. Measure the exact length of the belt in meters.

   a. Place a meterstick on the belt surface and mark a starting point.

   b. Advance the belt by hand, marking the belt 1 m at a time until you return to the starting point; record the value for belt length.
2. Place a small piece of tape near the edge of the belt surface.
3. Turn on the treadmill to a given speed by using the speed control.
4. Count 20 revolutions of the belt while tracking time with a stopwatch. Start your watch as the tape first moves past the fixed point, beginning counting with 0.
5. Convert the number of revolutions to revolutions per minute ($rev \cdot min^{-1}$). For example, if the belt made 20 complete revolutions in 35 sec, then

   $$35 \text{ sec} \div 60 \text{ sec} \cdot \text{min}^{-1} = 0.583 \text{ min.}$$

   So,

   $$20 \text{ rev} \div 0.583 \text{ min} = 34.3 \text{ rev} \cdot \text{min}^{-1}.$$
6. Multiply the calculated revolutions per minute (step 5) times the belt length (step 1). This gives the belt speed in meters per minute ($m \cdot min^{-1}$). For example, if the belt length is 5.025 m, then

   $$34.3 \text{ rev} \cdot \text{min}^{-1} \cdot 5.025 \text{ m} \cdot \text{rev}^{-1} = 172.35 \text{ m} \cdot \text{min}^{-1}.$$
7. To convert meters per minute to miles per hour, divide the answer in step 6 by 26.8 $(m \cdot min^{-1}) \cdot (mi \cdot hr^{-1})^{-1}$:

   $$\frac{172.35 \text{ m} \cdot \text{min}^{-1}}{26.8\ ([\text{m} \cdot \text{min}^{-1}] \cdot [\text{mi} \cdot \text{hr}^{-1}]^{-1})} = 6.43 \text{ mi} \cdot \text{hr}^{-1}$$
8. The value obtained in step 7 is the actual treadmill speed in miles per hour. If the speed indicator does not agree with this value, adjust the dial to the proper reading. Check the instruction manual for the location of the speed adjustment.
9. Repeat for a number of different speeds to ensure accuracy across the speeds used in test protocols.

Calibrating Elevation

Treadmill manuals describe how to calibrate the grade by using a simple carpenter's level and a square edge. This calibration procedure consists of three steps:

1. Use a carpenter's level to make sure that the treadmill is level, and check the zero setting on the grade meter under these conditions (with the treadmill electronics turned on). If the meter does not read zero, follow instructions to make the adjustment (usually by using the small screw on the face of the dial).
2. Elevate the treadmill so that the percentage grade dial reads approximately 20%. Measure the exact incline of the treadmill as shown in figure 5.7. When the level's bubble is exactly in the center of the tube, the rise measurement is obtained.
3. Calculate the grade from the rise over the run and adjust the treadmill meter to read that exact grade. For example, if the rise is 4.5 in. (11.4 cm) to the run's 22.5 in. (57.2 cm), the fractional grade is calculated as follows:

   $$\text{Grade} = \text{tangent } \mu = \text{rise} \div \text{run} = 4.5 \text{ in.} \div 22.5 \text{ in.} = 0.20 = 20\%$$

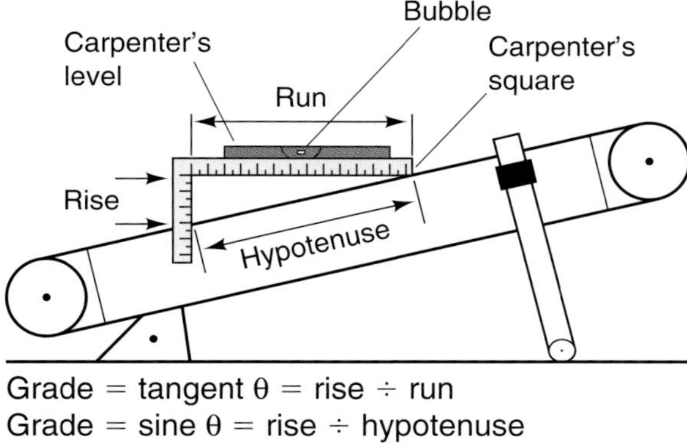

Figure 5.7 Calibrating grade by the tangent method (rise ÷ run) with a carpenter's square and level.

Reprinted, by permission, from E.T. Howley, 1988, The exercise testing laboratory. In *Resource manual for guidelines for exercise testing and prescription*, edited by S.N. Blair et al. (Philadelphia, PA: Lea & Febiger), 409.

4. The rise-over-run method is a typical engineering method for calculating grade, giving the tangent of the angle (the opposite side divided by the adjacent side of the right triangle, as shown in figure 5.7). Although the sine of the angle (opposite side divided by the hypotenuse) provides the most accurate setting of grade, table 5.9 shows that the tangent value is a good approximation of the sine value for grades less than 20%, or 12°. The rise-over-run method can also be used to calibrate steep grades: Obtain the tangent value as described previously and simply look across table 5.9 to obtain the correct sine value to set on the treadmill dial. For example, if the rise-over-run method yielded 0.268, or 26.8% (tangent), the correct setting would be 25.9% (sine). The latter value is set on the grade dial of the treadmill.

Key Point

Calibrating the treadmill includes checking both the speed and the elevation.

Calibrating the Cycle Ergometer

The cycle ergometer must be calibrated routinely to ensure that the work rate is accurate. Altering either the pedal rate or the load on the wheel varies the work rate on the mechanically braked cycle ergometer. Work equals force times the distance through which the force acts: $w = f \cdot d$. The kilopond (kp), defined as the force acting on a mass of 1 kg at the normal acceleration of gravity, is the proper unit for force. However, the kilopond and the kilogram typically are used interchangeably in exercise testing.

Table 5.9 Natural Sines and Tangents

Degrees	Sine	Grade (%)	Tangent	Grade (%)
0	0.0000	0.0	0.0000	0.0
1	0.0175	1.7	0.075	1.7
2	0.0349	3.5	0.0349	3.5
3	0.0523	5.2	0.0524	5.2
4	0.0698	7.0	0.0699	7.0
5	0.0872	8.7	0.0875	8.7
6	0.1045	10.4	0.1051	10.5
7	0.1219	12.2	0.1228	12.3
8	0.1392	13.9	0.1405	14.0
9	0.1564	15.6	0.1584	15.8
10	0.1736	17.4	0.1763	17.6
11	0.1908	19.1	0.1944	19.4
12	0.2079	20.8	0.2126	21.3
13	0.2250	22.5	0.2309	23.1
14	0.2419	24.2	0.2493	24.9
15	0.2588	25.9	0.2679	26.8
20	0.3420	34.2	0.3640	36.4
25	0.4067	40.7	0.4452	44.5

Reprinted, by permission, from E.T. Howley, 1988, The exercise testing laboratory. In *Resource manual for guidelines for exercise testing and prescription*, edited by S.N. Blair et al. (Philadelphia, PA: Lea & Febiger), 409.

On a mechanically braked cycle ergometer, the force (kilograms of weight on the wheel) is moved through a distance (in meters), so work is expressed in kilogram-meters (kgm). Because work is accomplished over time (e.g., minutes), the activity is referred to as a *work rate* or *power output* (kgm · min $^{-1}$), not a *workload.* On the Monark cycle ergometer, a point on the rim of the wheel travels 6 m per pedal revolution, so at 50 rev · min $^{-1}$, the wheel travels 300 m · min $^{-1}$. If a weight of 1 kg is hanging from that wheel, the work rate, or power output, is 300 kgm · min^{-1}. From these simple calculations you can see the importance of maintaining a correct pedal rate during the test—if the subject pedals at 60 rev · min^{-1}, the work rate is actually 20% higher (360 versus 300 kgm · min^{-1}) than it appears to be. The force setting (resistance on the wheel) also must be carefully set and checked because it tends to drift as the test progresses. It is crucial that the force (resistance) values on the scale are correct. The following four steps outline the procedure for calibrating the Monark cycle ergometer scale (4) (refer to figure 5.8):

1. Disconnect the belt at the spring.
2. Loosen the lock nut and use the adjusting screw on the front of the bike against which the force scale

rests so that the vertical mark on the pendulum weight matches with 0 kp on the weight scale (see figure 5.8*a*). The pendulum must be swinging freely. Lock the adjustment screw with the lock nut. To keep the calibration weights from touching the flywheel, it may be easier to elevate rear of the ergometer (with a 2 × 4 on edge), set the zero as described previously, and proceed to the next step.

3. Suspend a 4.0 kg weight from the spring so that it's not in contact with the flywheel, and see if the pendulum moves to the 4.0 kp mark (see figure 5.8*b*). If it doesn't, alter the position or size of the adjusting weight in the pendulum (see figure 5.8*c*). By loosening the lock screw on the back of the pendulum weight, the adjusting weight can be lowered, raised, or replaced. Check the force scale again and calibrate the ergometer through the range of values used in your tests. If you used the 2 × 4 to elevate the rear of the ergometer, remove it and reset the zero as described in step 2.
4. Reassemble the cycle ergometer.

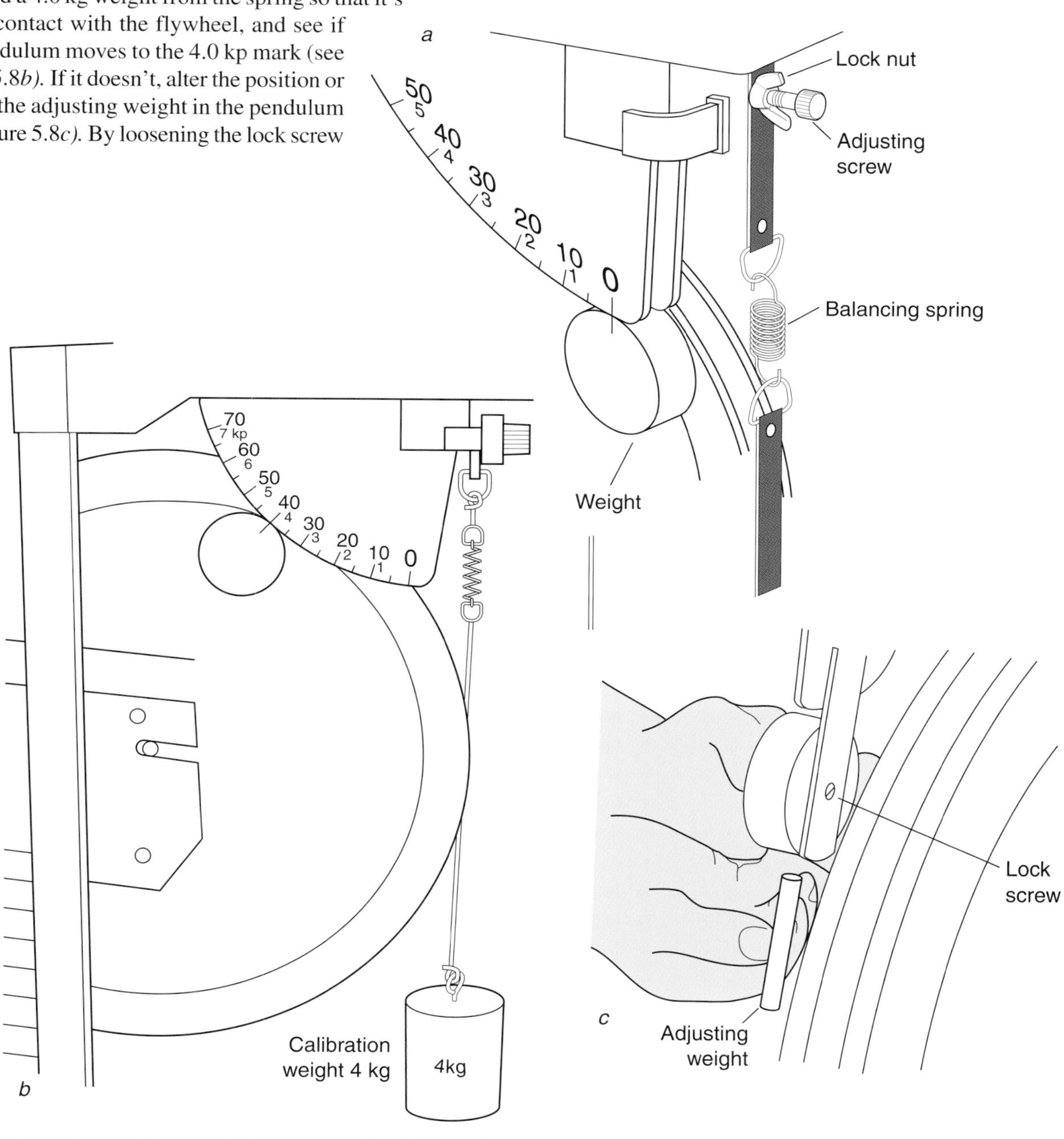

Figure 5.8 Calibrating the Monark cycle ergometer. *(a)* Adjust the pendulum to align with 0, *(b)* suspend a 4.0 kg weight from the spring, and *(c)* adjust the position or size of the weight in the pendulum.

Adapted, by permission, from Monark Sports and Medical, *Instruction manual, Monark model 818E* (Varberg, Sweden: Monark Exercise AB), 18.

Key Point

Calibrating the cycle ergometer involves establishing a true zero, hanging standard weights from the spring, and verifying that they line up with the readings on the scale.

Calibrating the Sphygmomanometer

A **sphygmomanometer** is a BP measurement system composed of an inflatable rubber bladder, an instrument that indicates the applied pressure, an inflation bulb that creates pressure, and an adjustable valve that deflates the system. The cuff and the measuring instrument are the most crucial for measurement accuracy. The cuff should be about 20% wider than the diameter of the limb to which it is applied, and when inflated, the bladder should not cause a bulging or displacement. If the bladder is too wide, blood pressure will be underestimated; if it is too narrow, pressure will be overestimated. Consequently, it is important to match cuff size to the subject being measured.

The device measuring the pressure, the manometer, can be a mercury or an aneroid type. The mercury type is the standard, and its calibration is easily maintained. The mercury column should rise and fall smoothly, form a clear meniscus, and read zero when the bladder is deflated. If the mercury sticks in the tube, remove the cap and swab out the inside. If it is very dirty, the tube should be removed and cleaned (with detergent, a water rinse, and alcohol for drying). If the mercury column falls below zero, add mercury to bring the meniscus exactly to the zero mark (10, 21, 24). Special care must be taken when handling toxic materials such as mercury; follow your institution's guidelines.

The aneroid gauge uses a metal bellows assembly that expands when pressure is applied, and the expansion moves the pointer on the indicator dial. A spring attached to the pointer moves the pointer downscale to zero when the bladder is deflated. This gauge should be calibrated at least once every 6 mo in a variety of settings, by using the mercury column just described. A simple Y tube (from the stethoscope) is used to connect the two systems (see figure 5.9). Readings should be taken with pressure falling to simulate the readings taken during an actual measurement (24).

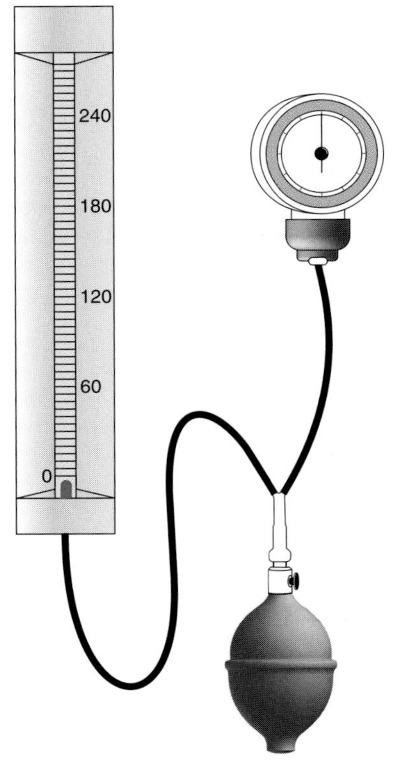

Figure 5.9 Calibrating an aneroid manometer with a mercury manometer.

Key Point

Using the correct size cuff is important when measuring blood pressure. The mercury sphygmomanometer is the standard, and the aneroid gauge should be calibrated against the mercury column every 6 mo.

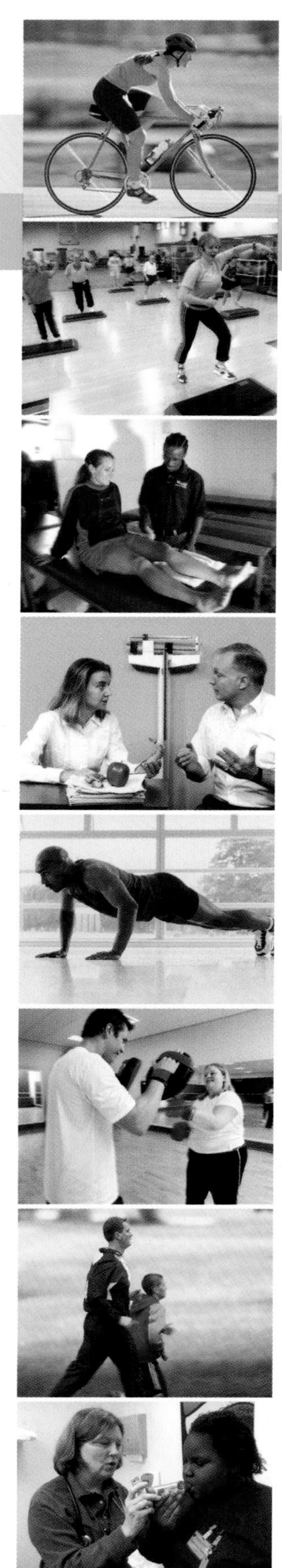

CHAPTER 6

Body Composition

Dixie L. Thompson

Objectives

The reader will be able to do the following:

1. Discuss how body composition affects health and describe the health implications of different patterns of body fat distribution.
2. Compare and contrast hydrostatic weighing, air displacement plethysmography, bioelectrical impedance analysis, and skinfold measurement as means for estimating body composition.
3. Identify common measurement sites for skinfolds and girths.
4. Calculate and interpret body mass index (BMI).
5. Assess body composition using a variety of techniques and describe the advantages and disadvantages of these techniques.

American media are filled with advertisements for programs designed to help people improve their health and fitness. Often the primary focus of these programs is weight loss. A healthy body weight and an appropriate amount of body fat are important aspects of a person's physical fitness. Fitness professionals need to understand the importance of appropriate body composition, become aware of the various means for assessing body fat, and become proficient at estimating body fat through skinfolds and girths. As with other aspects of fitness assessment, paying attention to detail and gaining experience with the techniques are necessary to become proficient at estimating body fatness. This chapter was written to assist fitness professionals in acquiring these skills.

Health and Body Composition

Body composition describes the component tissues of the body and is most often used to refer to the relative percentages of fat and fat-free tissues. **Fat-free mass (FFM), fat mass (FM),** and **percent body fat (%BF)** are the most frequently reported values in a body composition assessment. Percent body fat refers to the percentage of the total body mass that is composed of fat: %BF = fat mass ÷ body mass · 100%. Fat-free mass refers to the mass of the fat-free tissues of the body and often is used synonymously with the term **lean body mass.** Table 6.1 lists suggested age-based %BFs (17). Body composition is a vital aspect of overall fitness because of the ill effects related to excessively low or high body fatness. Various techniques are used to assess body composition, and fitness professionals should be skilled in their use.

Obesity is a condition in which a person has excess **adipose tissue,** or fat tissue. Obesity may be classified either by %BF or by the relationship of height and weight (see section on body mass index on page 97). Although classification systems vary, a %BF of >38% for females and >25% for males generally is considered in the obese range (17, 21). According to BMI standards, obesity is a value ≥30 kg · m^{-2} (26). **Overweight** is the condition in which a person is above the recommended weight range but is not yet in the obese category. A BMI of 25 to 29.9 kg · m^{-2} is considered in the overweight range. The **prevalence** of obesity and overweight among Americans is increasing at an alarming rate among adults and children (5, 9). For example, the percentage of American adults classified as obese in 1999 to 2000 was 30.5%, an increase from 22.9% in a survey conducted from 1988 to 1994 (5). According to recent estimates, nearly 65% of American adults are classified as overweight or obese (5, 9). Obesity has been documented as causing numerous negative health consequences including coronary artery disease, hypertension, stroke, type 2 diabetes, increased risk of various cancers, osteoarthritis, degenerative joint disease, abnormal blood lipid profile, and menstrual irregularities (26). Although precise estimates of the number of deaths that can be attributed to obesity vary considerably (6, 23, 25), hundreds of thousands of Americans die early each year because of conditions either directly or indirectly linked to obesity. Because of the link between obesity and poor health, fitness professionals must provide clients with an accurate assessment of this important fitness component.

When people gain excess fat, genetics determines where the adipose tissue accumulates. Researchers are quite interested in learning how **body fat distribution,** or **fat patterning,** affects health. **Android-type obesity** (i.e., male-pattern obesity, apple shape) is used to describe the excessive storage of fat in the trunk and abdominal areas. Excessive fat in the hips and thighs is labeled **gynoid-type obesity** (i.e., female-pattern obesity, pear shape). In terms of negative health consequences, android-type obesity appears to be the most dangerous, and it is closely linked with disease (7, 16). **Waist-to-hip ratio (WHR)** can be a useful tool for differentiating gynoid-type and android-type obesity. Waist circumference also is used to classify excessive trunk fat. Descriptions of how to make these measurements are presented later in this chapter.

Table 6.1 Suggested Age-Based Body Fat Percentage Standards for Adults (17)

Men	Recommended range[a]
18-34 yr	8-22
35-55 yr	10-25
56 yr or older	10-25
Women	
18-34 yr	20-35
35-55 yr	23-38
56 yr or older	25-38

[a]Values are %BF.

Key Point

The prevalence of obesity and overweight is approximately 65% among U.S. adults. Significant health consequences (e.g., cardiovascular disease, type 2 diabetes) may result from obesity. Disease risk is linked more closely with android-type obesity (apple shape) than with gynoid-type obesity (pear shape). Too little body fat also can lead to negative health outcomes.

Body Composition Techniques Used in Research Settings—Multicompartment Models

A disadvantage to using two-compartment models in calculating body composition is the need to make broad generalizations about the composition and density of various body tissues. To avoid this problem, researchers sometimes use models that combine measurements to estimate body composition. Although these techniques must still rely on some basic assumptions about the body's makeup, fewer broad generalizations about the body's component parts are made. Therefore, these multicompartment models more accurately assess body composition.

An example of a multicompartment model is Siri's three-compartment model, in which the body is divided into fat, water, and solids (protein and mineral) (29). This model requires measuring total body density and total body water. Total body water measurements are typically determined by having the participant ingest an isotope of hydrogen such as deuterium or tritium. After the ingested isotope spreads through the body's water, a fluid sample (e.g., urine, blood) can be used to calculate total body water. This model is particularly useful in clinical situations when patients have significantly altered body water. In cases where the bone mineral varies from what is assumed in a two-compartment model (e.g., in an osteoporotic patient), a technique requiring bone measurement is needed. Lohman (19) presented a model that divides the body into fat, mineral, and protein and water components. Both body density and bone mineral measurement (obtained via X ray imaging) are needed for this technique. Sometimes bone and water measurements are added separately to body density to provide a four-compartment model (i.e., protein, mineral, fat, and water) (10).

Multicompartment models provide important criterion measures of body composition for researchers. Data from these methodologies are used to develop better field methods for assessing body composition in diverse populations. However, the cost, time, and technical expertise required for these processes make them impractical in nonresearch settings.

volume is **air displacement plethysmography.** The Bod Pod (Life Measurement, Inc., Concord, CA) is a commercially available air displacement plethysmograph (see figure 6.2). In this method, body volume is estimated while the subject sits in a sealed chamber. During testing, a computer-controlled diaphragm moves, changing the volume of the chamber. Pressure changes in the chamber are related to the size of the person being measured. By examining the pressure–volume relationship, body volume and subsequently body density are calculated (3, 24). Once body density is known, the two-compartment equations listed in table 6.2 can be used to estimate %BF.

The primary advantage of air displacement plethysmography compared with hydrostatic weighing is that it is quicker and is less anxiety-producing for many individuals. Researchers continue to gather data on this device in an attempt to determine if it can be routinely substituted for hydrostatic weighing (4). The standard error of estimate for this technique is between 2.2% and 3.7% (17). The major disadvantage is the cost of the highly technical equipment needed to make the measurements. A major consideration for obtaining accurate measurements with the Bod Pod is that subjects must dress according to manufacturer's specifications (i.e., in a tight-fitting swimsuit and swim cap).

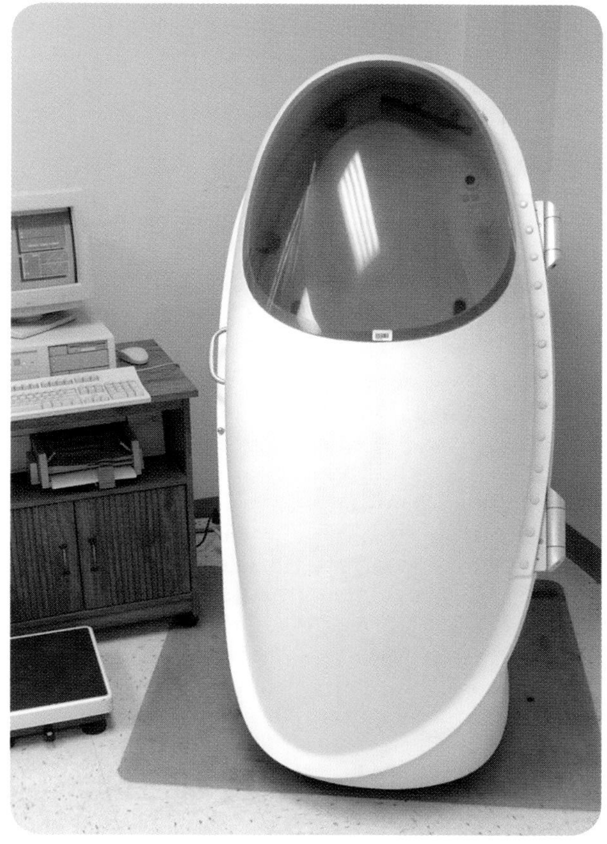

Figure 6.2 Bod Pod.

Bioelectrical Impedance Analysis

Bioelectrical impedance analysis (BIA) is a simple, quick, noninvasive method that can be used to estimate

%BF. This technique is based on the assumption that tissues high in water content conduct electrical currents with less resistance than those with little water (27). Because adipose tissue contains little water, fat impedes the flow of electrical current.

BIA requires that a small electrical current be sent through the body. This current is undetectable to the person being tested (27). There are several types of commercially available BIA devices. Some place electrodes on the hand and foot, some are handheld, and others, which look much like bathroom scales, have contact points for the bottom of the feet. Whatever the design of the machine, as the introduced current passes through the body, voltage decreases. This voltage drop (impedance) is used to calculate %BF. Typically, other information such as sex, height, and age are used in conjunction with impedance to predict %BF.

BIA has gained wide acceptance in the fitness industry because it is easy, inexpensive, and noninvasive. The accuracy of this technique depends on the type of equipment and equations used; however, a standard error of 3.5% to 5% commonly is reported (17). In other words, the %BF value from BIA is typically within 4% of that obtained using hydrostatic weighing. A problem with BIA is that the relationship between impedance and %BF varies among populations. This means that the best equation for predicting %BF depends on the person being tested. For more detailed information on choosing an appropriate BIA equation, refer to *Applied Body Composition Assessment* by Heyward and Wagner (11). BIA does not produce accurate results for individuals with amputations, significant muscular atrophy, severe obesity, or diseases that alter the state of hydration. It is recommended that people with implanted defibrillators avoid BIA assessment until the safety of BIA for these individuals has been determined (27).

A person's state of hydration can greatly alter BIA results; therefore, it is essential to follow standardized guidelines with this assessment technique (27). Following is a list of these guidelines.

- Remove oil and lotions from the skin with alcohol before placing electrodes.
- Place electrodes precisely as directed by the manufacturer of the impedance device. Incorrect electrode placement greatly reduces the accuracy of BIA.
- If required to measure height, mass, or both, measure height to the nearest 0.5 cm and body mass to the nearest 0.1 kg.
- Ask clients to avoid any substance that alters the body's hydration state, such as alcohol or diuretics, for at least 48 hr before BIA. (Diuretics being taken under a doctor's direction should not be stopped.)
- Inform clients that during the 4 hr before assessment they should avoid eating and should drink only enough water to maintain normal hydration.

Body Composition Techniques Used in Research Settings—Imaging Techniques

Dual-energy X-ray absorptiometry (DXA) was developed for measuring the density of bones. Although bone measurement remains the primary use of this methodology, software has been developed that can estimate %BF from DXA scans. To estimate %BF from DXA, a total-body X ray is performed with extremely low-dosage energy beams. As the X rays pass through the subject, the density of all parts of the body is determined. Because fat, bone, and nonbone lean tissue have different densities, these three compartments can be identified (18).

Although DXA requires a full-body X ray, the radiation exposure is minimal and is only a small fraction of the radiation exposure of a chest X ray. Some researchers claim DXA as the new criterion method for body composition assessment; however, there are still unresolved issues for this technology. For example, differences in DXA software packages may result in varied body fat outcomes. Also, variations in body segment thicknesses tend to alter DXA results (18). Studies investigating the error associated with this technique have reported errors ranging from 1.2% to 4.8% (20). This procedure is relatively quick (approximately 15 min) and has the potential for very accurate results regardless of the age, sex, or race of the individual being tested. The major prohibitive factors for using this procedure are cost and access to the equipment. Because of the radiation exposure involved, DXA equipment is housed in hospitals or clinically oriented research centers. At present, DXA is used most frequently as a research tool and in the clinical assessment of body composition.

Magnetic resonance imaging (MRI) and computed tomography (CT) are also imaging techniques that provide important information to clinicians and researchers. One of the common uses of these machines is to determine the amount of fat, particularly deep fat, found in the trunk. Because deep fat (visceral fat) is highly associated with disease, researchers use these techniques to quantify its distribution pattern. CT scans use X rays to produce images of the fat and nonfat tissues, whereas MRI uses a strong magnetic field for this purpose. The equipment necessary for this type of imaging is very expensive and is found in clinical settings.

Key Point

Two-compartment models divide the body into fat and fat-free components. Although the Siri two-compartment model is often used, other models are available. Both hydrostatic weighing and air displacement plethysmography use a two-compartment model. Bioelectrical impedance analysis is based on the principle that electrical currents will flow easier through more hydrated tissues (muscle) than through less hydrated tissues (fat). Although BIA is useful in body composition screening, steps should be taken to ensure that the client's hydration is normal at the time of testing. Multicompartment modeling and imaging techniques are used in research to assess body composition.

- Instruct clients to avoid exercise for 12 hr preceding BIA.
- Note menstrual cycle phase because of its ability to alter hydration levels.

Skinfolds

Measuring skinfold thickness is one of the most frequently performed tests to estimate %BF. This quick, noninvasive, inexpensive method can provide a fairly accurate assessment of %BF. The value obtained by skinfold equations is typically within 3.5% of the value measured with underwater weighing (17). Skinfold measurement is based on the assumption that, as a person gains adipose tissue, the increase in skinfold thickness will be proportional to the additional fat weight.

Because of the widespread use of skinfold measurement, fitness professionals should master the skills involved. Accurately assessing skinfold thickness requires that several steps be performed correctly: locating the skinfold site, pinching the skinfold away from the underlying tissue, measuring with the caliper, and choosing the proper equation. The following sections address each of these concerns.

Locating the Skinfold Site

It is critical to accurately determine the site of the skinfold measurement. To increase the accuracy of the measurement, especially for the inexperienced technician, the site should be located and then marked with a washable marker. This helps ensure that the calipers are placed in the correct position each time the skinfold is measured. All skinfold measurements should be taken on the right side of the body unless otherwise specified. Refer to table 6.3 for some of the most commonly used measurement sites. For a more complete description of determining skinfold sites, refer to the *Anthropometric Standardization Reference Manual* (22). Measuring skinfolds immediately after exercise should be avoided. Exercise can shift fluid volume and thus may lead to inaccurate results.

Pinching the Skinfold

Once the correct location for the skinfold measurement is determined, the tester gently but firmly pinches and lifts

Table 6.3 Locations of Commonly Used Skinfold Sites

Skinfold site	Description
Abdominal	Measure the vertical fold 2 cm to the right of and level with the umbilicus. Make sure the head of the caliper is not in the umbilicus.
Triceps	Measure the vertical fold over the belly of the triceps muscle. The arm should be relaxed. The specific site is the posterior midline of the upper arm, half the distance between the acromion and olecranon processes.
Chest	Measure a diagonal fold along the natural line of the skin one half (men) or one third (women) the distance between the anterior axillary line and the nipple.
Midaxillary	Measure the vertical fold at the level of the xiphoid process on the midaxillary line.
Subscapular	Measure 2 cm below the inferior angle of the scapula along the diagonal fold at a 45° angle.
Suprailiac	Measure the diagonal fold in line with the natural angle of the iliac crest. Measure along the anterior axillary line just above the iliac crest.
Thigh	Measure the vertical fold over the quadriceps muscle on the midline of the thigh. Measure half the distance between the top of the patella and the inguinal crease. Subject's leg should be relaxed.

the skinfold away from the underlying muscle in order to measure it. The following guidelines describe proper methods for measuring skinfolds:

1. Place the fingers perpendicular to the skinfold, approximately 1 cm from the site to be measured.
2. Gently yet firmly pinch the skinfold between the thumb and the first two fingers and lift away from the underlying tissues. Place the jaws of the caliper at the measurement site, perpendicular to the skinfold. The jaws of the caliper should be halfway between the bottom and the top of the fold. Maintain the pinch while taking the measurement.
3. Read the measurement on the caliper 1 to 2 sec after the jaws contact the skin.
4. Wait at least 15 sec before taking a subsequent measurement. To allow time for the fold to return to normal, take one measurement at each site and then repeat measurements. If the second measurement varies by more than 1 to 2 mm, repeat the measurement a third time.

Measuring the skinfolds of individuals who are obese can be difficult if not impossible. If the jaws of the caliper will not open wide enough to measure the skinfold, use an alternative method for assessing body composition. Girth measurements for predicting %BF (30, 31), BMI, and WHR may be used for individuals who are obese. These methods are described later in the chapter.

Measuring With the Caliper

Skinfold thickness is measured with a skinfold caliper. The numerous commercially available calipers vary in price and accuracy. The Lange and Harpenden calipers traditionally are the ones most often in research settings because of their precision and reliability; however, other calipers may also be used effectively (2). Obviously, if the calipers do not measure skinfolds accurately, they will compromise the estimate of body fat. Measure with calipers that closely match those used in the development of the equation you are using.

Choosing the Proper Equation

Most skinfold equations were developed by using underwater weighing as the criterion method and actually are designed to estimate body density. To develop skinfold equations, the body density of many people was measured (typically by using hydrostatic weighing), and this value was compared with skinfold thickness through a statistical method called *regression analysis.* This statistical technique results in the development of an equation that reflects the relationship between skinfolds and body density. Inserting a client's skinfold measurements (and sometimes other information such as age) into these equations produces an estimate of the client's body density. Body density then is converted to %BF by using a two-compartment model equation such as the Siri equation (table 6.2).

Both generalized and population-specific skinfold equations have been developed (14, 20). Generalized equations estimate body composition in groups of people who vary greatly in age, body composition, and fitness. An advantage of these equations is that they can be used to estimate body composition in most people; however, the equations lose accuracy when testing individuals who are dissimilar to those used to develop the equation. These equations are also typically less accurate for people at either end of the fatness continuum.

Population-specific equations predict body composition in a particular subgroup of the population, such as women runners. The advantage of using population-specific equations is that they tend to have higher accuracy when testing people that fit the physical profile of those in the subgroup of interest.

Because sex influences the areas where fat is stored, separate skinfold equations for men and women have been developed. The Jackson and Pollock (13) equations for men and the Jackson, Pollock, and Ward (15) equations for women are generalized equations that are used widely. Note that the client's age is used in these equations. This is because the relationship between total body fat and subcutaneous fat changes with age; as a person ages, proportionally less fat is stored subcutaneously. Equations from these authors that require 3 or 7 skinfold sites are listed on page 97. In addition, tables 6.4 and 6.5 provide quick references for estimating body fatness from skinfold thicknesses for men and women, respectively. To use these tables, total the sum of your client's skinfolds (chest, abdominal, and thigh sites for men; triceps, suprailiac, and thigh sites for women) and locate the corresponding value in the far left column. Then, locate the client's age in the top row. The intersection of the row and column is the client's estimated %BF.

Girth Measurements

Several girth measurements (body and limb circumferences) are used to either estimate body composition or describe body proportions. Girth measurements provide quick and reliable information about the individual. These measurements are sometimes used in equations to predict body composition and may also be used to track changes in body shape and size during weight loss. The major disadvantage is that they provide little information about the fat and fat-free components of the body. For example, a bodybuilder's thigh can have a larger circumference yet less fat than that of an individual who is obese. A list of several commonly measured girths follows; refer to the *Anthropometric Standardization Reference Manual* (22) for additional circumference sites.

Equations for Estimating Body Density From Skinfold Thicknesses (13-15)

Women

3 sites $D_b = 1.0994921 - 0.0009929\ (X1) + 0.0000023\ (X1)^2 - 0.0001392\ (X2)$

3 sites $D_b = 1.089733 - 0.0009245\ (X3) + 0.0000025\ (X3)^2 - 0.0000979\ (X2)$

7 sites $D_b = 1.097 - 0.00046971\ (X4) + 0.00000056\ (X4)^2 - 0.00012828\ (X2)$

X1 = sum of triceps, suprailiac, and thigh skinfolds

X2 = age in years

X3 = sum of triceps, suprailiac, and abdominal skinfolds

X4 = sum of triceps, abdominal, suprailiac, thigh, chest, subscapular, and midaxillary skinfolds

Men

3 sites $D_b = 1.10938 - 0.0008267\ (X1) + 0.0000016\ (X1)^2 - 0.0002574\ (X2)$

3 sites $D_b = 1.1125025 - 0.0013125\ (X3) + 0.0000055\ (X3)^2 - 0.0002440\ (X2)$

7 sites $D_b = 1.112 - 0.00043499\ (X4) + 0.00000055\ (X4)^2 - 0.00028826\ (X2)$

X1 = sum of chest, abdomen, and thigh skinfolds

X2 = age in years

X3 = sum of chest, triceps, and subscapular skinfolds

X4 = sum of triceps, abdominal, suprailiac, thigh, chest, subscapular, and midaxillary skinfolds

- Waist—narrowest part of the torso between the xiphoid process and the umbilicus
- Abdomen—circumference of the torso at the level of the umbilicus
- Hips—maximal circumference of the buttocks above the gluteal fold
- Thigh—largest circumference of the right thigh below the gluteal fold

The waist-to-hip ratio (WHR) is one of the most frequently used clinical applications of girth measurements. This value is often used to reflect the degree of abdominal, or android-type, obesity. A WHR greater than 0.95 for men or 0.86 for women classifies individuals as obese according to ACSM thresholds for CAD risk factors (1).

Waist circumference alone can also provide valuable information about disease risk (12, 16, 26). A waist circumference of 102 cm (40 in.) or greater in men or 88 cm (35 in.) or greater in women is considered to significantly increase the risk of obesity-related disease (1, 26).

When assessing girths, use the following procedures to standardize the measurements:

- Make sure that the measuring tape is horizontal when measuring trunk circumferences and is perpendicular to the long axis of the limb when measuring limbs. Using either a mirror or an assistant helps ensure that the tape is placed properly.
- Apply constant pressure to the tape without pinching the skin. Use a tape measure fitted with a handle that indicates the amount of tension exerted.
- When measuring limbs, measure on the right side of the body. Alternatively, measure on both sides and record the values for both right and left
- Ensure that the person stands erect, relaxed, and with feet together.
- When measuring girths of the trunk, take the measurement after the person exhales and before the next breath begins.

Body Mass Index

A widely used clinical assessment of the appropriateness of a person's weight is the **body mass index (BMI),** or Quetelet index. This value is calculated by dividing the weight in kilograms by height in meters squared.

BMI is a quick and easy method for determining if body weight is appropriate for body height. In the past, height–weight charts were used for this purpose, but BMI is the currently accepted method for interpreting the height–weight relationship. As is the case with girth measurements, BMI does not differentiate between fat and fat-free weight. This is problematic when testing athletic individuals with a large lean mass. For example, a football linebacker who is 6 ft 2 in. (1.9 m) and weighs 220 lb (100 kg) will be considered overweight according to BMI standards (BMI = $28.3\ kg \cdot m^{-2}$), when in fact he may have a very low %BF. On the other hand,

• Table 6.4 Estimating Percentage Body Fat for Men Using Age and the Sum of Chest, Abdominal, and Thigh Skinfolds •

Sum of skinfolds	Age to the last year								
(mm)	Under 22	23- 27	28-32	33-37	38-42	43-47	48-52	53-57	Over 57
8-10	1.3	1.8	2.3	2.9	3.4	3.9	4.5	5.0	5.5
11-13	2.2	2.8	3.3	3.9	4.4	4.9	5.5	6.0	6.5
14-16	3.2	3.8	4.3	4.8	5.4	5.9	6.4	7.0	7.5
17-19	4.2	4.7	5.3	5.8	6.3	6.9	7.4	8.0	8.5
20-22	5.1	5.7	6.2	6.8	7.3	7.9	8.4	8.9	9.5
23-25	6.1	6.6	7.2	7.7	8.3	8.8	9.4	9.9	10.5
26-28	7.0	7.6	8.1	8.7	9.2	9.8	10.3	10.9	11.4
29-31	8.0	8.5	9.1	9.6	10.2	10.7	11.3	11.8	12.4
32-34	8.9	9.4	10.0	10.5	11.1	11.6	12.2	12.8	13.3
35-37	9.8	10.4	10.9	11.5	12.0	12.6	13.1	13.7	14.3
38-40	10.7	11.3	11.8	12.4	12.9	13.5	14.1	14.6	15.2
41-43	11.6	12.2	12.7	13.3	13.8	14.4	15.0	15.5	16.1
44-46	12.5	13.1	13.6	14.2	14.7	15.3	15.9	16.4	17.0
47-49	13.4	13.9	14.5	15.1	15.6	16.2	16.8	17.3	17.9
50-52	14.3	14.8	15.4	15.9	16.5	17.1	17.6	18.2	18.8
53-55	15.1	15.7	16.2	16.8	17.4	17.9	18.5	19.1	19.7
56-58	16.0	16.5	17.1	17.7	18.2	18.8	19.4	20.0	20.5
59-61	16.9	17.4	17.9	18.5	19.1	19.7	20.2	20.8	21.4
62-64	17.6	18.2	18.8	19.4	19.9	20.5	21.1	21.7	22.2
65-67	18.5	19.0	19.6	20.2	20.8	21.3	21.9	22.5	23.1
68-70	19.3	19.9	20.4	21.0	21.6	22.2	22.7	23.3	23.9
71-73	20.1	20.7	21.2	21.8	22.4	23.0	23.6	24.1	24.7
74-76	20.9	21.5	22.0	22.6	23.2	23.8	24.4	25.0	25.5
77-79	21.7	22.2	22.8	23.4	24.0	24.6	25.2	25.8	26.3
80-82	22.4	23.0	23.6	24.2	24.8	25.4	25.9	26.5	27.1
83-85	23.2	23.8	24.4	25.0	25.5	26.1	26.7	27.3	27.9
86-88	24.0	24.5	25.1	25.7	26.3	26.9	27.5	28.1	28.7
89-91	24.7	25.3	25.9	26.5	27.1	27.6	28.2	28.8	29.4
92-94	25.4	26.0	26.6	27.2	27.8	28.4	29.0	29.6	30.2
95-97	26.1	26.7	27.3	27.9	28.5	29.1	29.7	30.3	30.9
98-100	26.9	27.4	28.0	28.6	29.2	29.8	30.4	31.0	31.6
101-103	27.5	28.1	28.7	29.3	29.9	30.5	31.1	31.7	32.3
104-106	28.2	28.8	29.4	30.0	30.6	31.2	31.8	32.4	33.0
107-109	28.9	29.5	30.1	30.7	31.3	31.9	32.5	33.1	33.7
110-112	29.6	30.2	30.8	31.4	32.0	32.6	33.2	33.8	34.4
113-115	30.2	30.8	31.4	32.0	32.6	33.2	33.8	34.5	35.1
116-118	30.9	31.5	32.1	32.7	33.3	33.9	34.5	35.1	35.7
119-121	31.5	32.1	32.7	33.3	33.9	34.5	35.1	35.7	36.4
122-124	32.1	32.7	33.3	33.9	34.5	35.1	35.8	36.4	37.0
125-127	32.7	33.3	33.9	34.5	35.1	35.8	36.4	37.0	37.6

Percentage of fat is calculated by the formula of Siri: $\%BF = [(4.95 \div D_b) - 4.5] \cdot 100$, where D_b = body density.

Adapted, by permission, from M.L. Pollock, D.H. Schmidt and A.S. Jackson, 1980, "Measurement of cardiorespiratory fitness and body composition in a clinical setting," *Comprehensive Therapy* 6(9): 12-27.

• Table 6.5 Estimating Percentage Body Fat for Women Using Age and Sum of Triceps, Suprailiac, and Thigh Skinfolds •

Sum of skinfolds	Age to last year								
(mm)	Under 22	23-27	28-32	33-37	38-42	43-47	48-52	53-57	Over 57
23-25	10.8	11.1	11.4	11.7	12.0	12.3	12.6	12.9	13.2
26-28	11.9	12.2	12.5	12.8	13.1	13.4	13.7	14.0	14.3
29-31	13.1	13.4	13.7	14.0	14.3	14.6	14.9	15.2	15.5
32-34	14.2	14.5	14.8	15.1	15.4	15.7	16.0	16.3	16.6
35-37	15.2	15.6	15.9	16.2	16.5	16.8	17.1	17.4	17.7
38-40	16.3	16.6	16.9	17.2	17.6	17.9	18.2	18.5	18.8
41-43	17.4	17.7	18.0	18.3	18.6	18.9	19.2	19.6	19.9
44-46	18.4	18.8	19.1	19.4	19.7	20.0	20.3	20.6	20.9
47-49	19.5	19.8	20.1	20.4	20.7	21.0	21.4	21.7	22.0
50-52	20.5	20.8	21.1	21.4	21.8	22.1	22.4	22.7	23.0
53-55	21.5	21.8	22.1	22.5	22.8	23.1	23.4	23.7	24.0
56-58	22.5	22.8	23.1	23.5	23.8	24.1	24.4	24.7	25.0
59-61	23.5	23.8	24.1	24.4	24.8	25.1	25.4	25.7	26.0
62-64	24.5	24.8	25.1	25.4	25.7	26.1	26.4	26.7	27.0
65-67	25.4	25.7	26.1	26.4	26.7	27.0	27.3	27.7	28.0
68-70	26.4	26.7	27.0	27.3	27.6	28.0	28.3	28.6	28.9
71-73	27.3	27.6	27.9	28.2	28.6	28.9	29.2	29.5	29.8
74-76	28.2	28.5	28.8	29.1	29.5	29.8	30.1	30.4	30.8
77-79	29.1	29.4	29.7	30.0	30.4	30.7	31.0	31.3	31.7
80-82	29.9	30.3	30.6	30.9	31.2	31.6	31.9	32.2	32.5
83-85	30.8	31.1	31.5	31.8	32.1	32.4	32.8	33.1	33.4
86-88	31.6	32.0	32.3	32.6	33.0	33.3	33.6	33.9	34.3
89-91	32.5	32.8	33.1	33.5	33.8	34.1	34.4	34.8	35.1
92-94	33.3	33.6	33.9	34.3	34.6	34.9	35.3	35.6	35.9
95-97	34.1	34.4	34.7	35.1	35.4	35.7	36.1	36.4	36.7
98-100	34.8	35.2	35.5	35.8	36.2	36.5	36.8	37.2	37.5
101-103	35.6	35.9	36.3	36.6	36.9	37.3	37.6	37.9	38.3
104-106	36.3	36.7	37.0	37.3	37.7	38.0	38.3	38.7	39.0
107-109	37.1	37.4	37.7	38.1	38.4	38.7	39.1	39.4	39.7
110-112	37.8	38.1	38.4	38.8	39.1	39.4	39.8	40.1	40.5
113-115	38.5	38.8	39.1	39.5	39.8	40.1	40.5	40.8	41.1
116-118	39.1	39.5	39.8	40.1	40.5	40.8	41.1	41.5	41.8
119-121	39.8	40.1	40.4	40.8	41.1	41.5	41.8	42.1	42.5
122-124	40.4	40.7	41.1	41.4	41.8	42.1	42.4	42.8	43.1
125-127	41.0	41.4	41.7	42.0	42.4	42.7	43.1	43.4	43.7
128-130	41.6	41.9	42.3	42.6	43.0	43.3	43.7	44.0	44.3

Percentage calculated using Jackson, Pollock, and Ward (15) and Siri (29) equations.

Adapted, by permission, from M.L. Pollock, D.H. Schmidt and A.S. Jackson, 1980, "Measurement of cardiorespiratory fitness and body composition in a clinical setting," *Comprehensive Therapy* 6(9): 12-27.

Table 6.6 Body Mass Index Classification (26)

Classification	BMI ($kg \cdot m^{-2}$)
Underweight	<18.5
Normal	18.5-24.9
Overweight	25.0-29.9
Obesity	
Class I	30.0-34.9
Class II	35.0-39.9
Class III (extreme obesity)	≥40.0

an inactive person with a similar height and weight is probably carrying excess adipose tissue. Even with the limitations of using BMI, for most adults there is a clear correlation between elevated BMI and negative health consequences (26). The recommended BMI range is from 18.5 to 24.9 $kg \cdot m^{-2}$. Overweight is classified as a BMI of 25 to 29.9 $kg \cdot m^{-2}$, and a BMI of 30 $kg \cdot m^{-2}$ or higher is considered obesity (1, 26). Table 6.6 lists all the BMI categories. In screening situations where estimating body fat is impossible or impractical, BMI can be useful for providing feedback to people about the appropriateness of their body weight.

Calculating Target Body Weight

As shown in table 6.1, healthy %BF ranges are quite different for females and males and cover a wide range. One of the important tasks of fitness professionals is helping clients determine an appropriate weight goal. Once an estimate of %BF has been obtained and %BF goals have been determined, the fitness professional can calculate an appropriate target weight. As discussed in chapter 11, setting reasonable goals for weight loss is a major factor in maintaining compliance. To calculate target body weight, you must know body weight, %BF, and the desired level of body fatness. An example of a calculation for target body weight is shown here.

Calculating Target Body Weight

Total body mass, fat mass, fat-free mass, and the desired %BF must be known in order to calculate target body weight. The following equations are needed for these calculations.

$$\text{Fat mass} = \text{body mass } (\%BF \div 100\%)$$

$$\text{Fat-free mass (FFM)} = \text{body mass} - \text{fat mass}$$

$$\text{Target body weight} = \frac{\text{FFM}}{1 - \left(\frac{\text{desired } \% \text{ BF}}{(100)}\right)}$$

Example: A 40-yr-old woman weighs 155 lb (70 kg) and has a %BF of 30. Her goal is to reach 23% body fat. What is her target weight?

$$\text{Fat mass} = 155 \text{ lb } (30 \div 100) = 46.5 \text{ lb}$$

$$\text{FFM} = 155 \text{ lb} - 46.5 \text{ lb} = 108.5 \text{ lb}$$

$$\text{Target body weight} = \frac{108.5}{1 - \left(\frac{23}{(100)}\right)} = 140.9 \text{ lb, or } 63.9 \text{ kg.}$$

Key Point

Skinfold measurements are a quick and relatively accurate method for estimating body fat percentage; however, care must be taken in making these measurements if the values are to be reliable. Girth measurements, particularly WHR and waist circumference, can be useful in assessing risk of obesity-related disease. BMI is useful for classifying individuals into overweight and obese categories. The recommended BMI range is from 18.5 to 24.9 $kg \cdot m^{-2}$. Target body weight can be calculated if current weight and body composition are known.

Case Studies

You can check your answers by referring to page 470 in appendix A.

1. You are the director of a work-site exercise facility. Mr. Jackson, a 37-yr-old man, has joined the exercise program. At his initial evaluation, you make the following measurements:

   Height = 5 ft 10 in. (1.78 m)

   Weight = 240 lb (109 kg)

   Hip circumference = 43 in. (1.09 m)

   Waist circumference = 44 in. (1.12 m)

   Skinfolds: Chest = 40 mm; abdomen = 55 mm; thigh = 26 mm

   a. Calculate and interpret BMI, WHR, and %BF.

   b. Mr. Jackson sets an initial %BF goal of 30%. Calculate his target body weight for his goal.

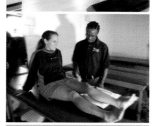

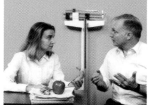

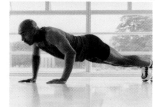

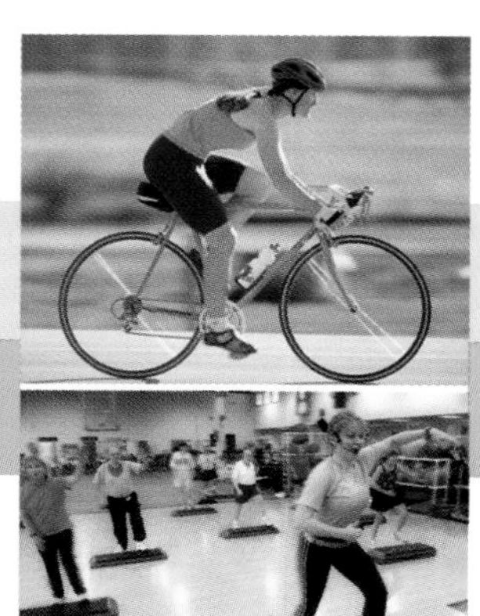

7
CHAPTER

Nutrition

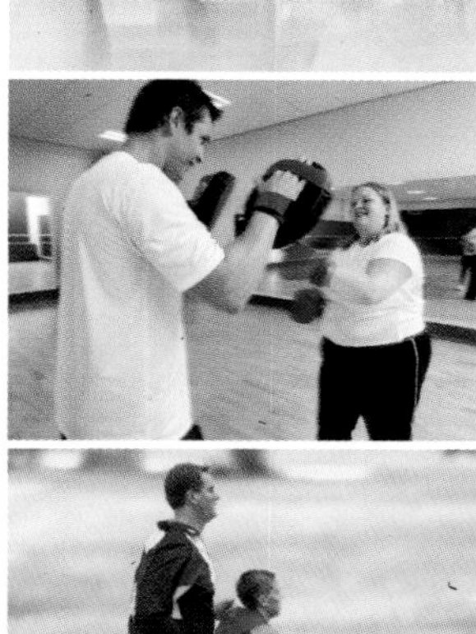

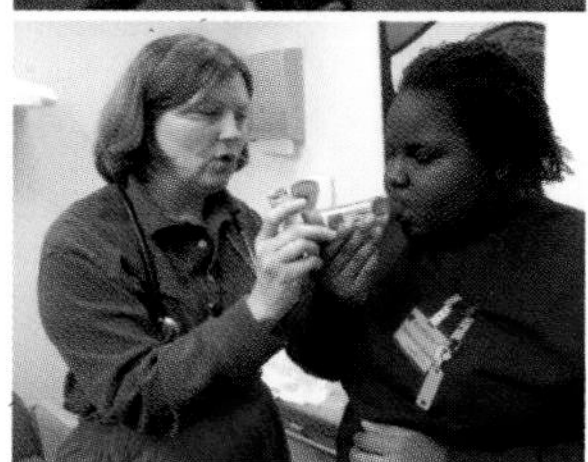

Dixie L. Thompson

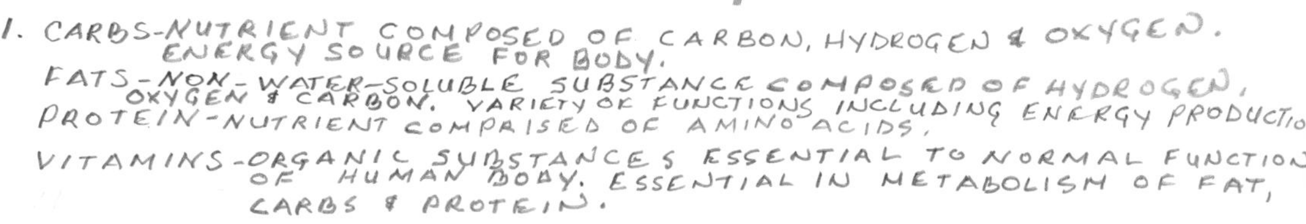

Objectives

The reader will be able to do the following:

1. List the six classes of essential nutrients and describe their role in the proper functioning of the body.
2. List the recommended percentage of calories from carbohydrate, fat, and protein.
3. Understand the importance of vitamins and minerals and how to optimize them in the typical diet.
4. Describe assessment of dietary intake for healthy adults.
5. Understand the role of the USDA Food Guide Pyramid and the U.S. dietary guidelines in making healthy nutritional choices.
6. Explain the relationship between blood lipid profile and cardiovascular disease and explain the role of diet and exercise in modifying blood lipids.
7. Know how to maintain hydration during exercise.
8. Discuss the protein, vitamin, and mineral needs of a physically active person.
9. Know how to maximize glycogen storage before competition.
10. List the three components of the female athlete triad.

Good nutrition results from eating foods in the proper quantities and with the needed distribution of nutrients to maintain good health in the present and in the future. **Malnutrition,** on the other hand, is the outcome of a diet in which there is an underconsumption, overconsumption, or unbalanced consumption of nutrients that leads to disease or increased susceptibility to disease. These definitions implicitly state that proper nutrition is essential to good health. A history of poor nutritional choices eventually leads to health consequences. Poor nutritional choices have been linked to chronic conditions including cardiovascular disease and cancer.

The public is bombarded with messages about nutrition, and it is often difficult for the layperson to distinguish good information from bad. Fitness professionals can play an important role in conveying basic nutritional information. However, a registered dietitian is the appropriate health care professional to counsel individuals with special nutrition needs.

Essential Nutrients

The body requires many **nutrients** for the maintenance, growth, and repair of tissues. Nutrients can be divided into six classes: carbohydrate, fat, protein, vitamins, minerals, and water. The Institute of Medicine has established **Dietary Reference Intakes (DRIs)** to help people achieve a healthy intake of nutrients (14). The DRIs consist of recommended intakes for nutrients, separated by age and sex, including the **Recommended Dietary Allowances (RDA),** or the amounts found to be adequate for approximately 97% of the population; **Adequate Intakes (AI),** or the amounts considered adequate although insufficient data exist to establish the appropriate RDA; and **Tolerable Upper Intake Levels (UL),** or the highest intake believed to pose no health risk. Additionally, **Acceptable Macronutrient Distribution Ranges (AMDR)** have been established for fat, carbohydrate, and protein. The Institute of Medicine reports can be accessed for free at the National Academies Press Web site (www.nap.edu).

Carbohydrate

Carbohydrate is a nutrient composed of carbon, hydrogen, and oxygen and is an essential source of energy in the body. Carbohydrate can be divided into three categories: monosaccharides, disaccharides, and polysaccharides. Examples of monosaccharides are glucose and fructose. Lactose and sucrose are two of the disaccharides, which are carbohydrates that form when monosaccharides combine. The monosaccharides and disaccharides are sometimes called **simple sugars.** Simple sugars contribute significantly to the caloric content of foods such as fruit juices, soft drinks, and candy. The most important simple sugar in the human body is **glucose.** The molecular formula for glucose is $C_6H_{12}O_6$. Polysaccharides are **complex carbohydrates** formed by combining three or more sugar molecules. Starches and fiber are polysaccharides found in plants. Rice, pasta, and whole grain breads are just a few examples of foods that are high in complex carbohydrates. When carbohydrate is stored in the body, glucose molecules are joined together to form large molecules called **glycogen.** Glycogen is stored in the liver and skeletal muscle.

Grains, vegetables, and fruits are excellent sources of carbohydrate. It is recommended that 45% to 65% of a person's daily calories come from carbohydrate (16) (see figure 7.1). The RDA for carbohydrate is 130 $g \cdot day^{-1}$ (16), but the average carbohydrate intake of Americans is well beyond this RDA. The majority of carbohydrate calories should come from complex carbohydrates; foods with added sugar should be limited (23). The reason for eating complex rather than simple carbohydrate is the higher **nutrient density** of complex carbohydrates. Nutrient density refers to the amount of essential nutrients in a food compared to the calories it contains. For example, a candy bar (containing simple sugars) has a low nutrient density, whereas a slice of whole grain bread (containing complex carbohydrates) contains a high nutrient density.

One of the benefits of consuming foods that are high in complex carbohydrate is that they also typically contain

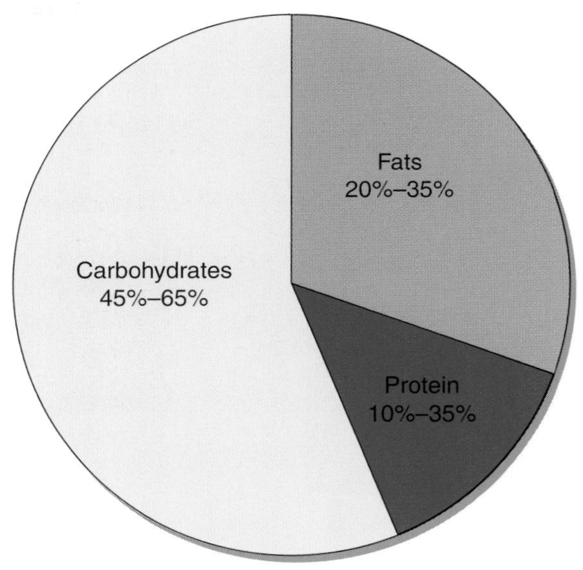

Figure 7.1 Acceptable macronutrient distribution for carbohydrate, fat, and protein (16).

Created from Food and Nutrition Board, Institute of Medicine, 2002, *Dietary reference intakes for energy, carbohydrates, fiber, fat, fatty acids, cholesterol, protein, and amino acids* (Washington, DC: National Academies Press).

dietary fiber. Fiber is nonstarch polysaccharide found in plants and cannot be broken down by the human digestive system. Although fiber cannot be digested, it helps prevent cancers of the digestive system, hemorrhoids, and constipation because it helps food move quickly and easily through the digestive system. Consuming some water-soluble fibers has been shown to lower cholesterol levels (6). Unfortunately, the typical American diet is low in fiber, with the average intake being approximately 15 g · day^{-1} (6). The fiber AI for men and women age 50 and younger is 38 g and 25 g · day^{-1}, respectively (16). For older men and women with lower calorie consumption, the daily recommended levels are 30 g and 21 g, respectively (16). *Dietary Guidelines for Americans* (23) recommends that adults consume approximately 10 g of fiber for every 1,000 kcal consumed. Excellent sources of dietary fiber are grains, vegetables, legumes, and fruit.

As mentioned earlier, carbohydrate is a vital source of energy in the human body. During high-intensity exercise, carbohydrate is the primary fuel source for ATP production. When carbohydrate is broken down in the human body, it yields approximately 4 kcal of energy per gram. This means that a person who eats 10 g of carbohydrate gains approximately 40 kcal of energy to use or store.

Fat

Fat is essential to a healthy diet and contributes to vital functions in the human body. Among the functions performed by fat are temperature regulation, protection of vital organs, distribution of some vitamins, energy production, and formation of cell membranes. Like carbohydrate, fat is composed of carbon, hydrogen, and oxygen; however, the chemical structure is different. **Triglycerides** are the primary storage form of fats in the body. These large molecules are composed of three fatty acid chains connected to a glycerol backbone. The majority of triglycerides are stored in adipose cells (i.e., fat cells). The aerobic metabolism of triglycerides provides much of the energy needed during rest and low-intensity exercise. When metabolized, 1 g of fat yields 9 kcal of energy. **Phospholipids** are another type of fat found in the body. As the name implies, these fats have phosphate groups attached to them. Phospholipids are important constituents of cell membranes. **Lipoproteins** are large molecules that allow fat to travel through the bloodstream. **Cholesterol** is a sterol, or a fatty substance in which the carbon, hydrogen, and oxygen atoms are arranged in rings. In addition to the cholesterol we consume in our diet, the body constantly produces cholesterol, which is

Focus on Glycemic Index

When carbohydrate is ingested, blood glucose rises and subsequently insulin is released from the pancreas. The rapidity with which blood glucose rises after food intake is represented by the **glycemic index.** Foods with a high glycemic index cause a rapid spike in blood glucose, whereas foods with a low glycemic index do not. A number of factors (biochemical composition, method of food preparation, fiber content) affect glycemic index. Examples of foods with a high glycemic index are baked potatoes, white rice, and soft drinks. Foods with a lower glycemic index include apples, kidney beans, and milk. For more information on the glycemic index of foods, see Walberg-Rankin (24).

Some evidence exists that a diet rich in foods with a low glycemic index helps fight cardiovascular disease, obesity, and type 2 diabetes (20). Proposed benefits of low glycemic index diets are increased satiety, lower triglycerides, higher high-density lipid cholesterol (HDL-C), and improved insulin sensitivity. Although some evidence exists that eating more foods with a lower glycemic index may improve health, this issue is still under investigation. In fact, recent dietary guidelines from the American Diabetes Association (ADA) do not emphasize using the glycemic index in making food choices. The ADA stresses attention to the total amount of carbohydrate rather than glycemic index. The ADA suggests that a diet that promotes a healthy weight and is low in fat is preferable for preventing and treating type 2 diabetes and its comorbidities (5).

Key Point

The six classes of nutrients are carbohydrate, fat, protein, vitamins, minerals, and water. The metabolism of 1 g of carbohydrate yields 4 kcal of energy. Carbohydrate should contribute 45% to 65% of one's daily calories, with limited calories coming from simple sugars.

used in forming cell membranes and making steroidal hormones. Meat and eggs are the major sources of cholesterol in the typical American diet, and it is recommended that people consume no more than 300 mg of cholesterol each day (23). However, for those attempting to lower blood lipids, limiting daily cholesterol intake to 200 mg is recommended (13).

Sources of dietary fat come from both animals and plants. The AMDR for fat is 20% to 35% (16) (figure 7.1). Saturated fats come primarily from animal sources and are typically solid at room temperature. Plant sources of saturated fats are palm oil, coconut oil, and cocoa butter. The chemical structure of saturated fats contains no double bonds between carbon atoms; in other words, the fat is saturated with hydrogen atoms. A high intake of saturated fat directly relates to increased cardiovascular disease. Therefore, one should limit consumption of saturated fat to no more than 10% of total calories (23). Unsaturated fats contain fewer hydrogen atoms because there are some double bonds between their carbon atoms. These fats are typically liquid at room temperature. Corn, peanut, canola, and soybean oil are sources of unsaturated fat. **Trans fat** is unsaturated fat that is common in many processed baked goods such as cookies and cakes. The intake of these fatty acids should be as low as possible because they are linked with negative health outcomes. The effects of various kinds of fats on health risk are discussed later in the chapter in the section "Diet, Exercise, and the Blood Lipid Profile."

Monounsaturated fatty acids, found in olive and canola oil, have a single double bond between carbon atoms in the fatty acid chain. **Polyunsaturated fatty acids** (e.g., fish, corn, soybean, and peanut oils) have two or more double bonds between carbon atoms. Two polyunsaturated fatty acids, alpha-linolenic acid (a type of omega-3 fatty acid) and linoleic acid (an omega-6 fatty acid) cannot be made by the body and must be consumed in the diet. The AI for alpha-linolenic acid is 1.6 g $\cdot$ day^{-1} for men and 1.1 g $\cdot$ day^{-1} for women (16). Fish, walnuts, and canola oil are sources of this fatty acid. The AI for linolenic acid is 17 g and 12 g $\cdot$ day^{-1} for men and women, respectively (16). Sources include vegetable oils, nuts, avocados, and soybeans.

Key Point

The AMDR for fat is 20% to 35%, and no more than 10% of calories should come from saturated fat. Cholesterol intake should be limited to 300 mg $\cdot$ day^{-1}. The breakdown of 1 g of fat yields 9 kcal of energy.

Protein

Protein is a substance composed of carbon, hydrogen, oxygen, and nitrogen. All forms of protein are combinations of **amino acids.** Amino acids are molecules composed of an amino group (NH_3), a carboxyl group (COO), a hydrogen atom, a central carbon atom, and a side chain. The differences in the side chains give unique characteristics to each amino acid. Amino acids can combine in innumerable ways to form proteins, and it is estimated that tens of thousands of different types of protein exist in the body. The order of the linked amino acids provides the unique structure and function of proteins. The unique chemical properties and structures of proteins allow them to serve many functions in the body. Some of their most common functions are the following:

- Carry oxygen (hemoglobin)
- Fight disease (antibodies)
- Catalyze reactions (enzymes)
- Allow muscle contraction (actin, myosin, and troponin)
- Act as a connective tissue (collagen)
- Clot blood (prothrombin)
- Act as a messenger (protein hormones such as growth hormone)

Of the 20 amino acids required by the human body, most can be constructed from other substances in the body; however, there are eight **essential amino acids** (nine essential for children and some older adults) that the body cannot synthesize and so must be a part of one's regular diet. Eating a variety of protein-containing foods typically meets this need. There is protein in both meat and plant products. Animal sources of protein such as meat, milk, and eggs contain the essential amino acids. Plant sources of protein such as beans, starchy vegetables, nuts, and grains do not always contain all essential amino acids. Because of this, vegetarians must consume a variety of protein-containing foods. Examples of foods that contain complementary proteins are legumes and grains, vegetables and nuts, and legumes and seeds (11). For more information on planning vegetarian diets, see the summary of the vegetarian food guide established by the American Dietetic Association and Dietitians of Canada (19).

The AMDR for protein is 10% to 35% (figure 7.1). This amount ensures adequate protein for the growth, maintenance, and repair of cells. The adult RDA for protein is 0.8 g of protein for each kilogram of body weight (16). As discussed later in this chapter, individuals who are training intensely may have higher protein requirements. In addition, children need more protein to support their continually growing bodies.

In addition to the functions listed previously, protein can be metabolized for energy production. The break-

Key Point

Protein is made of amino acids and serve numerous functions. To ensure that all needed amino acids are adequately available, people should eat a variety of protein-containing foods each day. The AMDR for protein is 10% to 35%. The breakdown of 1 g of protein yields 4 kcal of energy.

down of 1 g of protein yields approximately 4 kcal of energy for the body. The contribution of protein to resting energy needs or energy needs during exercise is quite small (<5%) in well-nourished individuals. During very long bouts of exercise (>1 hr) or when a person is not well nourished, protein may supply more of the body's energy needs, possibly up to 15%.

Vitamins

Vitamins are organic substances that are essential to the normal functioning of the human body. Although vitamins do not contain energy for the body, they are essential in the metabolism of fat, carbohydrate, and protein. The body needs 13 vitamins for numerous processes including blood clotting, protein synthesis, and bone formation. Because of the critical role vitamins play, it is necessary that they exist in proper quantities in the body. The major functions, important dietary sources, and recommended intakes of vitamins are listed in table 7.1. There are two major classifications of vitamins: fat soluble and water soluble.

The chemical structure of fat-soluble vitamins causes them to be transported and stored with lipids. The four fat-soluble vitamins are A, D, E, and K. Because these vitamins are stored, it is not necessary to continually ingest large amounts of them; however, a small daily intake of each is recommended.

The B vitamins and vitamin C are water-soluble vitamins. These vitamins are not stored in large quantities in the body and therefore must be consumed daily. Deficiencies related to water-soluble vitamins such as scurvy (vitamin C deficiency) and beriberi (thiamin deficiency) may occur rather quickly. Overconsuming either fat-soluble or water-soluble vitamins can lead to toxic effects; however, because fat-soluble vitamins are stored in the body, the potential for overdose with these substances is greater (11).

Minerals

Minerals are inorganic elements that serve a variety of functions in the human body. The minerals that appear in the largest quantities (calcium, phosphorus, potassium, sulfur, sodium, chloride, and magnesium) are often called *macrominerals* or *major minerals*. Other minerals are also essential to normal functioning of the body, but because they exist in smaller quantities, they are called *microminerals* or *trace elements*. The functions, dietary sources, and recommended intakes of minerals are listed in table 7.2.

Calcium is often inadequately consumed by Americans. Calcium is important in the mineralization of bone, in muscle contraction, and in transmission of nervous impulses. **Osteoporosis** is a disease characterized by a decrease in the total amount of bone mineral in the body and by a decrease in the strength of the remaining bone. This condition is most common in the elderly but also may exist in younger people who have diets inadequate in calcium, vitamin D, or both. It is estimated that in the United States, osteoporosis results in approximately 1.5 million fractures per year with resultant health care costs of $10 to $15 billion (21). Maximal bone density is achieved during the early adult years, and during older adult years bone density declines in everyone. Those who achieve the highest bone density and maintain adequate intakes of calcium and vitamin D are most protected from

Focus on Antioxidant Vitamins

During metabolic processes, molecules or fragments of molecules form that can damage the body's tissues. These **free radicals** have at least one unpaired electron in their outer shells; thus, they are very chemically reactive. Lipid-rich cell membranes and DNA are highly susceptible to free radicals, and cell damage can occur when free radicals accumulate. For example, atherosclerosis is linked with free radicals. Some vitamins can react with free radicals and diminish the damage they cause. These **antioxidant vitamins** are hypothesized to counteract the effects of aging and decrease the likelihood of developing cardiovascular disease and cancer and have received a great deal of media attention in the past few years. **Beta-carotene** (a precursor of vitamin A), vitamin C, and vitamin E are highly touted antioxidants. Recent results from several large epidemiological studies suggest that the cardioprotective benefits of antioxidant vitamins are minimal (18). However, studies continue to explore the potential health benefits of these vitamins. Because of the potential toxic effects from an overdose of antioxidants, it is wise to avoid overconsuming these substances (see table 7.1).

• Table 7.1 Vitamins: Functions, Sources, and Dietary Reference Intakes •

Vitamin	Function	Sources	Adult RDA[a] Men	Adult RDA[a] Women	UL[b]
Thiamin (B_1)	Functions as part of a coenzyme to aid utilization of energy	Whole grains, nuts, lean pork	1.2 mg	1.1 mg	ND
Riboflavin (B_2)	Involved in energy metabolism as part of a coenzyme	Milk, yogurt, cheese	1.3 mg	1.1 mg	ND
Niacin	Facilitates energy production in cells	Lean meat, fish, poultry, grains	16 mg	14 mg	35 mg
B_6	Absorbs and metabolizes protein, aids in red blood cell formation	Lean meat, vegetables, whole grains	1.3 mg	1.3 mg	100 mg
Pantothenic acid	Aids in metabolism of carbohydrate, fat, and protein	Whole grain cereals, bread, dark green vegetables	5 mg*	5 mg*	ND
Folic acid	Functions as coenzyme in synthesis of nucleic acids and protein	Green vegetables, beans, whole wheat products	400 µg	400 µg	1,000 µg
B_{12}	Involved in synthesis of nucleic acids, red blood cell formation	Only in animal foods, not plant foods	2.4 µg	2.4 µg	ND
Biotin	Functions as coenzyme in synthesis of fatty acids and glycogen	Egg yolk, dark green vegetables	30 µg*	30 µg*	ND
C	Aids intracellular maintenance of bone, capillaries, and teeth	Citrus fruits, green peppers, tomatoes	90 mg	75 mg	2,000 mg
A	Aids vision, formation and maintenance of skin and mucous membranes	Carrots, sweet potatoes, butter, liver	900 µg	700 µg	3,000 µg
D	Aids growth and formation of bones and teeth, aids calcium absorption	Eggs, tuna, liver, fortified milk	5 µg*	5 µg*	50 µg
E	Protects polyunsaturated fats, prevents damage to cell membrane	Whole grain cereals and breads, green leafy vegetables	15 mg	15 mg	1,000 mg
K	Important in blood clotting	Green leafy vegetables, peas, potatoes	120 µg*	90 µg*	ND

[a]Values are Recommended Daily Allowance (RDA) for adults ages 19 to 50, unless marked with an asterisk. The requirements may vary for children, older adults, and pregnant or lactating women. *Values are Adequate Intakes (AI), indicating that sufficient data to set the RDA are unavailable.

[b]Tolerable Upper Intake Levels (UL) for adults aged 19 to 50. Intakes above the UL may lead to negative health consequences.

ND = not yet determined.

Adapted from Franks and Howley, 1989, and Institute of Medicine.

• Table 7.2 Minerals: Functions, Sources, and Dietary Reference Intakes •

Mineral	Functions	Sources	Adult RDA[a] Men	Adult RDA[a] Women	UL[b]
Calcium	Bones, teeth, blood clotting, nerve and muscle function	Milk, sardines, dark green vegetables, nuts	1,000 mg*	1,000 mg*	2,500 mg
Chloride	Nerve and muscle function, water balance (with sodium)	Salt	2.3 g*	2.3 g*	3.6 g
Magnesium	Bone growth, nerve, muscle, and enzyme function	Nuts, seafood, whole grains, leafy green vegetables	420 mg	320 mg	350 mg[c]
Phosphorus	Bones, teeth, energy transfer	Meats, poultry, seafood, eggs, milk, beans	700 mg	700 mg	4,000 mg
Potassium	Nerve and muscle function	Fresh vegetables, bananas, citrus fruits, milk, meats, fish	4.7 g*	4.7 g*	ND
Sodium	Nerve and muscle function, water balance	Salt	1.5 g*	1.5 g*	2.3 g
Chromium	Glucose metabolism	Meats, liver, whole grains, dried beans	35 µg*	25 µg*	ND
Copper	Enzyme function, energy production	Meats, seafood, nuts, grains	900 µg	900 µg	10,000 µg
Fluoride	Bone and teeth growth	Fluoridated drinking water, fish, milk	4 mg	3 mg	10 mg
Iodine	Thyroid hormone formation	Iodized salt, seafood	150 µg	150 µg	1,100 µg
Iron	O_2 transport in red blood cells, enzyme function	Red meat, liver, eggs, beans, leafy vegetables, shellfish	8 mg	18 mg	45 mg
Manganese	Enzyme function	Whole grains, nuts, fruits, vegetables	2.3 mg*	1.8 mg*	11 mg
Molybdenum	Energy metabolism	Whole grains, organ meats, peas, beans	45 µg	45 µg	2,000 µg
Selenium	Works with vitamin E	Meat, fish, whole grains, eggs	55 µg	55 µg	400 µg
Zinc	Enzyme function, growth	Meat, shellfish, yeast, whole grains	11 mg	8 mg	40 mg

[a]Values are Recommended Daily Allowance (RDA) for adults aged 19 to 50, unless marked with an asterisk. The requirements may vary for children, older adults, and pregnant or lactating women. *Values are Adequate Intakes (AI), indicating that sufficient data to set the RDA are unavailable.

[b]Tolerable Upper Intake Levels (UL) for adults aged 19 to 50. Intakes above the UL may lead to negative health consequences.

[c]Refers to pharmacological agents only and not to amounts contained in food and water. No evidence of ill effects from ingesting naturally occurring amounts in food and water.

ND = not yet determined.

Adapted from Franks and Howley, 1989, and Institute of Medicine.

Table 7.3 Guidelines for Calcium Intake

Age	AI ($mg \cdot day^{-1}$)
0-6 mo	210
7-12 mo	270
1-3 yr	500
4-8 yr	800
9-13 yr	1,300
14-18 yr	1,300
19-50 yr	1,000
51 yr and older	1,200
Pregnant or lactating women (≤18 yr)	1,300
Pregnant or lactating women (19-50 yr)	1,000

Data from Institute of Medicine, 1997.

osteoporosis. The calcium AIs for different ages are listed in table 7.3 (14). The calcium AI for adults aged 19 to 50 is 1,000 $mg \cdot day^{-1}$, with higher values for older adults and adolescents. Milk, dark green vegetables, and nuts are excellent sources of calcium. One cup (8 oz or 237 ml) of 1% milk has approximately 300 mg of calcium, which is almost one third of the daily recommendation for a young adult.

Iron is another mineral that is often underconsumed by Americans, particularly women and children. In fact, the most prevalent nutrient deficiency in the United States is iron deficiency (11). In addition to being a critical component of hemoglobin and myoglobin, iron is necessary for the functioning of the immune system, the formation of brain neurotransmitters, and the functioning of the electron transport chain (11). The oxygen-carrying properties of hemoglobin depend on iron. There is a continual turnover of red blood cells in the body, and much of the iron used to form new hemoglobin comes from old red blood cells. However, there is a daily need for iron, and if iron reserves (liver, spleen, bone marrow) and iron intake are inadequate, hemoglobin cannot be formed and **iron-deficiency anemia** results. In this condition, the amount of hemoglobin in red blood cells falls, which decreases the capacity of the blood to transport oxygen. The recommended intake of iron for males and postmenopausal women is 8 $mg \cdot day^{-1}$ (15). For females during the childbearing years, the recommended daily intake is 18 $mg \cdot day^{-1}$ (15). Red meat and eggs are excellent sources of iron. Additionally, spinach, lima and navy beans, and prune juice are excellent vegetarian sources of iron. Consuming vitamin C with meals increases the body's ability to absorb iron.

Sodium, on the other hand, is a mineral that many Americans overconsume. High sodium intake has been linked with hypertension. The adult AI for sodium is 1.5 $g \cdot day^{-1}$ (17). It is suggested that adults should limit their daily sodium intake to no more than 2.3 g (17, 23). People can substantially reduce their sodium intake by consuming fewer processed foods and adding less salt to foods when cooking.

Water

Water is considered an essential nutrient because of its vital role in the normal functioning of the body. Water contributes approximately 60% of the total body weight (17) and is essential in creating the environment in which all metabolic processes occur. Water is necessary to regulate temperature and transport substances throughout the body.

AI for total water in adults is 3.7 $L \cdot day^{-1}$ for men and 2.7 $L \cdot day^{-1}$ for women (17). Approximately 80% of this amount comes from beverages. As discussed later in this chapter, the amount needed for good health may be higher for individuals exercising intensely. Environmental conditions may also increase the need for water. It is suggested that people should limit the intake of caffeinated beverages because of their diuretic effects.

Key Point

Vitamins, minerals, and water do not provide energy but are essential to the healthy functioning of the body. In general, Americans would benefit from limiting sodium consumption (to decrease blood pressure), increasing calcium intake (to improve bone strength), and increasing iron ingestion (to prevent anemia).

Assessing Dietary Intake

Examining people's dietary habits allows the fitness professional to suggest how they can better meet nutritional and weight loss or weight maintenance goals. Many methods can be used to gather information on dietary intake (9). A useful method for the fitness professional is a food diary in which the client records everything that is consumed. These records typically are kept for 3 or 7 days and provide a general idea of a person's nutritional habits. If the food diary is kept for 3 days, one of those days should be a weekend because many people eat differently on weekends than they do on weekdays (9). Once the records are completed, there are several software packages that can be used to analyze the diet. Although food diaries provide important information, they may pose some problems (25):

- People tend to underreport what they eat.
- People do not keep records that are specific enough to provide quality information.

- People often temporarily change how they eat when they record their food intake.

The fitness professional can take steps to minimize these problems. First, make sure that the clients understand the importance of completely and honestly recording what they eat. Emphasize to clients that the accuracy and usefulness of the feedback depend on the information they provide and that they are not going to be criticized or judged for what they have eaten. Additionally, provide clients with models or descriptions of how to accurately report food consumption. For more information on instructing clients on completing food diaries, see *ACSM's Resource Manual for Guidelines for Exercise Testing and Prescription* (9). Providing explicit instructions will allow the client to provide a more useful and accurate record. Additionally, the food diary should be user friendly and include cues to elicit complete responses. A sample food log with instructions is provided on form 7.1.

The fitness professional can provide general nutrition information to the public. Clients with special metabolic needs such as diabetes mellitus should be referred to a registered dietitian. Comparing dietary intake to DRIs can be particularly informative (14). For the typical client, the following intakes should be included in a nutritional profile:

- Total calories
- Percentage of calories from fat, carbohydrate, and protein
- Saturated fat, trans fat, and cholesterol
- Sodium
- Iron
- Calcium
- Fiber

Key Point

Food diaries record dietary practices. The client must provide detailed information for the dietary assessment to be accurate.

It also can be useful to examine the food diary for emotional or social cues to eating behaviors. For example, some people eat when depressed or only eat when alone. Such information can be helpful in making behavior changes needed for weight loss and weight maintenance. More information on weight management is covered in chapter 11.

Recommendations for Dietary Intake

Dietary Guidelines for Americans (23) is a joint effort of the U.S. Department of Health and Human Services and the U.S. Department of Agriculture (USDA). These recommendations can help people make healthy food choices, and they focus on lowering risk of chronic disease and promoting health. Because of the nutritional inadequacies common among Americans, the guidelines generally "encourage most Americans to eat fewer calories, be more active, and make wiser food choices" (23). The guidelines provide both general and specific recommendations. For example, all individuals are encouraged to "consume a variety of nutrient-dense foods and beverages within and among the basic food groups while choosing foods that limit the intake of saturated and trans fats, cholesterol, added sugars, salt, and alcohol" (23). Specific information is provided to pregnant women, including the recommendation to consume adequate amounts of folic acid. A complete copy of *Dietary Guidelines for Americans* (23) can be found at www.usda.gov.

Many different plans have been formulated to guide food intake. The USDA has suggested using the **Food Guide Pyramid** as a guide to eating (23). This program, called **My Pyramid,** uses a new approach to recommending food intake. My Pyramid bases personalized recommendations for intake of different food groups on sex, age, and level of physical activity (see figure 7.2). The food groups targeted are grains, vegetables, fruits, oils, milk, and meat and beans. Additionally, recommended levels of physical activity are provided. The amount of food suggested for each category depends on the caloric need of the individual. For example, a person consuming 2,000 kcal $\cdot$ day^{-1} should eat 2 cups (473 ml) of fruit each day, but people with a greater caloric need (e.g., athletes) should eat more. More information, including an interactive Web site for personalized dietary planning, can be found at www.MyPyramid.gov.

The U.S. Food and Drug Administration requires that all food be labeled with nutrition information. These labels, titled Nutrition Facts, list the serving size, total calories, fat (including saturated fat), cholesterol, sodium, carbohydrate (including dietary fiber), protein, and various vitamins and minerals contained in the food. **Daily Values (DVs)** indicate the percentage of daily recommended levels of nutrients that are contained in a food. The DVs were developed in an attempt to inform the public about the nutritional content of the foods they buy and are based on a calorie intake of 2,000 kcal $\cdot$ day^{-1}. The nutritional label contains the percentage of the recommended DVs provided by nutrients found in the food.

FORM 7.1 Sample Food Log

Instructions

1. Record everything you eat, including foods and beverages eaten at meals and snacks.
2. Record carefully how the food was prepared. Be as descriptive as possible (e.g., fried in corn oil, broiled in 1 tbsp. of margarine).
3. Be sure to indicate the amount of food eaten. Use typical household measures when possible (tsp. = teaspoon; tbsp. = tablespoon; cup = cup; oz = ounce).
4. Provide brand names and labels for packaged foods.
5. For composite foods such as sandwiches, casseroles, and soups, indicate the ingredients contained in the food. For example, a turkey sandwich might be described as 2 slices of whole wheat bread, 1 oz of baked turkey breast without skin, 1 slice of tomato, 2 leaves of iceberg lettuce, 1 tbsp. light mayonnaise.
6. Indicate where and with whom you were when you ate. Also, describe your feelings at the time—were you worried, content, lonely, stressed, hungry? (Be honest with yourself.)
7. Carry this form with you so that you can write down foods as you eat them. Do not wait until the end of the day to record your food intake.

Food/Drink	Description (e.g., amount, cooking method, brand name)	Location (e.g., place, people, alone)	Feelings (e.g., hunger, anger, joy)	Time

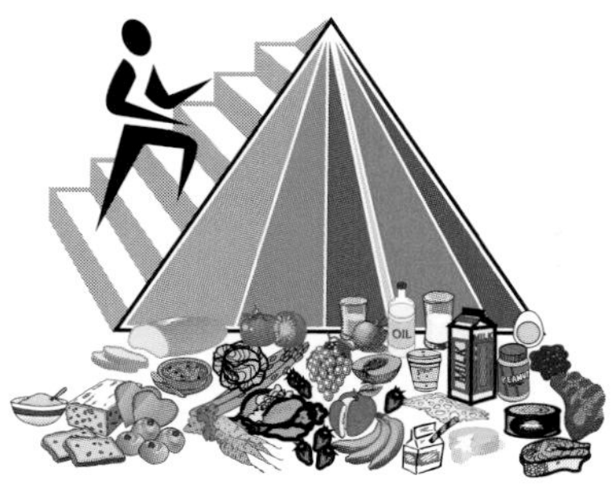

MyPyramid

STEPS TO A HEALTHIER YOU

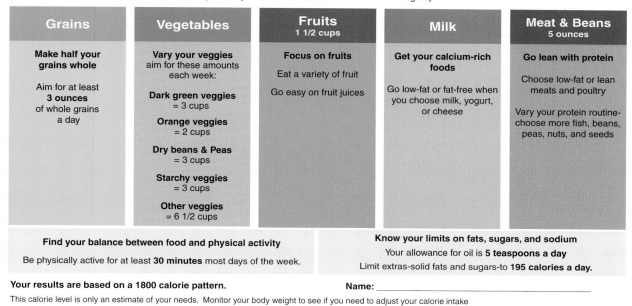

Based on the information you provided, this is your daily recommended amount from each food group

Grains	Vegetables	Fruits 1 1/2 cups	Milk	Meat & Beans 5 ounces
Make half your grains whole Aim for at least **3 ounces** of whole grains a day	**Vary your veggies** aim for these amounts each week: **Dark green veggies** = 3 cups **Orange veggies** = 2 cups **Dry beans & Peas** = 3 cups **Starchy veggies** = 3 cups **Other veggies** = 6 1/2 cups	**Focus on fruits** Eat a variety of fruit Go easy on fruit juices	**Get your calcium-rich foods** Go low-fat or fat-free when you choose milk, yogurt, or cheese	**Go lean with protein** Choose low-fat or lean meats and poultry Vary your protein routine-choose more fish, beans, peas, nuts, and seeds

Find your balance between food and physical activity

Be physically active for at least **30 minutes** most days of the week.

Know your limits on fats, sugars, and sodium

Your allowance for oil is **5 teaspoons a day**

Limit extras-solid fats and sugars-to **195 calories a day.**

Your results are based on a 1800 calorie pattern. **Name:** ______________

This calorie level is only an estimate of your needs. Monitor your body weight to see if you need to adjust your calorie intake

Figure 7.2 U.S. Food Guide Pyramid for a moderately active 58-yr-old female.

Reprinted, by permission, from V. Heyward, 2006, *Advanced fitness assessment and exercise prescription*, 5th ed. (Champaign, IL: Human Kinetics), 235. From www.mypyramid.gov.

For example, the suggested DV for cholesterol is 300 mg; therefore, if a food contains 15 mg of cholesterol, it will constitute 5% of the recommended daily intake of cholesterol. Additional information on food labels can be found at www.cfsan.fda.gov/label.html.

Key Point

Dietary Guidelines for Americans (23) encourages most Americans to eat fewer calories, be more active, and make wiser food choices. My Pyramid provides personalized information about the amount and types of food individuals should consume daily based on their age, gender, and activity pattern. Food labeling allows consumers to evaluate the nutritional content of foods.

Diet, Exercise, and the Blood Lipid Profile

Cardiovascular disease is the leading cause of death in the United States. One of the primary risk factors for cardiovascular disease is a poor blood lipid profile. Both diet and exercise can positively affect this crucial risk factor.

Lipoproteins and Risk of Cardiovascular Disease

Because lipids are hydrophobic (i.e., not water soluble), they need to bind with some other substance to be transported in the blood. Lipoproteins are macromolecules composed of cholesterol, triglycerides, protein, and phospholipids. Classifications for these molecules are based on their size and makeup. The two classes of lipoproteins most closely linked with cardiovascular disease are low-density lipoprotein (LDL) and high-density lipoprotein (HDL). LDL transports cholesterol and triglycerides from the liver to be used in various cellular processes. HDL retrieves cholesterol from the body's cells and returns it to the liver to be metabolized.

Elevated levels of **total cholesterol** (the sum of all forms of cholesterol) and **low-density lipoprotein cholesterol (LDL-C)** are linked with the development of atherosclerotic plaque in the arteries. Increased levels of **high-density lipoprotein cholesterol (HDL-C)** help prevent the atherosclerotic process. According to the 2001 National Cholesterol Education Program (NCEP) guidelines, total cholesterol levels below 200 mg · dL^{-1} and LDL-C values below 100 mg · dL^{-1} are desirable. Total cholesterol of 240 mg · dL^{-1} or higher and LDL-C of 160 mg · dL^{-1} or higher are considered high levels and are associated with greater risk of cardiovascular disease (see table 7.4). In addition, HDL-C below 40 mg · dL^{-1} is considered too low and HDL-C levels of 60 mg · dL^{-1} or higher are considered ideal (13).

Table 7.4 Blood Lipid Classifications (13)

Lipid level	Level rating
Total cholesterol	
<200	Desirable
200-239	Borderline high
≥240	High
HDL cholesterol	
<40	Low
≥60	High
LDL cholesterol	
<100	Optimal
100-129	Near or above optimal
130-159	Borderline high
160-189	High
≥190	Very high
Triglycerides	
<150	Normal
150-199	Borderline high
200-499	High
≥500	Very high

All values are mg · dL^{-1}.

Effects of Diet and Exercise on the Blood Lipid Profile

Consuming a diet low in saturated fat and cholesterol, losing weight, and participating in regular aerobic exercise all have been linked to positive changes in the blood lipid profile. The 2001 NCEP guidelines (13) recommend a therapeutic lifestyle changes (TLC) diet to improve the blood lipid profile. The TLC diet includes the following dietary practices:

- Limiting total fat intake to 25% to 35% of calories (if at the higher end of the range, care should be taken to ensure that most fats are monounsaturated)
- Limiting saturated fat to 7%, polyunsaturated fat to 10%, and monounsaturated fat to 20% of calories
- Limiting cholesterol intake to <200 mg · day^{-1}
- Limiting intake of trans fat

Consuming certain types of fat, such as omega-3 fatty acids, appears to benefit health. Omega-3 fatty acids are found in canola oil as well as in fish such as salmon and tuna. Omega-3 fatty acids are polyunsaturated fats that get their name from the site of the first double bond in the fatty acid chain. American diets are typically low in omega-3 fatty acids and higher in omega-6 fatty acids (e.g., peanut, corn, and soybean oils). Bringing the intake of these two types of fat into better balance appears to improve the lipoprotein profile and lower the risk of cardiovascular disease (18, 23).

People who engage in regular aerobic exercise and maintain a healthy weight typically have a better blood lipid profile than their sedentary counterparts have.

Focus on Trans Fat

Recent attention has focused on the health risks of trans fatty acids (i.e., trans fat). Although small amounts of trans fat are found in animal products, the majority of these hydrogenated fats are found in processed foods produced from fat in plants. The hydrogenation process chemically transforms the spatial orientation of hydrogen atoms in the fat. This hardens the liquid plant oil and leads to a more stable product that is better suited for cooking. Consequently, many processed foods (e.g., cookies, chips, doughnuts, french fries) are prepared with trans fat. Foods high in trans fat will have partially hydrogenated vegetable oils as a primary ingredient listed on their food label. The problem with trans fat is that, as saturated fat, it can harm the blood lipid profile. Trans fat elevates LDL-C and lowers HDL-C. Therefore, trans fat should be avoided to improve the lipid profile (23).

Key Point

Elevated total cholesterol and LDL-C and depressed HDL-C are risk factors for cardiovascular disease. Aerobic exercise, weight loss, and low intake of saturated fat, trans fat, and cholesterol effectively improve the blood lipid profile. A diet high in omega-3 fatty acids also has cardioprotective benefits.

It is difficult to ascertain which of these changes are attributable to the exercise and which relate to a healthy body weight. It appears that the primary blood lipid changes resulting from aerobic exercise are increases in HDL-C and decreases in blood levels of triglycerides (12). Weight loss has been linked with lower total cholesterol, LDL-C, and triglycerides as well as with higher HDL-C.

Nutrition for Physically Active Individuals

Nutrition plays an important role in health, and it is also essential for optimal performance during physical activity. The ACSM, American Dietetic Association, and the Dietitians of Canada released a joint position statement in 2000 that addresses the dietary needs of physically active adults (4). Fitness professionals should be familiar with these guidelines to provide basic nutritional advice to clients who exercise regularly.

Hydration Before, During, and After Exercise

Sweating is the body's primary mechanism for heat dissipation during exercise. The amount of sweat lost during exercise depends on environmental heat and humidity, type and intensity of exercise, and the characteristics of the exerciser. Dehydration reduces the body's capacity for sweating and can impair performance by decreasing strength, endurance, and coordination. In addition, dehydration increases the risk of heat cramps, heat exhaustion, and heat stroke (see chapter 25).

A person should consume 14 to 20 oz (400-600 ml) of water 2 hr before an endurance exercise bout (1, 4, 10) and then drink an additional 7 to 10 oz (200-300 ml) 10 to 20 min before beginning exercise (10). Fluid replacement during exercise is essential in activities that last an hour or longer, especially if they take place in hot, humid environments. During exercise a person should drink approximately 150 to 350 ml (6-12 oz) of water every 15 to 20 min (4). Water that is slightly chilled (5-10 °C) is suggested for increasing palatability and absorption (1).

In activities where large amounts of sweat are lost, fluid should be fully replaced. Weighing before and after these types of activities is recommended. The participant should drink approximately 16 to 24 oz (475-700 ml) of water for each pound of weight lost (4). If body weight has not returned to normal in the following days, additional water should be consumed before beginning exercise. For reviews of the hydration needs of athletes, refer to the position stands of NATA (10) and the ACSM (1).

Protein Intake for Athletes

Athletes who are training intensely may benefit from increasing their protein intake above the level recommended for a sedentary person (i.e., 0.8 g · kg^{-1}). An athlete training intensively in primarily endurance activities may benefit from consuming 1.2 to 1.4 g of protein per kilogram of body weight. For athletes engaging in high-intensity, high-volume resistance training, a protein intake of up to 1.7 g · kg^{-1} may be needed (4). To this point, most of the studies in this area have focused on male athletes, so little is known about the protein needs of female athletes.

Athletes should meet additional protein requirements through food choices, not through supplements. There is an upper limit to the rate at which muscle mass can be increased; therefore, excessive protein intake (i.e., above the recommendations) does not enhance performance or increase muscle mass (4). Because of the higher caloric intake of intensively training athletes, a diet with the normal distribution of macronutrients typically contains adequate amounts of protein, so purposefully consuming additional protein is usually not necessary (4, 26).

Another issue that sometimes arises is the adequacy of protein intake for vegetarian athletes. Because plant proteins are not digested as well as animal proteins, it is suggested that athletes following a strict vegetarian diet consume 1.3 to 1.8 g of protein per kilogram of body weight (4).

Ergogenic Aids

The search for nutritional and pharmacological agents that improve performance has led to the marketing of numerous products touted as **ergogenic aids.** Some of

Key Point

Adequate hydration is essential to performance. Water should be consumed before, during, and after extended bouts of exercise.

Focus on Creatine Supplementation

Creatine phosphate, a high-energy compound found in skeletal muscle, is a critical source of energy during bursts of high-intensity exercise. Athletes use creatine supplementation to increase the amounts of creatine phosphate in muscle in an effort to enhance high-intensity exercise performance. Studies demonstrate that creatine supplementation does improve high-intensity exercise performance, particularly repeated bouts of high-intensity cycling, under laboratory conditions. Less is known about its effect on performance under competitive conditions. Creatine supplementation also is associated with weight gain (~1 kg) as a result of water retention. It is unclear if this extra weight could impede, rather than enhance, performance in weight-bearing activities such as sprinting. There are some reports of muscle cramping and gastrointestinal distress with creatine use. No studies have examined the side effects of long-term creatine use. For more information on creatine supplementation, refer to the ACSM's roundtable report (3) and the review by Williams (26).

these products (e.g., bee pollen, brewer's yeast) provide no scientifically proven physiological advantage. Other products such as caffeine may improve performance in some instances (26) and have been regulated by various sporting agencies such as the International Olympic Committee. Some ergogenic aids must be strictly avoided, such as anabolic steroids, because of severe and sometimes fatal side effects (22). The ACSM has released a number of Current Comments (official statements concerning topics of interest) on potential ergogenic aids.

Athletes often consume vitamins and minerals in amounts higher than the RDA in an attempt to improve performance. There is no evidence that this practice enhances performance; however, if an athlete's diet provides inadequate amounts of any nutrient, health and performance could suffer (26). The two minerals that often need to be increased in the diet are iron and calcium (8). The most common mineral deficiency among athletes is iron deficiency (26). For athletes with anemia, increased iron consumption is advised and in many cases will improve performance (26). For female athletes with menstrual cycle irregularities, calcium supplementation often is prescribed to promote bone health. See chapter 17 for more information on issues specific to female athletes.

Key Point

The typical protein RDA for adults ($0.8\ g \cdot kg^{-1}$) may be inadequate for athletes. People who are training intensely should consume 1 to 1.5 g of protein per kilogram of body weight. Ergogenic aids are pharmacological or nutritional agents thought to improve athletic performance. Although some products may enhance performance, there are many highly touted products with unproven results. In healthy, well-nourished athletes, extra vitamins and minerals (i.e., above the RDAs) do not improve performance.

Carbohydrate Loading and Intake During Exercise

Adequate intake of carbohydrate is necessary for optimal athletic performance in endurance events. Glucose is the major source of energy during exercise; when blood glucose levels decline, the ability to continue exercise is limited. A physically active person should routinely consume a diet in which 60% to 65% of the calories are from carbohydrate. For an athlete who trains heavily on consecutive days or who engages in frequent exhaustive exercise bouts, a diet providing 6 to 10 g of carbohydrate per kilogram of body weight is recommended (4).

Carbohydrate loading is used to maximize glycogen storage before competition. This practice is most beneficial for athletes who compete in events requiring continuous activity lasting longer than an hour, such as marathon running. The American Dietetic Association recommends the following practices to enhance glycogen storage (7):

- Consume a diet in which 65% to 70% of the total calories are from carbohydrate.
- Decrease the duration of exercise bouts during the week before competition.
- Rest completely on the day before competition.

During events that involve continuous vigorous activity for 60 min or more, it is beneficial to consume easily absorbed forms of carbohydrate. The ACSM states that solutions containing 4% to 8% carbohydrate (glucose, sucrose, or starch) are best to balance the need for blood glucose maintenance and fluid replacement. The solution

Key Point

Adequate glycogen is necessary for optimal performance. Carbohydrate loading benefits extended bouts of exercise. Glucose intake during exercise can be beneficial if vigorous exercise lasts 60 min or more.

should be consumed in small to moderate amounts (150-350 ml) every 15 to 20 min (1).

Female Athlete Triad

The **female athlete triad** is a condition characterized by disordered eating, amenorrhea, and osteoporosis (2). As discussed in chapter 17, disordered eating is more common in female athletes than in the general population. It is thought that the pressure to succeed and the drive to be thin lead many female athletes to begin unhealthy eating practices such as severe caloric restriction (anorexia), purging of food after eating (bulimia), and compulsive overexercising. These unhealthy patterns interfere with normal hormone secretion and eventually can lead to irregular menses (**oligomenorrhea**) or a lack of menses altogether (**amenorrhea**). Because estrogen is essential in maintaining strong bones in women, the low estrogen levels observed in athletes with menstrual cycle irregularities can lead to a loss of bone. Weakening of the bones makes the athlete more susceptible to stress fractures and can lead to an early and severe onset of osteoporosis.

Fitness professionals should encourage all physically active people to consume adequate calories and nutrients to support their energy expenditure. Active females who begin to miss menstrual periods should be referred to a physician to evaluate the need for hormonal therapy or calcium supplementation. Some signs of disordered eating are listed in chapter 11. Athletes who exhibit these signs should be referred to a nutritionist or a psychologist (or both) who is qualified to counsel a person with eating disorders

Key Point

The female athlete triad (disordered eating, amenorrhea, and osteoporosis) can lead to serious health consequences. Athletes who exhibit signs of an eating disorder should be referred to a qualified nutritionist, psychologist, or both.

Case Studies

You can check your answers by referring to page 471 in appendix A.

1. A male college basketball player (weight = 190 lb, or 86.4 kg) with a daily caloric intake of 3,500 kcal is considering additional protein supplements. He currently consumes approximately 15% of his calories from protein. Is his protein intake adequate? Would you recommend that he increase his protein intake?

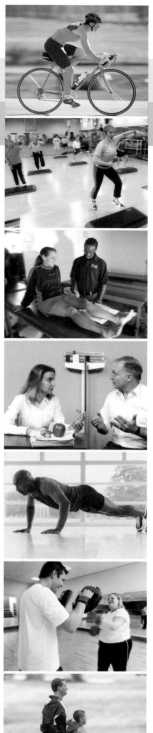

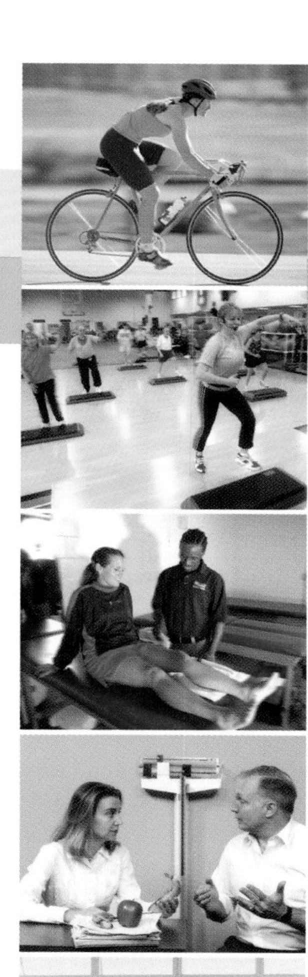

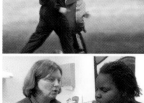

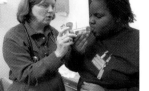

8 CHAPTER

Assessment of Muscular Fitness

Kyle McInnis and Avery Faigenbaum

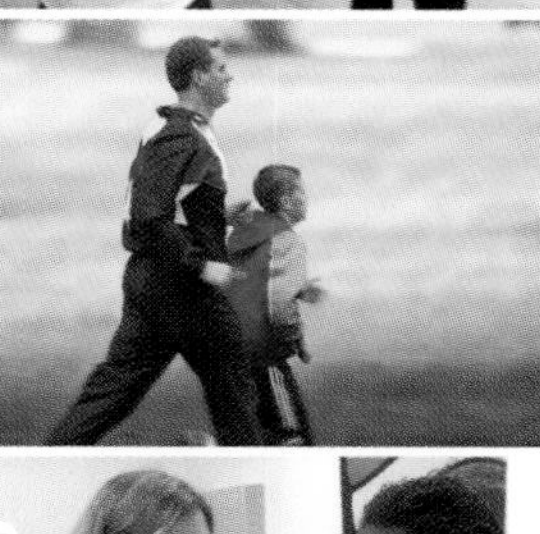

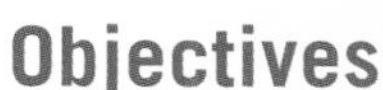

Objectives

The reader will be able to do the following:

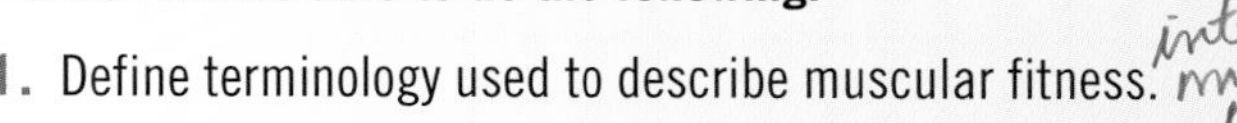

1. Define terminology used to describe muscular fitness.
2. Discuss precautions that enhance participant safety during muscular fitness assessments.
3. Describe methods of assessing muscular fitness, including the 1-repetition maximum (1RM) and 10-repetition maximum (10RM) tests, push-up test, abdominal curl-up test, and YMCA bench press test.
4. Identify methods for standardizing testing protocols.
5. Describe how to interpret the results from various muscular fitness tests as a component of a comprehensive health and fitness evaluation.
6. Describe how to assess muscular strength and endurance in older adults using the 30 sec chair stand test and single-arm curl test.
7. Describe the benefits, safety, and precautions for assessing muscular fitness in clients who are coronary prone.
8. Describe the benefits, safety, and precautions for assessing muscular fitness in children and adolescents.

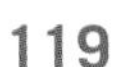

Muscular fitness refers to the integrated status of **muscular strength** (maximal force a muscle can generate) and **muscular endurance** (ability of a muscle to make repeated contractions or to resist muscular fatigue) (4, 16, 21). Muscular fitness is important in both promoting and maintaining health and enhancing athletic performance (3) (see box on page 121). Accordingly, in its position stand on the recommended quantity and quality of exercise to achieve and maintain fitness in healthy adults, the ACSM promotes routine resistance and strengthening exercise (3). In general, the ACSM recommends that resistance training of a moderate to high intensity, sufficient to develop and maintain muscle mass, become an integral part of a well-rounded fitness program (see chapter 12). This chapter describes tests commonly used in the health and fitness setting to assess muscular strength and endurance. Particular emphasis is given to strength tests that can be performed safely in the fitness setting, especially those that do not require specialized equipment or sophisticated procedures. Assessing muscular fitness and functional capabilities in special populations such as older adults, people at increased cardiovascular risk, and children or adolescents is described.

Preliminary Considerations

Muscular fitness often is assessed by the number of repetitions a person can perform with a given weight. This may be viewed as a continuum with strength at one end of the assessment scale and endurance at the other (figure 8.1) (4). Traditionally, tests allowing few repetitions (e.g., <5) before momentary muscle fatigue measure local muscular strength, whereas those that require high numbers of repetitions (e.g., >15) measure local muscular endurance.

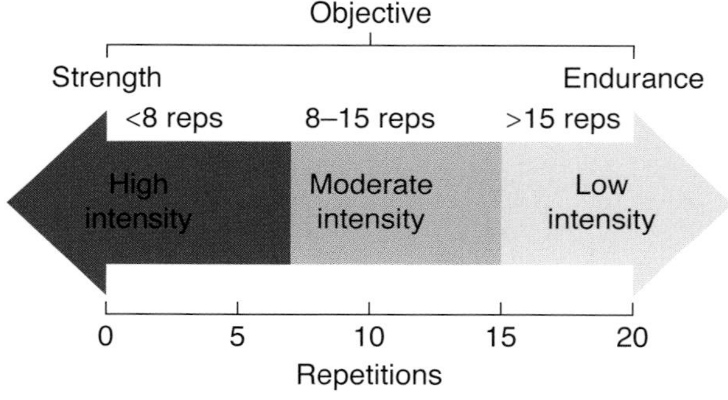

Figure 8.1 Classification of intensity of resistance exercise for training and assessment. Weight loads allowing few reps (e.g., <15) test for muscular strength, and weight loads that can be repeatedly lifted (e.g., 15 reps) assess muscular endurance.

Adapted from American College of Sports Medicine (ACSM), 2006, *ACSM's guidelines for exercise training and prescription*, 7th ed. (Philadelphia, PA: Lippincott, Williams & Wilkins).

However, the performance of a maximal repetition range (e.g., 4, 6, or 8 repetitions) also can assess strength. Performing fitness tests to assess muscular strength and local muscular endurance before commencing exercise training or as part of a fitness screening can provide valuable information on a client's baseline fitness. For example, results from a muscular fitness test can be compared with established standards and can help identify weaknesses in certain muscle groups or muscle imbalances that could be targeted in exercise training programs. The information obtained during baseline muscular fitness assessments also can serve as a basis for designing individualized exercise training programs. An equally useful application of fitness testing is to show a client's progressive improvements as a result of the training program and thus provide beneficial feedback that promotes long-term exercise adherence. For safety purposes, all participants who undergo fitness testing should first complete a medical history questionnaire. This questionnaire identifies individuals who may be at cardiovascular or orthopedic risk during testing and training. The ACSM's procedures for administering an appropriate health appraisal and subsequent risk stratification and for medical evaluation have been described in detail in this textbook (see chapter 3) and elsewhere (2).

- **Standardization of testing protocols.** According to the ACSM, individuals should participate in familiarization (practice) sessions, adhere to one test protocol, and perform a proper warm-up in order to obtain a reliable score that can be used to track true physiologic adaptations over time. Other standardized conditions that promote safe muscular fitness tests that yield valid and reproducible results include ensuring that the individual use a strict posture, a predetermined speed of contractions, and a full ROM on all lifts. Safety measures should be reviewed. Additionally, the muscular fitness tests should be specific to the training program.
- **Familiarization.** To obtain a reliable test score that can be used to track physiological adaptations over time, individuals should become familiar with the testing equipment and protocol by participating in one or more practice sessions with qualified instruction.
- **Warm-up.** A 5 to 10 min general warm-up including brief cardiovascular exercise, light stretching, and several light repetitions of the specific testing exercise should proceed muscular fitness testing. This increases muscle temperature and localized blood flow and promotes appropriate cardiovascular responses to exercise (3, 4).
- **Specificity.** Muscle strength and muscular endurance are specific to the muscle or muscle group, the type of muscular action (static or dynamic, concentric or eccentric), the speed of muscular action (slow or fast), and the joint angle being tested (16, 21). Accordingly,

muscular fitness tests should be similar to the exercises used during the training program.

- **Safety.** Safety measures related to the testing equipment and providing proper instruction should be employed prior to testing.
- **Interpretation of results.** The availability of health criteria or population-specific norms should be considered when you choose a test, particularly when classifying an individual's test data, such as when performing a fitness screening. However, availability of norms is less of a concern when the test is used primarily to detect improvements in muscular fitness, where the absolute strength values (e.g., kilograms lifted) or relative scores (e.g., kilograms lifted per kilogram of body weight) can be compared during repeated testing.

Muscular Strength

Muscular strength refers to the maximal force that can be generated by a specific muscle or muscle group. Isometric or static strength (constant muscle length during muscle activation) can be measured conveniently with a variety of devices, including cable tensiometers and handgrip dynamometers, which measure strength at one specific point in the range of motion. These tests and devices occasionally are used in research and academic settings but are not used routinely by most health and fitness practitioners. Thus, the procedures for these tests are described in detail elsewhere (5, 16). **Isokinetic testing** involves the assessment of maximal muscle tension throughout a range of joint motion at a constant angular velocity (e.g., $60° \cdot sec^{-1}$). Isokinetic testing devices measure peak rotational force, or torque, and data are obtained with specialized equipment that allows the tester to control the speed of rotation (degrees per second) around various joints (e.g., knee, hip, shoulder, elbow). Although the data collected from isokinetic strength assessments may be useful to health and fitness professionals, the necessary computerized equipment is expensive and therefore limits isokinetic testing almost entirely to rehabilitation and research settings. Consequently, isokinetic strength evaluations may not be a practical consideration for most health and fitness practitioners.

The most common type of strength assessment performed by fitness professionals is **dynamic testing,** which involves movement of the body (e.g., push-up) or an external load (e.g., bench press). Dynamic testing is typically inexpensive because it does not require sophisticated or specialized equipment. Moreover, dynamic assessments can be performed with different types of equipment, such as free weights (barbells and dumbbells) or weight-stack machines, and can test any major muscle or muscle group through a variety of different exercises.

Components of Muscular Fitness Related to Promoting or Maintaining Good Health, Fitness, and Athletic Performance (3)

Health Aspects of Muscular Fitness

- Preservation or enhancement of fat-free mass and resting metabolic rate
- Preservation or enhancement of bone mass with aging
- Improved glucose tolerance and insulin sensitivity
- Reduced HR and BP response while lifting any submaximal load (which reduces myocardial oxygen demand during activities requiring muscular force)
- Lowered risk of musculoskeletal injury, including low-back pain
- Improved ability to carry out activities of daily living in older age
- Improved balance and decreased risk of falls in older age
- Improved self-esteem

Performance Aspects of Muscular Fitness

- Enhanced muscular strength and muscular endurance
- Enhanced speed, power, agility, and balance
- Reduced risk for musculoskeletal injuries
- Improved body composition for various events or activities
- Improved confidence for performing certain athletic events and activities involving high levels of muscular fitness
- Enhanced performance in most athletic activities

Key Point

Muscular strength is best assessed by using a resistance that requires maximum or near-maximum tension with few repetitions, whereas local muscular endurance is assessed by using lighter resistance with a greater number of repetitions. In either case, muscular fitness can be assessed safely in the health and fitness setting and provides important information for individualized exercise prescription. An ideal application of these tests is to evaluate changes in muscular fitness over time using standardized testing procedures that ensure valid and reproducible results.

Exercises typically used for dynamic strength testing in fitness centers include the bench press, lat pull-down, and leg press.

Repetition Maximum Testing

The gold standard of dynamic strength testing is the **1-repetition maximum (1RM),** the heaviest weight that can be lifted only once using good form. Peak force development in such tests commonly is referred to as the **maximum voluntary contraction (MVC).** In general, 1RM tests are good indicators of strength and can be performed safely in the health and fitness setting with qualified supervision, for example, by fitness professionals who adhere to current guidelines of exercise leadership such as those described in this chapter and previously by the ACSM (3). Multiple RM tests that involve 8 to 12 repetitions can also safely and effectively assess strength in adults who are apparently healthy or have controlled chronic disease conditions (26). Moreover, when the purpose of testing is to define an initial training load, a multiple RM testing procedure minimizes the potential error compared with extrapolating the exercise intensity as a percentage of a 1RM. For example, the maximum weight a person can lift 10 times during testing can be used to identify an appropriate weight load for this number of repetitions performed during training and provides an index of strength changes over time, independent of the true 1RM. The procedures used to assess 1RM can be modified to test any given number of repetitions (e.g., 10RM).

Procedures for 1RM Testing

1. The subject performs a light warm-up of 5 to 10 repetitions at 40% to 60% of perceived maximum (e.g., light to moderate exertion).
2. After a 1 min rest with light stretching, the subject performs 3 to 5 repetitions at 60% to 80% of perceived maximum (e.g., moderate to hard exertion).
3. The subject attempts a 1RM lift. If the lift is successful, the subject rests 3 to 5 min.

   The goal is to find the 1RM within 3 to 5 maximal efforts. The process of increasing the weight to a true 1RM can be improved by familiarization sessions that approximate the 1RM. This process is continued until a failed attempt occurs.
4. The 1RM is reported as the weight of the last successfully completed lift.

Adapted from W. Kraemer and A. Fry, 1995, Strength testing development and evaluation of methodology. In *Physiological assessments of human fitness*, edited by P.J. Maud and C. Foster (Champaign, IL: Human Kinetics), 115-138. (21).

Interpreting Results

For comparing strength assessments of individuals who differ in body mass, such as when comparing men and women, it is best to express strength as a ratio of weight lifted during a single or multiple RM test relative to body weight. The following procedure describes how to determine a strength ratio from a 10RM test (21):

1. Determine the heaviest weight the client can lift for 10 good repetitions (10RM weight load).
2. Convert the 10RM weight load to a 1RM estimation by dividing the weight load by 0.75.
3. Divide the estimated 1RM by the client's body weight to obtain the strength ratio.

For example, a client who weighs 140 lb (63.5 kg) and completes 10 leg presses with 120 lb (54.4 kg) has an estimated 1RM of 120 ÷ 0.75, or 160 lb (72.6 kg). Her leg press weight ratio is 1.14 (160 ÷ 140).

Normative Data

Normative strength scores such as lower- or upper-body strength ratios for different age and sex categories have been published in *ACSM's Guidelines for Exercise Testing and Prescription* (4). However, most normative data to date have been derived from a relatively homogeneous sample of subjects (mostly middle- to upper-class Caucasians) using only certain types of resistance training equipment, which limits interpretation of test scores. For example, because equipment design can vary significantly from one manufacturer to another and because of inherent differences in using free weights versus machine weights, strength scores can vary widely with using different testing equipment. Thus, individual client scores can only be compared to norms generated from tests performed with the same type of equipment. Future research is needed to provide norms for different types of resistance training equipment as well as norms for diverse races, ethnicities, and age groups.

Comparing Pretraining and Posttraining

Often, the primary purpose of a muscular fitness test is to evaluate changes in strength over the course of a fitness program. Periodic muscle fitness testing is particularly appealing because it eliminates the need to compare individual data with data provided in normative tables. The frequency of follow-up testing depends on the quality and quantity of exercise training by the client as well as the client's desire and staff availability. When multiple tests are performed over time, useful feedback to the client should include the percentage improvement of strength or endurance (i.e., by dividing the pretraining score by posttraining score and multiplying by 100) and recommendations for improving or maintaining muscular fitness based on the client's individualized goals. For example, if Mrs. Smith performs a 10RM baseline of 40 lb (18.1 kg) on the chest press and improves to 60 lb (27.2 kg) during follow-up testing, she has demonstrated a 50% strength gain ([60 – 40 ÷ 40] · 100%) on that lift. This information can provide positive reinforcement about the efficacy of the training program. In cases when the client does not improve, recommendations for altering the exercise program can be made based on the client's individualized goals.

Local Muscular Endurance

Local muscular endurance, also called *local muscle endurance,* is the ability of a muscle group to repeatedly contract over a time long enough to cause muscular fatigue or to maintain a specific percentage of the maximum voluntary contraction for a prolonged time (4). Equipment (e.g., free weights or machines) for measuring strength can be used to assess local muscular endurance. In addition, simple field tests such as an abdominal curl-up (crunch) test (10, 12) or the maximum number of push-ups that can be performed without rest (8) can be used to evaluate the endurance of the abdominal or upper-body muscles. These field tests can be used either independently or in combination with other methods of strength or endurance assessment such as RM testing. Tests such as the abdominal curl-up or the push-up can screen for muscle weaknesses related to various health indicators. For example, scientific data suggest that poor abdominal strength or endurance predisposes muscular low-back pain and that the curl-up test can help identify individuals with abdominal strength or endurance weakness that may contribute to low-back pain (4, 19). Moreover, the muscles of the upper body, such as those tested by the push-up, are used in many daily activities such as raking or gardening, carrying luggage, or painting. Thus, these tests are a practical way to evaluate a client's muscular fitness and to provide useful feedback to the client about how muscular conditioning, or deconditioning, affects many common activities.

Push-Up and Curl-Up Tests

The procedures used to perform the push-up and curl-up tests as described by the ACSM are presented on page 124 and shown in figures 8.2 and 8.3 (push-up test) and 8.4 (curl-up test). The push-up test evaluates local muscular endurance of the upper body, including the triceps, anterior deltoid, and pectoral muscles. There are two standard push-up positions: one with the hands and toes in contact with the floor and the other with the hands and knees in contact with the floor (the modified push-up position). The procedures for administering the test are similar and either position may be used for men or women since the position should be based on strength and not on gender. However, the norms for the standard push-up are for men and the norms for the modified push-up are for women. When women perform the standard push-up and men the modified push-up, pre- and posttraining scores can be compared to evaluate improvement over time.

The bent-knee curl-up test evaluates abdominal muscle endurance. Full sit-up tests are unsatisfactory because hip flexor involvement during the sit-up motion may harm the low back (see chapter 9). Even though the traditional sit-up has been modified, as it is in the bent-knee position, the low back is still stressed during the motion. Consequently, the bent-knee curl-up test recently was modified to reduce the potential for low-back injury and to better assess abdominal muscle function (10).

Both the push-up and curl-up tests are relatively simple, inexpensive methods for assessing muscular endurance, and both can be used for men and women of various ages. Results of the standard push-up test for men and modified push-up test for women and curl-up tests for men and women can be compared with the standards in tables 8.1 and 8.2. As with RM testing, the push-up and curl-up tests can be performed serially to reliably assess changes in muscular endurance that occur with training. Finally, very deconditioned individuals, especially those who are overweight or obese, may find these tests difficult to perform. In such cases, poor results obtained during testing may discourage individuals from exercise participation. Thus, for each participant, the fitness professional must carefully consider whether these tests are appropriate and likely to yield useful information.

YMCA Bench Press Test

There are alternatives to the push-up and curl-up tests. The fitness professional can adapt resistance training equipment to measure muscular endurance by selecting an appropriate submaximal level of resistance and measuring the number of repetitions or the duration of static contraction before fatigue. For example, the YMCA bench press test involves performing standardized repetitions at a rate of 30 lifts · min^{-1} to test muscular endurance of the upper body (15). Men use an 80 lb (36.3 kg) barbell and women use a 35 lb (15.9 kg) barbell, and subjects are scored by the number of successful repetitions completed. The main disadvantage of the test is that it uses a fixed weight, which favors heavier clients over lighter clients. Also, the fixed weight may be too heavy for deconditioned or older clients to lift repeatedly. On the other hand, the load may be too light for very fit individuals, who may perform significantly more repetitions than typically used during training.

Despite these limitations, this test can be used independently or in combination with other tests in the overall

Push-Up and Curl-Up (Crunch) Test Procedures

Push-Up

1. Explain the purpose of the test to the client (to determine how many push-ups can be completed to reflect upper-body muscular strength and endurance).
2. Inform clients of proper breathing technique (to exhale with the effort, which occurs when pushing away from the floor).
3. The push-up test usually is administered with male subjects in the up position with hands shoulder-width apart, back straight, and head up, using the toes as the pivotal point. For female subjects, the modified knee push-up position often is used, with legs together, lower leg in contact with mat, ankles plantar flexed, back straight, hands shoulder width-apart, and head up. (Note: Some males will need to use the modified position, and some females can use the full body position).
4. The subject must lower the body until the chin touches the mat or until the chest touches the fist of the examiner. The stomach should not touch the mat.
5. For both men and women, the subject's back must be straight at all times and the subject must push up to a straight-arm position.
6. Demonstrate the test and allow clients to practice if desired.
7. Remind the client that a brief rest is allowed only in the up position.
8. Begin the test when the client is ready, and count the total number of push-ups the client completes before reaching the point of exhaustion.
9. The client's score is the total number of push-ups performed.

Curl-Up (Crunch)

1. Explain the purpose of the test to the client (to determine how many curl-ups can be completed to reflect abdominal muscular strength and endurance).
2. Explain proper breathing technique (to exhale with the effort, which occurs when curling up from the floor).
3. Have the individual assume a supine position on a mat, with the knees at 90°. The arms are at the side, with the tips of the fingers touching a piece of masking tape. A second piece of masking tape is placed 8 cm (for those who are ≥45 yr) or 12 cm (for those who are <45 yr) beyond the first. Clients slide arms along floor as they curl up, and stop the curl-up when their fingers reach the second piece of tape.*
4. Set a metronome to 40 beats · min^{-1}. Instruct the individual to perform slow, controlled curl-ups to lift the shoulder blades off the mat (the trunk makes a 30° angle with the mat) in time with the metronome (20 curl-ups · min^{-1}). The low back should be flattened before curling up.
5. Demonstrate the test and allow the client to practice if desired.
6. Have the individual perform as many curl-ups as possible without pausing, up to a maximum of 75.**

*Alternatives include (a) holding the hands across the chest and counting when the trunk reaches a 30° position and (b) placing the hands on the thighs and curling up until the hands reach the kneecaps. Elevating the trunk to 30° is the important aspect of the movement.

**An alternative includes doing as many curl-ups as possible in 1 min.

Descriptions of procedures are adapted from American College of Sports Medicine (ACSM), 2006, *ACSM's guidelines for exercise testing and prescription*, 7th ed. (Philadelphia, PA: Lippincott, Williams & Wilkins). (4).

assessment of muscular fitness. The procedures for this test are summarized next, and norms are shown in tables 8.3a and b.

1. Use a 35 lb (15.9 kg) straight barbell for women or an 80 lb (36.3 kg) straight barbell for men. A spotter should be present during the test.
2. Set a metronome to 60 beats · min^{-1}
3. Have the individual begin with the bar in the down position touching the chest, with the elbows flexed and hands shoulder-width apart.
4. Count 1 repetition when the elbows fully extend. After each extension, the participant should lower the bar to touch the chest.
5. Instruct the client to complete up or down movements in time to the 60 beats · min^{-1} rhythm, which should be 30 lifts per minute.
6. Count the total number of repetitions completed in good form.

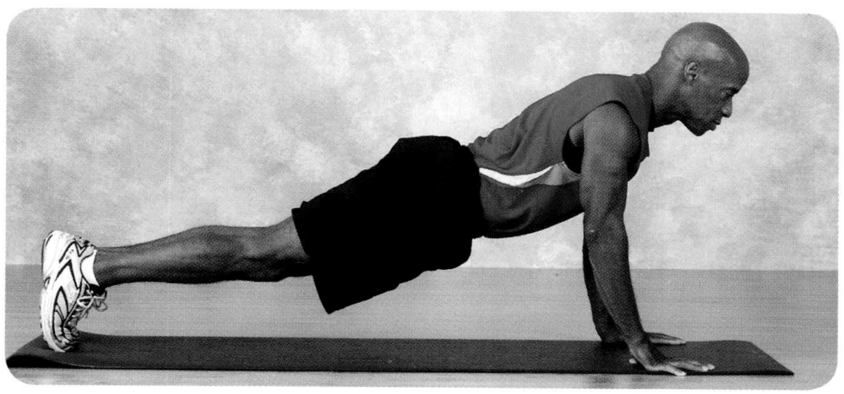

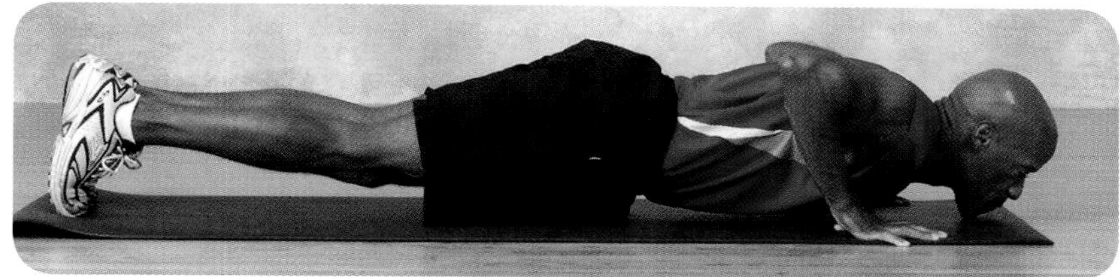

Figure 8.2 Proper form for the *(a)* starting position and *(b)* finishing position of the standard push-up test, as described by the ACSM (4).

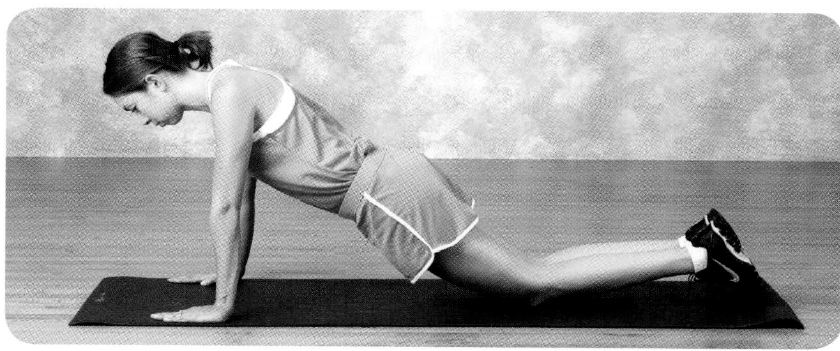

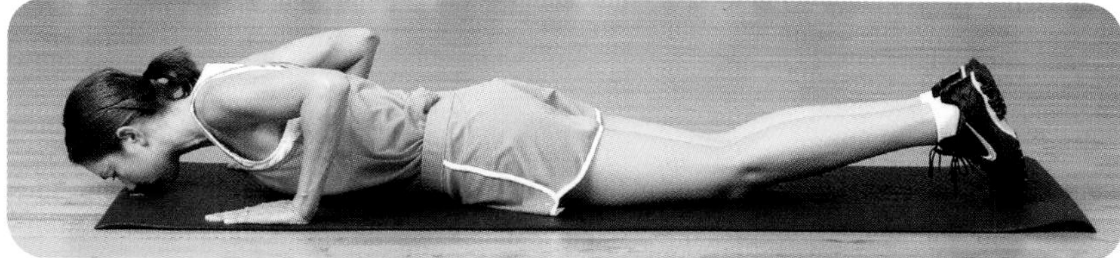

Figure 8.3 Proper form for the *(a)* starting position and *(b)* finishing position of the modified push-up test, as described by the ACSM (4).

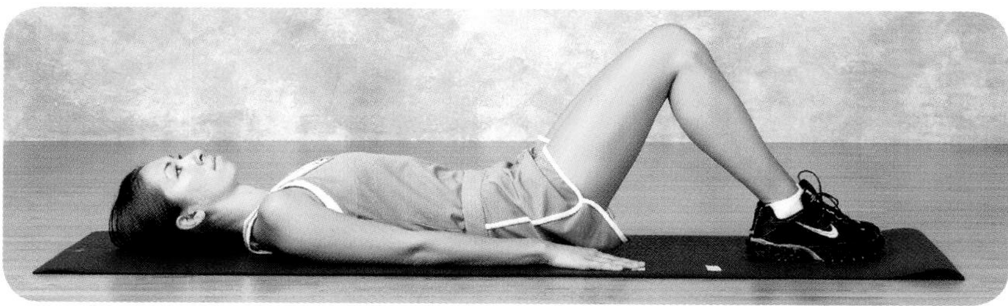

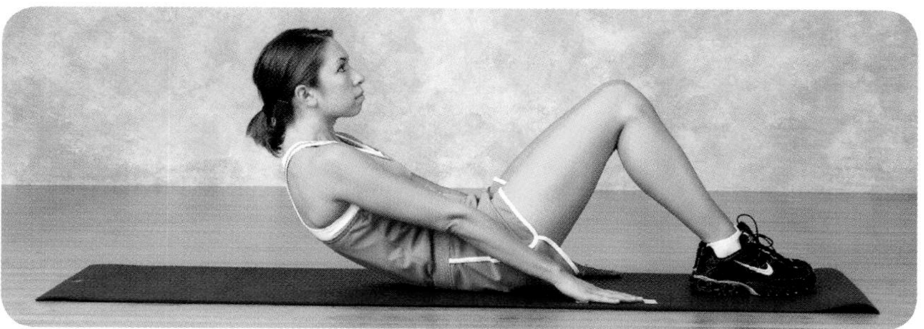

Figure 8.4 Proper form for the *(a)* starting position and *(b)* finishing position of the abdominal curl-up test, as described by the ACSM (4).

Table 8.1 Push-Up Norms for Men and Women by Age Groups Using Number Completed

	Age (yr)											
	(15-19)		(20-29)		(30-39)		(40-49)		(50-59)		(60-69)	
Fitness	**M**	**F**	**M**	**F**	**M**	**F**	**M**	**F**	**M**	**F**	**M**	**F**
Excellent	>39	>33	>36	>30	>30	>27	>22	>24	>21	>21	>18	>17
Above average	29-38	25-32	29-35	21-29	22-29	20-26	17-21	15-23	13-20	11-20	11-17	12-16
Average	23-28	18-24	22-28	15-20	17-21	13-19	13-16	11-14	10-12	7-10	8-10	5-11
Below average	18-22	12-17	17-21	10-14	12-16	8-12	10-12	5-10	7-9	2-6	5-7	1-4
Poor	<17	<11	<16	<9	<11	<7	<9	<4	<6	<1	<4	<1

The Canadian Standardized Test of Fitness was developed by and is reproduced with permission of the Government of Canada, Fitness and Amateur Sport (8).

Source: *Canadian Standardized Test of Fitness Operations Manual*, 3rd ed, Health Canada, 1986. Reproduced with permission from the Minister of Public Works and Government Services Canada, 2006.

Table 8.2 Curl-Up Norms by Age Group Using Number Completed

	Men			Women		
Fitness	**<35 yr**	**35-44 yr**	**45 yr**	**<35 yr**	**35-44 yr**	**45 yr**
Excellent	60	50	40	50	40	30
Good	45	40	25	40	30	15
Marginal	30	25	15	25	15	10
Needs work	15	10	5	10	6	4

From R.A. Faulkner, E.S. Springings, A. McQuarrie and R.D. Bell, 1989, "A partial curl-up protocol for adults based on an analysis of two procedures," *Canadian Journal of Sports Science* 14: 135-141. (12).

Table 8.3a YMCA Bench Press Norms for Number of Repetitions Completed for Men Using 80 Lb (36.3 kg)

	Age (yr)					
Fitness	**16-25**	**26-35**	**36-45**	**46-55**	**56-65**	**66+**
Excellent	>37	>33	>29	>23	>21	>17
Good	29-37	26-33	23-29	19-23	14-21	10-17
Above average	24-28	22-25	19-22	14-18	10-13	8-9
Average	21-23	18-21	15-18	10-13	7-9	5-7
Below average	15-20	13-17	11-14	7-9	4-6	3-4
Poor	9-14	6-12	6-10	3-6	1-3	1-2
Very poor	<9	<6	<6	<3	<1	0

Adapted from L.A. Golding, C.R. Myers and W.E. Sinning, 1989, *The Y's way to physical fitness*, 3rd ed. (Champaign, IL: Human Kinetics).

Key Point

The most common type of muscle fitness assessment in the fitness setting is dynamic strength testing with a single or multiple repetition maximum protocol. Although lack of adequate normative data often limits the evaluation of individual test data, such tests are valuable for tracking strength and endurance improvement. Field tests such as the push-up and abdominal curl-up tests provide a practical approach for evaluating muscular fitness, either alone or together with other types of muscular fitness evaluations.

Table 8.3b YMCA Bench Press Norms for Number of Repetitions Completed for Women Using 35 Lb (15.9 kg)

	Age (yr)					
Fitness	16-25	26-35	36-45	46-55	56-65	65+
Excellent	>35	>32	>27	>25	>21	>17
Good	27-35	24-32	21-27	19-25	16-21	12-17
Above average	22-26	19-23	16-20	13-18	11-15	9-11
Average	17-21	15-18	12-15	10-12	8-10	5-8
Below average	13-16	11-14	9-11	6-9	4-7	2-4
Poor	7-12	4-10	3-8	2-5	1-3	0-1
Very poor	<7	<4	<3	<2	0	0

Adapted from L.A. Golding, C.R. Myers and W.E. Sinning, 1989, *The Y's way to physical fitness*, 3rd ed. (Champaign, IL: Human Kinetics).

Testing Older Adults

The number of older adults in the United States is expected to increase exponentially over the next several decades. For instance, in 1990 there were 31.2 million U.S. adults (13%) aged 65 or older, but this number is expected to more than double to 70.3 million (20%) by the year 2030 (24). Because people are living longer, it is becoming increasingly important to find ways to extend active, healthy lifestyles and to reduce physical frailty in later years (2, 22). Assessing muscular strength and local muscular endurance as well as other aspects of physical fitness in older adults can reveal physical weaknesses and be used to design exercise programs that improve strength before serious functional limitations occur.

Senior Fitness Test

In response to the need for improved assessment for older adults, Rikli and Jones (28) developed a functional fitness test battery, the Senior Fitness Test (SFT). This test evaluates the key physiological parameters (e.g., strength, endurance, agility, and balance) needed to perform common everyday physical activities that are often difficult in later years. One aspect of the SFT is the 30 sec chair stand test (see Research Insight on page 128). This test, as well as others of the SFT, meets scientific standards for reliability and validity, is simple and easy to administer in the field setting, and has accompanying performance norms for men and women aged 60 to 94 based on a study of more than 7,000 older Americans (27). This test has been shown to correlate well with other strength tests such as the 1RM. The fitness professional can use the SFT to safely and effectively assess muscular strength and endurance in most older adults.

Assessing Muscular Fitness With the SFT

Before testing, all participants should warm up and follow other preliminary procedures as described earlier. In addition, for both the chair stand and arm curl test, the following instruction is recommended as a standardization procedure for administering tests on all clients:

> *Do the best you can on each test item but never push yourself to a point of overexertion or beyond what you think is safe for you.*

30 Sec Chair Stand Test

The 30 sec chair stand test, which reflects lower-body strength, involves counting the number of times within 30 sec that an individual can rise to a full stand from a seated position without pushing off with the arms (figure 8.5). Studies have shown that chair stand performance, a common method of assessing lower-body strength in older adults, correlates well with major criterion indicators of lower-body strength (e.g., isokinetic measured knee extensor and knee flexor strength), stair-climbing ability, walking speed, and risk of falling (6) and has been found to detect normal age-related declines in strength (9). Further, the chair stand has been found to be safe and sensitive in detecting the effects of physical training in older adults (17, 23). Table 8.4 summarizes the normal range of scores of participants ages 60 to 94. The normal range is defined as the middle 50% of the population tested for each age group, with the lower limits being equivalent to the 25th percentile rank and the upper limits equivalent to the 75th percentile rank within each 5 yr age group.

Single-Arm Curl Test

Upper-body function, including arm strength and local muscular endurance, is important in executing many

Research Insight

Measuring lower-body strength is critical in evaluating the functional performance of older adults. Jones, Rikli, and Beam's 1999 study (20) assessed the test–retest reliability and validity of a 30 sec chair stand as a measure of lower-body strength in adults over the age of 60. Seventy-six community-dwelling older adults (mean age = 70.5 yr) volunteered to participate in the study, which involved performing two 30 sec chair stand tests and two maximum leg press tests, each conducted on separate days 2 to 5 days apart. Test–retest interclass correlations of .84 for men and .92 for women, together with a nonsignificant change in scores from day 1 to day 2, indicated that the 30 sec chair stand has good stability reliability. A moderately high correlation between chair stand performance and maximum weight-adjusted leg press performance for both men and women ($r = .78$ and .71, respectively) supports the criterion-related validity of the chair stand as a measure of lower-body strength. Construct (or discriminant) validity of the chair stand was demonstrated by the ability of the test to detect differences among groups of various age and physical activity level. As expected, chair stand performance decreased significantly across age groups in decades—from the 60s to the 70s to the 80s ($p < .01$)—and was significantly lower for participants who were less active than for participants who were highly active ($p < .0001$). It was concluded that the 30 sec chair stand provides a reliable and valid indicator of lower-body strength in generally active, community-dwelling older adults.

normal everyday activities such as carrying groceries, lifting a suitcase, and picking up grandchildren (24). The 30 sec arm curl test, a measure of upper-body strength and endurance, determines the number of times a dumbbell (5 lb, or 2.3 kg, for women and 8 lb, or 3.6 kg, for men) can be curled through a full ROM in 30 sec. The prescribed protocol includes holding the weight in a handshake grip at full extension (to the side of the chair) and then supinating during flexion so that the palm of the hand faces the biceps at full flexion (figure 8.6). Results of studies indicate that the 30 sec arm curl test is a good predictor of both biceps strength and overall upper-body strength (27). Most participants, including those with arthritis, were able to perform the arm curl test without much discomfort and were less bothered performing the arm curl test described here than the maximum grip strength protocol commonly used as a strength measure in other studies (27). Results obtained from the 30 sec arm curl test can be compared with the norms presented in table 8.4.

Testing Clients With Coronary Heart Disease

Moderate resistance training performed just 2 days per wk improves muscular fitness, prevents and manages a variety of chronic medical conditions, modifies coronary risk factors, and enhances psychosocial well-being for persons with and without coronary heart disease (CHD) (14). Resistance training could benefit the majority of the approximately 13.5 million people in the United States living with CHD, because many cardiac patients lack the physical strength and self-confidence to perform common daily activities that require muscular effort (26). Consequently, authoritative professional health organizations including the AHA (26), the ACSM (4), and the AACPR (1) support resistance training as an adjunct to endurance exercise in their current recommendations and guidelines on exercise for individuals with cardiovascular disease. Resistance training is also recommended in the evidence-based clinical practice guidelines on cardiac rehabilitation (29).

Both moderate- or high-intensity (e.g., 40%-80% 1RM) resistance testing and training can be performed safely by cardiac patients deemed low risk (e.g., patients with absence of angina or serious ventricular arrhythmias during normal activities, with good left ventricular function, and with good exercise capacity) (26). Moreover, despite concerns that resistance exercise elicits abnormal cardiovascular pressor responses in patients with CHD or controlled hypertension, studies have found that strength tests and resistance training in these patients elicit clinically acceptable HR and BP responses (11, 25). Specific data on the benefits and safety of resistance training in women with CHD and patients with poor left ventricular function, such as those with congestive heart failure, are limited, and these areas require additional investigation. Contemporary exercise guidelines suggest that patients with uncontrolled hypertension (>160/90 mmHg), unstable angina pectoris, uncompensated congestive heart failure, poor left ventricular function (ejection fraction < 30%), abnormal hemodynamic responses during a clinical exercise test, severe orthopedic limitations, or uncontrolled metabolic diseases (e.g., uncontrolled diabetes or thyroid disease) should not undergo strength testing or training until their clinical status improves or stabilizes and until they receive appropriate medical clearance (26).

As with graded exercise testing, the risk of a serious cardiac event during strength testing can be minimized by proper preparticipation screening and close supervision by fitness professionals. When testing patients with

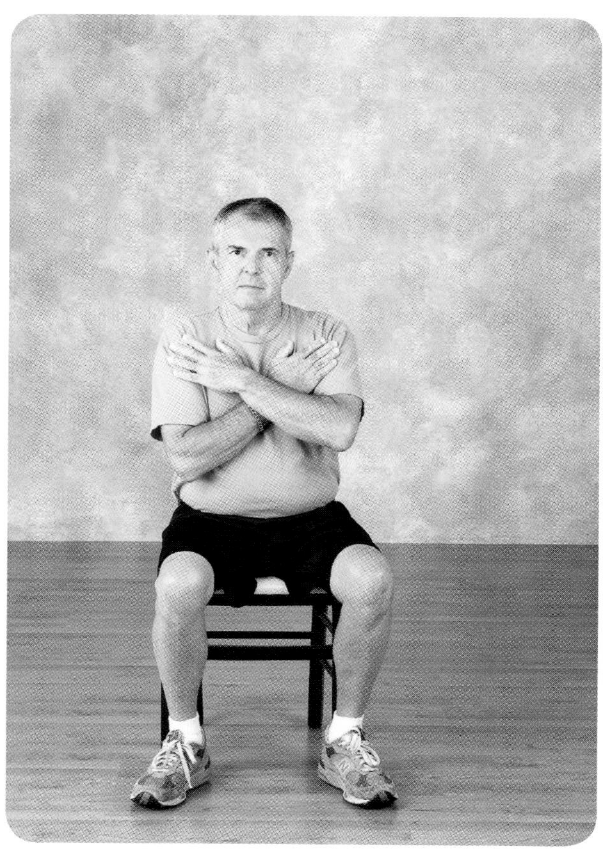
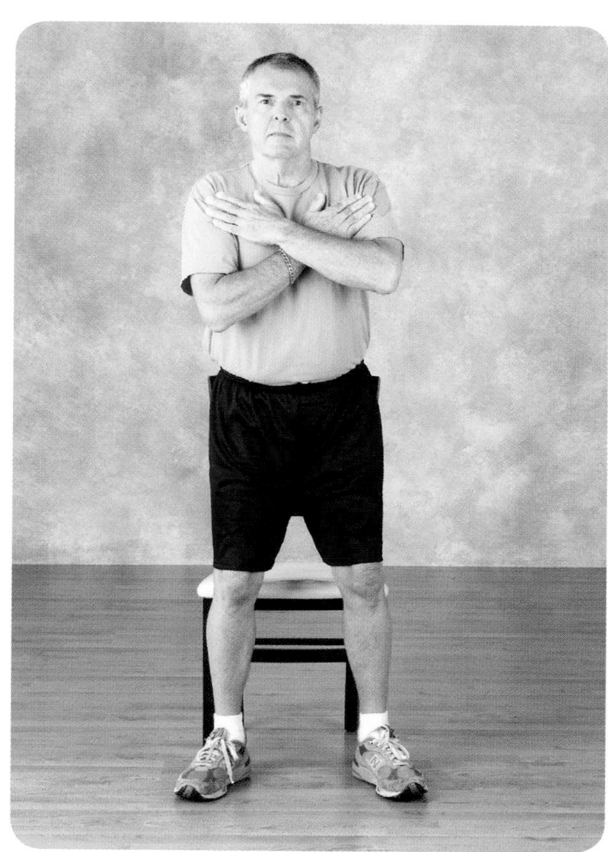

Figure 8.5 The 30 sec chair stand test (28).

Table 8.4 Normal Range of Scores on the 30 Sec Chair Stand and 30 Sec Arm Curl Tests for Older Adults

	Age (yr)						
	60-64	65-69	70-74	75-79	80-84	85-89	90-94
Chair stand (# of stands)							
Women	12-17	11-16	10-15	10-15	9-14	8-13	4-11
Men	14-19	12-18	12-17	11-17	10-15	8-14	7-12
Arm curl (# of reps)							
Women	13-19	12-18	12-17	11-17	10-16	10-15	8-13
Men	16-22	15-21	14-21	13-19	13-19	11-17	10-17

Normal is defined as the middle 50% of the population. Participants scoring above or below these ranges would be considered above normal or below normal for their age.

Reprinted, by permission, from R.E. Rikli and C.J. Jones, 2001, *Senior fitness test manual* (Champaign, IL: Human Kinetics), 143.

known or suspected CHD or hypertension, the fitness professional should do preliminary work to establish appropriate weight loads and instruct the participant on proper lifting techniques. This should include demonstrating proper ROM and speed of movement for each exercise as well as correct breathing patterns to avoid the Valsalva maneuver. The monitoring of resting and recovery BPs (e.g., every 1-3 min) and identification

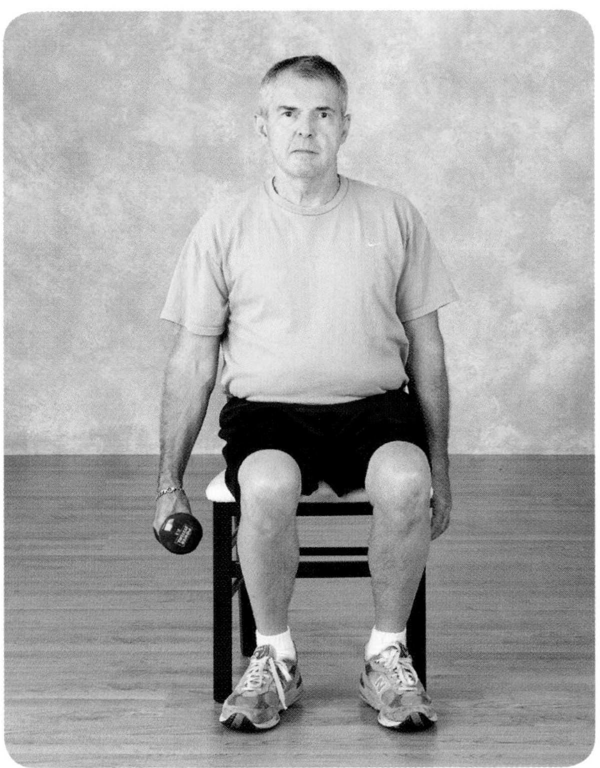

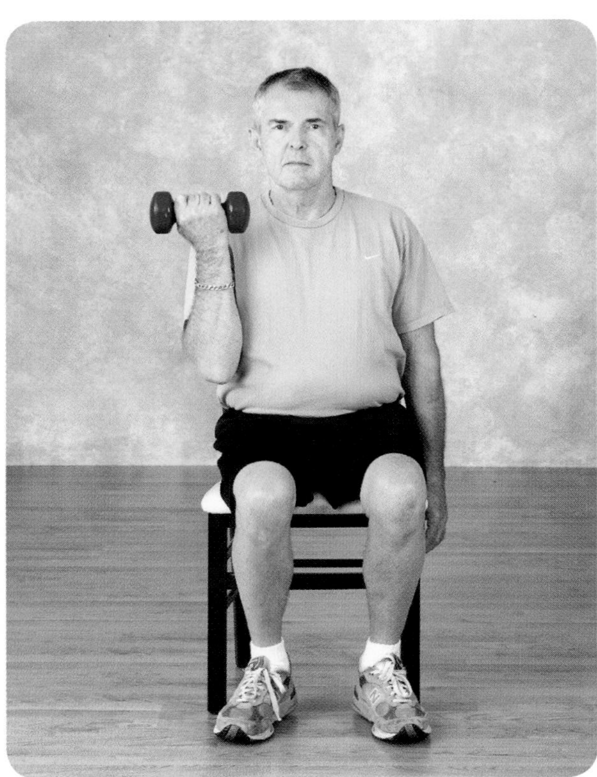

Figure 8.6 The 30 sec arm curl test (28).

and evaluation of abnormal signs and symptoms should be standard protocol during the initial evaluation of the cardiovascular response during testing. Exaggerated BP responses, clinical signs or symptoms of CHD, or any other abnormal findings as previously described by the ACSM that occur during resistance testing or training indicate to terminate the activity until further evaluation by a qualified health care provider (4). Because BP measured immediately postexercise tends to underestimate values during contractions, the fitness professional should act conservatively when evaluating the cardiovascular responses to testing in this population (13, 18).

Studies thus far have shown no adverse hemodynamic responses in low-risk cardiac patients who perform 1RM or multiple RM testing for upper- and lower-body exercises (11, 13). Moreover, there is no scientific evidence suggesting that 1RM testing is riskier than 10RM testing for low-risk cardiac patients. However, multiple repetition testing (e.g., 5RM or 10RM) is a more conservative and, therefore, sensible approach to testing clients with a history of cardiovascular disease. Regardless of the number of repetitions used during testing, the initial resistance or weight should be moderate to allow the participant to achieve the proper repetition range by working at a level that is somewhat hard (e.g., 13-15 on Borg's original RPE scale; see chapter 5) (7). Furthermore, the strength assessment procedures previously described in this chapter can be applied safely to clients with a history of known or occult CHD who are clinically stable and to clients with controlled hypertension, diabetes, or otherwise deemed higher cardiovascular risk. Careful screening and astute monitoring of abnormal signs or symptoms, such as angina, dizziness, or light-headedness, are paramount to minimize any potential risks while simultaneously maximizing the benefits of resistance testing or training for persons with and without known cardiovascular disease.

Testing Children and Adolescents

Along with cardiorespiratory fitness, flexibility, and body composition, muscular strength is an important component of health-related fitness in children and adolescents. Enhancing muscular strength helps young people develop proper posture, reduce the risk of injury, improve body composition, and enhance motor skills such as sprinting and jumping. Assessing muscular strength and local muscular endurance with the push-up and abdominal curl-up is common in most physical education programs, YMCA and YWCA recreation programs, and youth sport centers.

Standardized testing procedures have been developed for young people, and normative data for children and teenagers are available in most physical education textbooks. When properly administered, different fitness measures can be used to assess a child's strength and weaknesses, develop a personalized fitness program, track progress, and motivate participants. Conversely, unsupervised or poorly administered strength assessments may not only discourage young people from participating in fitness activities but also result in injury. Qualified fitness professionals should demonstrate how to properly perform each skill, allow each child to practice a few repetitions of each skill, and offer guidance and instruction when necessary. In addition, it is important and usually required to obtain informed consent from the parent or legal guardian before initiating muscular fitness testing or a formalized exercise program for children. The informed consent explains potential benefits and risks of resistance testing or training, the right to withdraw at any time, and issues regarding confidentiality.

When assessing fitness in young people, avoid the pass–fail mentality that may discourage some boys and girls from participating. Instead, refer to the assessment as a *challenge* in which all participants can feel good about their performance and get excited about monitoring their progress. Fitness professionals should also understand that children are not simply miniature adults. Since children are physically and psychologically less mature than adults, so evaluating any measure of physical fitness requires special considerations. Fitness professionals should develop a friendly rapport with each child, and the exercise area should be nonthreatening. Since most children have limited experience performing at maximum exertion, fitness professionals should reassure children that they can safely perform exercise at a high exertion. Moreover, positive encouragement can motivate children to help ensure a valid test outcome. Following the strength assessment, cool down afterward with gentle calisthenics and stretching exercises.

Key Point

Muscular fitness testing is useful for a variety of special populations including older adults, individuals at increased cardiovascular risk, and children and adolescents. While strength tests, particularly those involving maximal exertion, were once thought to evoke unsafe physiological responses in these populations, scientific evidence now supports the conclusion that such tests are safe and can provide valuable information for the resistance training prescription if properly administered and performed. For older adults and people at elevated cardiovascular risk, proper screening by a physician or other qualified health care professional is warranted to promote safe and effective muscular fitness evaluations.

Case Studies

Answers to questions 1 and 2 can be found in the tables and figures presented in this chapter. See details in the chapter for question 3.

A middle-aged female who recently joined your fitness facility would like to participate in an initial fitness assessment and receive advice about beginning an overall fitness program. She has not participated in a structured exercise program for several years, although she reports that she leads an active lifestyle that often includes accumulating moderate amounts of daily physical activity. Her preparticipation health history questionnaire reveals that she is without signs, symptoms, or diagnosis of any cardiovascular, metabolic, or musculoskeletal condition. With a classmate playing the role of this client, practice the procedures presented in this chapter:

1. Explain, demonstrate, and perform the procedures for one muscular strength test for the upper body and one for the lower body.
2. Explain, demonstrate, and perform the procedures for a muscular endurance test used to evaluate the abdominal muscles and for a test used in evaluating the upper body.
3. Explain the results of the tests performed in 1 and 2 to your client. Where appropriate, give specific reference to her level of muscular fitness and implications for subsequent training.

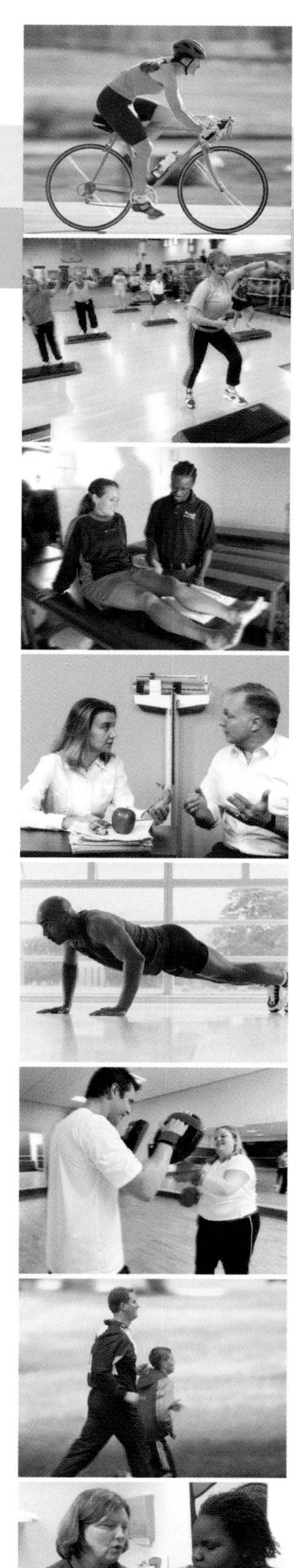

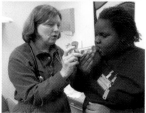

9 CHAPTER

Flexibility and Low-Back Function

Wendell Liemohn

Objectives

The reader will be able to do the following:

1. Describe the relationship between flexibility or range of motion (ROM) and low-back function.
2. List five factors that can affect an individual's flexibility or ROM.
3. Describe the amount of flexion that can occur between the rib cage and the sacrum and state a general rule for performing lumbar extension exercises.
4. Explain why having good ROM at the hip joint is important to having a healthy back.
5. Describe the pros and cons of the sit-and-reach test.

Flexibility relates to the ability to bend without breaking; **flexion** is the act of bending or being bent. In applied anatomy, *flexion* denotes a bending movement that occurs in the sagittal plane as two body segments are brought together (see chapter 27). When you bend over and touch your toes from the standing position, you demonstrate flexion at both iliofemoral (hip) joints and limited flexion in the lower intervertebral joints of the spine.[1] When you return to the standing position, the movement is called *extension;* moving the trunk further backward, beyond your normal standing posture, is called *hyperextension* (see chapter 27). Individuals may be called flexible if they can show an extreme amount of mobility in either forward bending (i.e., flexion) or backward bending (i.e., hyperextension) because both movements meet the criteria for the definition of flexion. Because there is potential confusion in describing a person's ability to hyperextend as flexibility, the term *range of motion (ROM)* frequently is used in place of *flexibility.* The two terms, however, often are interchanged.

Having functional ROM at all joints of the musculoskeletal system ensures efficient body movement; this is one reason why flexibility is a key component of physical fitness. Although some people might be considered to have very good ROM because they performed well in a flexibility test, flexibility is considered a joint-specific characteristic. In other words, having good ROM in trunk flexion does not guarantee having good ROM in trunk extension. Moreover, sometimes ROM relates to a person's genotype (i.e., is hereditary). In other cases, ROM relates more to the person's activities. For example, many years of ballet or gymnastics training should make a person more flexible than someone of the same age, same sex, and comparable genotype who did not participate in such training. Natural selection can also be a factor. A person without good innate flexibility might not strive to do well in ballet or gymnastics.

If the body is viewed as a kinetic chain, any asymmetrical tightness or looseness in the joints of the lower extremities could affect the spine. Good ROM is also usually considered desirable for low-back function. ROM at the hip joint is of particular concern because the position of the sacrum (and contiguous pelvis) is the foundation for the spine, and this position is controlled by muscles originating on the pelvis or spine and inserting on the femur. ROM of the spine itself is typically not viewed as problematic; however, too much mobility can contribute to instability. For example, if a disc and its supporting ligaments were damaged and the person's ability to control the supporting muscles was insufficient, further injury to the spine could occur. (Motor control issues of the spine are discussed further in chapter 13.)

Key Point

Flexibility and ROM are joint specific. Having good ROM at the hip joint can decrease the chances of having a low-back problem. Once a low-back problem has occurred, increasing ROM at the hip joint may be a goal in a therapeutic exercise program. However, in some cases a damaged motion segment may enable too much ROM and cause instability.

Factors Affecting ROM

Many different factors affect ROM. Although age, sex, and genotype may be good predictors, there are always exceptions.

Age and Sex

ROM depends on several demographic variables. For example, ROM typically decreases in adulthood; however, it is unknown how much of this diminution is attributable to aging or to the reduction in physical activity related to aging. Sex is another consideration; although females are generally considered to be more flexible than males, the opposite has been found in flexion and extension of the spine.

Nature and Nurture

Individuals may increase ROM by participating in good flexibility training programs; however, a person's genotype can limit flexibility. Some people have relatively poor flexibility; no matter how hard they train, their flexibility improves nominally. Although people with great flexibility may perform considerable numbers of stretching exercises, their genotype is important too. Some research suggests that improving ROM may relate more to the ability to tolerate pain than to actual changes in connective tissue length (15, 18). Moreover, McGill (17) makes a strong argument that tight hamstrings can enhance performance in sports such as basketball; obviously the issue is complex.

Posture

If individuals do not use their full ROM at a joint, tendinous tissue may compensate by shortening. It then

[1]The greatest amount of intervertebral movement occurs between the fifth lumbar vertebra (L5) and the fused sacrum (which begins with S1); this is referred to as the *lumbosacral joint.* The intervertebral joint between L4 and L5 also permits a substantial portion of the movement in the lower spine; however, the amount of movement permitted between L1 and L4 is nominal.

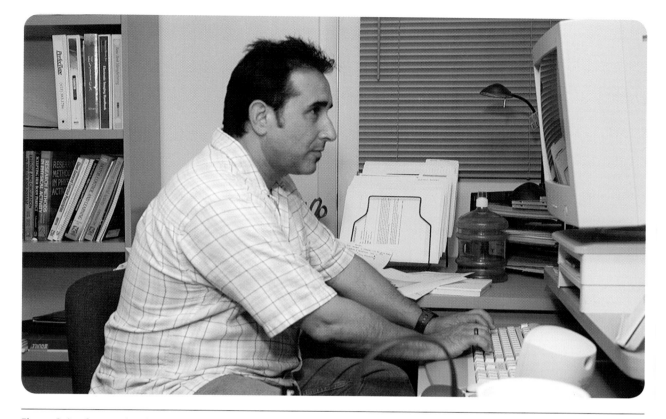

Figure 9.1 Connective tissue structures (e.g., ligaments and tendons) adapt to habitual poor sitting posture (e.g., rounding of the upper back or less lordotic curve in the lumbar region) by lengthening in response to stress; this adaptation is called *ligamentous creep* and *disc creep.* Without an attempt to remove these stresses or to develop counterbalancing ones, poor sitting postures can transfer to poor standing postures.

becomes difficult to make some of the movements needed in activities of daily living. For example, a person sitting at a computer terminal several hours each day without adequate postural support might develop a greater thoracic curve (e.g., a dorsal kyphosis) and rounded shoulders (see figure 9.1). If habitual postures such as this are maintained excessively, tendinous tissue that previously permitted good movement can shorten and impede movement. In the spine, injuries typically occur near the end of ROM; this factor should be considered especially when the spine moves while under load.

Disease

Disease can negatively affect a person's ROM. Arthritis and osteoporosis and their effect on ROM are discussed next.

Arthritis

Arthritis can have a debilitating effect on ROM because it affects articular cartilage. Articular cartilage, also called *hyaline cartilage,* is **avascular** (i.e., it does not have a blood supply); because of this, its healing capability is not good. Thus, if one or more joints are injured or diseased, the body's compensatory adaptations may work for a while but often become deficient with aging. Because articular cartilage does not repair itself well, fibrocartilage and bony spicules often replace the cartilage, which further diminishes joint movement. Two common types of arthritis are **rheumatoid arthritis** and **osteoarthritis.** Rheumatoid arthritis affects females more than males and can occur anytime in life but most often occurs between the ages of 25 and 60. It appears to be an autoimmune disease in some cases, but the exact cause is unknown; it can affect a few joints (pauciarticular) or many joints (polyarticular). Osteoarthritis is much more prevalent and accounts for 90% to 95% of arthritis cases. It can be considered a disease of aging, because after age 70 it may affect about 85% of the population. Its cause is usually some injury or mechanical derangement; however, in some cases the cause is unknown.

Lack of mobility attributable to arthritis often occurs in joints such as the fingers or the knee; however, arthritis also can decrease mobility in the spine if the site is a facet joint (see figure 9.2). Because articular cartilage is avascular, it depends on the diffusion of nutrients from tissue fluid, and so further deterioration

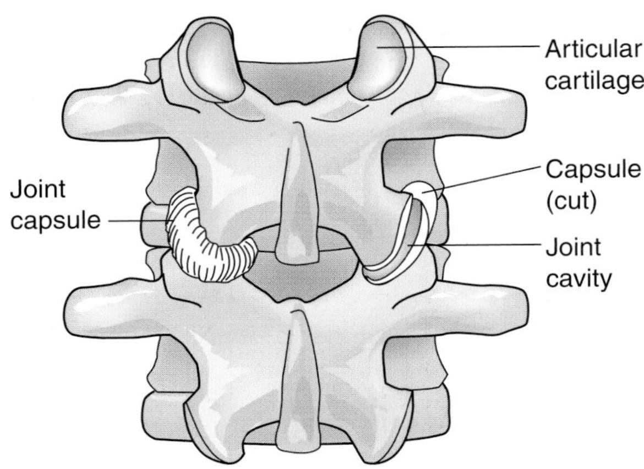

Figure 9.2 Posterior junctions between two vertebrae often are referred to as *facet joints.* Facet joints are synovial joints and have articular cartilage; if articular cartilage is damaged, arthritis can occur.

Adapted from W. Liemohn, 2001, *Exercise prescription and the back* (New York, NY: McGraw-Hill), 11, by permission of The McGraw-Hill Companies.

can result from lack of movement. Thus, it is desirable for people with arthritis to maintain as much ROM as possible.

Osteoporosis

Osteoporosis is characterized by a loss in bone mineral density or bone mass. Although it is seen particularly in women after menopause, it can also affect men and may be genetically influenced. Common osteoporotic sites include the hip, wrist, and vertebrae; a common characteristic of these sites is that cancellous bone predominates (see chapter 27). In the spine, osteoporosis can cause buckling and compression of vertebrae. A person with this condition may show extreme curves in the spine as well as loss of ROM. Fortunately, cancellous bone can become denser through weight-bearing activities and resistance training.

Key Point

Factors relating to ROM include age, sex, heredity, posture, and disease. If joint ROM is not used, it is lost; although declines in ROM relate to increased age, some declines in ROM result from a decline in physical activity or from injury. ROM relates to both nature and nurture. A person's genotype and activities can affect ROM. Habitual poor posture also can decrease ROM. Arthritis is a disease of the joints and thus tends to decrease joint ROM. Osteoporosis can reduce spine ROM because of its destructive effect on vertebral bodies.

ROM and Low-Back Function

Spinal carriage is functionally integrated with most movements because many movements emanate from the spine. An argument has been made that the spine and its associated tissues are the primary engine of locomotion in our species (6). Accepting this view demands an appreciation of the importance of maintaining good spinal mobility; however, this spine mobility must also be under muscle control.

Spine ROM

ROM deficiencies in the spine and particularly its supporting structures have been viewed as prognostic indicators of low-back pain (2, 21). ROM by itself, however, is not as good a predictor of impending low-back problems (3). In other words, although ROM can be a causal factor in some cases of low-back pain, more often two or more variables are jointly responsible for the problem. Individuals with chronic low-back pain often receive therapeutic stretching regimens to improve ROM at the hip; improving spine ROM is less often a goal (see chapter 13).

The flexion movement between the rib cage and the sacrum is, in essence, a straightening of the normal

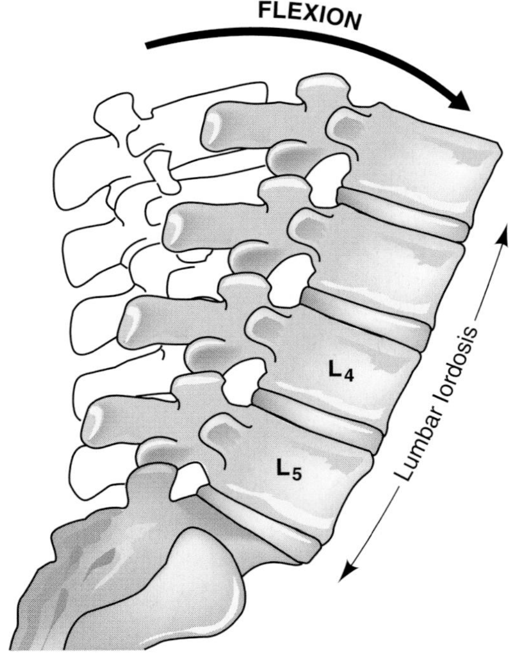

Figure 9.3 In forward movement of the trunk, lumbar flexion per se does not occur. What some may view as lumbar flexion is in essence a removal of the lordotic curve.

Adapted from W. Liemohn, 2001, *Exercise prescription and the back* (New York, NY: McGraw-Hill), 40, by permission of The McGraw-Hill Companies.

lumbar **lordotic curve** (figure 9.3). Although with aging spinal mobility may progressively decline in all planes, McKenzie (19) contended that greater decline occurs in extension because this movement is used less as a person ages. Unfortunately, spine extension is often ignored or misinterpreted in exercise programs (see chapter 13). Although ballistic extension movements of the spine (and ballistic rotation movements) are totally inappropriate, slow and controlled extension to maintain ROM and strengthen the erector spinae is appropriate in exercise programs. Nevertheless, if the back is actively extended, the person should not exceed the upper limit of the normal lumbar lordosis as seen in standing (22).

Scoliosis is an extreme lateral curvature; the fitness professional can use the Adam's test to get a better perception of the presence of scoliosis in a client (figure 9.4). Although there are many causes for scoliosis, usually the cause is unknown. A length discrepancy between the legs leading to a lateral tilt of the pelvis is associated with scoliosis and low-back pain; however, the evidence that scoliosis causes low-back pain is not conclusive. Depending on the degree of scoliosis, a person with this condition may present with a different posturing of the rib cage during abdominal strengthening exercises because of the spinal rotation that scoliosis may cause.

Iliofemoral Joint ROM

The muscles crossing the hip joint sometimes are viewed as guy-wires as they can limit movement of the pelvis by bracing it (see figure 9.5); if any of these guy-wires are too tight, the trunk musculature, regardless of how well it is developed, may have difficulty controlling pelvic position. Because the sacrum (in the pelvis) is the foundation for the 24 vertebrae stacked on it, pelvic positioning plays an important role in the integrity of the spine. For example, tightness in the hip flexors such as the psoas produces an anterior or forward pelvic tilt; tightness in the hip extensors such as the hamstrings produces a backward or posterior pelvic tilt (see figure 9.5). Thus, if either of these muscle groups is tight, the ability of

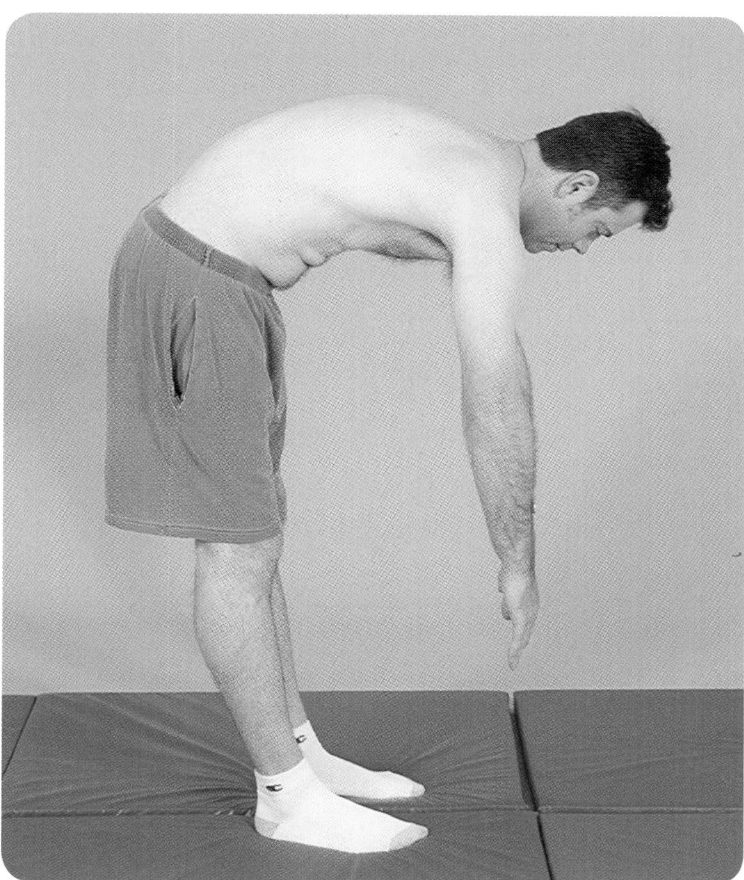

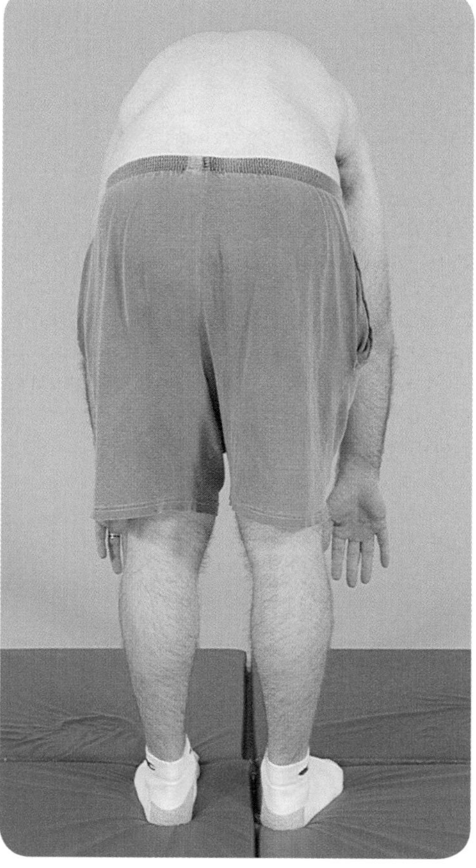

Figure 9.4 Adam's test. Viewing the spinous processes as the subject stands does not always reveal scoliotic curves even if present. However, it is much easier to see a scoliotic curve after the subject bends forward at the waist.

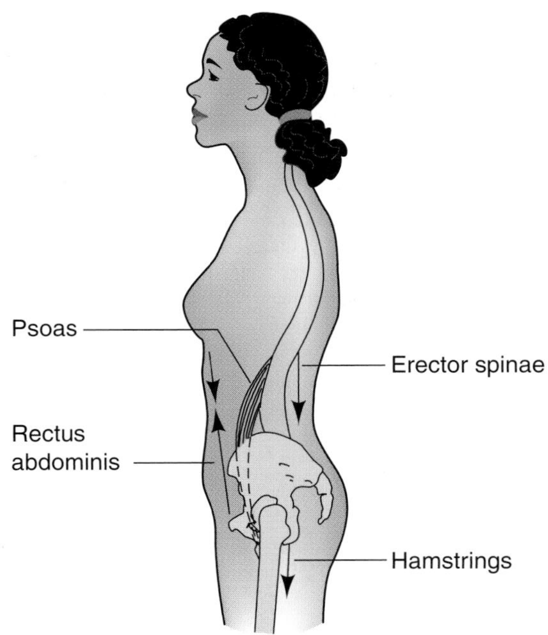

Figure 9.5 The muscles crossing the hip joint can be viewed as guy-wires. If, for example, the hamstring guy-wires are too tight, they will tend to posteriorly rotate the pelvis; under such a scenario the rectus abdominis will have difficulty controlling pelvic positioning. Inability to control pelvic positioning with the abdominal musculature predisposes a person to low-back problems.

the abdominal muscles to control pelvic positioning is adversely affected. Individuals who cannot control their pelvic positioning with their abdominal muscles are predisposed to low-back pain; this is one of the reasons why good ROM at the iliofemoral joint is important.

There may also be tightness in the iliotibial (IT) band; this can limit adduction movement of the thigh. Tightness in the piriformis muscle can limit movement in the transverse plane; this is a little more complex because such tightness can limit outward or inward rotation of the femur depending on the angle between hip and thigh (22).

Key Point

Spinal flexion between the rib cage and the sacrum is limited to the straightening of the normal lordotic curve. Although maintaining spine extension ROM is important, ballistic back extension movements should be avoided and back extension should not exceed the exerciser's normal lumbar lordosis. IT band and piriformis tightness also can have a deleterious effect on the biomechanics of the iliofemoral joint.

Measuring ROM of the Spine and at the Hip Joint

Some techniques used to measure ROM as it relates to low-back function are specific to the spine or to the hip joint; other techniques concurrently measure ROM of the spine and at the hip joint. Because certain techniques warrant more discussion than others, some are discussed here and others are shown in the chapter appendix.

Trunk Extension ROM

In Imrie and Barbuto's (9) test for back extension, the back musculature is not actively used. This test is considered a passive test of back ROM because the hyperextension movement in the spine results from arm and shoulder muscle contraction (see appendix). An active test of spine extension ROM, called the *trunk lift,* was developed by the Cooper Institute for Aerobics Research (5). It is an active test because muscles of the spine (i.e., erector spinae and multifidus) hyperextend the spine (see this chapter's appendix). Because both trunk extensor strength and ROM contribute to performance in the trunk lift and only ROM contributes to performance in the passive test, we used multiple regression analyses to further study performance on these tests by university students. Somewhat to our surprise, we found that the two tests in essence measure the same construct (13).

Hip Joint ROM

The Thomas test (see appendix) typically is used to measure tightness in the hip flexors. Two of the more popular tests used to measure this tightness are the relatively new active knee extension test (see appendix) and the often used passive straight leg raise test (see appendix). In some instances it may be desirable to check for tightness in the IT bands and in the piriformis muscles.

Combined Tests of ROM in Trunk and Hip Joint Flexion

The fingertips-to-floor and the sit-and-reach tests have often been used under the pretense that they measure

Key Point

Good ROM at the hip joint is important for good biomechanics of the spine. Although tightness in the hip flexors is not seen as often as tightness in the hip extensors, both are important factors in maintaining a healthy spine. Tightness in the muscles crossing the hip joint may predispose an individual to low-back problems.

flexibility in the low back as well as at the hip joint. It has been shown conclusively, however, that although both can be used to measure hip joint flexibility (e.g., hamstring length), in their conventional use neither effectively measures low-back ROM (16). Because the sit-and-reach is used more than the fingertips-to-floor test as a field test, it is examined here in greater detail. Most of the following comments apply to its use either as an exercise or as a test.

Using the sit-and-reach test as an exercise has been questioned clinically. For example, if the hamstrings are tight and the sitting stretch is performed ballistically, the structures of the spine may be obligated to absorb these stresses, and over time these repetitive motions may have a serious consequence on low-back function. Moreover, even if the sit-and-reach is done slowly, the static postures resulting during the stretching phase can place high compressive forces on the intervertebral discs (17, 20). Cailliet (4) cautioned that this exercise might damage ligaments of the spine, particularly if the participant's hamstrings are tight.

To reduce the stress on the spine incumbent in the sit-and-reach test, Cailliet (4) recommended what he called a *protective hamstring stretch* (see the appendix of this chapter). In this exercise, the hamstrings of each leg are alternately stretched while the nonstretched limb is bent at the knee joint with its foot flat on the floor next to the contralateral knee. Cailliet contended that lumbosacral stress is less in his hamstring stretch than in the more typical sit-and-reach test with both legs extended; if this is true, the same reasoning would warrant administering the sit-and-reach test with only one leg extended. However, we examined lumbosacral movement in university students tested with both legs extended as well as with just one leg extended and found that less flexion (which would imply less stress) was not seen in Cailliet's version of the sit and reach (14). Nevertheless, Cailliet's protective hamstring stretch has other advantages (e.g., permits checking for symmetry) and is deemed safer for the spine than the sit-and-reach test with both legs extended.

The sit-and-reach test has also been questioned because it does not allow for proportional differences between arm, trunk, and leg length. In response, Hopkins and Hoeger (7) developed a protocol that purportedly controls for some of this variance (see this chapter's appendix). More recent research by others suggests that the adjustment for limb length did not improve validity (8).

We noted that performance on the sit-and-reach test was significantly better with the ankle of the tested leg in passive plantar flexion as opposed to the fixed dorsiflexion posture usually required when the test is administered (12). Our research suggests that factors such as tightness in the connective tissue structures located behind the knee and tension on the **sciatic nerve** can affect performance on the sit and reach. (We used a sit-and-reach box that restrained only the heel of the tested leg and permitted the foot to plantar flex into the box.) Most recently, Hui and Yuen (8) reported on a test that also permits plantar flexion of the foot of the tested leg and that does not require a sit-and-reach box. Although their test appears to have some advantages to the sit-and-reach tests previously discussed (see appendix for description), the trunk

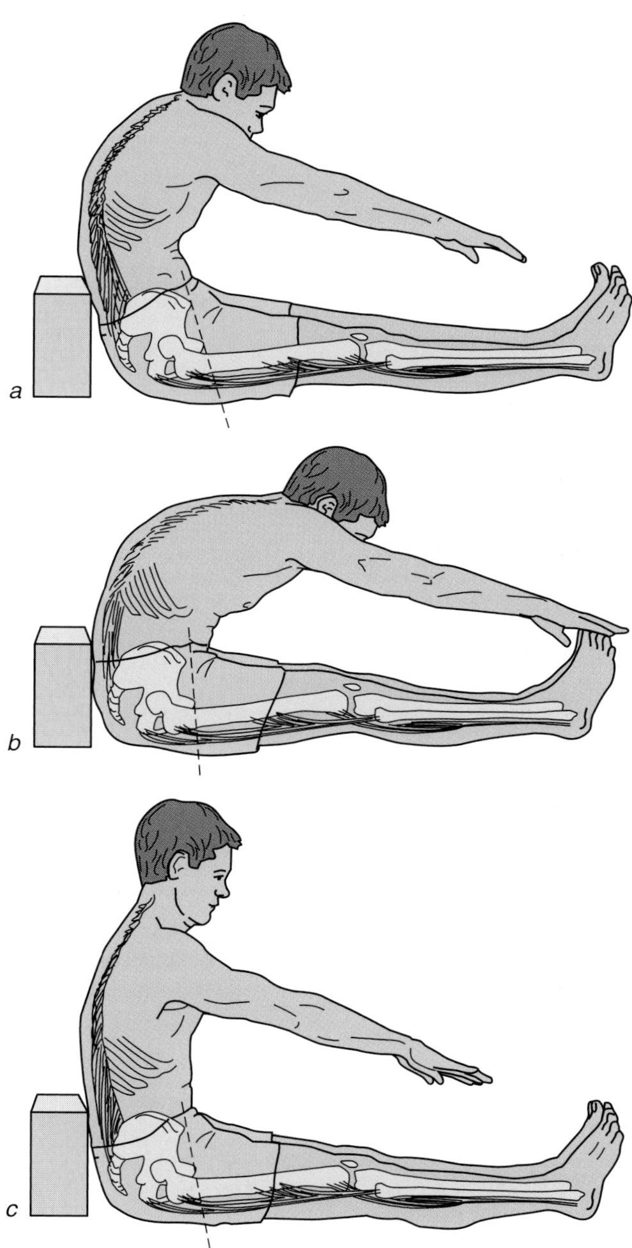

Figure 9.6 Sit-and-reach test. Quality points to look for include *(a)* tight hamstrings (note tilt of pelvis), tight low back, and stretched upper back; *(b)* normal length of hamstrings and low back; and *(c)* tight hamstrings (note tilt of pelvis) and tight low back.

posturing that this protocol permits might be problematic for some individuals who have disc disease, for extreme flexion moments can compromise their condition.

Even though the sit-and-reach activity has medical contraindications and a host of factors can affect its performance, it still has value as a field test provided that test users are aware of its shortcomings. Following are suggestions that can make the sit and reach a better test:

- It is argued that the number of centimeters reached is not the most valid indicator of performance. The test administrator is better advised to examine the quality of the movement of the individual being tested. Look for the angle of the sacrum (see figure 9.6) and the smoothness of the spinal curve. These relatively simple determinations can make the sit and reach a measure of low-back mobility as well as a measure of hamstring length. These and other quality points are delineated in figure 9.6.
- It is recommended that the individual extend only one leg during the sit-and-reach test. Although this technique doubles the number of measurements required, the tester will also be able to evaluate symmetry.
- If a sit-and-reach box is used to make measurements, it is recommended that it be altered to permit passive plantar flexion at the ankle joint. To alter the standard sit-and-reach box, simply replace the vertical surface under the cantilever extension with a 4 cm rod; this permits plantar flexion into the box but restrains the heel. This adjustment is not necessary if the protocol of Hui and Yuen (8) is followed.

Following are descriptions of two tests designed specifically to measure spine ROM; however, both require the ability to locate bony landmarks on the pelvis and spine. The inclinometer provides a relatively simple and reasonably reliable means for measuring the lumbar spine (1, 11). Although inclinometers are expensive (approximately \$100-\$150 each), they are much easier to use in measuring ROM of the spine than the goniometer is. Williams and colleagues (23) described a modification of the Schober technique that is used to measure spine ROM; although a tape measure is the only equipment required, this test is used primarily in clinical settings in part because the location of bony landmarks requires patients to remove their clothing.

Key Point

If a person with tight hamstrings practices the sit-and-reach maneuver with both legs extended, the soft-tissue structures of the spine can be damaged. In administering the sit-and-reach test, the fitness professional should consider the quality of the movement; it can be more important than the number of centimeters reached.

Case Studies

You can check your answers by referring to page 471 in appendix A.

1. After learning that one of the individuals participating in your physical fitness program was told that his hamstrings were tight, you administer the sit-and-reach test to get some baseline data on his tightness. Somewhat to your surprise you find that he can reach beyond his toes. What quality factors (other than centimeters reached) in his sit-and-reach performance might you further examine to explain this disparity? What other hamstring length test might you administer?
2. Another individual's record indicates that previous results from the Thomas test show she has very tight hip flexors. However, when you administer the Thomas test, you do not find evidence of tightness in the hip flexors. Assume that this person has done nothing to increase her ROM and that you are confident that you administered the Thomas test correctly. Explain how the previous administrator of the test might have erred.

Tests for Measuring ROM for Low-Back Function

Spine ROM

Passive Back ROM Test

While keeping the anterior part of the pelvis (i.e., anterior superior iliac spines) in contact with the floor, the subject elevates the torso with arm and shoulder muscles; the muscles of the back are not used in this movement. The score is the perpendicular distance from the suprasternal notch to the floor. From a geometric perspective it should be easy for individuals with longer trunks to have better scores. Scoring: 30 cm (12 in.) or more is excellent, 20 cm (8 in.) or more is good, and 10 cm (4 in.) or more is fair.

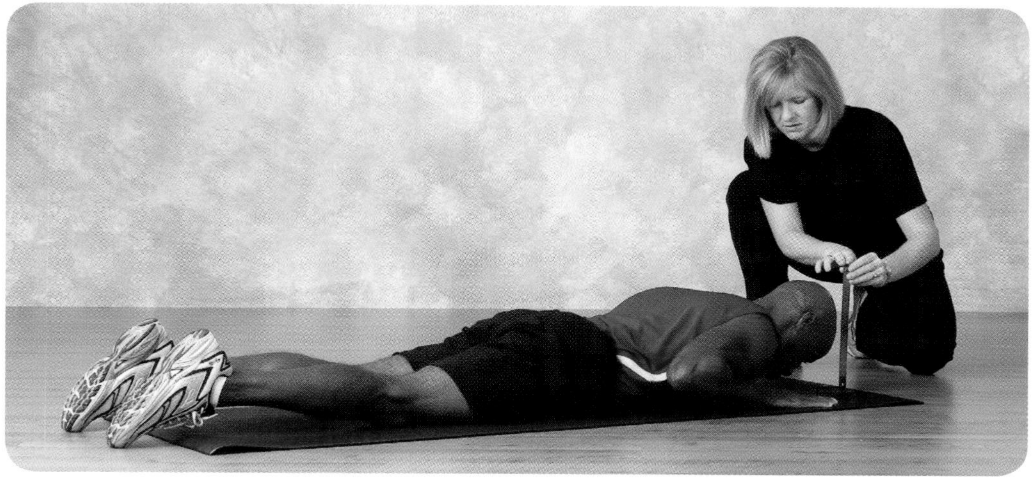

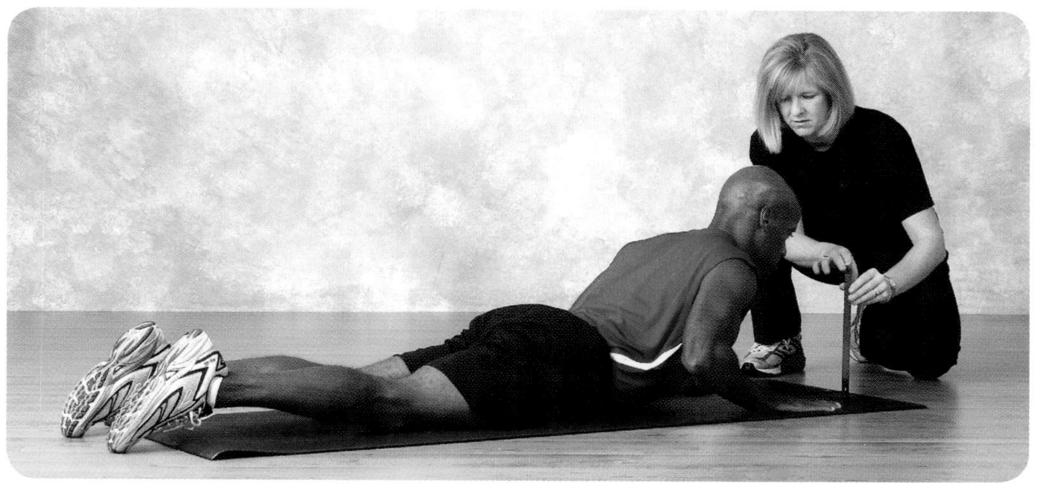

Active Back ROM and Strength Test

In this test, the individual slowly lifts the torso by contracting the erector spinae and multifidus muscle groups until the chin is a maximum of 30 cm (12 in.) from the mat. This test is from the Cooper Institute for Aerobics Research (5); although norms were not presented, most individuals tested should be able to raise the chin at least 15 cm (6 in.). (From a geometric perspective, it should be easier for individuals with longer trunks to have better scores; you should consider this factor when administering the test.)

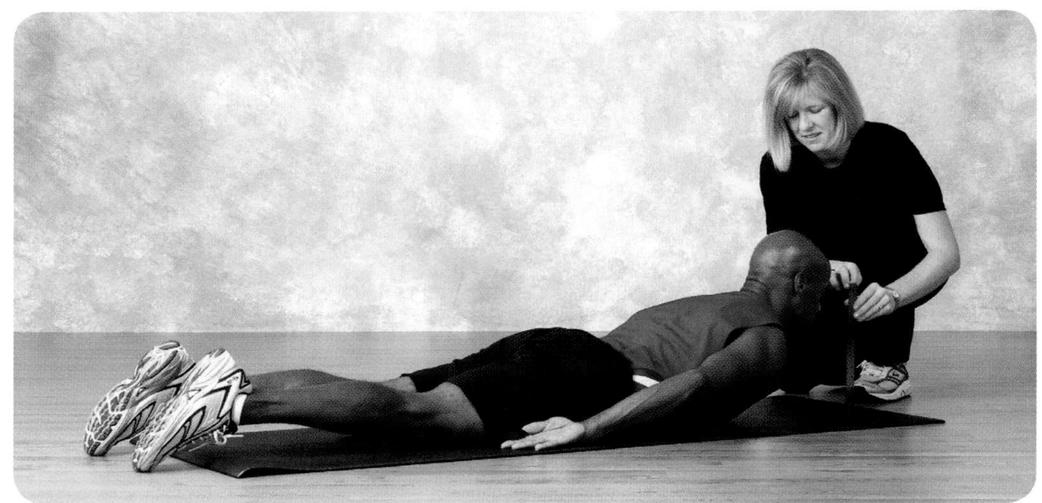

Hip Joint ROM

Thomas Test

The individual being tested pulls the contralateral leg toward the chest until the low back touches the testing surface. The test is successful if the thigh of the straight leg remains in contact with the table or floor (10). If it does not, the degree of elevation indicates the tightness of the hip flexors. The tester must ensure that there is not too much posterior rotation of the pelvis. Some subjects may be able to posteriorly rotate the pelvis beyond the point where the low back touches the testing surface, which could suggest a false positive (i.e., with too much posterior rotation of the pelvis, anyone's hip flexors might look tight).

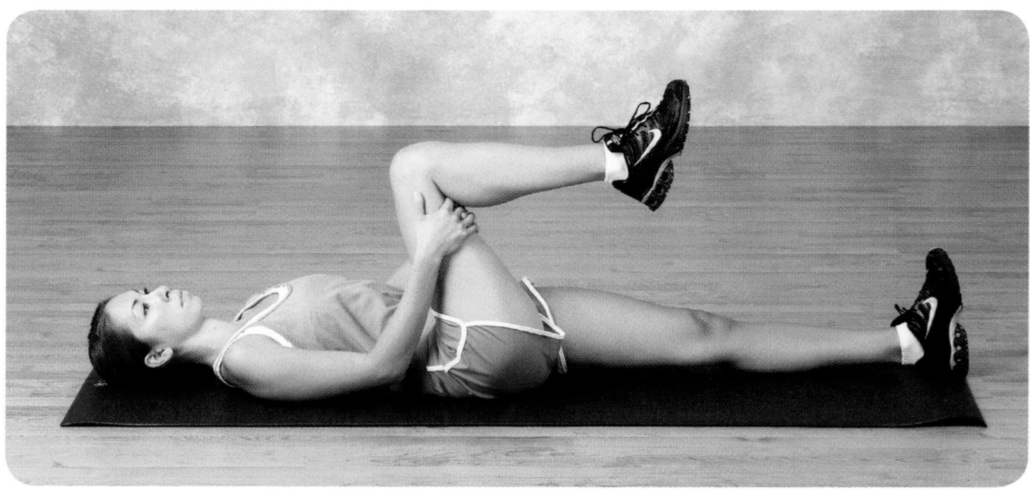

Ober's Test (IT Band Tightness)

The pelvis is in the neutral position with the hips stacked. The score is the number of finger breadths that the medial femoral condyle remains elevated from the testing surface (24). This test can be helpful in determining the effect of exercise programming on IT band tightness, a problem seen in runner's knee (also referred to as *patellofemoral syndrome* or *chondromalacia patella).*

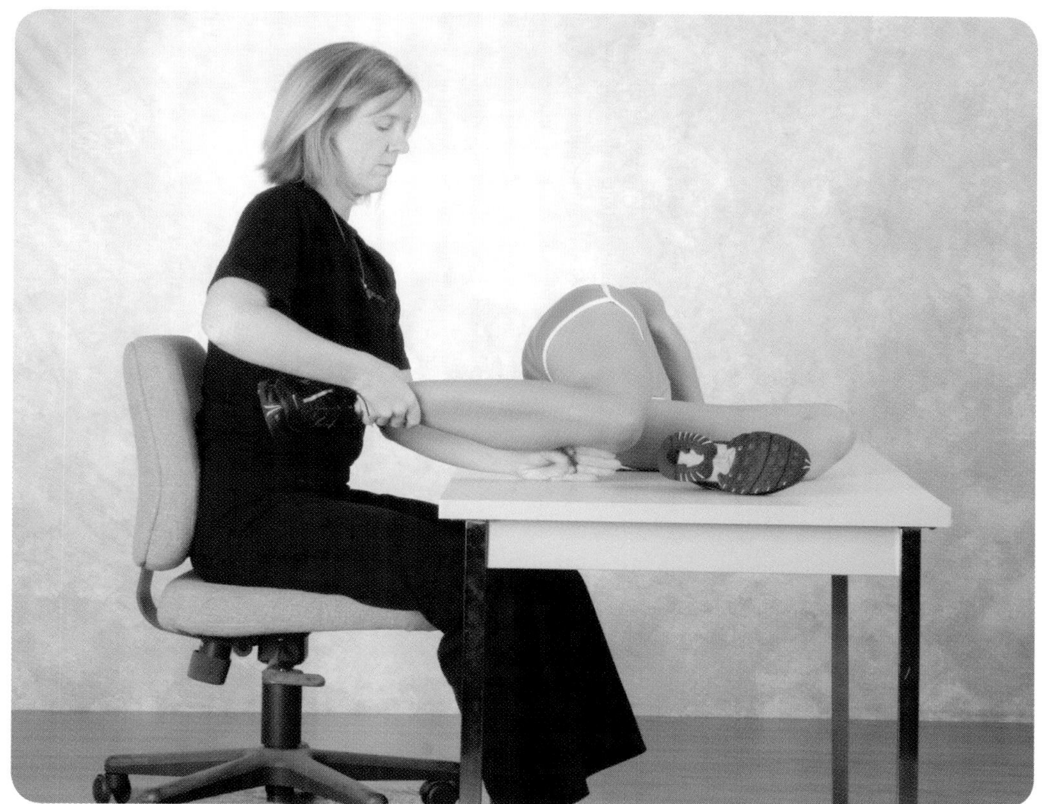

Piriformis ROM

Examining piriformis ROM is difficult and thus should be done only by those with appropriate experience. It includes (a) assessment below 90° of hip flexion (in this position it is an external rotator and abductor) and (b) assessment above 90° of hip flexion (in this position it is an internal rotator and adductor) (24). This test can help determine the effect of exercise programming on piriformis tightness.

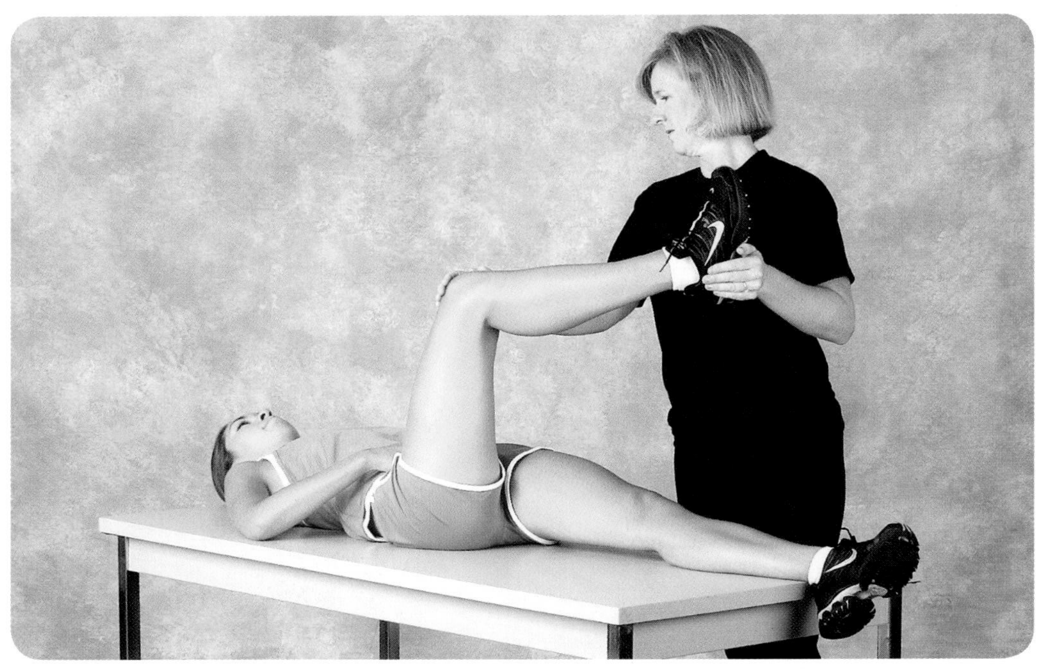

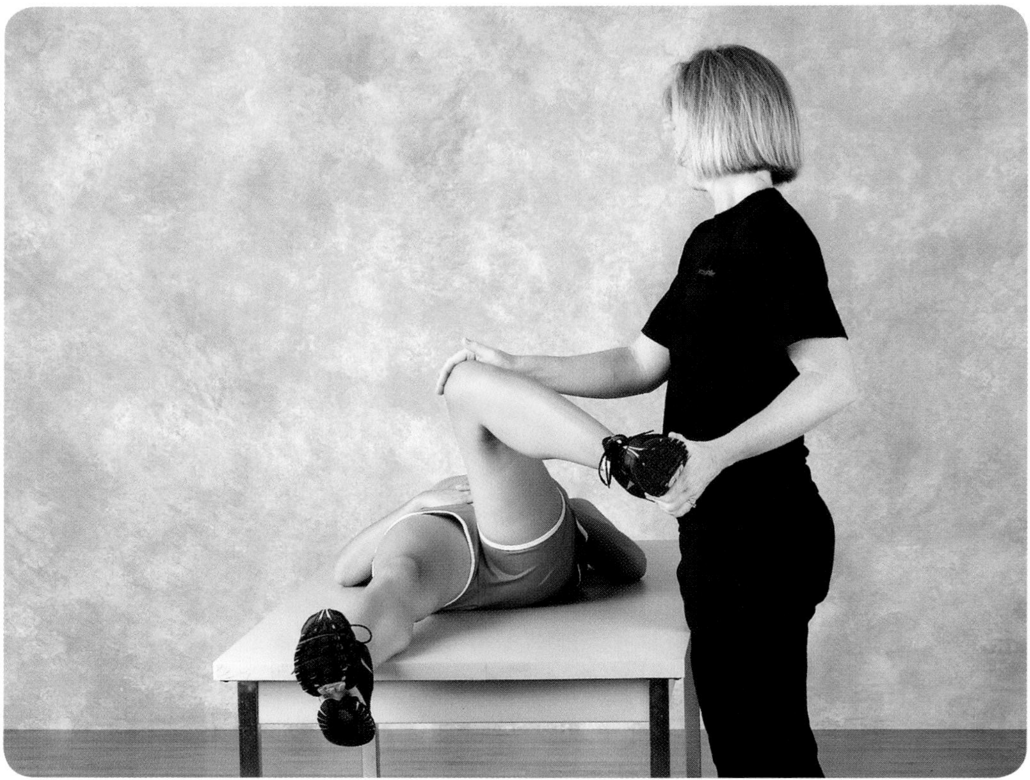

Passive Straight Leg Raise Test

In the straight leg raise test that is recommended, the pelvis is first posteriorly rotated until the low back is snug against the table; one leg is then raised by the tester while ensuring that the other one remains extended and flat on the testing surface. ROM in flexion can be determined with a goniometer placed on its axis on the greater trochanter or an inclinometer placed just below the tibial tubercle. A minimum of 80° is desirable on the passive straight leg raise; however, most therapists would like to see 90°. If large numbers of subjects are being tested, a protractor-type device can be contrived (e.g., marked on wall) to speed up the testing process; however, the measurement will not be as precise. (Although the Leighton Flexometer can be used for measuring ROM of the extremities in a test such as this one, its use was not seen in the literature reviewed.)

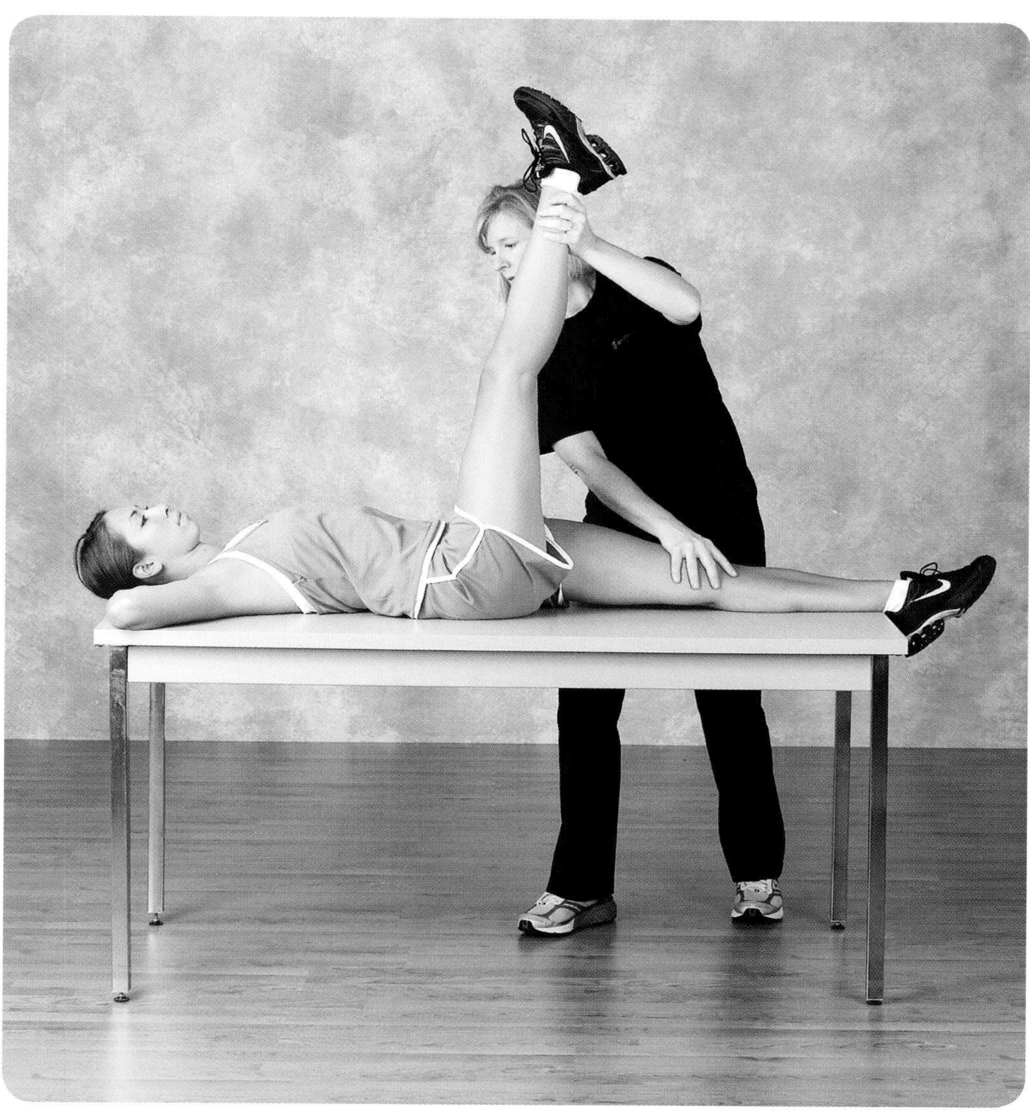

Active Knee Extension (AKE) Test, or the 90/90 Test

In this test, the thigh of one leg is raised perpendicular (i.e., 90° to the floor) with the lower leg 90° to the thigh (the tester will have to hold it in this position). The subject then actively extends this lower leg. A score of zero indicates that the leg was moved 90° (i.e., perpendicular to the table and in line with the thigh); a score of 10 indicates that the leg was moved 80°. A score of 5 to 15 is desirable. Many therapists like this test because the individual being tested controls the amount of movement. (Some therapists determine passing ROM using the 90/90 starting position.)

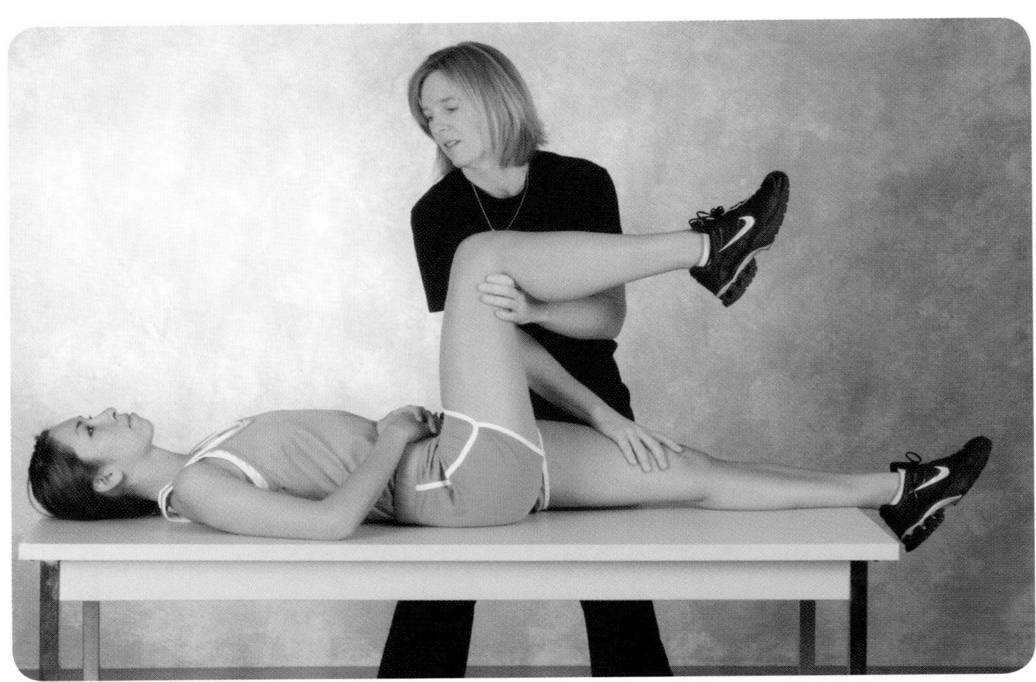

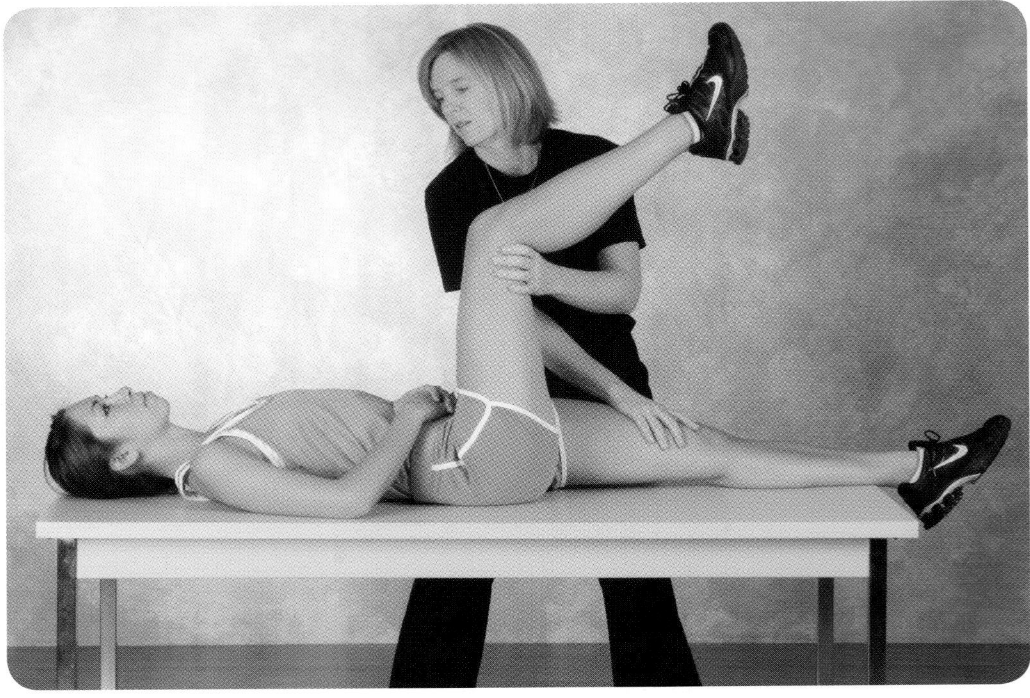

Combined Tests of Trunk and Hip Joint Flexion

Cailliet Protective Hamstring Stretch

As the participant flexes the hip and knee of the contralateral leg, the attendant posterior rotation of the pelvis decreases the turning moment of inertia of the torso; this is one reason why some believe that this exercise or test is safer than the bilateral sit-and-reach activity (4).

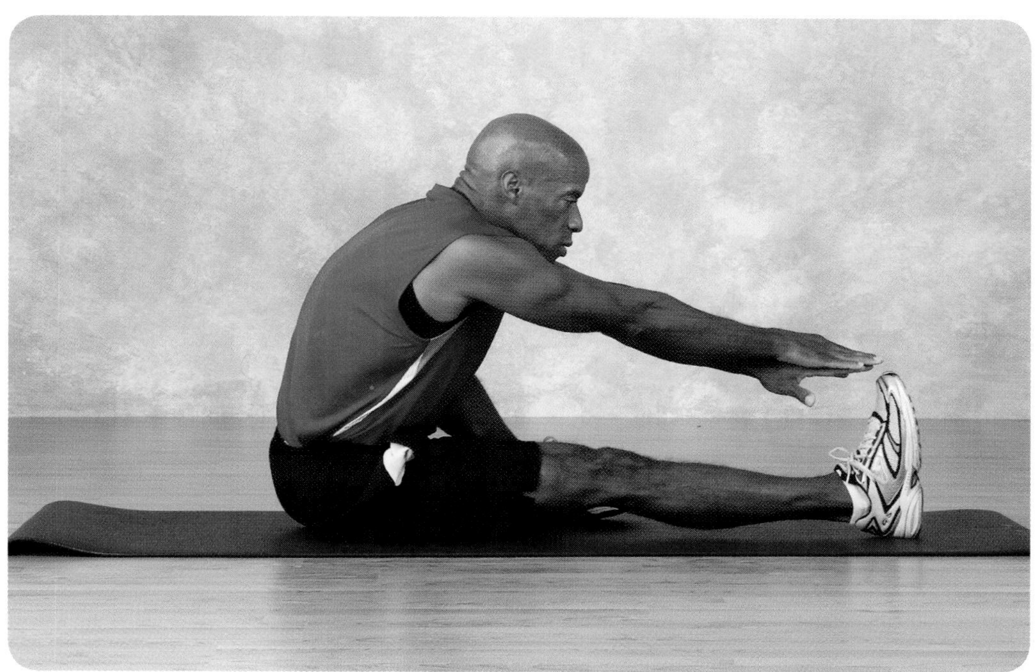

Hopkins and Hoeger Sit and Reach

A reach score is first determined with the back against the wall; this score is then subtracted from the maximum reach score (7). Recent research has questioned its validity in adjusting for arm- and leg-length discrepancies. If this test is administered, a sit-and-reach box with a lengthened cantilever extension would be required for many subjects.

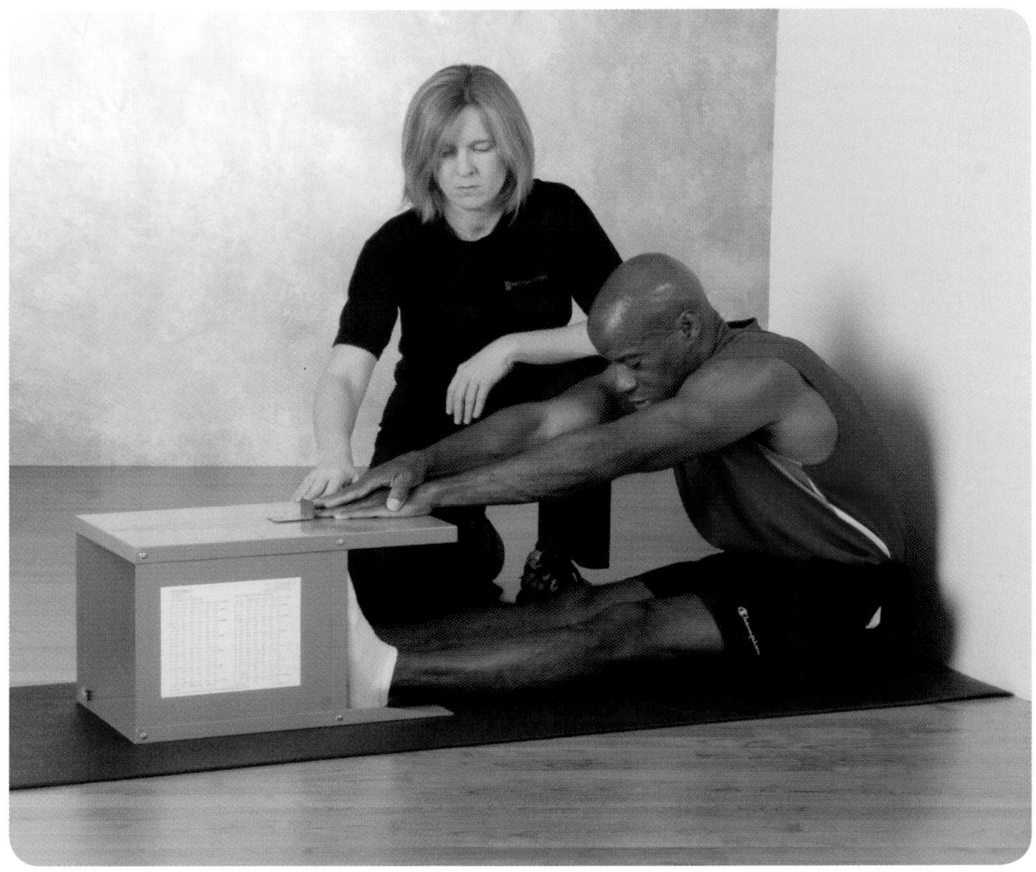

Modified Back-Saver Sit and Reach

The only equipment required for this test is a meterstick and a bench. Because the ankle is permitted to passively plantar flex, connective tissue tightness behind the knee, as well as other factors such as sciatic nerve tension, does not affect performance (8).

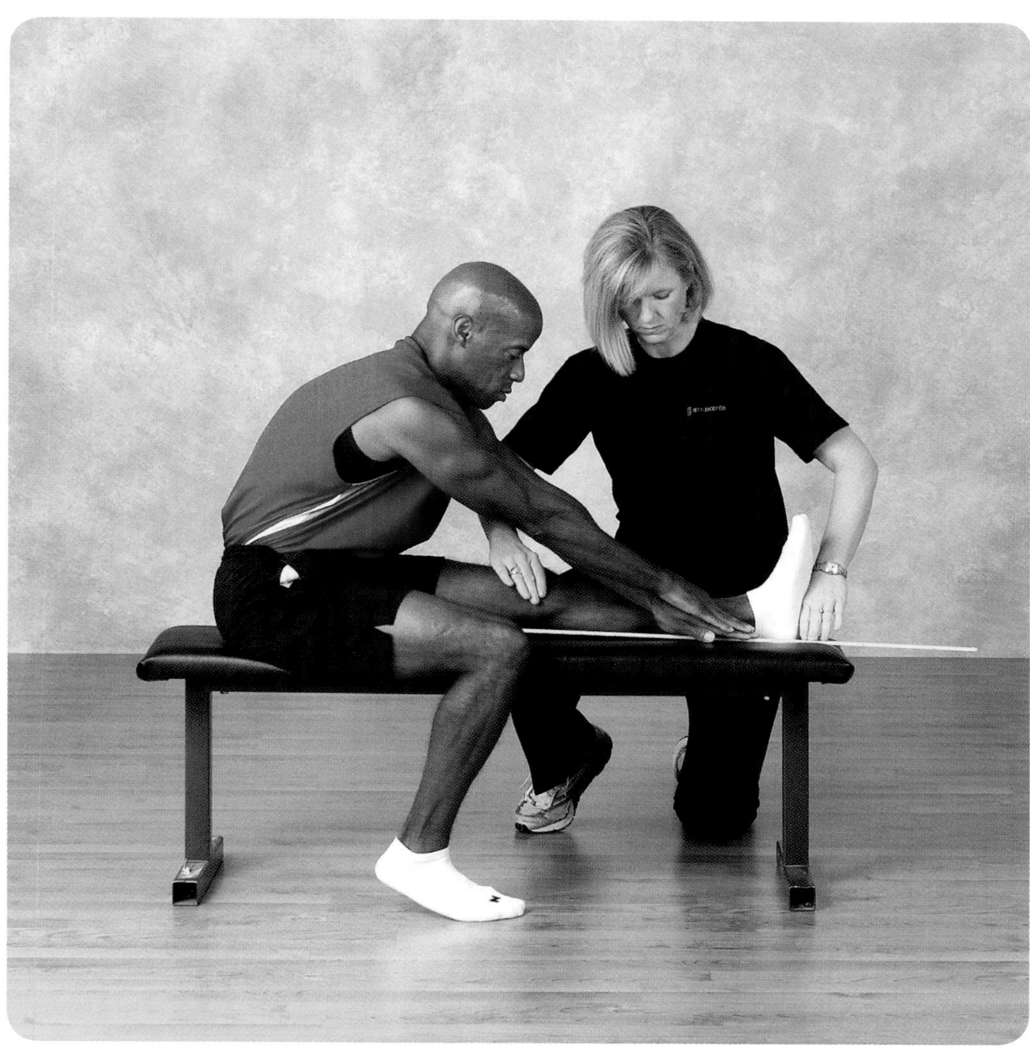

PART III

Exercise Prescription for Health and Fitness

In part III we provide guidelines for exercise programming for each of the fitness components: cardiorespiratory fitness (chapter 10), weight management (chapter 11), muscular strength and endurance (chapter 12), and flexibility and low-back function (chapter 13). We describe exercise leadership and include examples of a variety of activities in chapter 14. The degree to which a tissue such as bone, skeletal muscle, or cardiac muscle functions depends on the activity to which it is exposed. This statement summarizes the two major principles underlying training programs: overload and specificity.

The principle of overload describes a dynamic characteristic of living creatures: Use increases functional capacity. If a tissue or organ system is required to work against a load to which it is not accustomed, it becomes stronger instead of wearing out and becoming

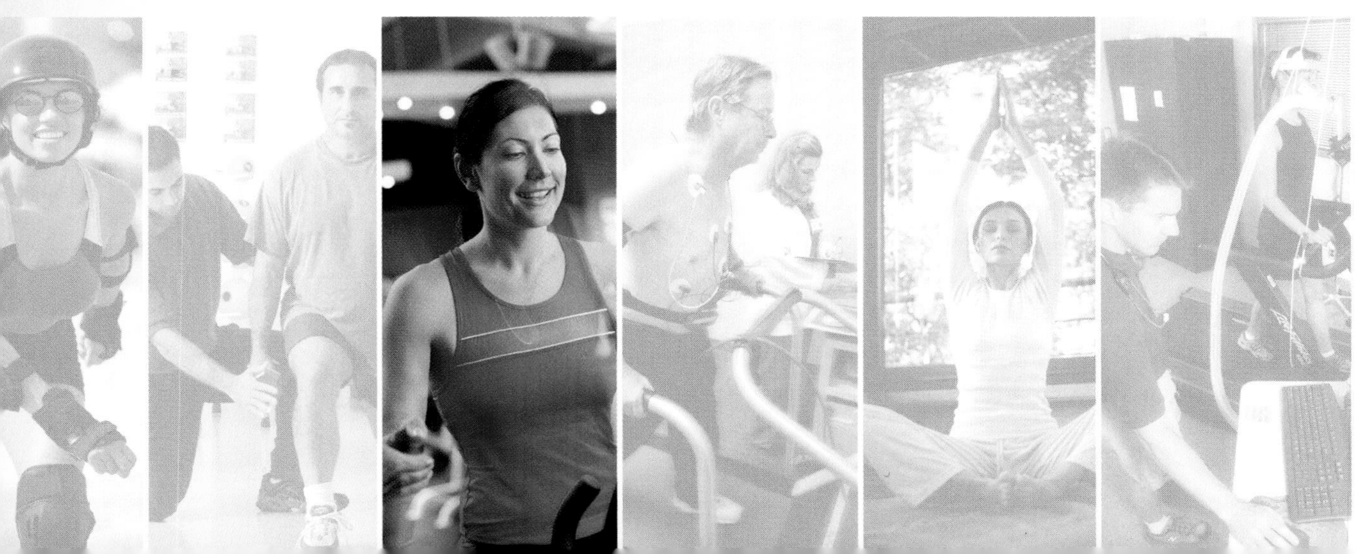

weaker. The common adage for this principle is "Use it or lose it." The corollary of the overload principle is the principle of reversibility, which indicates that physiological gains are lost when a tissue or organ system is not used. The variables that contribute to overload in an exercise program include intensity, duration, and frequency of exercise. As we will see, it is the combination of these elements that results in a sufficient amount of total work, or energy expenditure, to increase the functional capacity of the cardiorespiratory systems.

The principle of specificity states that the training effects derived from an exercise program are specific to the exercise performed and the muscles involved. For example, a person who runs for exercise shows little change in the arm muscles. A person who exercises at a low intensity that recruits only slow-twitch muscle fibers will see little or no training effect in the fast-twitch fibers. If muscle fibers are not used, they cannot adapt, and thus they will not become trained. The type of adaptation that occurs as a result of training is specific to the type of training taking place (e.g., endurance versus heavy resistance training). Running increases the number of capillaries and mitochondria in the muscle fibers involved in the exercise, which makes them more resistant to fatigue. Resistance training causes hypertrophy of the muscles involved, due to an increase in the amount of contractile proteins, actin and myosin, in the muscle.

Following is a summary of overload and specificity:

- Tissues adapt to the load to which they are exposed.
- To increase the functional capacity of a tissue, it must be overloaded (i.e., subjected to a load to which it is not accustomed).
- The type of adaptation is specific to the muscle fibers involved and the type of exercise.
- Endurance exercise increases mitochondria and capillary numbers.
- Resistance training increases the contractile proteins and the size of the muscle.

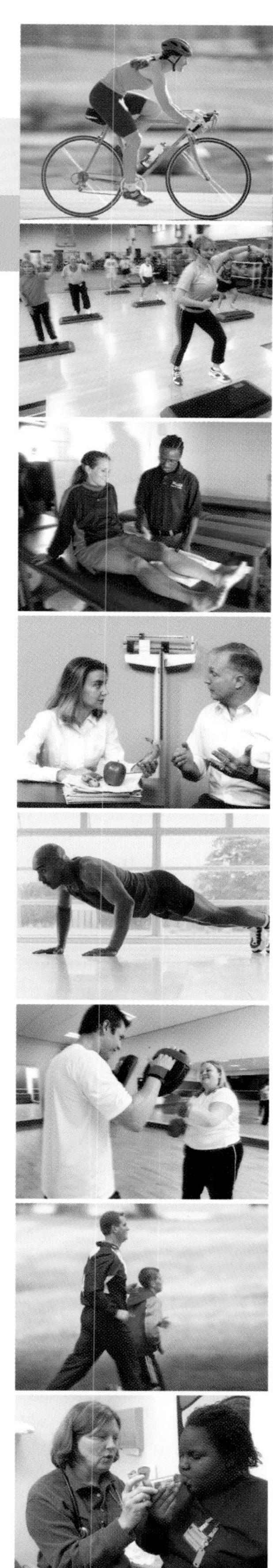

10 CHAPTER

Exercise Prescription for Cardiorespiratory Fitness

Objectives

The reader will be able to do the following:

1. Characterize the dose of exercise in an exercise prescription and identify means by which a health-related effect might occur.
2. Describe the public health recommendation for physical activity.
3. Explain the concepts of overload and specificity as they relate to training programs.
4. Describe general guidelines related to cardiorespiratory fitness programs, including those related to warm-up and cool-down.
5. Develop an exercise prescription with the exercise intensity, duration, and frequency needed to achieve and maintain cardiorespiratory fitness goals.
6. Express exercise intensity in terms of energy production, HR, and RPE.
7. Contrast the approaches used for developing exercise prescriptions for the general public, for the fit population, and for people whose complete GXT results are available.
8. Describe the differences between a supervised and an unsupervised program.
9. Describe how temperature and humidity, altitude, and pollution affect the exercise prescription.

The *Surgeon General's Report on Physical Activity and Health* (63) concluded that physical inactivity is a major risk factor for cardiovascular, respiratory, and metabolic diseases. Of more than 450 health objectives for the nation, *Healthy People 2010* (64) selected physical activity as one of the top 10 health indicators. A symposium on dose–response issues concerning physical activity and health concluded that regular physical activity reduces all-cause mortality, fatal and nonfatal total CVD, and CHD. Physical activity also was linked to a lower incidence of obesity and type 2 diabetes and to an improvement in metabolic control in individuals with type 2 diabetes (14, 39). The reader is directed to chapters 11, 19, and 20 for details on prescribing exercise for weight management, obesity, and diabetes, respectively. This chapter deals with the important question of how much activity is needed to improve cardiorespiratory fitness (CRF).

Prescribing Exercise

There is a close parallel between the fitness professional's desire to know the proper **dose** of exercise needed to bring about a desired **effect** (response) and the physician's need to know the type and quantity of a drug needed to cure a disease. For example, there is a difference between what is needed to cure a headache and what is needed to cure tuberculosis. In the same way, there is no question that the dose of physical activity required to achieve a high level of performance is different from that required to improve a health-related outcome (e.g., lowered BP, reduced risk of CHD). Similarities can be drawn between the dose–response relationship for medications and that for exercise, which is shown in figure 10.1 (19).

- **Potency.** The potency of a drug is a relatively unimportant characteristic in that it makes little difference whether the effective dose is 1 mg or 100 mg as long as the drug can be administered in an appropriate dosage (19). Likewise in exercise prescriptions, walking 4 mi (6.4 km) at a moderate pace is as effective in expending calories as running 2 mi (3.2 km).

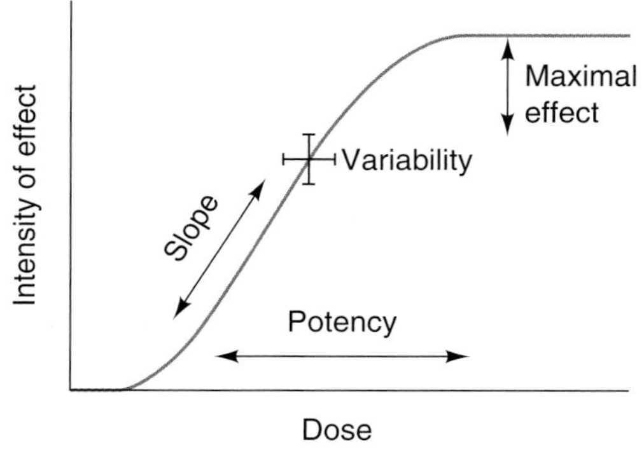

Figure 10.1 Representative dose–effect curve illustrating its four characterizing parameters.

Reprinted from A. Goodman, 1975, *Pharmacological basis of therapeutics* (New York, NY: McGraw-Hill), 25 by permission of the McGraw-Hill Companies.

- **Slope.** The slope of the curve describes how much of an effect comes from a change in dose (19). Some physiological measures such as HR and lactate response to a fixed exercise task change quickly (in days) for a dose of exercise, whereas some health-related effects (e.g., changes in serum cholesterol) are realized only after many months of exercise.

- **Maximal effect.** The maximal effect (efficacy) of a drug varies with the type of drug. For example, morphine can relieve pain of all intensities, whereas aspirin is effective against only mild to moderate pain (19). Similarly, strenuous exercise can increase $\dot{V}O_2$max and modify risk factors, whereas light to moderate exercise can improve risk factors while minimally affecting $\dot{V}O_2$max.

- **Variability.** The effect of a drug varies between individuals and within individuals depending on the circumstances. The point where the slope changes in figure 10.1 indicates the variability in the dose required to bring about a particular effect and the variability in the effect associated with a given dose (19). For example, gains in $\dot{V}O_2$max attributable to endurance training show considerable variation, even when the initial $\dot{V}O_2$max value is controlled for (12).

- **Side effect.** No drug produces a single effect (19). The effects might include adverse (side) effects that limit the usefulness of the drug. For exercise, the side effects might include an increased risk of injury.

Unlike most drugs, which people stop taking when a disease is cured, physical activity is needed throughout life to promote its health-related and fitness effects.

The exercise dose usually is characterized by the intensity, frequency, duration, and type of activity; we discuss each of these in detail later in this chapter. However, in contrast to what we know about the role of each of these variables in improving $\dot{V}O_2$max, less is known about the minimum or optimal quantities of each variable related to achieving health outcomes (27). In the symposium on dose–response issues related to physical activity and health, it was concluded that there was strong evidence of an inverse and generally linear relationship between physical activity and the rates of all-cause mortality, total CVD, CHD incidence and mortality, and type 2 diabetes. On the other hand, it was more difficult to determine a dose–response relationship for other health outcomes (14, 39). The following Research Insight provides more information.

The response (effect) generated by a particular dose of exercise can include changes in $\dot{V}O_2max$, resting BP, insulin sensitivity, body weight (percentage body fat), and depression. However, as Haskell (26, 27) pointed out, we may have to reexamine our understanding of cause and effect when we study how a dose of physical activity relates to the responses of physical fitness and health. Physical activity could bring about favorable changes by improving

- fitness (especially cardiovascular fitness) and thereby health,
- fitness and health simultaneously and separately,
- fitness but not a specific health outcome, or
- a specific health outcome but not fitness.

Improvements in a variety of health-related concerns do not depend on an increase in $\dot{V}O_2max$; this distinction is important to mention at the beginning of this chapter, which concerns itself with ways to improve $\dot{V}O_2max$.

Key Point

An exercise dose reflects the interaction of the intensity, frequency, duration, and type of exercise. The cause of the health-related response may relate to an improved $\dot{V}O_2max$ or may act through some other mechanism, making health-related outcomes and gains in $\dot{V}O_2max$ independent of each other.

Short- and Long-Term Responses to Exercise

Haskell indicated that in addition to understanding the cause-and-effect connection between physical activity and specific outcomes, we need to distinguish between short-term (acute) and long-term (training) responses (25, 28). The responses in the days and weeks following the initiation of a dose of exercise can vary substantially, depending on the variable being measured:

- Acute responses—Responses occur with one or several exercise bouts but do not improve further.
- Rapid responses—Benefits occur early and plateau.
- Linear responses—Gains are made continuously over time.
- Delayed responses—Responses occur only after weeks of training.

The need for such distinctions can be seen in figure 10.2 (37), which shows proposed dose–response relationships between physical activity, defined as minutes of exercise per week at 60% to 70% of maximal work capacity, and a variety of physiological responses:

- BP and insulin sensitivity are most responsive to exercise.
- Changes in $\dot{V}O_2max$ and resting HR are intermediate.
- Serum lipid changes such as increases in HDL are delayed.

The dose–response relationship of exercise has important implications when exercise is used alone or in

Research Insight

Although physical activity is known to favorably affect many health-related problems, some people question as to whether evidence exists to support a dose–response relationship. To address this issue, scientists examined both the quality and the quantity of evidence linking physical activity to a wide variety of health-related problems. The results of their deliberations were published in a special supplement of *Medicine and Science in Sports and Exercise* (14).The consensus statement (39) from that meeting found that more activity was associated with lower rates of the following:

- All-cause mortality
- Total CVD
- CHD and mortality
- Type 2 diabetes
- Total fat
- Colon and breast cancer
- Osteoporosis

More (of certain types) activity may cause problems:

- Low-back pain
- Osteoarthritis

Although physical activity helps prevent or treat the following health problems, the symposium found no evidence of a dose–response effect for physical activity in the following problems:

- Blood pressure
- Stroke
- Glucose control in type 2 diabetes
- Blood lipids
- Abdominal and visceral fat
- Depression
- Anxiety
- Independent living in older adults

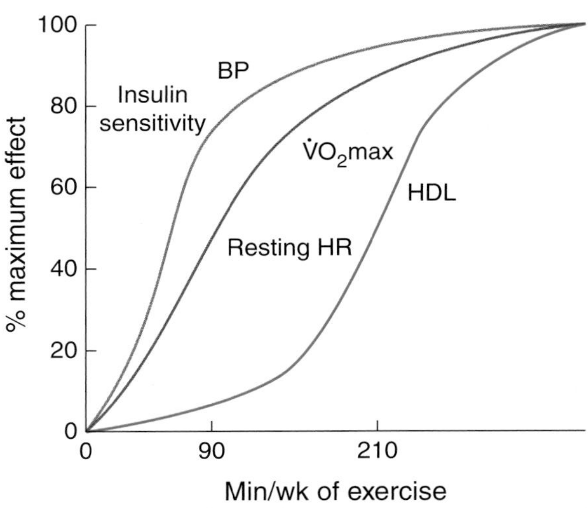

Figure 10.2 Proposed dose–response relationships between amount of exercise performed per week at 60% to 70% maximum work capacity and changes in BP and insulin sensitivity (curve on left), which appear most sensitive to exercise; maximum oxygen consumption ($\dot{V}O_2max$) and resting HR, which are parameters of physical fitness (middle curve); and lipid changes, such as increases in HDL (curve on right).

Reprinted from G.L. Jennings, G. Deakin, P. Korner, I. Meredith, B. Kingwell and L. Nelson, 1991, "What is the dose-response relationship between exercise training and blood pressure?," *Annals of Medicine* 23: 313-318, by permission of Taylor & Francis, Ltd. www.tandfco.uk/journals, .

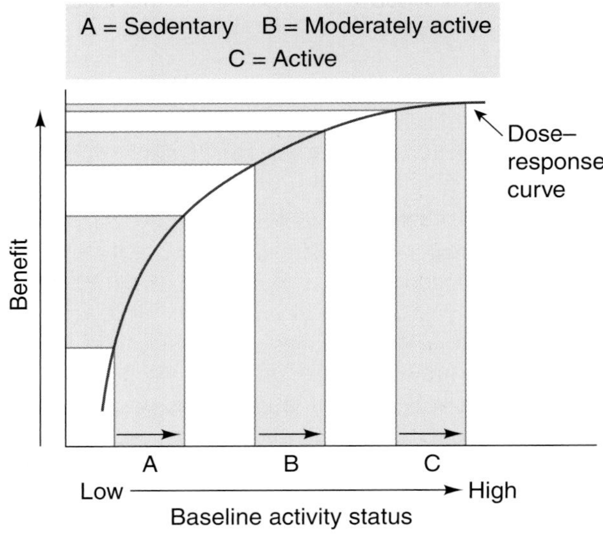

Figure 10.3 The dose–response curve that represents the best estimate of the relationship between physical activity (dose) and health benefit (response).The lower the baseline physical activity status, the greater will be the health benefit associated with a given increase in physical activity (arrows A, B, and C).

From R.R. Pate et al., 1995, "Physical activity and public health," *Journal of the American Medical Association* 273(5): 404.

concert with medication to control disease; we discuss this further in chapter 24.

Public Health Recommendations for Physical Activity

It should be no surprise, given the previous discussion, that it is difficult to provide a single exercise prescription that addresses all the issues related to preventing and treating various diseases. Despite this, there has been a great need to provide a general exercise recommendation to improve the health status of all adults in the United States. The ACSM and the CDC responded to this need by publishing guidelines for physical activity (45): Every U.S. adult should accumulate 30 min or more of moderate-intensity (3-6 METs) physical activity on most, preferably all, days of the week.

These guidelines were based on a comprehensive review of the literature dealing with health-related aspects of physical activity; the dose–response curve in figure 10.3 summarizes the findings. By moving the most sedentary group (A) up just one level of physical activity, the greatest gains in health-related benefits can be realized. These physical activity recommendations were based on the finding that caloric expenditure and total time of physical activity are associated with reduced CVD and mortality. Further, doing the activity in multiple intermittent bouts (e.g., 10 min each) is an alternative way of meeting the 30 min goal (45, 64).

The preceding physical activity recommendations are appropriate for individuals taking the first step from being sedentary to becoming active. However, individuals who expend more than 2,000 kcal · wk^{-1} or who have a high $\dot{V}O_2max$ show the lowest death rate from all causes (6, 44). Greater energy expenditure also helps individuals achieve and maintain a normal body weight (see chapters 11 and 19). Consequently, benefits are gained not only when a sedentary person becomes active but also when a moderately active person engages in more vigorous exercise that increases functional capacity ($\dot{V}O_2max$). This chapter leads you through the steps for developing

Key Point

The basis for the public health physical activity recommendation is that the health-related benefits of physical activity correlate more with the total number of calories expended than with the intensity level of the exercise. The goal is to have sedentary individuals participate in 30 min of moderate-intensity physical activity on most, preferably all, days of the week.

an exercise prescription to improve CRF in apparently healthy individuals.

General Guidelines for CRF Programs

To apply the principles of overload and specificity (see the introduction to part III) to CRF, activities that overload the heart and respiratory systems need to be used in exercise programs. Activities that involve the large muscle groups contracting in a rhythmic and continuous manner can overload the cardiorespiratory systems. Activities involving a small muscle mass and resistance training exercises are less appropriate because they tend to generate very high cardiovascular loads relative to energy expenditure (see chapter 28). Activities that improve CRF are high in caloric cost and therefore help to achieve a goal of relative leanness. So how do you get someone started in a CRF program?

Screen Participants

If the person has not already done so, have her fill out one of the health status forms. Chapter 3 provides guidelines for who should and should not seek medical clearance before exercising.

Encourage Regular Participation

Exercise must become a valuable part of a person's lifestyle. It is not something that can be done sporadically, nor will doing it for only a few months or years build up a fitness reserve. Dramatic gains accomplished through fitness activities are lost quickly with inactivity (see chapter 28). Only people who continue activity as a way of life enjoy its long-term benefits.

Provide Different Types of Activities

A fitness program starts with easily quantified activities, such as walking or cycling, so that the proper exercise intensity can be achieved. After a minimum level of fitness is achieved, a variety of activities are included in the program. Chapter 14 outlines three phases of physical activity: (a) work up to walking briskly each day; (b) gradually begin jogging and work up to jogging continuously for 2 to 3 mi (3.2-4.8 km); and (c) introduce a variety of activities, including exercise to music.

Program for Progression

Given the importance of helping sedentary people become active, the emphasis in any health-related fitness program that includes such individuals should be to start slowly and, when in doubt, do too little rather than too much. Participants should begin at work levels that can be easily completed and should be encouraged to gradually increase the amount of work they can do during a workout. For example, sedentary participants who are interested in jogging should begin a training program by walking a distance that they can complete without feeling fatigued or sore. With time, the participants will be able to walk farther and faster without discomfort. After they can walk several miles briskly without stopping, they can gradually work up to jogging 2 to 3 mi (3.2-4.8 km) continuously during each workout. When these participants are first ready to begin jogging, you might introduce the interval workout (walking, jogging, walking, jogging). As individuals adapt to the interval workouts, they will be able to gradually increase the amount of jogging while decreasing the distance walked (see the walking and jogging programs in chapter 14).

Adhere to Format for a Fitness Workout

The main body of the fitness workout consists of dynamic activities using large muscle groups at an intensity high enough and a duration long enough to accomplish enough total work to specifically overload the cardiorespiratory systems. Stretching and light endurance activities are included before the workout (warm-up) and after the workout (cool-down) for safety and for improving low-back function.

There are physiological, psychological, and safety reasons for including the warm-up and cool-down. In general, the warm-up and cool-down should consist of the following:

- Activities similar to those in the main body of the workout but at a lower intensity (e.g., walking, jogging, or cycling below THR)
- Stretching exercises for the muscles involved in the activity as well as for those in the midtrunk area
- Muscular endurance exercises, especially for the muscles in the abdominal region

These activities help participants ease into and out of a workout and promote a healthy low back. If a workout is going to be shorter than usual, the main body of the workout is the part that should be adjusted so that 5 to 10 min are retained for the warm-up and cool-down.

Conduct Periodic CRF Tests

Routine health-related fitness testing to determine a participant's progress can be motivational and may help alter programs that are not achieving desired results. The fitness professional can help by setting realistic goals for the next testing session when discussing test results. A general rule would be a 10% improvement in 3 mo in

> **Key Point**
>
> People interested in a fitness program should be screened for risk factors and encouraged to exercise regularly. The program should provide different types of activities that use large muscle groups and overload the heart and respiratory systems, and the individual should start slowly and progress gradually to higher levels of work. The workout should have a warm-up and a cool-down, including stretching and muscular endurance exercises for the midtrunk. Periodic CRF tests can be used to alter the exercise prescription.

the test scores that need to change. Once the person has reached a desirable fitness level, the goal is to maintain that level.

Formulating the Exercise Prescription

The CRF training effect depends on the degree to which the systems are overloaded; that is, it depends on the intensity, duration, and frequency of training. **Intensity** generally is expressed as a percentage of some maximal physiological response, typically, oxygen uptake (%$\dot{V}O_2$max) or HR (%HRmax) or derivatives of these—oxygen uptake reserve ($\dot{V}O_2$R) or HR reserve (HRR). These are described in detail in the next section. The interaction of intensity (low to high), duration (short to long), and frequency (seldom to often) should result in an energy expenditure (total work) of 150 to 400 kcal · day^{-1}. The lower end of this range is a little over the 1,000 kcal · wk^{-1} recommended for previously sedentary individuals to gain health benefits (3).

Intensity

How hard does a person have to work to sufficiently overload the cardiovascular and respiratory systems to increase CRF? To answer this question, we must first define the different expressions of exercise intensity and show how they relate to each other.

- **Percentage of maximal oxygen uptake (%$\dot{V}O_2$max).** Across a broad range of CRF levels, many physiological responses are normalized (i.e., made similar between individuals) when the intensity of exercise is expressed as a percentage of $\dot{V}O_2$max (%$\dot{V}O_2$max). A person who is working at 24.5 ml · kg^{-1} · min^{-1} and has a $\dot{V}O_2$max of 35 ml · kg^{-1} · min^{-1} is working at 70% $\dot{V}O_2$max. This approach has been used extensively to develop exercise guidelines, as can be seen in the *ACSM's Guidelines for Exercise Testing and Prescription* and its position stands. However, in the most recent updates of both of these documents, the relative intensity is expressed as the percentage of oxygen uptake reserve (%$\dot{V}O_2$R) (2, 3).
- **Percentage of oxygen uptake reserve (%$\dot{V}O_2$R).** $\dot{V}O_2$R is calculated by subtracting 1 MET (3.5 ml · kg^{-1} · min^{-1}) from the subject's $\dot{V}O_2$max. The %$\dot{V}O_2$R is a percentage of the difference between resting $\dot{V}O_2$ and $\dot{V}O_2$max and is calculated by subtracting 1 MET from the exercise oxygen uptake, dividing by the subject's $\dot{V}O_2$R, and multiplying by 100%. For example, an individual with a $\dot{V}O_2$max of 35 ml · kg^{-1} · min^{-1} who is exercising at 24.5 ml · kg^{-1} · min^{-1} is at 67% $\dot{V}O_2$R: (24.5 – 3.5) ÷ (35 – 3.5) · 100%. The %$\dot{V}O_2$R equals the HR response when HR is expressed as a percentage of the HRR (59, 60).
- **Percentage of HRR (%HRR).** The HRR is calculated by subtracting resting HR from maximal HR. The %HRR is a percentage of the difference between resting and maximal HR and is calculated by subtracting resting HR from the exercise HR, dividing by the HRR, and multiplying by 100%. An individual exercising at 160 beats · min^{-1} who has a maximal HR of 200 beats · min^{-1} and a resting HR of 60 beats · min^{-1} is working at 71% of the HRR: (160 – 60) ÷ (200 – 60) · 100%. For many years the %HRR was believed to be linked to the %$\dot{V}O_2$max on a one-to-one basis; that is, 70% HRR = 70% $\dot{V}O_2$max. However, Swain and colleagues (59, 60) pointed out that although this is the case when fit individuals exercise vigorously, it is not the case for low intensities of exercise, especially when they are performed by people with low fitness levels. For example, a 3 MET activity for someone with a 5 MET maximal aerobic power is 60% $\dot{V}O_2$max but only 50% of $\dot{V}O_2$R: 2 METs ÷ (5 METs – 1 MET) · 100%. An advantage of expressing exercise intensity as %HHR is that the %$\dot{V}O_2$R is numerically identical to the %HRR across the fitness continuum.
- **Percentage of maximal HR (%HRmax).** Because of the linear relationship between HR (above 110 beats · min^{-1}) and $\dot{V}O_2$ during dynamic exercise, investigators and clinicians have long used a simple percentage of maximal HR (%HRmax) to estimate %$\dot{V}O_2$max in setting exercise intensity. This method of expressing exercise intensity is easier to teach than is the %HRR.
- **Rating of perceived exertion (RPE).** The RPE is not viewed as a substitute for prescribing exercise intensity by HR, but once the relationship between the HR and RPE has been established, RPE can be used in its place (2). However, the RPE may not consistently translate to the same intensity for different modes of exercise, so do not expect the RPE to exactly match to a %HRmax or %HRR (3).

Table 10.1 shows the categories of exercise intensity as described in the 1998 ACSM position stand, with

Table 10.1 Classification of Physical Activity Intensity

	Endurance activity										
	Relative intensity			Intensity (METs and $\%\dot{V}O_2max$) in healthy adults differing in $\dot{V}O_2$							
	$\%\dot{V}O_2R$*										
Intensity	%HRR	$\%HR_{max}$ [y]	RPE [‡]	$\dot{V}O_2max$ = 12 METs		$\dot{V}O_2max$ = 10 METs		$\dot{V}O_2max$ = 8 METs		$\dot{V}O_2max$ = 5 METs	
				METs	$\%\dot{V}O_2max$	METs	$\%\dot{V}O_2max$	METs	$\%\dot{V}O_2max$	METs	$\%\dot{V}O_2max$
Very light	<20	<50	<10	<3.2	<27	<2.8	<28	<2.4	<30	<1.8	<36
Light	20-39	50-63	10-11	2.3-5.3	27-44	2.8-4.5	28-45	2.4-3.7	30-47	1.8-2.5	36-51
Moderate	40-59	64-76	12-13	5.4-7.5	45-62	4.6-6.3	46-63	3.8-5.1	48-64	2.6-3.3	52-67
Hard	60-84	77-93	14-16	7.4-10.2	63-85	6.4-8.6	64-86	5.2-6.9	65-86	3.4-4.3	68-87
Very hard	≥85	≥94	17-19	≥10.3	≥86	≥8.7	≥87	≥7.0	≥87	≥4.4	≥88
Maximal	100	100	20	12	100	10	100	8	100	5	100

* $\%\dot{V}O_2R$ = percent of oxygen uptake reserve; %HRR = percent of heart rate reserve.
[y] %HRmax = 0.7305 ($\%\dot{V}O_2max$) + 29.95 (Londeree and Ames 1976); values based on 10 MET group.
[‡] Borg Rating of Perceived Exertion 6-20 Scale (Borg 1988).
$\%\dot{V}O_2max = [(100\% - 90\% \dot{V}O_2 R) \text{ MET max}^{-1}] + \% \dot{V}O_2 R$ (personal communication, Dave Swain, 2000).
Modified from Table 1 of ACSM Position Stand (ACSM 1998), and Howley (2001).

$\%\dot{V}O_2R$ and %HRR used to set the standard for the other expressions of exercise intensity (2). These are shown on the left side of the table, with intensities ranging from very light to maximal.

The RPE values are based on the Borg RPE 6-20 scale (7). The values in table 10.1 for %HRmax and $\%\dot{V}O_2max$ have been updated to more accurately reflect the relationship between them and $\%\dot{V}O_2R$ (%HRR) (35). Further, Table 10.1 provides the absolute exercise intensities (in METs) for each of the intensity classifications for four groups that vary in $\dot{V}O_2max$. As you can see, by looking across the table from the 12 MET to the 5 MET column, the difference between $\%\dot{V}O_2max$ and $\%\dot{V}O_2R$ grows larger as $\dot{V}O_2max$ becomes smaller, with the difference more obvious for the very light to moderate range of exercise intensities. For people with $\dot{V}O_2max$ values of 10 METs, there is little practical difference between $\%\dot{V}O_2R$ and $\%\dot{V}O_2max$ values. The MET values listed for each fitness level equal the stated $\%\dot{V}O_2max$ and $\%\dot{V}O_2R$ values. The $\%\dot{V}O_2R$ can be converted to $\%\dot{V}O_2max$ by using the following equation (D.P. Swain, personal communication, 2000):

$$\%\dot{V}O_2max = [(100\% - \%\dot{V}O_2R) \text{ METmax}^{-1}] + \%\dot{V}O_2R$$

The %HRmax values listed in table 10.1 were derived from an equation by Londeree and Ames (40).

$$\%HRmax = 0.7305\ (\%\dot{V}O_2max) + 29.95$$

This equation is similar to those of Swain and colleagues (58) and of Hellerstein and Franklin (30). There was little difference in the %HRmax values across the four fitness groups for each of the intensity classifications, so the $\%\dot{V}O_2max$ values for the 10 MET fitness group were used to provide the %HRmax values for table 10.1.

Table 10.1 allows the fitness professional to consistently classify data on exercise intensity, whether data are expressed in oxygen uptake (METs), HR, or RPE. From a practical standpoint, for people with average CRF who exercise at moderate to hard intensities, there is little practical difference between $\%\dot{V}O_2max$ and $\%\dot{V}O_2R$.

The 1998 ACSM position stand recommended a range of exercise intensities of 40% or 50% to 85% of $\dot{V}O_2R$ (%HRR) to achieve CRF goals. However, the position stand also indicated that the lower end of this continuum of intensities (i.e., 40%-49% $\dot{V}O_2R$) was appropriate for people who are quite unfit (2). That indication is consistent with the need of this group to focus on moderate exercise that can be carried out long enough to achieve health-related benefits and perhaps gains in CRF. Consequently, for the average sedentary individual, the appropriate range of exercise intensities for achieving CRF goals is 50% to 85% of $\dot{V}O_2R$ (% HRR). As you can see in table 10.1, for an individual with a CRF of 10 METs, there is, at most, a 6% difference between the values for $\%\dot{V}O_2max$ and for $\%\dot{V}O_2R$ (% HRR) at moderate to very hard exercise intensities. For that reason we will use $\%\dot{V}O_2max$ and $\%\dot{V}O_2R$ interchangeably, except where special attention is warranted. The following Research Insight provides more information on oxygen uptake reserve.

Research Insight

Traditionally, the intensity of the exercise prescription was based on a percentage of the individual's maximal oxygen uptake, expressed in ml · kg^{-1} · min^{-1} or in METs. Estimates of the percentage of $\dot{V}O_2$max were derived from the percentage of maximal HR or percentage of HRR. The 1998 ACSM position statement (2) recommended that a percentage of oxygen uptake reserve ($\dot{V}O_2$R) be used. The oxygen uptake reserve uses the same principle as the HRR uses; that is, the resting oxygen intake is taken into account. Thus, to determine the exercise intensity of 60% $\dot{V}O_2$R in an individual with a $\dot{V}O_2$max of 40 ml · kg^{-1} · min^{-1}, the following calculation would be made:

$$\dot{V}O_2R = \dot{V}O_2max - \text{resting } \dot{V}O_2$$

In this example, 40 – 3.5 ml · kg^{-1} · min^{-1} = 36.5 ml · kg^{-1} · min^{-1}.

$$60\% \text{ of } 36.5 \text{ ml} \cdot \text{kg}^{-1} \cdot \text{min}^{-1} = 21.9 \text{ ml} \cdot \text{kg}^{-1} \cdot \text{min}^{-1}$$

This number is added to the resting oxygen uptake:

$$\dot{V}O_2 = 21.9 + 3.5 = 25.4 \text{ ml} \cdot \text{kg}^{-1} \cdot \text{min}^{-1}$$

As table 10.2 shows, using $\dot{V}O_2$R results in the person working at a slightly higher target $\dot{V}O_2$ (ml · kg^{-1} · min^{-1}) than that found by simply taking the percentage of the person's $\dot{V}O_2$max without regard to the resting $\dot{V}O_2$. In the preceding example, the individual would be working at 25.4 ml · kg^{-1} · min^{-1} for 60% of $\dot{V}O_2$R, whereas it would be 24 ml · kg^{-1} · min^{-1} for the direct percentage of $\dot{V}O_2$max.The difference between %$\dot{V}O_2$R and %$\dot{V}O_2$max is greater at lower intensity levels and for individuals with lower $\dot{V}O_2$max levels.

Table 10.2 Differences in $\dot{V}O_2$ When Training Intensities Are Expressed as %$\dot{V}O_2$R Versus %$\dot{V}O_2$max for Individuals With Different $\dot{V}O_2$max Values

	$\dot{V}O_2$max — Target $\dot{V}O_2$ (ml · kg^{-1} · min^{-1})					
	20 ml · kg^{-1} · min^{-1}		40 ml · kg^{-1} · min^{-1}		60 ml · kg^{-1} · min^{-1}	
%	%$\dot{V}O_2$max	%$\dot{V}O_2$R	%$\dot{V}O_2$max	%$\dot{V}O_2$R	%$\dot{V}O_2$max	%$\dot{V}O_2$R
40	8	10.1	16	18.1	24	26.1
50	10	11.75	20	21.75	30	31.75
60	12	13.4	24	25.4	36	37.4
70	14	15.05	28	29.05	42	43.05
80	16	16.7	32	32.7	48	48.7

To recap, it generally is believed that the intensity threshold for a training effect is at the low end of the intensity continuum for people who are sedentary and at the high end of the scale for people who are fit (3). For older, deconditioned adults, 40% to 60% $\dot{V}O_2$max is a good place to start, and for adults who are physically active and at the high end of the fitness scale, intensities >80% $\dot{V}O_2$max are appropriate. However, for most people who are cleared to participate in a structured exercise program, 60% to 80% $\dot{V}O_2$max seems to be the optimum range of exercise intensities. Figure 10.4 shows that exercise at the high end of the scale has been associated with more cardiac complications (11, 30). Exercise intensity must be balanced against the duration so that the person can exercise long enough to expend 150 to 400 kcal · day^{-1}, an expenditure that is consistent with achieving CRF and body composition goals. If the exercise intensity is too high, the person may not be able to exercise long enough to achieve the total work goal.

Duration

How many minutes of exercise should a person do per session? Figure 10.4 shows that improvements in $\dot{V}O_2$max

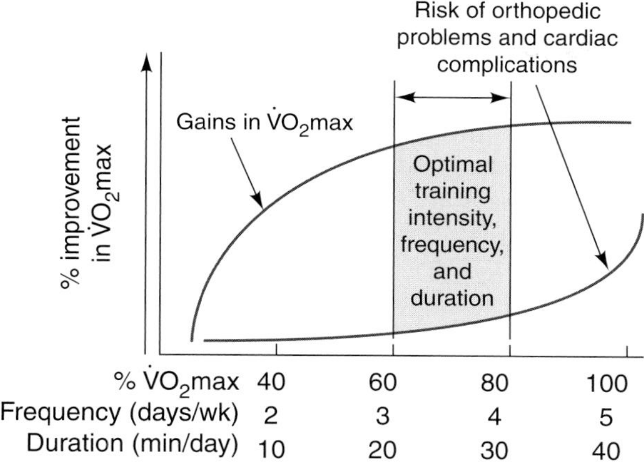

Figure 10.4 Effects of increasing the frequency, duration, and intensity of exercise on the increase in $\dot{V}O_2$max. This figure demonstrates the increasing risk of orthopedic problems attributable to exercise sessions that are too long or conducted too many times per week. The probability of cardiac complications increases with exercise intensity beyond that recommended for improving cardiorespiratory fitness.

From Powers and Howley, 1997. Drawing based on Dehn and Mullins, 1977, and Hellerstein and Franklin, 1984.

increase with the **duration** of the exercise session. However, the optimum duration of an exercise session depends on the intensity. The **total work** accomplished in a session is the most important variable determining CRF gains, once the minimal intensity **threshold** is achieved (3). If the goal were to accomplish 300 kcal of total work in an exercise session in which the individual works at 10 kcal · min^{-1} (2 L of oxygen per min), the duration of the session would have to be 30 min. If the person were working at half that intensity, 5 kcal · min^{-1}, the duration would have to be twice as long. Thirty minutes of exercise can be taken as one 30 min session, two 15 min sessions, or three 10 min sessions. Figure 10.4 also shows that when the duration of hard exercise (75% $\dot{V}O_2$max) exceeds 30 min, the risk of orthopedic injury increases (46).

Frequency

Why recommend that a person do 3 to 5 workouts each week, if 2 would suffice? Figure 10.4 shows that gains in CRF increase with the frequency of exercise but begin to level off at 4 days per wk. People who start a fitness program should plan to exercise 3 or 4 times per week. The long recommended work-a-day-then-rest-a-day routine has been validated by improvements in CRF, low incidence of injuries, and achievement of weight loss goals. Although exercising for fewer than 3 days per wk can improve CRF, the participant would have to exercise at a higher intensity, and weight loss goals may be difficult to achieve (46). Exercising for more than 4 days

> **Key Point**
>
> CRF improves with exercise intensities of 40% to 85% $\dot{V}O_2$R. The intensity threshold for a training effect is lower (40%-60% $\dot{V}O_2$R) for people who are sedentary and higher (>80% $\dot{V}O_2$R) for people who are physically active and have high CRF. The optimal training intensity for the average individual is approximately 60% to 80% $\dot{V}O_2$R. The duration of an exercise session should balance the exercise intensity to result in an energy expenditure of 150 to 400 kcal · day^{-1} (minimum of 1,000 kcal · wk^{-1}). The optimum frequency of training, based on improvement in CRF and a low risk of injuries, is 3 to 4 times each week for exercise intensities rated as hard.

per week for previously sedentary people seems to be too much and results in more dropouts and injuries and less psychological adjustment to the exercise (11, 46).

Determining Intensity

How is exercise intensity set for a particular individual? This section reviews direct and indirect methods to determine appropriate exercise intensity, with a focus on the typically sedentary individual. The approach would be the same for people with very low or very high levels of physical activity and CRF but different intensity guidelines would be used.

Metabolic Load

The most direct way to determine the appropriate exercise intensity is to use a percentage of the measured maximal oxygen consumption. Remember, the optimum range of exercise intensities associated with improved CRF in typically sedentary individuals is 60% to 80% $\dot{V}O_2$max. The advantage of measuring oxygen consumption to determine exercise intensity is that the method is based on the criterion test for CRF—maximal oxygen consumption. The major disadvantages are the expense and difficulty of measuring oxygen consumption for each individual and trying to suit specific fitness activities to meet the specific metabolic demand for each person.

QUESTION: A 75 kg man completes a maximal GXT, and his $\dot{V}O_2$max is 3.0 L · min^{-1}. This equals 15 kcal · min^{-1} (5 kcal · L^{-1} · 3 L · min^{-1}), 40 ml · kg^{-1} · min^{-1}, and 11.4 METs. At what exercise intensities should he work to be at 60% to 80% $\dot{V}O_2$max?

1. 60% of 3.0 L · min^{-1} = 1.8 L · min^{-1}; 80% of 3.0 L · min^{-1} = 2.4 L · min^{-1}.

2. 60% of 15 kcal · min^{-1} = 9 kcal · min^{-1}; 80% of 15 kcal · min^{-1} = 12 kcal · min^{-1}.
3. 60% of 40 ml · kg^{-1} · min^{-1} = 24 ml · kg^{-1} · min^{-1}; 80% of 40 ml · kg^{-1} · min^{-1} = 32 ml · kg^{-1} · min^{-1}.
4. 60% of 11.4 METs = 6.8 METs; 80% of 11.4 METs = 9.1 METs.

Answer: He should use activities that require the following:

1.8 to 2.4 L · min^{-1}

9 to 12 kcal · min^{-1}

24 to 32 ml · kg^{-1} · min^{-1}

6.8 to 9.1 METs

At what exercise intensities does he work to be at 60% and 80% $\dot{V}O_2R$? Using the preceding data, we find that 60% to 80% of $\dot{V}O_2R$ = 60% (40 ml · kg^{-1} · min^{-1} – 3.5 ml · kg^{-1} · min^{-1}) + 3.5 ml · kg^{-1} · min^{-1}.

Target $\dot{V}O_2$= 0.6 (36.5 ml · kg^{-1} · min^{-1}) + 3.5 ml · kg^{-1} · min^{-1}

Target $\dot{V}O_2$ = 21.9 + 3.5 = 25.4 ml · kg^{-1} · min^{-1} = 7.3 METs (i.e., 25.4 ÷ 3.5)

80% (40 ml · kg^{-1} · min^{-1} – 3.5 ml · kg^{-1} · min^{-1}) + 3.5 ml · kg^{-1} · min^{-1}.

Target $\dot{V}O_2$ = 0.8 (36.5 ml · kg^{-1} · min^{-1})+ 3.5 ml · kg^{-1} · min^{-1}

Target $\dot{V}O_2$ = 29.2 + 3.5 = 32.7 ml · kg^{-1} · min^{-1} = 9.3 METs (i.e., 32.7 ÷ 3.5).

Answer: He should use activities that require the following:

25.4 to 32.7 ml · kg^{-1} · min^{-1}

7.3 to 9.3 METs

When these exercise intensity values are known, appropriate exercises can be selected from tables listing the energy costs of various activities (see appendix C for these tables). However, all this is a very cumbersome method for prescribing exercise. Prescribing on the basis of the caloric cost of the activity does not take into consideration the effect that environmental (e.g., heat, humidity, altitude, cold, pollution), dietary (e.g., hydration state), and other variables have on a person's response to some absolute exercise intensity. The ability of participants to complete a workout depends on their physiological responses and perception of effort rather than the metabolic cost of the activity itself. Fortunately, by using specific HR values that are approximately equal to 60% to 80% $\dot{V}O_2max$, you can formulate an exercise prescription that takes many of these factors into consideration. These HR values are called the **target heart rate (THR)** range. How is the THR range determined?

THR: Direct Method

As described in chapters 5 and 28, HR increases linearly with the metabolic load. In the direct method for determining THR, HR is monitored at each stage of a maximal GXT. HR is then plotted on a graph against the $\dot{V}O_2$ (or MET) equivalents of each stage of the test. The fitness professional determines the THR range by taking the percentages of $\dot{V}O_2max$ (%$\dot{V}O_2max$) at which the person should train and finding what the HR responses were at those points. Figure 10.5 shows this method being used for a subject with a functional capacity of 10.5 METs. Work rates of 60% to 80% of maximal METs demanded HR responses of 132 to 156 beats · min^{-1}, respectively. The HR values become the intensity guide for the subject and represent the THR range (2).

THR: Indirect Methods

In contrast to the direct method, which requires the participant to complete a maximal GXT, two indirect methods have been developed to estimate an appropriate THR.

HRR Method

The HRR is the difference between resting and maximal HR. For a maximal HR of 200 beats · min^{-1} and a resting HR of 60 beats · min^{-1}, the HRR is 140 beats · min^{-1}. As shown in figure 10.6, the percentage of the HRR equals the percentage of $\dot{V}O_2R$ across the range of exercise intensities (59, 60). For participants with average to high levels of CRF, the %HRR approximately equals the %$\dot{V}O_2max$.

The HRR method of determining the THR range, made popular by Karvonen, requires a few simple calculations (38):

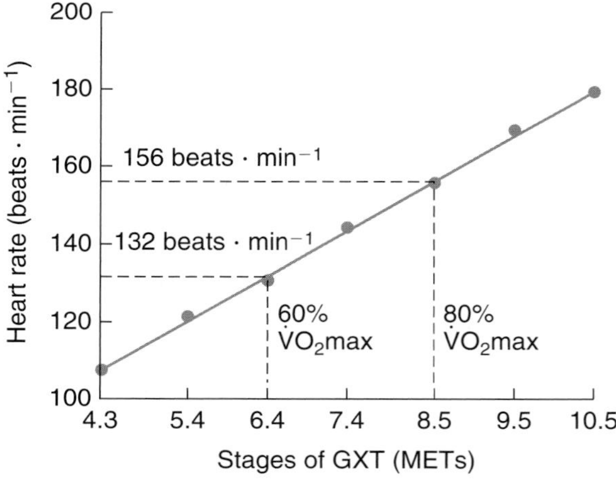

Figure 10.5 Direct method of determining the THR zone when maximal aerobic power (functional capacity) is measured during a GXT.

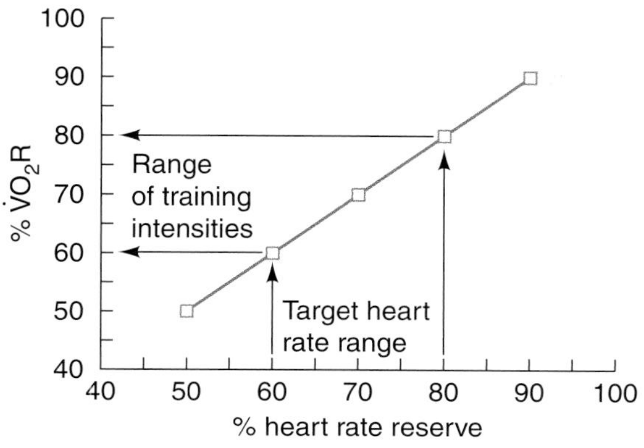

Figure 10.6 Relationship of percentage HRR and percentage of oxygen uptake reserve (%$\dot{V}O_2R$).
From D.P. Swain, B.C. Leutholtz, M.E. King, L.A. Haas and J.D. Branch, 1998, "Relationship between % heart rate reserve and % $\dot{V}O_2$ reserve in treadmill exercise," *Medicine and Science in Sports and Exercise* 30: 318-321.

1. Subtract the resting HR from the maximal HR to obtain the HRR.
2. Calculate 60% and 80% of the HRR.
3. Add each value to the resting HR to obtain the THR range.

QUESTION: A 40-yr-old male participant has a measured maximal HR of 175 beats · min^{-1} and a resting HR of 75 beats · min $^{-1}$. What is his THR range, calculated by the Karvonen (HRR) method?

Answer:

1. HRR = 175 beats · min^{-1} – 75 beats · min^{-1} = 100 beats · min^{-1}
2. 60% of 100 beats · min^{-1} = 60 beats · min^{-1}, and 80% of 100 beats · min^{-1} = 80 beats · min^{-1}
3. 60 beats · min^{-1} + 75 beats · min^{-1} = 135 beats · min^{-1} for 60% $\dot{V}O_2max$

   80 beats · min^{-1} + 75 beats · min^{-1} = 155 beats · min^{-1} for 80% $\dot{V}O_2max$

The advantages of using this procedure to determine exercise intensity are that the recommended THR is always between the person's resting and maximal HRs and that the %HRR equals the %$\dot{V}O_2R$ across the entire range of CRF. Although the resting HR varies and can be influenced by factors such as caffeine, lack of sleep, dehydration, emotional state, and training, this variation does not introduce serious errors into calculating the THR by the Karvonen method (24). Consider the following example:

QUESTION: The 40-yr-old subject mentioned previously participates in an endurance training program, and his resting HR decreases by 10 beats · min^{-1}. Because maximal HR (175 beats · min^{-1}) is not affected by training, what happens to his THR range?

Answer:

1. The HRR now equals 175 beats · min^{-1} – 65 beats · min^{-1} = 110 beats · min^{-1}
2. 60% of 110 beats · min^{-1} = 66 beats · min^{-1} + 65 beats · min^{-1} = 131 beats · min^{-1}
3. 80% of 110 beats · min^{-1} = 88 beats · min^{-1} + 65 beats · min^{-1} = 153 beats · min^{-1}

Consequently, the change in resting HR had only a minimal effect on the THR range.

Percentage of Maximal HR Method

Another method of determining THR range is to use a fixed percentage of the maximal HR (%HRmax). The advantage of this method is its simplicity and the fact that it has been validated across many populations (30, 41, 58). Figure 10.7 shows the relationship between %HRmax and %$\dot{V}O_2max$.

It is clear that %HRmax and %$\dot{V}O_2max$ are linearly related and that the %HRmax can be used to estimate the metabolic load in training programs. The usual guideline to estimate reasonable exercise intensity for the typically sedentary individual is 70% to 85% HRmax. This THR range equals approximately 55% to 75% $\dot{V}O_2max$ and results in an intensity prescription that is slightly more conservative than that generated by the HRR method when 60% to 80% of HRR is used. The range of 75% to 90% HRmax is more similar to 60% to 80% $\dot{V}O_2max$ and HRR; the following example shows how to use the %HRmax method to calculate the THR range.

QUESTION: How can I calculate a THR range if I don't know what the resting HR is? Use the data from the 40-yr-old subject mentioned previously, who had a measured maximal HR of 175 beats · min^{-1}.

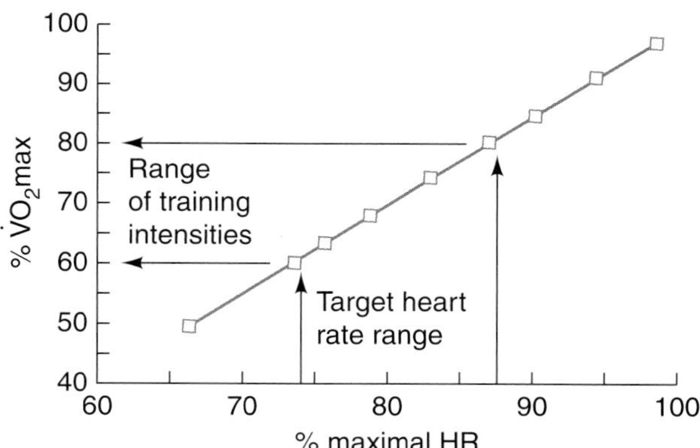

Figure 10.7 Relationship of percentage of maximal heart rate (%HRmax) and percentage of maximal aerobic power (%$\dot{V}O_2max$).
From B.R. Londeree and S.A. Ames, 1979, "Trend analysis of the % $\dot{V}O_2$max-HRregression," *Medicine and Science in Sports and Exercise* 8: 122-125.

Table 10.3 Relationship of %HRmax and %$\dot{V}O_2$max

%$\dot{V}O_2$max	%HRmax
50	66
55	70
60	74
65	77
70	81
75	85
80	88
85	92

From Londeree and Ames, 1976.

Answer: Take 75% and 90% of the maximal HR:

75% of 175 beats · min^{-1} = 131 beats · min^{-1}, and

90% of 175 beats · min^{-1} = 158 beats · min^{-1}.

These values are similar to those calculated by using the HRR method described earlier. Table 10.3 shows the relationship between %$\dot{V}O_2$max and %HRmax across the range of exercise intensities from 50% to 85% $\dot{V}O_2$max. Using this table simplifies the process of making specific exercise intensity recommendations by using the %HRmax method.

Threshold

As mentioned earlier, the intensity of exercise that provides an adequate stimulus for cardiorespiratory improvement varies with activity level and age and spans the range of 40% to 85% $\dot{V}O_2$R and $\dot{V}O_2$max. In a systematic review of the literature, Swain and Franklin verified the low end of the threshold range. They found that the threshold for an improvement in $\dot{V}O_2$max was only 30% HRR for people with $\dot{V}O_2$max values less than 40 ml · kg^{-1} · min^{-1} and only 46% HRR for individuals with higher $\dot{V}O_2$max values; however, higher intensities more effectively increased $\dot{V}O_2$max (61). Consequently, for most of the population, the optimal intensity threshold is in the following ranges:

- 60% to 80% of $\dot{V}O_2$max, HRR, and $\dot{V}O_2$R
- 75% to 90% of HRmax

As we mentioned at the beginning of this section, the threshold is toward the lower part of the range (50%-60% HRR) for older, sedentary populations and toward the upper part of the range (>80% HRR) for younger, more fit populations. The middle of the range (70% HRR, 70% $\dot{V}O_2$max, or 80% HRmax) is an *average* training intensity and is appropriate for the typical apparently healthy person who wishes to be involved in a regular fitness program. Participating in activities at these intensities constitutes an overload on the cardiorespiratory system, resulting in an adaptation over time.

HRmax

The indirect methods for determining exercise intensity use HRmax. It is recommended that the HRmax be measured directly (by maximal GXT) when possible. If it cannot be measured, then any estimation must consider the effect of age on HRmax. Previously, HRmax had been estimated with the formula HRmax = 220 – age. However, this formula underestimates HRmax for older individuals (see the Research Insight).

Any estimate of HRmax is a potential source of error for both the HRR and the %HRmax methods of calculating a THR. For example, given that 1 SD of this estimate of HRmax is about 10 beats · min^{-1}, a 45-yr-old's true HRmax may be anywhere between 145 and 205 beats · min^{-1} (3 SD) rather than the estimated 175. However, 68% (1 SD) of the population would be between 165 and 185 beats · min^{-1}. If the HRmax is known (e.g., from a GXT), the fitness professional should use this measured HRmax to determine THR rather than using the estimate with its potential error (41). Estimating HRmax is another reason for using caution when relying solely on the THR range as an indicator of exercise intensity. The potential for error exists both in the estimate of HRmax and in the equations in which various percentages of HRmax are used to predict %$\dot{V}O_2$max The intensity levels should only be considered as guidelines (see the Research Insight on page 165).

Research Insight

Tanaka, Monahan, and Seals (62) evaluated the validity of the classic 220 – age formula for estimating HRmax. They analyzed 351 published studies and cross-validated these findings with a well-controlled laboratory study. They found almost identical results for both approaches: HRmax = 208 – 0.7 · age. This new formula yields HRmax values that are 6 beats · min^{-1} lower for 20-yr-olds and 6 beats · min^{-1} higher for 60-yr-olds. Although the new formula yields better estimates of HRmax on average, the investigators emphasize the fact that the estimated HRmax for a given individual is still associated with a standard deviation of 10 beats · min^{-1}.

Research Insight

The two indirect HR methods for estimating exercise intensity provide guidelines to use in an exercise program, and small differences between methods are not important. Both approaches must be used as guidelines because, as for any prediction equation, an error is involved in the resulting estimation. For example, 2 SDs of the estimate of % $\dot{V}O_2$max determined from HR equal 11.4% $\dot{V}O_2$max (40). Therefore, for 95% of participants, when we use %HRR or %HRmax to predict a work intensity that is 60% $\dot{V}O_2$max, the true intensity is somewhere between 48.6% and 71.4% $\dot{V}O_2$max! This is why these calculated THR values should be used as guidelines in helping individuals increase or maintain CRF. The fitness professional needs other indicators of exercise intensity to compensate for some of the inherent variability in the THR prescription (see later in this chapter).

Use of THR

The concept of an intensity threshold provides the basis for regular fitness workouts. Low-intensity activity around the house, yard, and office should be encouraged, but specific workouts above the intensity threshold are necessary to achieve optimum CRF results. At the other extreme, people who push themselves near their maximum do not have a fitness advantage because similar results can be obtained at any lower intensity that is above the threshold.

The THR can be used as an intensity guide for large muscle group, continuous, whole-body types of activities such as walking, running, swimming, rowing, cycling, skiing, and dancing. However, the same training results may not occur from activities using small muscle groups or resistance exercises, because these exercises elevate the HR much higher for the same metabolic load.

People who are less active and have more risk factors should use the lower end of the THR range. More active people with fewer risk factors should use the upper end of the THR range. The THR can be divided by 6 to provide the desired 10 sec THR. If the person's HRmax is unknown, the estimated THR for 10 sec, by age and activity level, can be found in table 10.4. People can learn to exercise at their THRs by walking or jogging for several minutes and then stopping and immediately taking a 10 sec HR. If the person's HR is not within the target range, then the individual should adjust the intensity by going slower or faster for a few minutes and then taking another 10 sec count. Using the THR to set exercise intensity has many advantages:

- It has a built-in individualized progression (i.e., as people increase their fitness, they have to work harder to achieve the THR).
- It accounts for environmental conditions (e.g., a person decreases the intensity while working in very hot temperatures).
- It is easily determined, learned, and monitored.

These recommendations are appropriate for most people, but individuals differ in terms of the threshold

Table 10.4 Estimated 10 Sec Target Heart Rate for People Whose Maximal Heart Rate Is Unknown

	Intensity	Age (yr)						
Population	%$\dot{V}O_2$max	20	30	40	50	60	70	80
Inactive with several risk factors	50	22	21	20	18	17	16	15
	55	23	22	21	19	18	17	16
Normal activity with few risk factors	60	24	23	22	20	19	18	17
	65	25	24	23	21	20	19	18
	70	26	25	24	22	21	20	18
	75	28	26	25	24	22	21	19
	80	29	28	26	25	23	22	20
Very active with low risk	85	30	29	27	26	24	23	21
	90	31	30	28	27	25	24	22

Data from Londeree and Ames, 1976.

needed for a training effect, the rate of adaptation to the training, and how exercise feels to them. The fitness professional must use subjective judgment, based on observations of the person exercising, to determine whether the intensity should be higher or lower. If the work is so easy that the person experiences little or no increase in ventilation and is able to work without effort, then the intensity should be increased. At the other extreme, if a person shows signs of doing very hard work and is still unable to reach THR, then a lower intensity should be chosen. In this case, the top part of the THR range might be above the person's true HRmax because the 220 – age formula only roughly estimates the true value. The fitness professional should not rely on the THR as the only method of judging whether the participant is exercising at the correct intensity. Attention should be paid to other signs and symptoms of overexertion; the Borg RPE scale might be useful in this regard (see box below).

RPE

The Borg RPE scale that is used to indicate the subjective sensation of effort experienced during a GXT (see chapter 5) can be used in prescribing exercise for the apparently healthy individual (7). Exercise perceived as just below somewhat hard to just above hard, a rating of 12 to 16 on the original RPE scale, approximates 40% or 50% to 85% of $\dot{V}O_2R$ or 60% or 65% to 90% of HRmax (2, 3). As mentioned earlier, the RPE is not viewed as a substitute for prescribing exercise intensity by HR (2). However, if the HRmax is not known and the THR range is perceived as too low or too high, an RPE rating can estimate the overall effort experienced by the individual; the exercise intensity can then be adjusted accordingly. Further, as a participant becomes accustomed to the physical sensations experienced when exercising at the THR range, there will be less need for frequently measuring the pulse rate.

Key Point

The exercise intensity for a CRF training effect can be described in a variety of ways: 40% or 50% to 85% $\dot{V}O_2R$ (HRR), 60% or 65% to 90% HRmax, and 12 to 16 on the original RPE scale.

When Moderate-Intensity Exercise May Be Hard

The ACSM and CDC have recommended that every U.S. adult accumulate 30 min or more of moderate-intensity (3-6 METs) physical activity on most, preferably all, days of the week. The fitness professional must recognize that the range of 3 to 6 METs, while being moderate exercise for some, may be hard exercise for others. Figure 10.8 shows the relative intensity for a fixed exercise to vary considerably across the range of $\dot{V}O_2max$ values (35). Consequently, some individuals with low $\dot{V}O_2max$ values would function in the intensity range consistent with achieving gains in $\dot{V}O_2max$, whereas those with higher CRF values would not. This example emphasizes the need to consider the THR range and the RPE when following recommendations that specify absolute exercise intensities (e.g., METs).

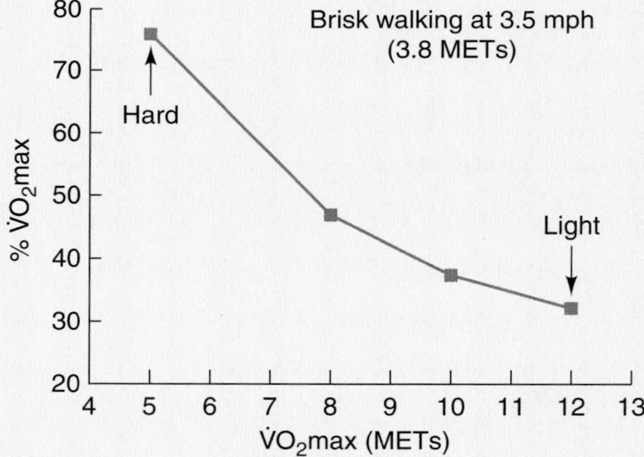

Figure 10.8 Changes in the relative intensity of exercise (% $\dot{V}O_2max$) when the same absolute intensity of exercise is performed by groups differing in $\dot{V}O_2max$ (METs).

Reprinted, by permission, from E.T. Howley, 2001, "Type of activity: Resistance, aerobic and leisure versus occupational physical activity," *Medicine and Science in Sports and Exercise* 33: S364-369.

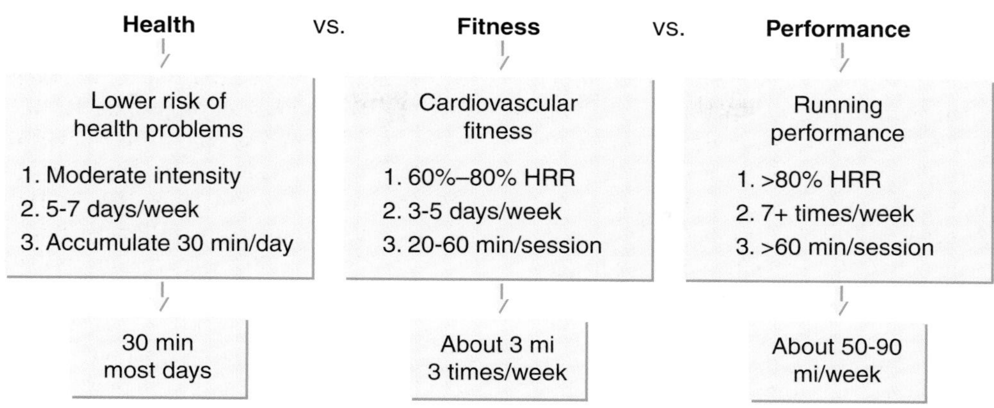

Figure 10.9 Contrasting recommendations for achieving health, fitness, and performance goals.

Exercise Recommendations for the Untested Masses

Certain general recommendations can be made for any person wanting to begin a fitness program. Although the fitness professional might wish to have each individual undergo a complete testing protocol before beginning exercise, that simply is not realistic. In addition, people without known health problems who follow the general guidelines mentioned before can begin to exercise at low risk. In fact, the CHD risks of continuing not to exercise are greater than those of beginning a modest exercise program. Figure 10.9 summarizes the recommendations for achieving health, fitness, and performance goals.

Exercise Programming for the Fit Population

Exercise recommendations written for people who are reasonably physically fit tend to be associated with less risk, and these participants require less supervision. In fact, people in this group may focus on performance, in contrast to health and fitness, as the primary goal. A wide variety of programs, activities, races, and competitions is available to address the needs of this group.

The THR range will be calculated as described before, but very fit individuals will work at the top part of the range (>85% of $\dot{V}O_2$max or >90% of HRmax). As was mentioned earlier, a person who is less fit can start working out at the low end of the range and still experience a training effect. The individual who is more fit needs to work at the top end of the range to maintain a high level of fitness.

Training for competition demands more than the training intensity needed for CRF. Individuals who do interval-type training programs have peak HRs close to maximum during the intervals. The recovery period between the intervals should include some work at a lower intensity (near 40%-50% $\dot{V}O_2$max) to help metabolize the lactate produced during the interval (13) and to reduce the chance of cardiovascular complications that can occur when a person comes to a complete rest at the end of a strenuous exercise bout (47).

For people who participate in sports that are intermittent in nature but that still require high levels of aerobic fitness for success, a running and jogging program is a good way to maintain general conditioning when not participating in the primary sport. However, given the specificity of training, there is no substitute for the real activity when conditioning for a sport.

As figure 10.9 shows, people interested in performance who work at the top end of the THR range, who exercise 5 to 7 or more times each week, and who exercise for longer than 60 min each exercise session are doing much more than the person interested in fitness, and it should be no surprise that they tend to experience more injuries. When the risk of injury during exercise is coupled with the inherent risks associated with competitive activities, it is clear that alternative activities should be planned that can be done when participation in the primary activity is not possible. This planning reduces the chance of becoming detrained when injuries do occur.

Exercise Prescriptions Using Complete GXT Results

In the previous sections, the exercise recommendation was made on the basis of little or no specific information about the person involved. In many adult fitness programs, potential participants have had a general medical exam or a maximal GXT with appropriate monitoring of the HR, BP, and possibly ECG responses. Unfortunately, this information sometimes is not used in designing the exercise program; instead, the measured HRmax is used in the THR formulas and the rest of the data are ignored. This section outlines the steps that should be followed when the fitness professional assists in making the exercise recommendation using information about the person's functional capacity and cardiovascular responses to graded exercise. The fitness professional is not generally involved in the clinical evaluation of a GXT, but understanding the procedures used to make clinical judgments clearly enhances communication with the program director, exercise specialist, and physician. The following information on using GXTs for exercise prescription and programming was written with this intent.

Program Selection

Exercise program options include exercising alone, in small groups, in fitness clubs, and in clinically oriented settings. The fitness professional must consider a variety of factors before recommending participation in a supervised or an unsupervised program.

Supervised Program

The risk factors, the response to the GXT, the health and activity history, and personal preference influence the type of program in which an individual should participate. Generally, the higher the risk, the more important it is that the person participate in a supervised program. People at high risk for CHD and those who have diseases such as diabetes, hypertension, asthma, and CHD should be encouraged to participate under supervision, at least at the beginning of an exercise program. The personnel in the supervised program are trained to provide the necessary instruction in the appropriate activities, to help monitor the participant's response to the activity, and to administer appropriate first aid or emergency care.

Supervised programs run the gamut from those conducted within a hospital for patients with CHD and other diseases to programs conducted in fitness clubs for people at low risk for CHD. In general, as a person moves along the continuum from inpatient to outpatient, less formal monitoring is required. In addition, the background and training of the personnel tend to vary. The exercise programs aimed at maintaining the fitness level of the CHD patients who went through a hospital-based program have medical personnel and emergency equipment appropriate for the population being served. Supervised fitness programs for the apparently healthy have a fitness professional who can focus more on the appropriate exercise, diet, and other lifestyle behaviors needed to improve health.

Using GXTs for Exercise Prescription and Programming

Analyzing GXT for Exercise Prescription

1. Analyze the person's history and list the known risk factors for CHD; also, identify those factors that might have a direct bearing on the exercise program, such as orthopedic problems, previous physical activity, and current interests.
2. Determine if the functional capacity is a true maximum or if it is limited by a sign or symptom. Express the functional capacity in METs, and record the highest HR and RPE achieved without significant signs or symptoms.
3. If ECG was monitored, itemize the person's ECG changes as indicated by the physician.
4. Examine the HR and BP responses to see if they are normal.
5. List the symptoms reported at each stage.
6. List the reasons why the test was stopped (e.g., ECG changes, falling SBP, dizziness).

Designing an Exercise Program From a GXT

1. Given the overall response to the GXT, decide to either refer for additional medical care or initiate an exercise program.
2. Identify the THR range and approximate MET intensities of selected activities needed to be within that THR range.
3. Specify the frequency and duration of activity needed to meet the goals of increased CRF and weight loss.
4. Recommend that the person (a) participate in either a supervised or an unsupervised program, (b) be monitored or unmonitored, and (c) do group or individual activities.
5. Select a variety of activities at the appropriate MET level that allow the person to achieve THR. Consider environmental factors, medication, and any physical limitations of the participant when making this recommendation.

The supervised program offers a socially supportive environment for individuals to become and stay active. This is important, given the difficulty of changing lifestyle behaviors. The group program allows for more variety in the activities used (e.g., group games) and reduces the chance of boredom. For the program to be effective in the long run the program leader should try to wean the participants from the group in a way that encourages them to maintain their activity patterns when they are no longer in the program.

Unsupervised Program

Despite the risks just described, the vast majority of people at risk for or already having CHD participate in unsupervised exercise programs. Reasons for this include the limited number of supervised programs, the level of interest of the participant and physician in such programs, and the financial resources required to participate in such programs.

Participation in an unsupervised exercise program requires the fitness professional or physician to clearly communicate how to begin and maintain the exercise program. The emphasis in beginning an unsupervised exercise program is on low intensity (e.g., 40%-50% $\dot{V}O_2R$, ~50% $\dot{V}O_2max$, or ~65% HRmax), because the threshold for a training effect is lower in deconditioned people. The goal is to increase the duration of the activity, with exercise frequency approaching every day. This reduces the chance of muscular, skeletal, or cardiovascular problems caused by the exercise intensity and increases muscle function with the expenditure of a relatively large number of calories. In addition, the regularity of the exercise program encourages a positive habit. The outcome of such programs results in the individual being able to conduct her daily affairs with more comfort and sets the stage for people who would like to exercise at higher levels.

In an unsupervised exercise program, the person should be provided explicit information about the intensity (THR), duration, and frequency of exercise so that no doubt remains about what should be done. For example, the exercise recommendation might read, "Walk 1 mi (1.6 km) in 30 min each day for 2 wk. Monitor and record your heart rate." The person must be told how to take the pulse rate and be encouraged to follow through on the recording.

Updating the Exercise Program

During participation in an endurance training program, an individual's capacity for work increases. The best sign of this is that the recommended exercise is no longer sufficient to reach THR; clearly the person is adapting to the exercise. Taking the HR during a regular activity session provides a sound basis for upgrading the intensity or duration of the exercise session.

The exercise program, including the THR, should be updated periodically. The need to update is greater for those with a lower initial level of fitness and a greater number of risk factors. An individual who has a low functional capacity because of heart disease, orthopedic limitations, or chronic inactivity (which might include prolonged bed rest) has difficulty reaching a true maximum on a first treadmill test. Further, he experiences the greatest improvements in the shortest time during the fitness program. This individual benefits from frequent retesting because the test allows progress (or the lack thereof) to be monitored, and it may give new information that influences the exercise prescription. If the person has had a change in medication that influences the HR response to exercise, the exercise program must be reevaluated.

For people who reach a true maximum in the first test, actual THR will change little during a fitness program because the HRmax is affected very little by regular endurance exercise. However, these people still benefit from a regular evaluation of the overall exercise program, given that their activity interests may change or they may develop orthopedic problems that did not exist before. The reevaluation allows fitness professionals to probe for information that may enable them to refer the person for treatment at a time when treatment will do the most good. Such contact increases the

Key Point

Exercise recommendations for the general public emphasize low intensity and regular participation; see the public health physical activity recommendations on page 167. Exercise performed at 60% to 80% $\dot{V}O_2R$ for 20 to 40 min 3 or 4 times · wk^{-1} increases and maintains CRF. Exercise recommendations for very fit individuals emphasize the top end of the training intensity (>80% $\dot{V}O_2R$) and frequent (almost daily) participation. The potential for injury is greater for such performance-driven workouts. For people who undergo a comprehensive, diagnostic GXT with ECG monitoring, all test results are used to select an optimal and safe exercise prescription. Participants with multiple risk factors for CHD and those with existing diseases benefit from participating in a supervised program. However, most of such individuals will participate in an unsupervised program, necessitating clear communication about the exercise prescription and safety concerns.

chance that the person will stay involved in an activity program—which is the most important factor in maintaining aerobic fitness.

Environmental Concerns

THR is used to indicate the proper exercise intensity in health-related fitness programs. However, environmental factors such as heat, humidity, pollution, and altitude can elevate HR and RPE during an exercise session. This could shorten the exercise session and reduce the participant's chance of expending sufficient calories to meet energy balance goals. Fortunately, by decreasing the exercise intensity we can "control" these environmental problems to provide a safe and effective exercise prescription. This section discusses the effects that different environmental factors have on the exercise prescription and what we can do about them.

Environmental Heat and Humidity

Chapter 28 describes the increases in body temperature that occur with exercise, the mechanisms of heat loss called into play, and the benefits of becoming acclimatized to the heat. Our core temperature (37 °C, or 98.6 °F) is within a few degrees of a value that could lead to death by heat injury. As described in chapter 25, however, to prevent a progression from the least to the most serious heat injury, individuals should recognize and attend to a series of stages from heat cramps to heatstroke. Although treating these problems is important, prevention is a better approach.

Each of the following factors influences susceptibility to heat injury and can alter the HR and metabolic responses to exercise:

- **Fitness.** Fit people have a lower risk of heat injury (18), can tolerate more work in the heat (15), and acclimatize to heat faster (9).
- **Acclimatization.** Exercising for 7 to 14 days in the heat increases our capacity to sweat, initiates sweating at a lower body temperature, and reduces salt loss. Body temperature and HR responses are lower during exercise, and the chance of salt depletion is reduced (3, 9).
- **Hydration.** Inadequate hydration reduces sweat rate and increases the chance of heat injury (9, 53, 54). Generally, during exercise the focus should be on replacing water, not salt or carbohydrate stores.
- **Environmental temperature.** Exercising in temperatures greater than skin temperatures results in a heat gain by convection and radiation. Evaporation of sweat must compensate for this gain if body temperature is to remain at a safe level.
- **Clothing.** As much skin surface as possible should be exposed to encourage evaporation, although the skin should be protected by sunblock from too much exposure to the sun. Materials should be chosen that will wick sweat to the surface for evaporation; materials impermeable to water will increase the risk of heat injury and should be avoided.
- **Humidity (water vapor pressure).** Evaporation of sweat depends on the water vapor pressure gradient between skin and environment. In warm and hot environments, the relative humidity is a good index of the water vapor pressure, with a lower relative humidity facilitating the evaporation of sweat.
- **Metabolic rate.** During times of high heat and humidity, decreasing the exercise intensity decreases the heat load as well as the strain on the physiological systems that must deal with it.
- **Wind.** Wind places more air molecules into contact with the skin and can influence heat loss in two ways: If there is a temperature gradient for heat loss between the skin and the air, wind will increase the rate of heat loss by convection. In a similar manner, wind increases the rate of evaporation, assuming the air can accept moisture.

Recommendations for Fitness

The members of a fitness program should be educated about all of the heat-related factors just mentioned. The fitness professional might suggest the following:

- Learning about heat-illness symptoms (e.g., cramps, lightheadedness) and how to deal with them (see chapter 25)
- Exercising in the cooler parts of the day to avoid heat gain from the sun or from building or road surfaces heated by the sun
- Gradually increasing exposure to high heat and humidity over 7 to 14 days to safely acclimatize to these environmental conditions
- Drinking water before, during, and after exercise and weighing in each day to monitor hydration
- Wearing only shorts and a tank top in order to expose as much skin as possible, but being careful to use a sunblock to reduce the chance of skin cancer
- Taking HR measurements several times during the activity and reducing exercise intensity to stay in the THR zone

The last recommendation, regarding THR, is most important. HR is a sensitive indicator of dehydration, environmental heat load, and acclimatization. Variation in any of these factors will modify the HR response to any fixed submaximal exercise. It is therefore important for fitness participants to monitor HR regularly and slow down to stay within the THR zone. The RPE also can be used in circumstances of extreme heat to provide an index of the overall physiological strain that the participant is experiencing.

Implications for Performance

Any athlete performing in an environment that is not conducive to heat loss is at an increased risk of heat injury. This has been a major problem for football, where clothing and equipment prevent heat loss, but the increased number of people participating in 10K races, marathons, and triathlons has shifted our focus to them (21, 36). In the latter cases, the athlete has a very high metabolic rate while exercising in direct exposure to the sun. In response to this problem and on the basis of sound research, the ACSM developed its position stand on thermal injuries (both heat and cold) during distance running (1). The elements in this position stand are consistent with the information presented at the beginning of this section.

Environmental Heat Stress

The preceding discussion mentioned high temperature and relative humidity as factors increasing the risk of heat injuries. To quantify the overall heat stress associated with any environment, a **wet-bulb globe temperature (WBGT)** guide has been developed (1). This overall heat stress index is composed of the following measurements:

- **Dry-bulb temperature (T_{db})**—Ordinary measure of air temperature taken in the shade.
- **Black-globe temperature (T_g)**—Measure of the radiant heat load in direct sunlight; temperature is measured inside a 15 cm diameter of a copper globe painted flat black.
- **Wet-bulb temperature (T_{wb})**—Measurement of air temperature with a thermometer whose mercury bulb is covered with a wet cotton wick, which makes it sensitive to the relative humidity (water vapor pressure) and provides an index of the ability to evaporate sweat.

The formula used to calculate the WBGT temperature shows the importance of the wet-bulb temperature, which makes up 70% (0.7) of the WBGT index, in determining heat stress (1). This is related to the role the wet-bulb temperature plays in estimating the ability to evaporate sweat, the most important heat-loss mechanism in most situations. The formula is as follows:

$$\text{WBGT} = 0.7\ T_{wb} + 0.2\ T_g + 0.1\ T_{db}$$

The risk of heat illness (**hyperthermia**) attributable to environmental stress while wearing shorts, socks, shoes, and a T-shirt is rated on the following scale:

Very high risk: WBGT exceeds 28 °C (82 °F)
High risk: WBGT = 23 to 28 °C (73-82 °F)
Moderate risk: WBGT = 18 to 23 °C (65-73 °F)
Low risk: WBGT less than 18 °C (less than 65 °F)

The risk of **hypothermia** while wearing shorts, socks, shoes, and a T-shirt also must be considered in distance running. A WBGT index of less than 10 °C (less than 50 °F) is associated with an increased risk of hypothermia, especially in wet and windy conditions.

Table 10.5 provides an estimate of the WBGT using just air temperature and relative humidity. Because this table does not include radiant heat load (globe temperature), 4 °F should be added to the estimated WBGT if exercise is conducted in direct sunlight (5).

Table 10.5 Estimate of Wet-Bulb Globe Temperature (WBGT) (°F) From Air Temperature and Relative Humidity (RH%)

	WBGT (°F)										
RH%	60	65	70	75	80	85	90	95	100	105	110
90	60	64	69	74	79	85	90	95	100	105	110
80	59	63	68	72	77	82	88	93	99	105	110
70	58	62	66	71	76	80	85	90	96	102	108
60	57	60	66	69	73	78	83	87	93	98	103
50	55	59	63	67	71	75	80	84	89	94	99
40	54	58	62	65	69	73	77	82	88	90	95
30	53	57	60	64	67	71	76	79	83	87	91
20	52	55	58	62	65	69	72	76	79	83	87
10	51	54	57	60	63	68	69	73	76	79	82

For inside or outside, WBGT can be estimated from air temperature at the time and place of exercise. Relative humidity is very sensitive to air temperature. If the exercise occurs in direct sunlight, add 4 °F to the estimated WBGT. To convert °F to °C, subtract 32 and divide by 1.8.

Adapted, by permission, from American College of Sports Medicine (ACSM), 2001, *ACSM's resource manual for guidelines for exercise testing and prescription*, 4th ed. (Philadelphia, PA: Lippincott, Williams & Wilkins), 209-216.

Exercise and Cold Exposure

Exercising in the cold can create problems if certain precautions are not taken. As mentioned previously, a WBGT of 10 °C (50 °F) or less is associated with hypothermia. Hypothermia is a decrease in body temperature that occurs when heat loss exceeds heat production. In cold air, there is a larger gradient for convective heat loss from the skin; cold air also is dryer (has a low water vapor pressure) and facilitates the evaporation of moisture from the skin to further cool the body. The combined effects can be deadly, as shown in Pugh's report of three deaths during a walking competition of 45 mi (72 km) that was performed in very cold temperatures (49).

Factors related to hypothermia include environmental factors, such as temperature, water vapor pressure, wind, and whether air or water are involved; insulating factors, such as clothing and subcutaneous fat; and the capacity for sustained energy production. Each of these factors is discussed in the following paragraphs.

Environmental Factors

Conduction, convection, and radiation depend on a temperature gradient between the skin and the environment; the larger the gradient, the greater the rate of heat loss. What surprises many is that the environmental temperature does not have to be below freezing to cause hypothermia. Other environmental factors interact with temperature to facilitate heat loss: namely, wind and water.

Windchill Index

The rate of heat loss at any given temperature is influenced directly by wind speed. Wind increases the number of cold air molecules coming into contact with the skin, increasing the rate of heat loss. The **windchill index** indicates the temperature equivalent (under calm air conditions) for any combination of temperature and wind speed (see figure 10.10). The windchill index allows the fitness professional to properly gauge the cold stress associated with a variety of wind velocities and temperatures. Keep in mind that for activities such as running, riding, or cross-country skiing into the wind, the speed of the activity must be added to the wind speed to evaluate the full impact of the windchill. For example, cycling at 20 mi · hr^{-1} (32 km · hr^{-1}) into calm air at 0 °F (–17.8 °C) has a windchill value of –22 °F (–30.0 °C)! However, wind is not the only factor that can increase the rate of heat loss at any given temperature.

Water

Heat is lost 25 times faster in water than in air of the same temperature. Unlike air, water offers little or no insulation

Windchill Chart
Temperature (°F)

Wind (mph)																		
Calm	40	35	30	25	20	15	10	5	0	−5	−10	−15	−20	−25	−30	−35	−40	−45
5	36	31	25	19	13	7	1	−5	−11	−16	−22	−28	−34	−40	−46	−52	−57	−63
10	34	27	21	15	9	3	−4	−10	−16	−22	−28	−35	−41	−47	−53	−59	−66	−72
15	32	25	19	13	6	0	−7	−13	−19	−26	−32	−39	−45	−51	−58	−64	−71	−77
20	30	24	17	11	4	−2	−9	−15	−22	−29	−35	−42	−48	−55	−61	−68	−74	−81
25	29	23	16	9	3	−4	−11	−17	−24	−31	−37	−44	−51	−58	−64	−71	−78	−84
30	28	22	15	8	1	−5	−12	−19	−26	−33	−39	−46	−53	−60	−67	−73	−80	−87
35	28	21	14	7	0	−7	−14	−21	−27	−34	−41	−48	−55	−62	−69	−76	−82	−89
40	27	20	13	6	−1	−8	−15	−22	−29	−36	−43	−50	−57	−64	−71	−78	−84	−91
45	26	19	12	5	−2	−9	−16	−23	−30	−37	−44	−51	−58	−65	−72	−79	−86	−93
50	26	19	12	4	−3	−10	−17	−24	−31	−38	−45	−52	−60	−67	−74	−81	−88	−95
55	25	18	11	4	−3	−11	−18	−25	−32	−39	−46	−54	−61	−68	−75	−82	−89	−97
60	25	17	10	3	−4	−11	−19	−26	−33	−40	−48	−55	−62	−69	−76	−84	−91	−98
Frostbite occurs in:							30 min		10 min					5 min				

$$\text{Windchill (°F)} = 35.74 + 0.6215T - 35.75(V^{0.16}) + 0.4275T(V^{0.16})$$

T = air temperature (°F) V = wind speed (mph)

Figure 10.10 Windchill index.
Courtesy of the NOAA National Weather Service
www.nws.noaa.gov

where it meets the skin, so heat is lost rapidly from the body. Movement in cold water increases heat loss from the arms and legs (32), so it is better to stay as still as possible in long-term unplanned immersions or to wear a wetsuit for anticipated activities in cold water.

Insulating Factors

The rate at which heat is lost from the body is related inversely to the insulation between the body and the environment. The insulating quality is related to the thickness of subcutaneous fat, the ability of clothing to trap air, and whether the clothing is wet or dry.

Body Fat

Subcutaneous fat thickness is an excellent indicator of total body insulation per unit surface area through which heat is lost (29). For example, in one report an obese man was able to swim for 7 hr in 16 °C water with no change in body temperature, but a thinner man had to leave the water in 30 min with a core temperature of 34.5 °C (50). For this reason, long-distance swimmers tend to have more body fat than short-distance swimmers; the higher body fatness provides more buoyancy, requiring less energy to swim at any set speed (31).

Clothing

Clothing can extend our natural subcutaneous fat insulation, allowing us to endure very cold environments. The insulation quality of clothing is given in clo units, where 1 clo unit is the insulation needed at rest (1 MET) to maintain core temperature when the environmental temperature is 21 °C (70 °F), the relative humidity is 50%, and the air movement is 6 mi · hr^{-1} (9.7 km · hr^{-1}) (8). As the air temperature falls, clothing with a higher clo value must be worn to maintain core temperature because the gradient between skin and environment is increasing. Figure 10.11 shows the insulation needed at different energy expenditures across a broad range of environmental temperatures, from –60 to +80 °F (–51.1 to 26.7 °C) (8). As energy production increases, insulation must decrease to maintain core temperature. When clothing is worn in layers, insulation can be removed as needed to maintain core temperature. By following these steps, the sweat rate will be reduced and the clothing will retain more of its insulating value. If the clothing becomes wet, the insulating quality decreases because the water can now conduct heat away from the body about 25 times better than air can (32). A primary goal, then, is to avoid wetness caused by either sweat or weather. This problem is exacerbated by the cold environment's very dry air, which causes a greater evaporation of moisture. When this problem of cold, dry air and wet clothing is coupled with windy conditions, the risk is even greater. The wind not only provides for greater convective heat

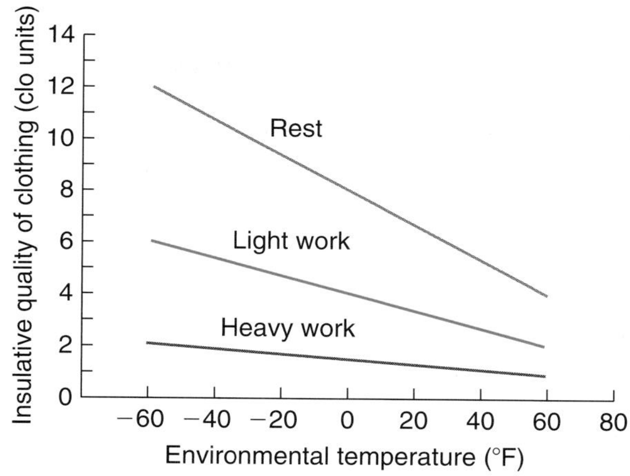

Figure 10.11 As work intensity increases, less insulation is needed to maintain core temperature.
From A.C. Burton and O.G. Edholm, 1955, *Man in a cold environment* (London: Edward Arnold).

loss, as described in the windchill section, but it also accelerates evaporation (22).

Energy Production

Energy production can modify the amount of insulation needed to maintain core temperature and prevent hypothermia (see figure 10.11). When thin (less than 16.8% fat) male subjects were immersed in cold water, the drop in body temperature that occurred at rest was prevented when they did exercise at an energy expenditure of about 8.5 kcal · min^{-1} (42, 43).

Table 10.6 shows the progression of signs and symptoms of hypothermia that occur as body temperature decreases (57). It is important to deal with these problems on site rather than wait until the person can be taken to an emergency room. According to Sharkey (56), you should do the following to help a person with hypothermia:

- Get the person out of the cold, wind, and rain.
- Remove all wet clothing.
- Provide warm drinks, dry clothing, and a warm dry sleeping bag for a mildly impaired person.
- Keep the person awake; if semiconscious, undress the person and put him into a sleeping bag with another person.
- Find a heat source, such as a campfire.

Effect of Air Pollution

Air pollution includes gases and particulates that are products of the combustion of fossil fuels. The smog that results when these pollutants are highly concentrated can have detrimental effects on health and performance. The

Table 10.6 Clinical Symptoms of Hypothermia

Core temperature (°C)	Symptoms and signs
37	Feeling of cold Skin cooling Decreased social interaction
36	Goose pimples
35	Shivering Muscle tension Fatigue
34.5	Deep cold Numbness Loss of coordination Stumbling Dysarthria Muscle rigidity
32	Disorientation Decreased visual acuity
31-30	Semicoma or coma
28	Ventricular fibrillation and cardiovascular death

Reprinted from *Cardiology clinics*, Vol 5, L.E. Hart and J.R. Sutton, "Environmental considerations for exercise," p. 246, Copyright 1987, with permission from Elsevier.

gases can affect performance by decreasing the capacity to transport oxygen, increasing airway resistance, and altering the perception of effort required when the eyes burn and the chest hurts.

Physiological responses to these pollutants are related to the amount, or dose, received. Several major factors determine the dose:

- Concentration of the pollutant
- Duration of the exposure to the pollutant
- Volume of air inhaled

The volume of air inhaled is large during exercise, and this is one reason why physical activity should be curtailed during times of peak pollution levels (16). The following discussion focuses on the major air pollutants: particulate matter, ozone, sulfur dioxide, and carbon monoxide.

Particulate Matter

The air is full of microscopic and submicroscopic particles, many of which can be tied to motor vehicles (especially diesels) and industrial sources. Over the past several years, more attention has been directed on the very small particles because of their potential to promote pulmonary infection and actually cross the epithelium to enter the circulation (17). Fine-particle pollution elevates BP in people with preexisting cardiovascular disease and may contribute to an increased risk of cardiac mortality and morbidity (55, 65).

Ozone

The **ozone** in the air we breathe is generated by the reaction between ultraviolet (UV) light and emissions from internal combustion engines. There is evidence that a single 2 hr exposure to a high ozone concentration, 0.75 parts per million (PPM), decreases $\dot{V}O_2$max; further, recent studies show that a 6 to 12 hr exposure to a concentration of only 0.12 PPM (the U.S. air-quality standard) decreases lung function and increases respiratory symptoms. Interestingly, people can adapt to ozone exposure, showing diminished responses to subsequent exposures during the ozone season. Concern about long-term lung health suggests, however, that it would be prudent to avoid heavy exercise during the time of day when ozone and other pollutants are elevated (16).

Sulfur Dioxide

Sulfur dioxide (SO_2) is produced by smelters, refineries, and electrical utilities that use fossil fuel for energy generation. SO_2 does not affect lung function in normal individuals, but it causes bronchoconstriction in people who have asthma—a response influenced by the temperature and humidity of the inspired air. Nose breathing is encouraged to scrub the SO_2, and drugs like cromolyn sodium and beta-agonists can partially block the response to SO_2 (16).

Carbon Monoxide

Carbon monoxide (CO) is derived from the burning of fossil fuel, coal, oil, gasoline, and wood, as well as from cigarette smoke. CO can bind to hemoglobin (HbCO) and decrease the capacity for oxygen transport. The CO concentration in blood is generally less than 1% in nonsmokers but may be as high as 10% in smokers (52). As mentioned in chapter 28, beyond an HbCO concentration of 4.3% there is a 1% reduction in $\dot{V}O_2$max for each 1% increase in the HbCO concentration. In contrast, when one exercises at about 40% $\dot{V}O_2$max, the HbCO concentration can be as high as 15% before endurance is affected. The cardiovascular system simply has a greater capacity to respond with a larger cardiac output when the oxygen concentration of the blood is reduced during submaximal work (33, 51, 52). This, of course, requires a higher HR for the same work task, and a participant needs to reduce the intensity of exercise during exposure to CO to stay in the THR range. Because it takes about 2 to 4 hr to remove half the CO from the blood once the exposure has been removed, CO can have a lasting effect on performance (16). Unfortunately, it is difficult to predict what the actual CO concentration will be in any given environment. Because we must consider the previous exposure to the pollutant, as well as the length of time and rate of ventilation associated with the current exposure, the following guidelines are provided for exercising in an area with air pollution (52):

- Reduce exposure to the pollutant before exercise because the physiological effects are time and dose dependent.
- Stay away from areas where you might receive a high dose of CO: smoking areas, high traffic areas, and urban environments.
- Do not schedule activities during the times when pollutants are at their highest levels because of traffic: 7 to 10 a.m. and 4 to 7 p.m.

Air Quality Index

The air quality index (AQI) is a measure of the quality of the air for five major air pollutants regulated by the Clean Air Act: ground-level ozone, particulate matter, carbon monoxide, sulfur dioxide, and nitrogen dioxide. The AQI scale runs from 0 to 500, with values of 0 to 50 being good, 51-100 moderate, 101-150 unhealthy for sensitive groups, 151-200 unhealthy, and so forth. This information is generally provided in a local community's weather forecast. The fitness professional should suit the AQI information to the individual—some people experience symptoms at lower levels of pollution than others do (10).

Effect of Altitude

An increase in altitude decreases the partial pressure of oxygen and reduces the amount of oxygen bound to hemoglobin. As a result, the volume of oxygen carried in each liter of blood decreases. As mentioned in chapter 4, maximal aerobic power steadily decreases with increasing altitude so that by 2,300 m (7,500 ft) the value is only 88% of that measured at sea level. This means that an activity that demanded 88% of $\dot{V}O_2$max at sea level now requires 100% of the "new" $\dot{V}O_2$max.

More than maximal aerobic power is affected by altitude exposure. Any submaximal work rate is going to demand a higher HR at altitude compared with sea level (shown in figure 10.12). The reason is quite simple. Because each liter of blood has less oxygen at altitude, more blood is required to deliver the same quantity of oxygen to the tissues. Consequently, the HR response is elevated at any given submaximal work rate. To stay within the THR range, a person must decrease the intensity of the exercise when at altitude. As with exercising in high heat and humidity, monitoring the THR allows the exerciser to modify the intensity of the activity relative to any additional environmental demand (34).

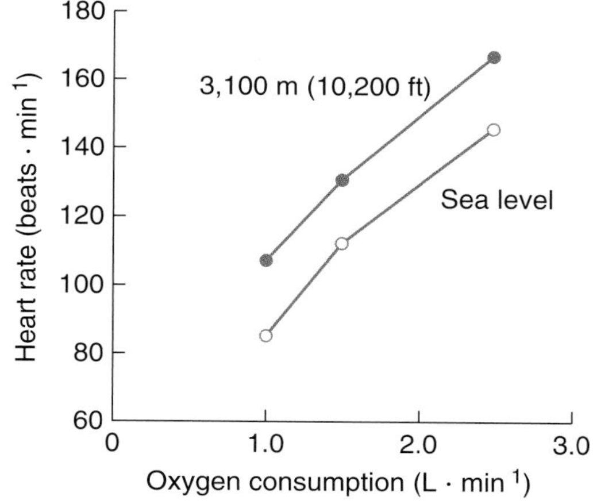

Figure 10.12 The effect of altitude on the HR response to submaximal exercise.

Based on data from R. Grover, J. Reeves, E. Grover and J. Leathers, 1967, "Muscular exercise in young men native to 3,100 m altitude," *Journal of Applied Physiology* 22: 555-564.

Key Point

In conditions of high heat and humidity, the exerciser should decrease the work rate to stay in the THR zone. Exercisers should acclimatize to heat over 7 to 14 days to reduce the risk of heat injury. Advise participants to drink water before, during, and after exercise and to exercise in the early morning to reduce environmental heat load. When exercising in cold weather, participants should wear clothing in layers and remove layers to minimize sweating and to stay dry. Participants should become aware of the AQI readings in their communities and avoid exercising at times and in places in which air pollution is a problem. When exercising at altitude, participants should decrease work intensity to stay in the THR zone.

Case Studies

In the following case studies you are given general information about an individual, data on risk factors, and the results of an exercise test. Analyze each case, delineate the risk factors, and react to the person's responses to the test (whether normal or not). Then, on the basis of your analysis, make some recommendations for the individual relative to an exercise program and risk-factor reduction program. You can check your answers on page 471 in appendix A.

1. Paul, a Caucasian male, is 36 yr of age, weighs 88 kg, is 178 cm tall, and has 28% body fat. Blood chemistry values indicate that his total cholesterol is 270 mg · dl^{-1} and HDL cholesterol is 38 mg · dl^{-1}. His mother died of a heart attack at the age of 63, and his father had a heart attack at the age of 68. He is sedentary and has engaged in no endurance training program since college. The following are the results of a maximal GXT conducted by his physician.

• Test: Balke, 3 mi · hr^{-1} (4.8 km · hr^{-1}); 2.5% every 2 min •

% Grade	METs	SBP (mmHg)	DBP (mmHg)	HR (beats · min^{-1})	ECG	Symptoms
	Rest	126	88	70	Normal	—
2.5	4.3	142	86	142	Normal	—
5	5.4	184	88	150	Normal	—
7.5	6.4	162	86	160	Normal	—
10	7.4	174	84	168	Normal	—
12.5	8.5	186	84	176	Normal	—
15	9.5	194	84	190	Normal	Calf tight
17.5	10.5	198	84	198	Normal	Fatigue

2. Mary is a 38-yr-old Hispanic American female and is 170 cm tall, weighs 61.4 kg, and has 30% body fat. Blood chemistry values indicate a total cholesterol of 188 mg · dl^{-1} and an HDL-C of 59 mg · dl^{-1}. Her resting blood pressure is 124/80 mmHg. Family history indicates that her father had a nonfatal heart attack at the age of 67. She has smoked one pack of cigarettes per day for the past 13 yr, and her lifestyle is sedentary. The following is the result of her submaximal cycle ergometer test.

• Test: YMCA cycle test •

Work rate (kpm · min^{-1})	HR (min 2)	HR (min 3)
150	118	120
300	134	136

Pedal rate = 50 rev · min^{-1}; predicted HRmax = 182 beats · min^{-1}; seat height = 6; and 85% HRmax = 155 beats · min^{-1}.

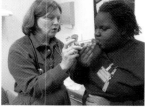

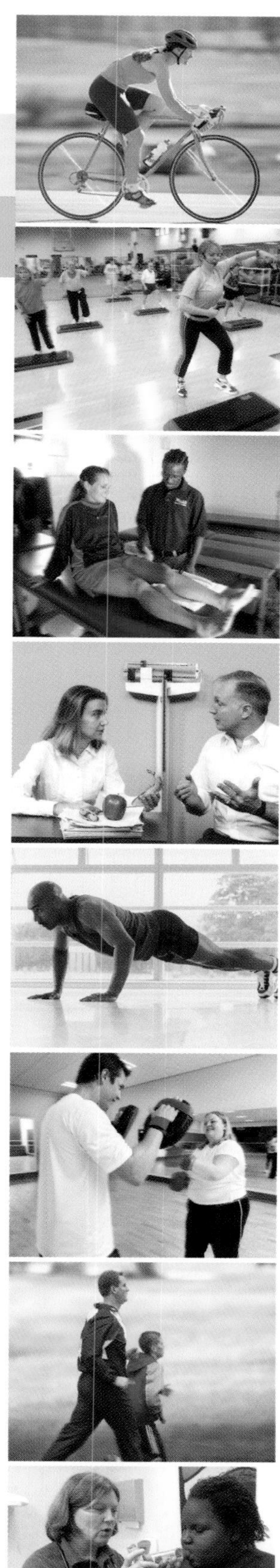

CHAPTER 11

Exercise Prescription for Weight Management

Dixie L. Thompson

Objectives

The reader will be able to do the following:

1. Identify factors that contribute to obesity.
2. Describe the role that energy balance plays in weight loss and weight maintenance.
3. Provide guidelines for caloric intake to facilitate appropriate weight loss.
4. Discuss the role of exercise in weight loss and weight maintenance.
5. Prescribe safe and effective exercise programs for weight management.
6. Describe strategies for behavioral change for weight control.
7. Be aware of the fallacy of quick-fix weight loss.
8. Recognize signs of eating disorders.
9. Provide healthy guidelines for gaining weight.

Americans spend billions of dollars each year on weight loss. The weight loss industry provides a broad spectrum of goods and services, including over-the-counter and prescription drugs, motivational and educational books, and weight loss clinics. Weight loss groups have sprung up in many environments, ranging from schools to health clinics to churches. Despite this multibillion dollar industry, Americans are getting fatter. Nearly two thirds of American adults are classified as either overweight or obese (10). Unfortunately, this same trend is found among U.S. children (11, 14). Although many Americans lose the fight against obesity, some manage to maintain a healthy weight throughout their lives, and many successfully lose excess weight. The lessons from these people provide a road map for successful weight control (15, 36).

Increasing Prevalence of Obesity in the United States

In the early 1960s, 13.4% of American adults were obese (i.e., had a BMI $\geq$ 30 kg · m^{-2}) (10). Recent national statistics (from 1999-2000) revealed that obesity has soared to 30.9 % (10). Figure 11.1 shows the increasing prevalence of obesity during the past four decades for both men and women. Some segments of the population have even more dramatic values. For example, obesity prevalence for non-Hispanic Black women is currently approximately 50%, an 11.5% increase since the early 1990s (10). Because of the rapid changes in obesity prevalence, this trend does not appear to be causally linked to genetics. As discussed later, lifestyle changes seem to be the major culprit.

> **Key Point**
>
> Although Americans spend billions of dollars each year on weight loss, the prevalence of obesity is increasing. Nearly two thirds of adults are overweight or obese. People tend to accumulate fat as they age, but excessive fat accumulation is unhealthy.

Adults commonly accumulate additional adipose tissue as they age. This gradual accumulation of fat is sometimes called **creeping obesity.** Part of this change in body composition is attributable to a natural loss of muscle caused by aging. A decreasing metabolic rate, a more sedentary lifestyle, and unadjusted eating patterns, however, appear to be the most important factors contributing to the increased body fat (7). Although some fat accumulation is acceptable (see chapter 6, table 6.1), when BMI climbs to obese levels, negative health consequences follow (25, 26).

Etiology of Obesity

The cause of obesity cannot be described simply, because many factors contribute to its development. Ultimately, **positive caloric balance** (i.e., taking in more calories than are expended) leads to obesity. Factors contributing to obesity can be discussed under two broad categories: genetics and lifestyle.

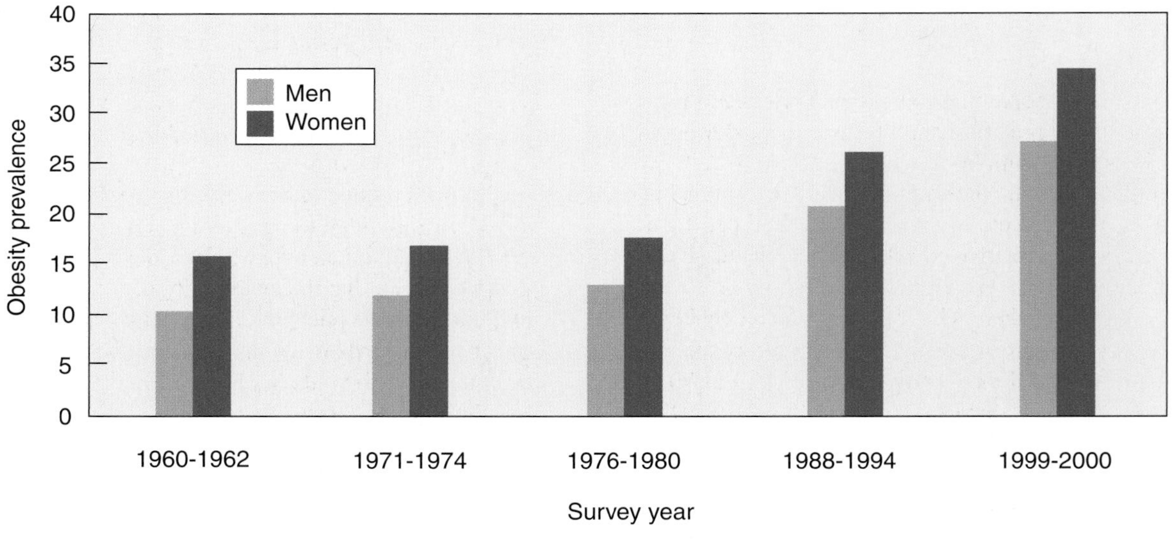

Figure 11.1 Prevalence of obesity among American adults

Data from K.M. Flegal, 1999, "The obesity epidemic in children and adults: Current evidence and research issues," *Medicine and Science in Sports and Exercise* 31: S509-S514. (10).

Genetics

Evidence exists that inheritance contributes to the development of obesity (15, 29). In evaluating the effect of genetics, researchers have attempted to differentiate among factors that are genetic and sociocultural and are passed down through the generations. Bouchard and colleagues (6) estimated that approximately 25% of the variance in percent body fat is attributable to genetics. Interestingly, these authors found that inheritance has a larger effect on total fat and deep deposits of adipose tissue than on subcutaneous fat. Additional evidence on the importance of genetics comes from data demonstrating that the BMI of adopted children is more similar to that of their biological parents than to that of their adoptive parents (30). The recent discoveries of genes linked with obesity provide additional evidence that genetic factors help determine the likelihood of being obese and developing diseases that accompany obesity. Research continues in an attempt to understand the link between genetics and obesity.

Many genes are linked with obesity, and the expression of each gene depends on environmental factors (e.g., availability of fatty foods, social influences); therefore, the genetics of obesity is complex and much is yet to be learned (5). A negative consequence of our growing knowledge of the genetic link to obesity is that people with many overweight family members may become discouraged and believe that they can do nothing about their weight status. Although genetics can contribute to the development of obesity, a primary reason that people become obese is lifestyle. Fitness professionals must emphasize to clients that genetics may predispose certain people to obesity, but those people still can significantly affect their body weight.

Lifestyle

The choices people make about energy expenditure and caloric intake predominantly influence the development of obesity. The number of calories consumed, the types of foods eaten, and the amount of daily activity all affect body weight. If more calories are consumed than are expended, the positive caloric balance results in weight (fat) gain. To lose fat weight, a **negative caloric balance** must be established. This balance can be achieved by decreasing caloric intake, increasing caloric expenditure, or both. National data comparing 1971 to 2000 show that the daily calorie intake increased by 168 kcal $\cdot$ day^{-1} for men and 335 kcal $\cdot$ day^{-1} for women (37), and daily physical activity rates during these same years did not increase to offset the change in energy intake. Thus the typical American today weighs just over 24 lb (11 kg) more than the typical American of 40 yr ago (27).

Food Intake

When excess calories (particularly fat calories) are consumed, the energy is stored as fat. From an evolutionary standpoint, fat storage is a positive adaptation to variations in food availability. In other words, fat accumulation occurs during times of plenty, and this stored energy is used when food supplies are low. In populations that have a constant abundance of food with high caloric density, this mechanism often results in excessive fat accumulation.

Health professionals sometimes question whether individuals who are obese typically consume more calories than their counterparts who are average weight. Dietary recall studies provide little clear information about this issue because people tend to underreport dietary intake and overestimate physical activity (22). Some research suggests that subjects who are obese particularly underreport consumption of high-fat and snack foods (34). Highly advanced research procedures in which people ingest isotopes of oxygen and hydrogen (doubly labeled water) indicate that individuals who are overweight expend and consume more calories than persons of normal weight (33). The higher energy expenditure is caused by the metabolic cost of supporting excess body weight. The reasons extra calories are consumed are not known.

Types of Food Eaten and Obesity

When fat is consumed, it is stored as adipose tissue more readily than either protein or carbohydrate is. From a theoretical perspective, the low thermic effect of fat (i.e., the energy needed to digest, absorb, transport, and store fat), the ease with which fat is stored as adipose tissue, and the high caloric density of high-fat foods make fat a likely culprit in the development of obesity. National data indicate that during the past 30 yr, the percentage of calories from fat in the typical American diet has gone down (37). However, since the total energy intake has increased, the actual number of calories from fat intake has changed very little.

Several studies indicate that people who are obese and overweight tend to consume a higher percentage of calories from fat than people of normal weight consume (34). It appears that the availability of foods high in fat and simple sugars puts individuals at higher risk for obesity. In cultures where the majority of calories consumed are complex carbohydrate, the rates of obesity are lower than those in the United States.

Daily Energy Expenditure

Researchers have found a relationship between low physical activity and an increased likelihood of obesity (35). Amish adults who live an active life that is comparable to what was typical in the late 19th century have much lower rates of obesity compared to the average American (4). Additionally, women who walk more daily have a lower BMI, waist circumference, and body fat percentage compared to women who are less active (17, 20, 31). Because these studies are cross-sectional, it is impossible to determine whether low physical activity leads to obesity or obesity causes people to reduce their activity levels.

The role of regular exercise in weight loss is complex and has been reviewed by several authors (13, 26, 28). Certainly increasing physical activity can help create a negative caloric balance. Additionally, some studies have supported the role of exercise in maintaining fat-free mass and metabolic rate during weight loss. Although studies sometimes differ in their findings on the short-term effects of exercise on weight loss, the long-term positive consequences of physical activity on weight maintenance are clear. Exercise appears to be one of the strongest predictors of long-term weight maintenance (21, 35, 36). Additionally, regular physical activity attenuates age-related weight gain (9).

Key Point

Both genetics and lifestyle contribute to obesity. Caloric intake, food choices, and daily physical activity are all aspects of lifestyle that affect fat accumulation. A positive caloric balance results in weight gain; a negative caloric balance results in weight loss.

Maintaining a Healthy Weight

Numerous methods can be used to maintain a healthy weight or to lose weight when necessary. Fitness professionals should encourage clients to choose weight maintenance or weight loss techniques that are effective yet pose little threat to overall health. The following sections outline practices that most adults can implement safely.

Assessing Daily Caloric Need

Whether planning individualized weight loss or weight maintenance programs, it is helpful to know the number of calories the client needs to sustain her current body weight. You can gain this knowledge by estimating daily caloric need. **Daily caloric need** is the number of calories a person needs to sustain current body weight, assuming that activity levels remain constant. The resting metabolic rate, **thermic effect of food,** and energy consumed by daily activities determine the daily caloric need (figure 11.2).

Resting metabolic rate (RMR) is the number of calories expended to maintain the body during resting conditions. For most people, RMR is 60% to 70% of the daily caloric need. For people who engage in regular, vigorous exercise, the RMR may account for a smaller proportion of daily caloric need because the energy requirements of exercise account for a larger percentage. RMR can be measured in a laboratory using indirect calorimetry. To accurately measure RMR, assess the client when he has not eaten for several hours, has not exercised vigorously for the past 12 hr, and has been in a resting, reclined position for 30 min (23). Because of the cost of indirect calorimetry and the strict control needed to obtain accurate results, measuring RMR is not always practical; therefore, a number of equations have been developed to predict RMR. These RMR equations are based on the following principles:

- RMR is proportional to body size.
- RMR decreases with age.
- Muscle is more metabolically active than fat.

The larger the body, the more calories needed to sustain it. This relationship is reflected in all RMR equations. In addition to body size, age significantly affects RMR. As a person ages RMR decreases, meaning that a person's daily caloric need decreases with age. Generally RMR equations are sex specific because males often have more fat-free mass than females have, and fat-free mass requires more energy than fat tissue requires; therefore, different equations are needed for men and women.

If a client's fat-free mass is known, the following equation can be used to predict RMR (8). There is no need for sex-specific equations when fat-free mass

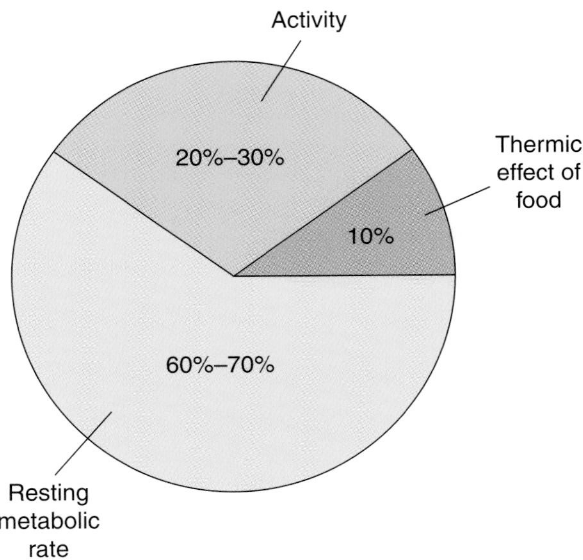

Figure 11.2 Contributors to daily caloric need.

is known, because a gram of muscle has the same metabolic need whether it resides in a male or female body.

$$\text{RMR (kcal} \cdot \text{day}^{-1}) = 370 + (21.6 \cdot \text{fat-free mass in kg})$$

When determining daily caloric need, an estimate of the calories burned in physical activity is needed. This assessment requires information about work and leisure activity. Although there are numerous ways to gather information about daily activity, one typical method is an activity log in which the client records work and leisure activity. Once the activity pattern is established, the caloric cost of various activities can be calculated (see chapter 4) and used to estimate the energy burned in activity. Estimating this energy is especially important if working with an individual who trains extensively. Alternately, you can estimate daily caloric need by using the methods outlined in the following sidebar.

The smallest part of the daily caloric need comes from the thermic effect of food. This is the energy needed to digest, absorb, transport, and store the food that is eaten. Although this value may vary slightly depending on the food eaten, the thermic effect of food typically accounts for 10% of the daily caloric need (24).

Changing Lifestyle to Promote a Healthy Weight

Although each individual must assess which areas of his lifestyle contribute to excessive weight accumulation, common steps that benefit the majority of people who are attempting to lose weight include the following:

- Reduce total calories.
- Reduce fat intake.
- Increase physical activity.
- Change eating behaviors.

As previously mentioned, a negative caloric balance must be established for weight loss. The number of calories consumed while attempting to lose weight should be determined by the client's health, caloric need, and ultimate weight loss goals. Most healthy adults who need to lose weight can institute a short-term, low-calorie diet (LCD) consisting of 800 to 1500 kcal · day^{-1} without major adverse consequences. However, it is not recommended that people institute a very low-calorie diet (VLCD) in which caloric intake is less than 800 kcal · day^{-1} (26). Weight loss studies show that VLCDs may result in greater initial weight loss but at 1 yr show no better success than that seen with LCDs (26).

The ACSM recommends that weekly weight loss goals should not exceed 1 kg (about 2.2 lb) a week (2). A general guideline is to establish a caloric deficit of 3,500 to 7,000 kcal · wk^{-1} (500-1,000 kcal · day^{-1}), which theoretically results in a 1 to 2 lb (0.5-0.9 kg) loss of fat each week (1 lb or 0.5 kg of fat = 3,500 kcal). The ACSM also recommends that people restricting their caloric intake limit their fat intake to less than 30% of total calories (1). These are general recommendations, and people

Calculating Daily Energy Needs

The Institute of Medicine (12) recommends the following equations for calculating a person's daily caloric need or estimated energy requirement (EER). These formulas require knowing the client's age in years, height in meters, weight in kilograms, and level of physical activity.

Adult Man

EER = 662 – 9.53 (age) + PA [15.91 (weight) + 539.6 (height)]

Adult Woman

EER = 354 – 6.91 (age) + PA [9.36 (weight) + 726 (height)]

PA reflects a person's level of daily physical activity. Use the following table to choose the appropriate PA value.

Activity level	PA value (men)	PA value (women)
Sedentary—extremely limited activity	1.0	1.0
Low active—typical activities of daily living only	1.11	1.12
Active—regular moderate physical activity	1.25	1.27
Very active—regular vigorous exercise	1.45	1.45

with special needs (e.g., athletes, the elderly, people with metabolic disorders) may require a different approach to weight loss. Any caloric restriction can be expected to lead to decreased RMR and fat-free mass. The decrease in RMR and loss of fat-free mass will be greater in dieters with large daily caloric deficits (26).

Exercise Prescription for Weight Management

The ACSM recommends a combined approach of exercise and moderate caloric restriction for people attempting weight loss (1, 2). Although debate continues over the precise contribution of exercise to weight management, the recommended combination of exercise and moderate calorie restriction appears to be most effective in maintaining lean mass and avoiding excessive decreases in RMR. Existing data clearly demonstrate that people who are successful in maintaining weight loss engage in regular aerobic activity (36). Studies also show that regular exercise helps prevent weight gain (9, 18). From a theoretical perspective, adding exercise to everyday life can significantly alter body weight. For example, expending just 100 kcal · day^{-1} beyond daily caloric need for a year creates a caloric deficit of 36,500 kcal. The ACSM recommends that individuals engage in a minimum of 150 min of moderate-intensity exercise per week and further states that additional exercise (200-300 min · wk^{-1}) is more likely to be associated with successful weight control (1, 2). The following are specific recommendations for weight loss with exercise (2):

- Frequency: 5-7 days each week
- Intensity: initially moderate (40%-60% heart rate reserve [HRR]), then progressing to higher intensity (50%-75% HRR)
- Duration: progress from short, easily tolerated bouts to 45 to 60 min daily

Key Point

Daily caloric need is determined by RMR, the thermic effect of food, and activity levels. Reducing total calories, decreasing fat intake, increasing physical activity, and changing eating behaviors are some common steps that will benefit many people who are attempting to lose weight. The exercise prescription for weight management should involve regular aerobic activity of at least 150 min each week. When weight reduction is needed, most healthy adults can safely initiate weight loss goals of 1 to 2 lb (0.5-0.9 kg) a week.

In addition to the physical benefits, psychological variables improve with exercise. Improvements in self-esteem and self-efficacy are commonly reported outcomes of engaging in regular exercise. The empowerment that comes from becoming more fit can add to the resolve to live a healthy lifestyle and maintain a healthy weight.

Behavior Modification for Weight Loss and Maintenance

The majority of attempts to lose weight and maintain weight loss are unsuccessful. Behavior modification (changes in lifestyle habits) is an important component of successful weight loss and maintenance programs (26). For additional information on behavior modification, see chapter 22.

When people are committed to changing eating and activity patterns, a number of strategies can improve the chances of long-term success. During the initial phase of weight loss (the action stage; see chapter 22), implementing these strategies requires a great deal of effort and there is a significant chance of failure (i.e., relapse). After 6 mo or more of using these strategies (the maintenance stage; see chapter 22), changes in diet and lifestyle become more natural. Some strategies effective for losing weight and maintaining weight loss are discussed next. Not every client responds well to the same techniques. Each client should be considered separately, and an individualized plan should be developed for each client.

Keeping Records

Before implementing a weight loss or weight maintenance program, it is wise to examine current eating patterns. This is most easily done with an eating diary or food log. A sample food log is provided in chapter 7. Remember, it is important to gather information about the types and quantities of food eaten as well as the social and emotional circumstances surrounding eating.

Careful record keeping accomplishes several objectives. First, food logs document the problem areas of food intake. Many people are unaware of the total calories or the amount of fat they consume daily. Second, eating diaries document the social and emotional cues to eating. After keeping records for a while, individuals begin to recognize the factors, other than hunger, that lead to eating (e.g., socializing with friends, watching television, feeling stressed). To combat these cues to eating, the social and emotional situations that trigger overeating must be recognized and strategies developed to overcome them. Third, recording food intake makes eating a cognitive process. For many people, eating is a habit, and they automatically choose how much and what to eat without conscious consideration. As discussed next, appropriately planning meals and snacks is an important component of successful weight loss.

Planning Meals and Snacks

Weight loss does not occur by accident; it takes a concerted effort. Purchasing appropriate foods and planning meals are imperative for success. One of the most helpful practices in controlling food intake is not purchasing high-fat and calorie-dense food. Substituting low-calorie and low-fat foods for high-calorie and high-fat foods also can substantially affect weight loss. For example, substituting a cup (8 fl oz, or 237 ml) of 1% milk for a cup of whole milk decreases caloric intake by approximately 50 kcal. If a person drinks 2 c of milk per day, this substitution will reduce caloric intake by 36,500 kcal in 1 yr!

Meal planning is also essential. In busy households, planning healthy meals often becomes a low priority, and this can lead to meals that are easy to prepare but may not promote health or weight control. One technique for overcoming time constraints is buying breakfast foods that are quick to prepare, yet are nutritious and relatively low in calories (e.g., fresh fruit, bagels, low-fat yogurt, whole grain cereals). These foods provide a morning meal that offsets hunger and includes important nutrients.

Because many Americans are not at home for the noon meal, they often try to eat at restaurants that are convenient, affordable, and quick. This leads many to visit fast-food restaurants. Although several fast-food chains have added lower fat items to their menus, the majority of fast food is high in both fat and calories. Individuals who choose to eat fast food are less successful at maintaining weight loss than are those who avoid these food choices (16). Planning ahead might allow some people to carry their lunch to work and ensure that they can choose from a variety of healthy, low-fat, low-calorie foods for this important meal.

The evening meal contributes a significant percentage of the daily caloric intake of many Americans. It is not uncommon for people who have limited their food intake during the day to overindulge at night. Because of the effort required to cook a meal, many people eat at restaurants or purchase packaged meals that tend to be high in fat and calories. The effort necessary for cooking nutritious meals can be reduced by doing the following:

- Cook and store meals ahead of time.
- Find a variety of low-calorie meals that are quick and easy to prepare.
- Purchase food items ahead of time to avoid unnecessary shopping.
- Keep a variety of fresh vegetables on hand.

It is also important to consider the foods available for snacks. Although avoiding food between meals may be ideal for many, there are times when snacks are necessary. Foods that are nutritious and also low in calories are the best choices (e.g., fresh fruit, raw vegetables, low-fat yogurt).

Establishing a Support System

Studies have shown the benefit of having a support system when trying to lose weight (26). The source of the support, however, will vary depending on the client. A support system may be a friend, spouse, significant other, parent, coworker, therapist, or support group. Fitness professionals should encourage clients in a weight loss or weight maintenance program to seek out other people to encourage them in their efforts.

Many people are encouraged by supporting others who also are attempting to lose weight. Many commercial weight loss centers provide support groups. These groups serve several functions: They provide a group to whom participants are accountable, a setting in which helpful hints and success stories can be shared, and a nonthreatening environment where all of the participants are pursuing the same objective. For some people, the reasons for overeating are emotional and deeply rooted. In these cases, a trained therapist may be needed.

Committing to Behavioral as Well as Outcome-Oriented Goals

Clients must develop goals that encourage healthy eating practices. Goal setting is important to help individuals remain focused on weight loss or weight maintenance. Goal setting should be a mutual exchange between the fitness professional and the client. The fitness professional provides information about healthy weight loss or management practices; the client identifies the behavioral goals to which she is willing to commit.

Typically, weight loss is outcome oriented (i.e., the end result is the measure of success). Weight loss goals should be reasonable for the client and should follow the guidelines listed previously in this chapter. In contrast to outcome goals, behavioral goals focus on the process of weight loss, not the final outcome. Behavioral goals can help the client make behavior and lifestyle changes that will affect weight loss or weight maintenance. These goals may target altering eating patterns, making wise food choices, and increasing daily energy expenditure. An example of a behavioral goal is, "I will walk the stairs to my office daily rather than riding the elevator." More specific information on goal setting can be found in chapter 22.

Designing a Reward System

Part of human nature is the desire to be rewarded for accomplishing goals. When designing a weight loss or weight maintenance program, it is wise to provide motivation by rewarding success. As with goal setting, it is vital that the client be involved in developing the rewards that will be used. One rule that fitness professionals should encourage, however, is to avoid using food as a reward. The reward program should recognize the achievement of both outcome-oriented and behavioral goals. This is important because attaining an outcome goal may take a substantial amount of time and much longer than it may take to change certain behaviors. Also, there will be times when a person's weight plateaus; behavioral goals should be rewarded during these times. Here are some examples of rewards:

- Purchasing new clothes
- Purchasing hobby items (e.g., books, compact discs, tools)
- Taking a trip
- Attending special events (movies, music and dance concerts, lectures)

Avoiding Self-Defeating Behaviors

Certain situations increase the likelihood of overeating. A client trying to lose weight needs to acknowledge these situations and institute measures to minimize the chance of succumbing to self-defeating behaviors. For example, a person who snacks on high-calorie foods late at night might avoid purchasing such foods and also implement a behavioral objective of not eating after 7:00 p.m. A person who loves pizza but tends to overindulge when going out to a restaurant might make pizza at home using low-fat ingredients and vegetables as toppings.

There are special times (birthdays, holiday dinners) when people will want to eat foods that are not a part of their weight management plan. Fitness professionals should emphasize to clients that a lapse in eating (or activity) should not mean an end to the weight management plan. Clients should be encouraged to immediately return to their healthy eating and exercise plan after the lapse. Fitness professionals might help clients who feel guilty by suggesting they view the lapse not as a failure but as an opportunity for renewing the commitment to weight loss or weight maintenance.

Combining Moderate Caloric Restriction and Aerobic Exercise

Regular exercise is an important facet of successful weight loss and weight maintenance. As mentioned previously, the ACSM (1, 2) and National Institutes of Health (26) support the use of exercise for weight loss and maintenance. The majority of weight loss studies that compare diet with diet plus exercise show that the combined approach leads to greater weight loss (26). Regular aerobic activity at least 150 $min \cdot wk^{-1}$ is recommended for people attempting to lose or maintain weight (1, 2). See previous comments in this chapter and also chapter 19 for more information on exercise prescription for weight loss or weight maintenance.

Changing Unhealthy Eating Patterns

Specific eating patterns have been linked with excessive weight gain (7). Being aware of these behaviors and implementing plans to avoid them increase the likelihood of successful weight management. These four changes in eating patterns are recommended:

- Slow down.
- Make wise substitutions.
- Consume a variety of nutritious foods.
- Eat smaller and fewer portions.

People often eat rapidly and then feel uncomfortably full several minutes after they finish eating. When food is eaten rapidly, inadequate time is allowed for the satiety mechanisms to help curb hunger. This results in people overeating before they realize that they are no longer hungry. To help slow their eating, people can put down eating utensils between bites, pause at least 30 sec between bites, and chew food completely and swallow before taking another bite (7).

Substituting foods that contain less fat and calories for foods that are high in fat and calories can significantly reduce caloric intake. For example, a person who eats a roasted chicken breast without the skin instead of a fried chicken breast with the skin will save approximately 160 kcal. The wise consumer looks closely at the total calories in a food as well as the calories that are contributed by fat. Reducing fat intake not only helps with weight control but also may help improve the blood lipid profile.

One problem that people face when trying to manage weight is diet burnout. It is not uncommon to find dieters who consume only certain foods. To help avoid becoming bored and frustrated with a diet, it is important to consume a variety of healthy, low-calorie, and tasty foods. This objective is linked to the planning process. Maintaining variety in the diet not only helps avoid boredom but also provides nutritional balance.

When attempting to lose weight, one of the most helpful changes is to decrease the portion size as well as the number of portions consumed. Many people are in the habit of completely filling their plates and eating everything on the plate. Additionally, Americans demonstrate to their hosts that they enjoy the provided food by eating extra portions. Taking smaller portions of foods as well as avoiding seconds contribute significantly to caloric restriction.

Committing to Lifelong Maintenance

Weight loss is only temporary unless a plan is in place to maintain the loss. In examining the variables that predict success in maintaining weight loss, Lavery and Loewy (21) concluded, "There are no quick-fix, easy solutions to obesity. The solution is the harsh realization of the need for permanent lifestyle changes to maintain a desired weight status." Fitness professionals should help clients understand the need to commit to long-term lifestyle changes rather than focus solely on short-term weight loss goals. It is encouraging, however, to learn that long-term maintenance of weight loss is much more likely once people have kept the weight off for 2 to 5 yr (36).

Key Point

Some strategies for successful weight management are keeping records, planning meals and snacks, developing a support system, designing a reward system, committing to both outcome-oriented and behavioral goals, avoiding self-defeating behaviors, combining moderate caloric restriction with aerobic exercise, changing unhealthy eating patterns, and committing to lifelong weight maintenance.

Gimmicks and Gadgets for Weight Loss

Over the years numerous devices have been marketed for weight loss. The majority of these devices are ineffective, and, unfortunately, some are potentially harmful.

Saunas and sweat suits have, at times, been recommended to help weight loss by burning off or melting away fat. This is a false claim. These devices may induce short-term (i.e., a few hours) loss of weight by dehydration. These devices do not burn fat but can cause people to sweat profusely. Overusing saunas and sweat suits can lead to severe dehydration. Further, the warmer core temperature that is caused by these devices could harm fetuses during the first trimester of pregnancy.

Other devices such as vibrating belts, body wraps, and electrical stimulators have been used in attempted weight loss. Although these devices may not be harmful, they do not lead to weight loss. The money spent on these useless devices would be better spent on proven techniques. Additionally, people who put faith and effort into these unproven techniques may delay making lifestyle changes that lead to long-term weight loss and maintenance.

A widely held myth is that exercise emphasizing a particular body part will cause that area to lose fat faster than the rest of the body. This false theory is called **spot reduction.** People commonly perform curl-ups in an attempt to decrease their waistlines. Although curl-ups are terrific for increasing the muscular strength and endurance of the abdominal muscles, they are not very effective for burning fat. As a person establishes a caloric deficit through regular aerobic exercise, fat loss occurs all over the body, not just at the parts he would like to see the decrease.

Programs that advertise rapid, large weight losses are typically deceptive. The rapid weight losses seen at the beginning of such programs primarily result from lost water weight. Also, dietary plans that establish extremely large caloric deficits substantially reduce RMR and lean body mass and do not establish healthy, lifelong eating habits. As stated earlier, diets consisting of less than 800 kcal $\cdot$ day^{-1} are not recommended (26). Useful information about fad diets is highlighted below.

Focus on Fad Diets

Dietary plans that promise incredible results can be found easily on bookshelves, in media ads, and on the Internet. Many people are looking for quick, easy ways to lose weight, and entrepreneurs are eager to supply them. No one description summarizes all fad diets. Many focus on eating one food or food group, whereas others emphasize avoiding certain foods. Most of these plans are low in calories and may result in weight loss. However, the majority of these diets do not emphasize a balanced diet with an adequate supply of essential nutrients. Over time, these nutritional deficiencies can lead to serious health consequences. Because of the potential for negative health consequences, the AHA has declared war on fad diets. Another problem with these diets is that they do not lead to lifestyle changes that result in permanent weight loss. Many people follow these diets for a brief time and then regain their excess weight when they return to their previous pattern of overconsuming calories. These diets typically focus on food rather than on behavior change (e.g., increasing physical activity, using food substitution). For more information on making healthy diet choices, see the Web sites of the American Dietetic Association (www.eatright.org) and National Institute of Diabetes and Digestive and Kidney Diseases (www.niddk.nih.gov).

Key Point

A number of quick fixes for weight loss are marketed, but these products are often ineffective and sometimes dangerous.

Disordered Eating Patterns

There are conditions in which an eating pattern can have a serious negative effect on health. **Eating disorders** are clinically diagnosed conditions in which the unhealthy eating patterns may lead to severe declines in health and even to death. **Anorexia nervosa, bulimia nervosa,** and **binge eating disorder** are three of the eating disorders recognized by the American Psychiatric Association (APA) (3). **Disordered eating** refers to subclinical, unhealthy eating patterns that are often the precursors of eating disorders.

In the United States, anorexia nervosa occurs at a rate of 0.5% to 1% and bulimia nervosa occurs at a rate of 2% to 4% (19). No single mechanism has been identified as the primary cause of disordered eating or eating disorders. It appears that genetic, psychological, and sociocultural factors may predispose a person to these conditions. In American populations, these conditions are most common in young women from middle and high socioeconomic environments and female athletes in sports that emphasize extreme leanness. It is hypothesized that the social pressure to be thin as well as discomfort with sexual development contribute to unhealthy eating patterns in young women. For female athletes, the pressure to perform in some sports is linked with extremely low body weights. For example, it has been reported that more than 60% of female gymnasts exhibit a disordered eating pattern (19).

In anorexia nervosa, a preoccupation with body weight leads to self-starvation. People with anorexia nervosa typically view themselves as overweight even when their weight is substantially below normal. The APA lists the following criteria for diagnosis of anorexia nervosa (3):

- Purposefully maintaining weight at less than 85% of expected weight for age and height
- Extreme fear of gaining weight or fat
- Unhealthy body image in which the person feels overweight even when underweight; often associated with a severe intertwining of body image and self-esteem and a disregard for the seriousness of maintaining an extremely low body weight
- Absence of at least three consecutive menstrual cycles in postmenarchal women

Signs of Disordered Eating

- A preoccupation with food, calories, and weight
- Repeatedly expressed concerns about being or feeling fat, even when weight is average or below average
- Increasing self-criticism about the body
- Secretly eating or stealing food
- Eating large meals, then disappearing or making trips to the bathroom
- Consuming large amounts of food not consistent with current body weight
- Bloodshot eyes, especially after trips to the bathroom
- Swollen parotid glands at the angle of the jaw, giving a chipmunk-like appearance
- Vomitus or odor of vomitus in the bathroom
- Wide fluctuations in weight over a short time
- Bouts of severe caloric restriction
- Excessive laxative use
- Compulsive, excessive exercise that is not part of the planned training regimen
- Unwillingness to eat in front of others
- Expression of self-deprecating thoughts after eating
- Wearing baggy or layered clothing
- Mood swings
- Appearing preoccupied with the eating behavior of others
- Continuous drinking of diet soda or water

Adapted from M.D. Johnson, 1994, Disordered eating. In *Medical and orthopedic issues of active and athletic women,* edited by R. Agostini (Philadelphia, PA: Hanley and Belfus), 141-151. (19).

Bulimia nervosa is characterized by consuming large amounts of food followed by food purging (3). Misuse of laxatives, self-induced vomiting, and excessive exercise are among the methods that may be used to purge. To meet the diagnostic criteria established by the APA, a person must engage in this behavior at least two times a week for 3 mo. Patients with bulimia nervosa, similarly to those with anorexia nervosa, have an impaired body image and fear losing control over their body weight. Both anorexia nervosa and bulimia nervosa should be considered life-threatening disorders.

Binge eating disorder is characterized by consuming large amounts of food in a short time (3). Unlike bulimia nervosa, binge eating is not associated with purging. Binge episodes are often initiated by emotional or psychological cues (e.g., loneliness, anxiety) rather than by physical hunger. These binges typically occur when the person is alone and may be followed by shame, guilt, and depression. To be clinically diagnosed with binge eating disorder, a person must engage in at least two binges per week for 6 mo (3). The prevalence of binge eating disorder in the general population has been estimated at 2%. In contrast, 25% to 70% of obese individuals seeking treatment for weight loss may have this disorder (32).

Recognizing the signs of disordered eating is necessary for successful intervention. Some of the common signs of disordered eating are listed on page 186. Fitness professionals who observe these signs should discuss the issue in a nonconfrontational manner with the client. However, when approached, many people will deny the existence of a problem. Asking gentle questions about the client's health (e.g., "How are you feeling?" or "Are you a little tired?") is one way to attempt to break the ice on this delicate subject. Successful intervention for eating disorders requires a multidisciplinary approach combining medical, nutritional, and psychological professionals. Knowledge of local support groups or professionals who work with patients who have eating disorders will allow fitness professionals to recommend places for clients to receive help.

Key Point

Eating disorders can significantly impair health and may even result in death. Anorexia nervosa, bulimia nervosa, and binge eating disorder are three eating disorders recognized by the APA. Intervention for eating disorders should be multidisciplinary and should include psychological counseling.

Strategies for Gaining Weight

Before concluding this chapter we must mention that some individuals struggle to increase their body weight. Fitness professionals should encourage these individuals to accumulate fat-free mass rather than all fat weight. This will necessitate adding resistance training to the exercise routine. Various nutritional supplements are touted as "guaranteed" ways to increase muscle mass. However, as mentioned in chapter 7, even those who are training intensely need only about 1.5 g of protein per kilogram of body weight. Supplements such as creatine monohydrate may contribute somewhat to weight gain, but much of the change comes from greater water retention in the muscle.

The following are tips for increasing weight over time. When individuals continually lose weight or struggle to gain weight, a physician should be consulted about the possibility of underlying conditions.

- Increase caloric intake by 200 to 1,000 kcal $\cdot$ day^{-1} by increasing the meal size, number of meals, or number of between-meal snacks.
- Increase the number of healthy snacks consumed. Choose bread, fruit, granola, and other nutritious foods.
- Consume complex carbohydrate (e.g., whole wheat pasta, whole grain bread, brown rice, potatoes) to get the majority of additional calories.
- Add resistance training to the daily routine. Weight training is an effective means for increasing the body's fat-free mass.
- When training intensely, make sure each day to consume 1.5 g of protein for each kilogram of body weight.
- Increase consumption of milk and fruit juices. These excellent choices not only provide additional calories but also provide essential nutrients.

Key Point

The additional calories needed to increase weight should come from increasing the number of healthy snacks or the size of meals. Adding resistance training to the exercise routine may help increase muscle mass.

Case Studies

You can check your answers by referring to page 471 in appendix A.

1. A 52-yr-old female comes to your facility for an initial evaluation. She complains that she has gained 15 lb (6.8 kg) in the last 3 yr, and she wants to lose that extra weight. She is 5 ft 5 in. (1.65 m) and weighs 160 lb (72.6 kg). She currently does not exercise and has a sedentary job, but she is beginning an exercise program that will expend about 200 $kcal \cdot day^{-1}$. Calculate her estimated daily energy requirements. In order for her to lose approximately 1 lb (0.5 kg) a week, what calorie intake would you recommend?

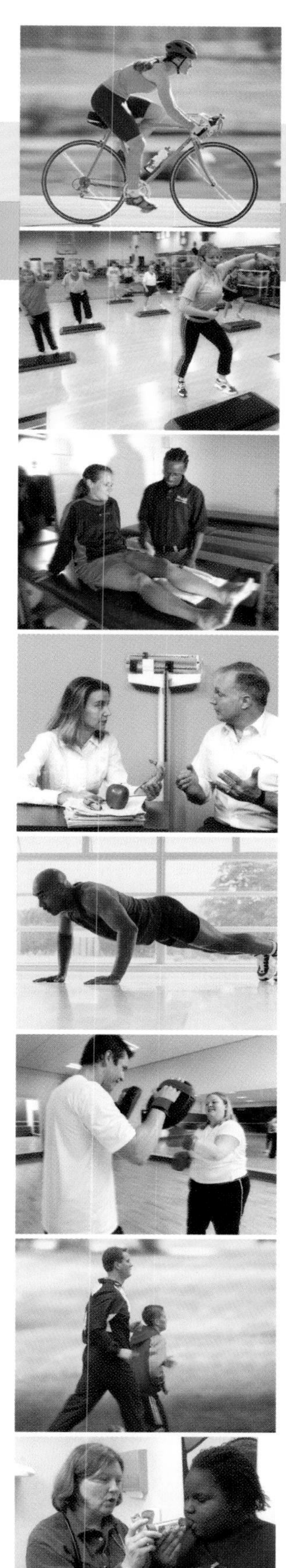

12

CHAPTER

Exercise Prescription for Resistance Training

Avery Faigenbaum and Kyle McInnis

Objectives

The reader will be able to do the following:

1. Explain the physiological principles of overload, specificity, and progressive resistance and how they relate to exercise programming.
2. Describe the following methods of resistance training: isometrics, dynamic constant external resistance training, variable resistance training, isokinetics, and plyometrics.
3. Describe the different modes of resistance training.
4. Discuss the health and fitness benefits of resistance training and understand precautions that enhance participant safety.
5. Describe the program variables that are used to design resistance training programs and discuss the relationship among the amount of resistance used, the training volume, the repetition velocity, and the rest intervals between sets and exercises.

(continued)

Objectives *(continued)*

6. Understand periodization and its application in the design of exercise programs, and differentiate between overreaching and overtraining.
7. Describe the following systems of resistance training: single set, multiple set, circuit training, preexhaustion, and assisted training.
8. Design resistance training programs for untrained and trained individuals.
9. Discuss the safety, benefits, and recommendations of resistance training for young people, older people, pregnant women, and adults with CHD.
10. Identify safe and effective exercises that enhance the fitness of specific muscle groups.

Traditionally, **resistance training** was used primarily by adult athletes to enhance sport performance and increase muscle size. Today, resistance training is recognized as a method of enhancing the health and fitness of men and women of all ages and abilities (6, 52). Like aerobic training, moderate-intensity resistance training provides a variety of health and fitness benefits (see table 12.1). Resistance training is recommended by national health organizations such as the ACSM and is performed by everyone from children to older adults, pregnant women, and patients with chronic disease. For fitness professionals, the ability to design safe and effective resistance training programs for people of all ages, fitness levels, and health conditions is a valuable professional asset. This chapter focuses on principles of resistance training that can be used in designing exercise programs for enhancing muscular fitness in untrained and trained individuals. Advanced resistance training programs for developing speed, strength, and power for elite athletes are available elsewhere (7, 14, 66).

In this chapter, the term *resistance training* refers to a method of conditioning designed to increase a person's ability to exert or resist force. This term encompasses a wide range of resistive loads (from light manual resistance to plyometric jumps) and a variety of training modalities, including free weights (barbells and dumbbells), weight machines, elastic tubing, medicine balls, stability balls, and body weight. Resistance training should be distinguished from the competitive sports of **weightlifting, powerlifting,** and **bodybuilding.** Weightlifting and powerlifting are sports in which athletes attempt to lift maximal amounts of weight, and bodybuilding is a sport in which the goal is muscle size and symmetry. **Local muscular endurance** refers to the ability of a muscle or muscle group to perform repeated contractions against a submaximal resistance. **Strength** is defined as the maximal force that a muscle or muscle group can generate at a specified velocity. **Power** refers to the rate of performing work and is the product of strength and speed of movement. For ease of discussion, the terms *children* and *youth* are broadly defined in this chapter to include the preadolescent and adolescent years, and the terms *older* and *senior* have been defined to include individuals over 65 yr of age.

Principles of Training

A key factor in the design of any resistance training program is appropriate program design. Since the act of resistance training itself does not ensure gains in muscular performance, the resistance training program needs to be based on sound training principles and must be carefully prescribed in order to maximize training outcomes. Although factors such as initial fitness level, heredity, nutritional status (e.g., diet composition and hydration), health habits (e.g., sleep), and motivation influence the rate and magnitude of the adaptation that occurs, there are four principles that determine the effectiveness of all resistance training programs: progression, regularity, **overload,** and **specificity.** These principles of resistance training can be remembered as the PROS.

Principle of Progression

According to the principle of progression, the demands placed on the body must continually and progressively increase over time in order to result in long-term fitness gains. This does not mean that heavier weights should be used in every workout, but rather that over time exercise sessions should become more challenging in order to create a more effective exercise stimulus. Without a more challenging stimulus that is consistent with individual needs, goals, and abilities, the human body has no reason to adapt any further. This principle is particularly important after the first 2 or 3 mo of resistance training, when the threshold for training-induced adaptations in conditioned individuals is higher (47, 48).

• Table 12.1 Effects of Aerobic Endurance Training and Resistance Training on Health and Fitness Variables •

Variable	Aerobic exercise	Resistance exercise
Bone mineral density	↑↑	↑↑
Body composition		
% Fat	↓↓	↓
LBM	↔	↑↑
Strength	↔	↑↑↑
Glucose metabolism		
Insulin response to glucose challenge	↓↓	↓↓
Basal insulin levels	↓	↓
Insulin sensitivity	↑↑	↑↑
Serum lipids		
HDL-C	↑↔	↑↑↔
LDL-C	↓↔	↓↔
Resting HR	↓↓	↔
Stroke volume, resting and maximal	↑↑	↔
BP at rest		
Systolic	↓↔	↔
Diastolic	↓↔	↓↔
$\dot{V}O_2max$	↑↑↑	↑↑↔
Submaximal and maximal endurance time	↑↑↑	↑↑
Basal metabolism	↑	↑↑

↑= values increase; ↓ = values decrease; ↔ = values remain unchanged; single arrow = small effect; double arrows = medium effect; triple arrows = large effect; LBM = lean body mass; HDL-C = high-density lipoprotein cholesterol; LDL-C = low-density lipoprotein cholesterol; HR = heart rate; BP = blood pressure.

Adapted, by permission, from Pollock et al., 2000, "Resistance exercise in individuals with and without cardiovascular disease," *Circulation* 101: 828-833.

The training stimulus should increase at a rate that is compatible with the training-induced adaptations. Beginners can progress relatively fast whereas slower rates of improvement are appropriate for individuals with experience in resistance training. A reasonable guideline for a beginner is to increase the training weight about 5% to 10% and decrease the **repetitions** (the number of times a movement is completed) by 2 to 4 once a given load can be performed for the desired number of repetitions with proper exercise technique. For example, if an adult female can easily perform 12 repetitions of the chest press exercise using 100 lb (45 kg), she should increase the weight to 110 lb (50 kg) and decrease the repetitions to 8 if she wants to continually gain muscular strength. Alternatively, she could increase the number of sets, increase the number of repetitions, or add another chest exercise to her routine. The decision on how this person will progress should be based on her training experience and personal goals.

Principle of Regularity

In order to make continual gains in muscular fitness, resistance training must be performed regularly several times per week. Inconsistent training will result in only modest training adaptations, and prolonged inactivity will result in a loss of muscular strength and size. The adage, "Use it or lose it," is appropriate for exercise programming because training-induced adaptations cannot be stored. Although adequate recovery is needed between training sessions, the principle of regularity states that long-term gains in muscle strength and performance will be realized only if the program is performed on a regular basis.

Principle of Overload

For more than a century, the overload principle has been a tenet of resistance training. The overload principle states that to enhance muscular performance, the body must exercise at a level beyond that at which it is normally stressed. For example, an adult male who can easily complete 10 repetitions with 20 lb (9 kg) while performing a barbell curl must increase the weight, the repetitions, or the number of **sets** (a group of repetitions) if he wants to increase his arm strength. If the training stimulus is not increased beyond the level to which the muscles are accustomed, training adaptations will not occur. Overload is typically manipulated by changing the exercise intensity, duration, or frequency over the course of a training program. This process is often referred to as *progressive overload* and is the basis for maximizing long-term training adaptations.

Principle of Specificity

The principle of specificity refers to the adaptations that take place as a result of a training program. The adaptations to resistance training are specific to the muscle actions, velocity of movement, exercise ROM, muscle groups, energy systems, and intensity and volume involved in training (50). Specificity is often referred to as the *SAID principle,* which stands for Specific Adaptations to Imposed Demands. In essence, every muscle or muscle group must be trained to make gains in strength and local muscular endurance. Exercises such as the squat and leg press can enhance lower-body strength, but these exercises will not affect upper-body strength.

The adaptations that take place in a muscle or muscle group will be as simple or as complex as the stress placed on them. For example, because basketball requires multijoint and multiplanar movements (e.g., in the frontal, sagittal, and transverse planes), basketball players should perform complex exercises that closely mimic the movements of their sport. The specificity principle also can be applied to designing resistance training programs for people who want to enhance their ability to perform activities of daily life such as stair-climbing and house cleaning, which also require multijoint and multiplanar movements.

Key Point

Gains in muscular strength and local muscular endurance will occur only if the overload is greater than that to which the muscle or muscle group is normally accustomed. To make continual gains, training must progress gradually and be performed regularly. The program design will influence the training-induced adaptations that occur. The most beneficial resistance training programs are designed to meet individual needs, goals, and abilities.

Program Design Considerations

Similarly to exercise programs that enhance cardiorespiratory fitness, resistance training programs should be based on the participant's interests, current fitness level, health needs, clinical status, and personal goals as well as on the principles of resistance training. By assessing the needs of each participant and applying principles of training to the program design, safe and effective resistance training programs can be developed for each person. However, because the magnitude of adaptation to a given exercise stimulus varies among individuals, fitness professionals must be aware of interindividual differences and be prepared to alter the program to reduce the risk of injury and to optimize gains.

Health Status

The health status of each person should be assessed before the resistance training begins. As discussed in chapter 3, each participant should complete a health and medical questionnaire, and the fitness professional should review it to make decisions about further medical evaluation. Additional questions on the HSQ regarding past resistance training experiences, previous musculoskeletal injuries, and personal goals can also help with designing the resistance training program.

Fitness Level

An important factor to consider when designing resistance training programs is the participant's previous experience with resistance training, or training age. Those who are the least experienced in resistance training tend to have a greater capacity for improvement compared with those who have been resistance training for several years. Although any reasonable program can increase the strength of untrained individuals, more comprehensive programs are often needed to produce desirable adaptations in trained individuals. For example, a 32-yr-old person with 5 yr of resistance training experience (i.e., a training age of 5 yr) may not achieve the same strength gains in a given time as a 25-yr-old person who has no experience with resistance training (i.e., a training age of 0 yr). The potential for adaptation gradually decreases as training age increases. Thus, as people gain experience with resistance training, they need more advanced programs so that they may continue to gain muscular strength (47, 48).

Training Goals

After the preexercise screening, participants should establish realistic short- and long-term goals. The results of a muscular fitness evaluation (see chapter 8) along with the participant's interests can be used to help set realistic and measurable goals. To improve compliance, these goals ideally are set by the individual with guidance from a knowledgeable fitness professional. Typical goals are to increase muscle strength and decrease body fat. An effort to establish realistic goals and increase confidence to achieve those goals is important because it may help people avoid unrealistic expectations that ultimately can lead to discouragement and poor adherence. Testing fitness periodically and reviewing individualized workout logs can help the fitness professional assess training progress and modify the program. Understanding that resistance training programs designed to improve health and fitness are quite different from training programs designed to enhance sport performance will further promote the development of and adherence to programs suited to an individual's needs.

Types of Resistance Training

Different types of resistance training can be used to enhance muscular strength and local muscular endurance. Although each method has advantages and disadvantages, there are several factors to consider when selecting one type of training over another or including multiple types of training within a given program. The most common types of resistance training include isometrics, dynamic constant external resistance training, variable resistance training, isokinetics, and plyometrics.

Isometrics

Isometric training, or static resistance training, refers to muscle actions in which muscle length does not change. This type of training is usually performed against an immovable object such as a wall or a weight machine loaded with a heavy weight. The concept of isometric training was popularized in the 1950s when Hettinger and Muller reported remarkable gains in muscle strength resulting from one daily 6 sec isometric contraction at two thirds of maximal force (35). Although subsequent studies also reported gains in strength resulting from isometric training, the reported gains were substantially less than those reported earlier (28).

An advantage of isometric training is that specialized equipment is not required and the cost is minimal. Increases in strength and muscle **hypertrophy** (an increase in size or mass) can occur from this type of training; however, a major limitation is that the strength gains are specific to the joint angle at which the training occurred. For example, if isometric training of the elbow flexors is performed at a joint angle of 90°, muscle strength will increase at this joint angle but not necessarily at other angles. Even though there seems to be about 20° of carryover on either side of the joint angle, to increase strength throughout the full ROM the same isometric exercise must be performed at varying joint angles. Isometric training may help to maintain muscle strength and prevent muscle **atrophy** (a decrease in size or mass) when a limb is immobilized in a cast, but gains in functional strength (e.g., stair-climbing) and motor performance (e.g., sprinting and jumping) as a result of isometric training are unlikely to occur if isometric training takes place only at one joint angle.

Factors such as the number of repetitions performed, duration of contractions, intensity of contractions, and frequency of training can influence the strength gains resulting from isometric training. In general, isometric training characterized by maximal voluntary muscle actions performed for 3 to 5 sec for 15 to 20 repetitions at least 3 times $\cdot$ wk^{-1} tends to optimize strength gains (28). Because of the nature of isometric training, it is particularly important to avoid the breath-holding Valsalva maneuver, which reduces venous return to the heart and increases SBP and DBP. During all types of resistance training, regular breathing patterns (i.e., exhale while lifting and inhale while lowering) should be encouraged.

Dynamic Constant External Resistance (DCER) Training

Resistance training that involves a lifting and lowering phase is called *dynamic*. Exercises using free weights (e.g., barbells and dumbbells) and weight machines are dynamic because the weight is lifted and lowered through a predetermined ROM. Although the term *isotonic* traditionally was used to describe this type of training, this term literally means constant *(iso)* tension *(tonic)*. Because tension exerted by a muscle as it shortens varies with the mechanical advantage of the joint and the length of the muscle fibers at a particular joint angle, the term *isotonic* does not accurately describe this training method. As shown in figure 12.1, during a barbell curl, the elbow flexors are strongest at approximately 100° and weakest at 60° (elbows fully flexed) and at 180° (elbows fully extended). The same principle applies to other muscle groups. DCER better describes resistance training in which the weight does not change during the lifting (**concentric**) and lowering (**eccentric**) phase of an exercise.

DCER training is the most common method of resistance training for enhancing health and fitness. Endless combinations of sets and repetitions and different types of training equipment can be used for DCER training. Although there is not enough scientific evidence to make any specific recommendations regarding the most effective speed for DCER training (e.g., 4 sec or 14 sec per repetition), proper form and technique should be used on all exercises. Weight machines generally limit the user to fixed planes of motion. However, they are easy to use

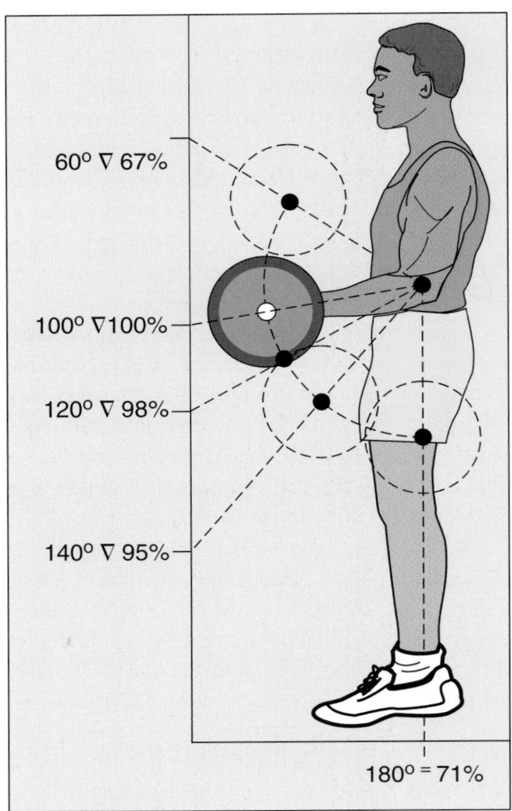

Figure 12.1 Variation in strength relative to the angle of the elbow flexors during the biceps curl.

Reprinted, by permission, from J.H. Wilmore and D.L. Costill, 2004, *Physiology of sport and exercise*, 3rd ed. (Champaign, IL: Human Kinetics), 105.

and are ideal for isolating muscle groups. Free weights are less expensive and can be used for a wide variety of different exercises that require greater proprioception, balance, and coordination. Several free weight exercises (e.g., barbell squat and bench press) require the use of a spotter who can assist the lifter in case of a failed repetition. In addition to improving health and fitness, DCER training is also used to enhance motor performance skills and sport performance.

During DCER training, the weight lifted does not change throughout the ROM. Because muscle tension can vary significantly during a DCER exercise, the heaviest weight that can be lifted throughout a full ROM is limited by the strength of a muscle at the weakest joint angle. As a result, DCER exercise provides enough resistance in some parts of the movement range but not enough resistance in others. For example, during the barbell bench press, more weight can be lifted during the last part of the exercise than in the first part of the movement when the barbell is being pressed off the chest. This is a limitation of DCER training that should be recognized when choosing starting weights for beginners.

In an attempt to overcome this limitation, mechanical devices that operate through a lever arm or cam have been designed to vary the resistance throughout the ROM of an exercise (see figure 12.2). These devices, called variable resistance machines, theoretically force the muscle to contract maximally throughout the ROM by varying the resistance to match the exercise strength curve. These machines can be used to train all the major muscle groups, and by automatically changing the resistive force throughout the movement range, they provide proportionally less resistance in weaker segments of the movement and more resistance in stronger segments of the movement. Like all weight machines, variable resistance machines provide a specific movement path, which makes the exercise easier to perform compared with free weight exercises, which require balance, coordination, and the involvement of stabilizing muscle groups. These features make variable resistance machines a popular mode of resistance training for people who desire safe and simple exercise sessions.

Isokinetics

The term *isokinetics* refers to muscular actions performed at a constant angular limb velocity. Isokinetic training involves specialized and expensive equipment, and most isokinetic devices are designed to train only single-joint movements. Isokinetic machines generally are not used in fitness centers, but they are used by physical therapists and athletic trainers for injury rehabilitation. Unlike other types of resistance training, in isokinetics the speed of movement—rather than the resistance—is controlled. During isokinetic training, any force applied to the isokinetic machine is met with an equal reaction

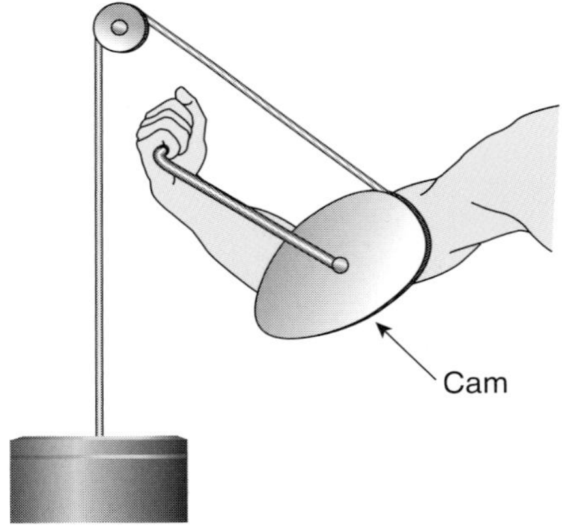

Figure 12.2 Variable resistance device for the biceps muscle in which a cam alters the resistance throughout the ROM.

Adapted, by permission, from D. Wathen and F. Roll, 1994, Training methods and modes. In *Essentials of strength training and conditioning*, edited by T.R. Baechle (Champaign, IL: Human Kinetics), 408

force. Although it is theoretically possible for a muscle to contract maximally through the full ROM of an exercise, this seems unlikely during isokinetic training because of the acceleration at the beginning and deceleration at the end of the ROM.

Isokinetic training studies have generally found that strength gains are specific to the training velocity (11). Isokinetic training at a slow movement velocity (e.g., $60° \cdot sec^{-1}$) will increase strength at that velocity, but strength gains at faster velocities are unlikely to occur. If the purpose of the training program is to increase strength at higher velocities (e.g., for enhanced sport performance), high-speed isokinetic training appears prudent. Although further research is warranted, the best approach may be to perform isokinetic training at slow, intermediate, and fast velocities to develop strength and power at different movement speeds.

Plyometrics

Plyometric training, first known simply as *jump training*, refers to a specialized method of conditioning designed to enable a muscle to reach maximal force in the shortest possible time (14). Unlike an exercise such as the bench press, plyometric training is characterized by quick, powerful movements that involve rapid stretching of a muscle (eccentric muscle action) immediately followed by rapid shortening (concentric muscle action). This type of muscle action, sometimes called stretch–shortening cycle exercise, provides a physiological advantage because the muscle force generated during the concentric muscle action is potentiated by the preceding eccentric muscle action (46). Although both muscle actions are important, the amount of time it takes to change direction from the eccentric to the concentric muscle action is a critical factor in plyometric training. This amount of time is called the **amortization phase** and should be as short as possible (<0.1 sec) in order to maximize training adaptations. Both mechanical factors (i.e., increased stored elastic energy) and neurophysiological factors (i.e., change in the muscle's force velocity) contribute to the increased force production resulting from plyometric training (68).

Exercises that involve explosive jumping, skipping, hopping, and throwing can be considered plyometric exercise. Although plyometric exercises often are associated with high-intensity drills such as depth jumps (i.e., jumping from a box to the ground and then immediately jumping upward), common activities such as jumping jacks and hopscotch are also plyometric exercises because every time the feet hit the ground, the quadriceps go through a stretch–shortening cycle. Strength and power athletes in sports such as football, volleyball, and track and field regularly perform plyometric exercises as part of their conditioning program. More recently, this type of training has become popular in group exercise classes and fitness programs.

Since plyometric exercises can greatly stress muscles, connective tissues, and joints, they need to be carefully prescribed to reduce the likelihood of musculoskeletal injury. In some cases, the risks of performing plyometric exercises may outweigh the potential benefits for untrained or overweight individuals who may lack the strength and coordination to perform the exercises properly. In other cases, plyometrics may be a worthwhile addition to the exercise program of a trained individual who wants to join a recreational basketball league. Clearly, the prescription of plyometric exercises needs to be individualized and based on a person's health history, training experience, and personal goals. It seems prudent to restrict plyometric training to people who have developed a foundation of muscle strength by first participating in a general resistance training program. It is also reasonable to begin plyometric training with lower-intensity drills and gradually progress to higher-intensity drills as technique and performance improve.

Other considerations for plyometric training include proper footwear, adequate space, shock-absorbing landing surfaces (e.g., suspended floor or grass playing field), and training frequency. Although research has yet to determine the minimal training threshold for maximizing training adaptations from plyometric exercise, it is always better to undertrain than overtrain and risk an injury. It seems reasonable to begin plyometric training with 1 to 3 sets of 6 to 10 repetitions on several low-intensity exercises for the upper and lower body twice per week on nonconsecutive days. Fitness professionals who have experience with plyometric training should provide demonstrations and coaching cues in order to enhance learning, improve technique, and reduce the likelihood of injury. Additional training guidelines and examples of plyometric drills are available elsewhere (14).

Key Point

Different types of resistance training can increase muscular strength, local muscular endurance, and power. The effects of isometric training are generally limited to the joint angle at which the training occurs. DCER training refers to exercises performed throughout a ROM with free weights and weight machines. Isokinetic training occurs at a constant limb velocity with maximal force exerted throughout the ROM of the joint. Plyometric training exploits the muscle cycle of lengthening and shortening to increase speed of movement and muscle power.

Modes of Resistance Training

Different modes of resistance training can be used to accommodate the needs of youth, adults, and seniors. Provided that the principles of training are adhered to, almost any mode of resistance training can be used to enhance muscular fitness. Some types of equipment are relatively easy to use, while others require balance, coordination, and high levels of skill. The decision to use a certain mode of resistance training should be based on each client's needs, goals, and abilities. The major modes of resistance training are weight machines; free weights (barbells and dumbbells); body weight exercises; and a broadly defined category of balls, bands, and elastic tubing.

Single-joint exercises such as the biceps curl target a specific muscle group and require less skill. Multijoint exercises such as the bench press involve more than one joint or major muscle group and require more balance and coordination. Although both single- and multijoint exercises enhance muscular fitness, multijoint exercises are generally considered to be more effective for increasing muscle strength because they involve a greater amount of muscle mass and therefore enable a heavier weight to be lifted (50). Multijoint exercises have also been shown to have the greatest acute metabolic and anabolic (e.g., testosterone and growth hormone) hormonal response, which could favorably influence resistance training that targets improvements in muscle size and body composition (51). Table 12.2 summarizes the advantages and disadvantages of weight machines; free weights (barbells and dumbbells); body weight exercises; and balls, bands, and elastic tubing.

Weight machines are designed to train all the major muscle groups and can be found in most fitness centers. Both single-joint (e.g., leg extension) and multijoint (e.g., leg press) exercises can be performed on weight machines, which are relatively easy to use because the exercise motion is controlled by the machine and typically occurs in only one anatomical plane. This may be particularly important when designing resistance training programs for sedentary or inexperienced individuals. Also, several weight machine exercises such as the lat pull-down and leg curl are difficult to mimic with free weights. Weight machines are designed to fit the average male or female, so smaller individuals may not be able to properly position themselves on the equipment. A seat pad or back pad can be used to adjust body position to allow for a better fit. Some companies now manufacture weight machines specifically for children. These machines are smaller versions of adult-sized machines and have weight increments that are appropriate for younger populations.

Free weights are also popular in fitness centers and come in a variety of shapes and sizes. Although it may take longer to master proper exercise technique when using free weights compared with weight machines, free weights have several advantages. For example, proper fit is not an issue with adjustable barbells and dumbbells because one size fits all. Free weights also offer a greater variety of exercises than weight machines because they can be moved in many different directions. Another benefit of free weights is that they require the use of stabilizing and assisting muscles to hold the correct body position during an exercise. As such, free weight training can occur in different planes. This is particularly true with dumbbells because they train each side of the body independently.

In general, free weights allow the participant to train functionally by encouraging different muscle groups to work together while performing exercises that are very similar to the individual's sport or activity. However, unlike weight machines, several free weight exercises require the aid of a spotter who can assist the lifter in case of a failed repetition. Using a spotter is particularly important when performing the bench press. Tragically, at least six documented deaths have been associated with weight training equipment, and at least half involved the home bench press or other supine free weight exercises (56). Accidents such as these underscore the importance of close supervision and an appropriate progression of training loads when training with free weights.

Table 12.2 Comparison of Different Modes of Resistance Training

	Weight machines	Free weights	Body weight	Ball and cords[a]
Cost	High	Low	None	Very low
Portability	Limited	Variable	Excellent	Excellent
Ease of use	Excellent	Variable	Variable	Variable
Muscle isolation	Excellent	Variable	Variable	Variable
Functionality	Limited	Excellent	Excellent	Excellent
Exercise variety	Limited	Excellent	Excellent	Excellent
Space requirements	High	Variable	Low	Low

[a]Medicine balls, stability balls, and elastic cords.

Body weight exercises such as push-ups, pull-ups, and curl-ups are some of the oldest modes of resistance training. Obviously, a major advantage of body weight training is that equipment is not needed and a variety of exercises can be performed. Conversely, a limitation of body weight training is the difficulty in adjusting the body weight to the individual's strength level. Sedentary or overweight participants may not be strong enough to perform even one push-up or pull-up. In such cases, body weight exercises not only may be ineffective, they may have a negative effect on program compliance. Exercise machines that allow people to perform body weight exercises such as pull-ups and dips by using a predetermined percentage of their body weight are available. These machines provide an opportunity for participants of all abilities to incorporate body weight exercises into their resistance training program.

Stability balls, medicine balls, and elastic tubing are safe and effective alternatives to weight machines and free weights. Medicine balls first became popular in the 1950s, and stability balls and elastic tubing have been used by therapists for many years. Now fitness professionals are using balls and bands for resistance training and conditioning. Not only are stability balls, medicine balls, and elastic tubing relatively inexpensive, they can also be used to enhance strength, local muscular endurance, and power. In addition, exercises performed with balls and tubing can challenge proprioception, which carries added benefit including gains in agility, balance, and coordination.

Stability balls are lightweight, inflatable balls about 45 to 75 cm in diameter that add the elements of balance and coordination to any exercise while targeting selected muscle groups. Although many exercises can be performed with stability balls, they are often used to develop core (i.e., abdominal and low-back) strength and improve posture. When participants sit on a stability ball, their feet should be at a 90° angle. The firmer the ball, the more difficult the exercise will be. Since proper body alignment is crucial when performing an exercise on a stability ball, fitness professionals should know how to perform each exercise correctly and when to modify an exercise to meet individual needs and abilities. Different types of exercise programs using stability balls can be created to enhance strength, local muscular endurance, and flexibility (15). Figure 12.3 illustrates the performance of abdominal curls on a stability ball.

Medicine balls come in different shapes and sizes (about 1 kg to more than 10 kg) and are a safe and effective alternative to free weights and weight machines. In addition to squatting or chest pressing with a medicine ball, participants can use the ball in throwing drills—such as throwing from participant to instructor or against the wall—to enhance upper-body explosive power. High-speed medicine ball training can add a new dimension to resistance training that can benefit men and women of all ages. Further, since medicine ball training typically requires the body to function as a unit instead of as separate parts, it is particularly effective for mimicking natural body positions and movement speeds that occur in daily life and game situations. Progressive medicine ball training that can be used in one-on-one settings or group fitness classes is available (60). Figure 12.4 illustrates the medicine ball squat.

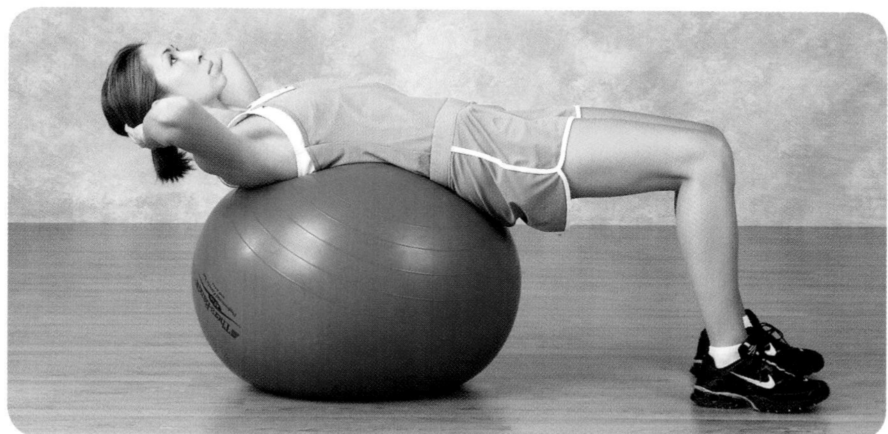

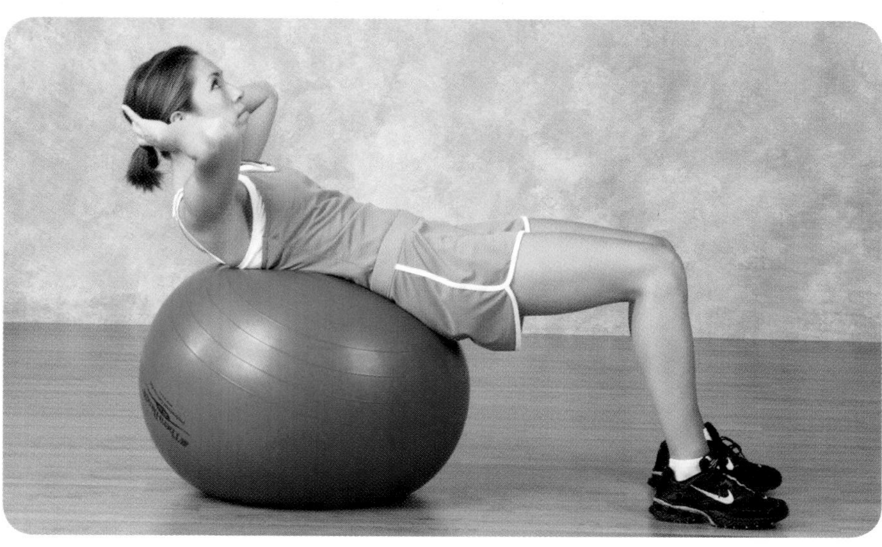

Figure 12.3 Abdominal curl on a stability ball.

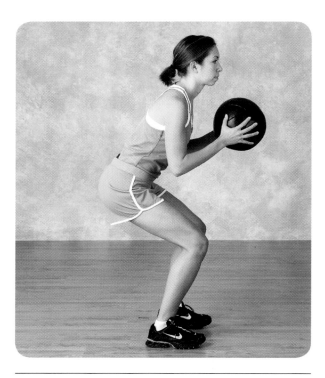

Figure 12.4 Medicine ball squat.

Resistance training with an elastic band involves performing an exercise against the force required to stretch the band and then return it to its unstretched state. A variety of exercises can be performed by holding the ends of the cord with both hands or attaching one end of the cord to a fixed object. For safety reasons, fitness professionals should ensure that the cord is secured under both feet or to a fixed object before performing any exercise. Incorporating exercises with stability balls, medicine balls, and elastic tubing into a workout session can be challenging, motivating, beneficial, and fun. Figure 12.5 illustrates a chest press with an elastic band.

Key Point

Weight machines, free weights, body weight exercises, medicine balls, stability balls, and elastic bands can be used to enhance muscular fitness. When designing resistance training programs, fitness professionals should evaluate the advantages and disadvantages of each training mode to meet individual needs, goals, and abilities.

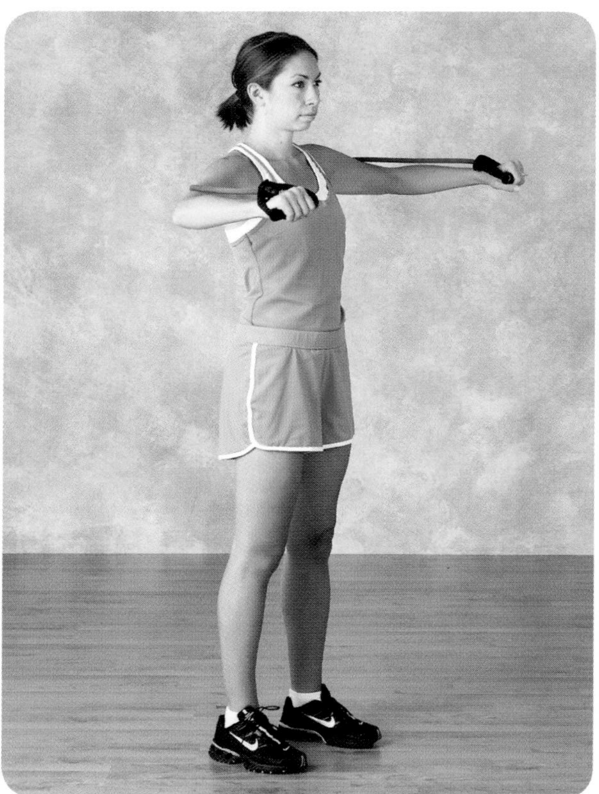

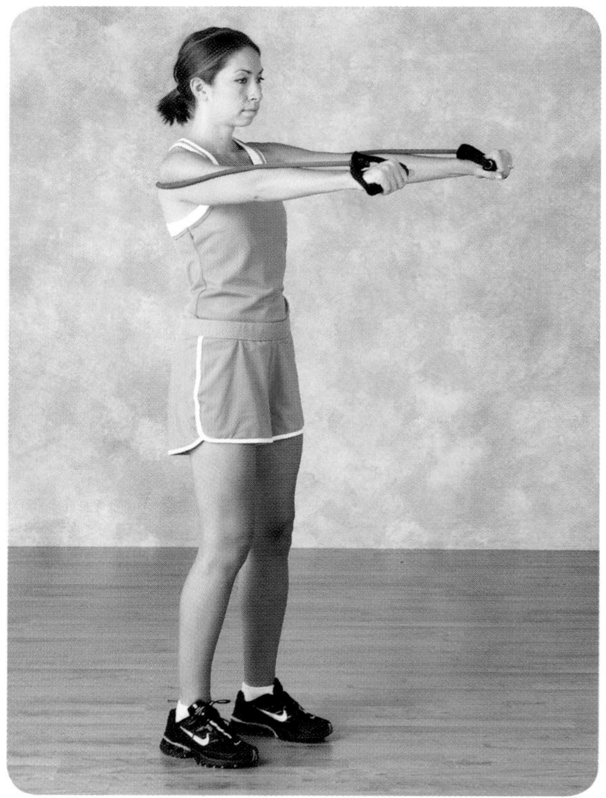

Figure 12.5 Chest press with elastic band.

Safety Issues

Resistance training programs should be designed by fitness professionals who are knowledgeable about safe and effective training methods. Although all resistance training activities have some degree of medical risk, the chance of injury can be reduced by following established training guidelines and safety procedures. Without proper supervision and instruction, injuries that require medical attention may occur. In fact, a retrospective 20 yr survey of resistance training injuries indicated that about 1 in 4 injuries occurred from misuse of resistance training equipment (40). Clearly, people who resistance train should receive instruction on appropriate training guidelines and equipment use. General safety recommendations for designing and instructing resistance training programs are given below.

Supervision and Instruction

People who want to participate in resistance training should first receive guidance and instruction from qualified fitness professionals who understand principles of resistance training and appreciate individual differences. Fitness professionals should be able to correctly perform the exercises they prescribe and should be able to modify exercise form and technique if necessary. Fitness professionals should know which exercises require spotters and should be prepared to offer assistance in case of a failed repetition. When working in a health or fitness facility, the staff should be attentive and should try to position themselves with a clear view of the training center so that they can have quick access to people who need assistance. In addition, the fitness staff is responsible for enforcing safety rules (e.g., wear proper footwear, store weights safely, no foolish play in the fitness center) and safe training procedures (e.g., emphasizing proper exercise technique rather than the amount of weight lifted). Not only can fitness professionals enhance the safety of resistance training, but they can help clients maximize strength gains (59) when they develop and supervise personalized programs.

Training Environment

If exercise is to take place in a public, community, work site, or school-based fitness center, the training area should be well lit and large enough to handle the number of people exercising in the facility at any given time. The facility should be clean and the equipment should be well maintained. Equipment pads that come in contact with the skin should be cleaned daily, and cables, guide rods, and chains on machines should be checked weekly. Equipment should be spaced to allow easy access to each resistance training exercise, and equipment such as free weights and collars should be returned to the proper storage area after each use. Recommended temperature (68-72 °F, or 20.0-22.2 °C), humidity (60% or less), and air circulation (at least 8 air exchanges per hour) should be maintained in the resistance training area (4). Additional recommendations for fitness facility maintenance and risk management are available elsewhere (5).

Safety Recommendations for Resistance Training

- Review participants' health history questionnaires before they begin resistance training.
- Provide adequate supervision and instruction when necessary.
- Regularly practice emergency procedures.
- Encourage participation in warm-up and cool-down activities.
- Move carefully around the resistance training area, and don't back up without looking first.
- Fix broken or malfunctioning equipment immediately or put an out-of-order sign on it.
- Use collars on all plate-loaded barbells and dumbbells.
- Be aware of proper spotting procedures and offer assistance when needed.
- Model appropriate behavior and do not allow horseplay in the fitness center.
- Demonstrate correct exercise technique and do not allow participants to train improperly.
- Periodically check all resistance training equipment.
- Ensure the training environment is free of clutter and appropriately maintained.
- Stay up to date with current resistance training guidelines and safety procedures for special populations.

Warm-Up and Cool-Down

Resistance training should be preceded by warm-up activities. A proper warm-up increases body and muscle temperature, increases blood flow, and may enhance performance (38). A general warm-up typically includes 5 to 10 min of low- to moderate-intensity aerobic exercise such as slow jogging or stationary cycling. Dynamic warm-up protocols that include low- to moderate-intensity hops, skips, and jumps and various movement-based exercises for the upper and lower body are also effective (57). A general or dynamic warm-up before stretching is recommended to enhance the benefits of stretching. The increase in muscle temperature resulting from the warm-up will allow for greater flexibility.

A specific warm-up involves movements that are similar to the resistance training exercises that are about to be performed. For example, after a general warm-up, a lifter could perform a light set of 10 repetitions on the bench press exercise before performing the training set with a heavier weight. It makes sense to physically and mentally prepare for the demands of resistance training by spending a few minutes warming up. After a resistance workout, it's a good idea to cool down with general calisthenics and static stretching exercises. A cool-down can help to relax the body and possibly reduce muscle stiffness and soreness.

Key Point

Qualified supervision and instruction, a safe training environment, and adherence to established training guidelines will help minimize the risk of injury during resistance training. Fitness professionals should educate participants about safe training procedures and design programs that are consistent with each person's needs and abilities. Warm-up and cool-down activities can enhance performance and reduce the likelihood of muscle soreness and injury.

Resistance Training Guidelines

Guidelines for resistance training are not as universally accepted as recommendations for enhancing aerobic fitness. Although sports medicine organizations recognize the importance of resistance training for health and fitness, there has been considerable debate regarding training volume (i.e., sets · repetitions · weight lifted). In particular, the efficacy of performing either single or multiple sets has captured the interest of some exercise scientists (12, 28, 69). Yet, despite various claims about the best training approach, there does not appear to be one optimal combination of sets, repetitions, and exercises that will promote long-term adaptations in muscular fitness for all individuals. Rather, many program variables may be altered to achieve desirable outcomes provided that the tenets of resistance exercise are followed. Clearly, resistance training programs need to be individualized and based on a person's training history and personal goals.

There are many factors to consider when designing a resistance training program, including the following (28):

1. Choice of exercise
2. Order of exercise
3. Resistance used
4. Training volume (total number of sets and repetitions)
5. Rest intervals between sets and exercises
6. Repetition velocity
7. Training frequency

Summary of the ACSM's Resistance Training Guidelines for Apparently Healthy Adults

- Perform a minimum of 8 separate exercises for each of the major muscle groups.
- Perform 1 set of each exercise to a point of volitional fatigue.
- Choose a repetition range between 3 and 20 (e.g., 8-12).
- Perform each repetition at a moderate velocity through the full range of motion.
- Perform each exercise with proper technique.
- Maintain a normal breathing pattern.
- Resistance train 2 or 3 nonconsecutive days per week.
- If possible, exercise with a partner who can provide feedback, assistance, and motivation.

Adapted, by permission, from American College of Sports Medicine (ACSM), 2006, *ACSM's guidelines for exercise testing and prescription,* 7th ed. (Philadelphia, PA: Lippincott, Williams & Wilkins) 158.

By varying one or more of these variables, endless resistance training programs can be designed. But since different people will respond differently to the same resistance training program, decisions must be based on an understanding of exercise science, individual needs, and personal goals. The ACSM's resistance training guidelines for apparently healthy adults are summarized on page 200.

Choice of Exercise

A limitless number of exercises can be used to enhance muscular strength, power, and local muscular endurance. Selected exercises should be appropriate for an individual's exercise experience and training goals. Also, the choice of exercises should promote muscle balance across joints and between opposing muscle groups (e.g., quadriceps and hamstrings). Selected weight machine and free weight exercises and the primary muscle groups strengthened are listed in table 12.3.

Exercises generally can be classified as single joint (i.e., body-part specific) or multijoint (i.e., structural). Dumbbell biceps curls and leg extensions are examples of single-joint exercises that isolate a specific body part (biceps and quadriceps, respectively), whereas squats and deadlifts are multijoint exercises that involve two or more primary joints. Exercises also can be classified as closed kinetic chain or open kinetic chain. Closed kinetic chain exercises are those in which the distal joint segment is stationary (e.g., squats), whereas open chain exercises are those in which the terminal joint is free to move (e.g., leg extensions). Closed kinetic chain exercises more closely mimic everyday activities and include more functional movement patterns (16).

Single-joint exercises and many machine exercises are often used by people who have limited experience resistance training or by those who simply enjoy this mode of training. This mode is also beneficial in activating specific muscles (e.g., during injury rehabilitation). With most machines, the path of movement is fixed and therefore the movement is stabilized. Conversely, exercises with free weights require additional muscles to stabilize the movement and are therefore more challenging. Also, dual-limb exercises with free weights (e.g., dumbbell lateral raises) may be particularly beneficial for people who need to strengthen a weaker limb. It is important to eventually incorporate multijoint exercises into a resistance training program to promote the coordinated use of multijoint movements. When participants learn a new multijoint exercise, such as the squat, they should start with a light weight (e.g., unloaded barbell or wooden dowel) so that they can master the exercise technique before adding weight to the bar. Regardless of the exercise type, the concentric and eccentric phases of each lift should be performed in a controlled manner with proper technique.

Another issue concerning choice of exercise is including exercises for abdominal and low-back musculature. It is not uncommon for beginners to focus on strengthening the chest and biceps and not spend enough time strengthening their abdominal muscles and low back. Strengthening the midsection not only may improve force output and enhance body control during free weight exercises such as the squat, it also may decrease the risk of injury. Thus, prehabilitation exercises for the low back and abdominal muscles should be included in all resistance training programs. In other words, as a preventive health measure, exercises that may be prescribed for the rehabilitation of an injury should be performed before injury occurs. Exercises such as abdominal curl-ups and back extensions are useful, but they only train the muscles that control trunk flexion and extension. Multidirectional exercises that involve rotational movements and diagonal

• Table 12.3 Selected Weight Machine and Free Weight Exercises and the Primary Muscle Group(s) Strengthened •

Weight machine exercise	Free weight exercise	Primary muscle group(s) strengthened
Leg press	Barbell squat	Quadriceps, gluteus maximus
Leg extension	Dumbbell lunge	Quadriceps
Leg curl	Barbell standing hip extension	Hamstrings
Chest press	Barbell bench press	Pectoralis major
Pec dec	Dumbbell fly	Pectoralis major
Front pull-down	Dumbbell pullover	Latissimus dorsi
Seated rows	Dumbbell one-arm row	Latissimus dorsi
Overhead press	Dumbbell press	Deltoids
Biceps curl	Barbell curl	Biceps
Triceps extension	Lying triceps extension	Triceps

A description of the proper exercise technique for each exercise is available elsewhere (7, 8).

patterns performed with body weight or a medicine ball can effectively strengthen the abdominal muscles and the low back. Depending on the needs and goals of the individual, other prehabilitation exercises (e.g., internal and external rotation for the rotator cuff musculature) can be incorporated into the exercise session.

Order of Exercise

There are many ways to sequence the exercises in a training session. Traditionally, exercises for large muscle groups are performed before exercises for smaller muscle groups, and multijoint exercises are performed before single-joint exercises. Following this order will allow participants to use heavier weights on the multijoint exercises because fatigue will be less of a factor. It is also helpful to perform more challenging exercises earlier in the workout when the neuromuscular system is less fatigued. However, in some cases (injury prevention or rehabilitation), it may be appropriate to reverse this order so that the smaller muscle groups are trained first. In general, it seems reasonable to follow the priority system of training in which exercises that will most enhance health and fitness are performed early in the training session. Also, participants should perform power exercises such as plyometrics before strength exercises so that they can train for maximal power without undue fatigue. A sample resistance training program is illustrated below.

Resistance Used

One of the most important variables in designing a resistance training program is the amount of weight used for an exercise (63). Gains in muscular strength and performance are influenced by the amount of weight lifted, which is highly dependent upon program variables such as exercise order, training volume, repetition velocity, and rest interval length (50, 51). By definition, the amount of weight that can be lifted with proper technique for only 1 repetition is the 1-repetition maximum (or 1RM). Similarly, the amount of weight that can be lifted with proper technique for 10 but not 11 repetitions is called the 10-repetition maximum (or 10RM). To maximize gains in muscle strength and performance, it is recommended that training sets be performed to volitional fatigue (defined as the inability to complete a repetition because of temporary fatigue) using the appropriate resistance.

The use of RM loads is a relatively simple method to prescribe resistance training intensity. Research studies suggest that RM loads of 6 or fewer have the greatest effect on developing muscle strength, whereas RM loads of 20 or more have the greatest effect on developing local muscular endurance (13, 28). Although beginners can make significant gains in muscle strength with lighter loads, it is believed that people with resistance training experience may need to train with a heavier resistance (28). Accordingly, the ACSM recommends

Weekly Resistance Training Log

	10/23			10/25			10/27			
Name: ______________	**Wt**	**Rep**	**Set**	**Wt**	**Rep**	**Set**	**Wt**	**Rep**	**Set**	**Comments**
Leg extension	90	10	2	90	11	2	90	12	2	
Leg curl	55	10	2	55	11	2	55	12	2	
Chest press	80	10	2	80	11	2	80	12	2	
Lat pull-down	80	10	2	80	11	2	80	12	2	
Biceps curl	30	10	2	30	11	2	30	11	2	
Triceps extension	40	10	2	40	11	2	40	12	2	Slight soreness in triceps
Kneeling trunk extension	No wt	10	2	No wt	11	2	No wt	12	2	
Abdominal curl	No wt	10	2	No wt	11	2	No wt	11	2	

Wt = weight.
Rep = repetitions.

a repetition range between 3 and 20 depending on individual goals and training experience (6). RM loads in the middle of this continuum (e.g., 8RM-12RM) are commonly used to enhance muscle strength and performance (see figure 12.6). Using weights that exceed a person's 6RM capacity minimally affects local muscular endurance, whereas training with very light weights (e.g., above 20RM) results in only small gains in maximal muscle strength. Since each repetition zone (e.g., 3-6, 8-12, or 15-20) has its advantages, the best approach is to systematically vary the resistance used in order to avoid training plateaus and to optimize training adaptations.

A percentage of an individual's 1RM also can be used to determine the resistance training intensity. If the 1RM on the chest press is 100 lb (45 kg), a training intensity of 70% would be 70 lb (32 kg). It is reasonable for beginners to use a training resistance of approximately 60% to 70% 1RM because they are mostly improving motor performance at this stage (47). As participants get stronger and gain training experience, heavier resistances (70%-80% 1RM) will be needed to make continual gains in muscular strength and performance (47). Obviously, this method of prescribing resistance exercise requires testing the 1RM on all exercises in the training program. In many cases this is not realistic because of the time required to correctly perform 1RM testing on 8 to 10 different exercises. Furthermore, maximal resistance testing for small muscle group assistance exercises (e.g., biceps curls and lying triceps extensions) typically is not performed.

Fitness professionals should also be knowledgeable of the relationship between the percentage of the 1RM and the number of repetitions that can be performed. In general, most people can perform about 10 repetitions using 75% of their 1RM. However, the number of repetitions that can be performed at a given percentage of the 1RM varies with the amount of muscle mass required to perform the exercise. For example, studies have shown that at a given percentage of the 1RM (e.g., 60%), adults can perform more repetitions of an exercise for large muscle groups such as the leg press compared with an exercise for smaller muscle groups such as the leg curl (37). Therefore, prescribing a resistance training intensity of 70% of 1RM on all exercises warrants additional consideration because at 70% of the 1RM,

Research Insight

While it is known that different types of resistance training result in specific adaptations, there is little information concerning specific intramuscular adaptations to different set and repetition combinations. Campos and colleagues (13) compared the effects of three different 8 wk resistance training programs on adaptations in the vastus lateralis muscle in untrained men. Subjects were divided into four groups: low repetition (3RM-5RM for 4 sets with a 3 min rest interval), intermediate repetition (9RM-11RM for 3 sets with a 2 min rest interval), high repetition (20RM-28RM for 2 sets with a 1 min rest interval), and the nonexercising control. Performance measures and muscle biopsy samples were measured pre- and posttraining. Maximal strength improved significantly more for the low-repetition group, and local muscular endurance improved significantly more for the high-repetition group. Muscle fibers hypertrophied following low and intermediate repetitions only. These data demonstrate that physiological adaptations to resistance training are linked to the intensity and volume of training.

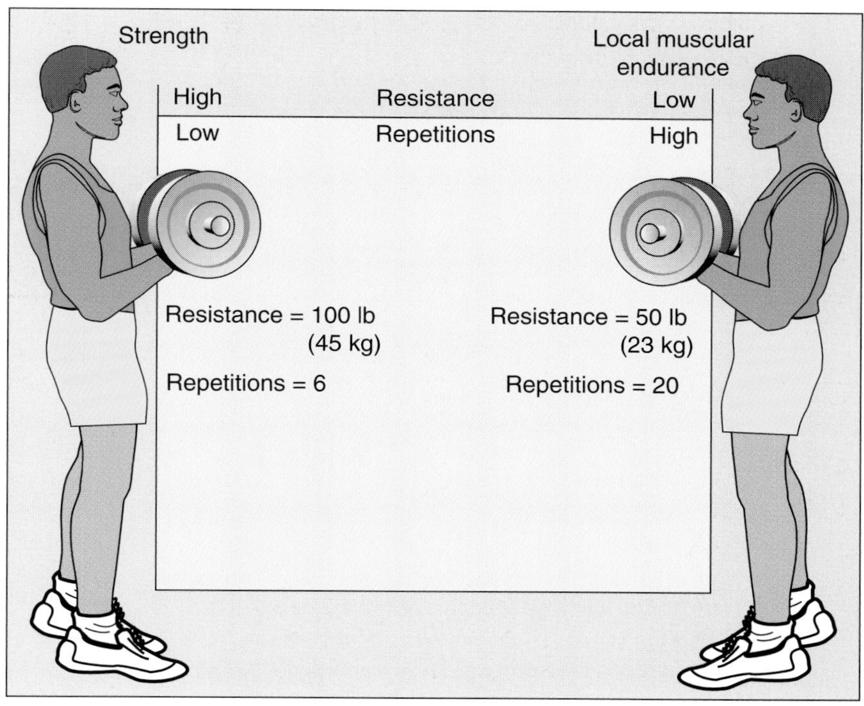

Figure 12.6 The strength–endurance continuum. The use of heavy weights and low repetitions has the greatest effect on strength and power, whereas the use of light weights and high repetitions has the greatest effect on local muscular endurance.

an individual may be able to perform 20 or more repetitions on a large muscle group exercise, which may not be ideal for enhancing muscle strength. If a percentage of the 1RM is used for prescribing resistance training, the prescribed percentage of the 1RM for each exercise may need to vary to maintain a desired training range (e.g., 8RM-10RM).

Training Volume

The number of exercises performed per session, the repetitions performed per set, and the number of sets performed per exercise all influence the training volume (50). For example, if an individual performs 3 sets of 10 repetitions with 100 lb (45 kg) on the bench press, the training volume for this exercise is 3,000 lb (3 · 10 · 100 = 3,000), or 1,361 kg. Although there has been much debate regarding training volume, it is important to remember that every training session does not need to be characterized by the same number of sets, repetitions, and exercises.

The ACSM recommends that apparently healthy adults perform 1 set of each exercise to achieve muscular fitness goals (6). In general, protocols using 1, 2, or 3 sets have proven to be equally effective for untrained individuals during the first 2 to 3 mo of training if the programs are not periodized or varied over time (32, 39, 58, 62, 73). Thus it appears that single- or multiple-set protocols may be effective during this introductory stage. However, the results from most (53, 54, 58)—but not all (33)—studies suggest that multiple-set periodized programs result in superior gains in muscular strength and performance in individuals with resistance training experience. Although additional long-term training studies are needed to explore the effects of different training volumes on muscular strength and performance in trained and untrained subjects, a multiple-set training protocol is considered to be more effective than a single-set protocol for maximizing training adaptations in individuals with resistance training experience.

When fitness professionals design a resistance training program, they need to consider the person's training status and goals because of the numerous possibilities for program design. It seems reasonable for beginners to start with a single-set program and gradually increase the number of sets depending on personal goals and time available for training. A single-set protocol reduces training time and may therefore provide a practical approach for people who do not train regularly. However, it is also possible that a multiple-set protocol can be a time-efficient method of training. For example, instead of performing 1 set for each of 12 different exercises during every workout, individuals can perform 2 sets for each of 6 exercises or 3 sets for each of 4 exercises. With a careful selection of multijoint exercises, all muscle groups can be trained each exercise session regardless of the number of sets or exercises performed. By periodically varying the sets, repetitions, and number of exercises (i.e., training volume), the training stimulus will remain effective and therefore the adaptations to the training program will be maximized. Periods of low-volume or single-set training can provide a needed variation for people who have been participating in a high-volume or multiple-set conditioning program for a prolonged time

Research Insight

A quantifiable relationship between program variables and strength improvements has been somewhat controversial. Rhea and colleagues (69) used meta-analytical techniques to combine and evaluate the treatment effects from 140 studies that included strength measures before and after a resistance training intervention. They reported that a training intensity of 60% 1RM elicits maximal strength gains in untrained individuals, whereas 80% 1RM is most effective in trained individuals. In addition, they found that 4 sets per muscle group elicited maximal gains in trained and untrained individuals. While the importance of gradually increasing the demands placed on the body must not be overlooked, fitness professionals can use this information to make an informed decision regarding the time and effort needed to achieve training goals.

Rests Between Sets and Exercises

The rest interval between sets and exercises is an important but often overlooked training variable. In general, the length of the rest influences energy recovery and the training adaptations that take place. For example, if the primary goal of the program is to maximize gains in muscular strength, heavier weights and longer rests (e.g., 2-3 min) are needed, whereas if the goal is local muscular endurance, lighter weights and shorter rests (e.g., <1 min) are required. Obviously, training intensity, training goals, and fitness level will influence the length of the rest interval. For example, it has been shown that individuals could complete 3 sets of 10 repetitions with a 10RM load if they were allowed to rest 3 min between sets. However, they only performed 10, 8, and 7 repetitions, respectively, when they rested only 1 min between sets (45).

As previously noted for the other program variables, the same rest interval does not need to be used for all exercises. In addition, fatigue resulting from a previous exercise should be considered when prescribing the rest interval. In general, resting 1 to 2 min between sets is appropriate for most beginners, although those with resistance training experience may want to rest 2 to 3 min between sets depending upon the resistance used and training goal (47). Short rests (<30 sec between sets and exercises) are not recommended for beginners because of the discomfort and high blood lactate concentrations (10-14 mmol $\cdot$ L^{-1}) associated with this type of training (49). However, the rests can be shortened gradually over time to provide ample opportunity for the body to tolerate increased muscle and blood acid levels.

Repetition Velocity

The velocity or cadence at which a resistance exercise is performed can affect the adaptations to a training program. According to the principle of training specificity, gains in muscle strength and performance are specific to the training velocity (28). For example, fast-velocity plyometric training is more likely to enhance speed and power than slow-velocity exercises on weight machines. However, there are two types of slow-velocity training (50). *Unintentional* slow velocities are used when a heavy resistance is lifted and the velocity is slow despite an individual's attempt to exert maximal force. On the other hand, *intentional* slow velocities are used when an individual trains with a submaximal load and purposefully performs the exercise at a slow velocity. Given that concentric force production is lower for an intentionally slower velocity compared to a moderate velocity, it appears that lighter loads performed at a slower velocity may not be optimal for maximizing strength development (43).

Since beginners need to learn how to perform each exercise correctly with a light resistance, it is generally recommended that untrained individuals perform exercises at a slow to moderate velocity (47). As they gain experience, they may use unintentional slow velocities with a heavier resistance to optimize strength gains. Depending on training goals and experience, individuals can also perform moderate- to fast-velocity training (e.g., plyometrics) in order to maximize performance adaptations. It is likely that the performance of different velocities within a training program may provide the most effective stimulus.

Training Frequency

Training frequency typically refers to the number of training sessions per week. In general, a training frequency of 2 to 3 times each week on nonconsecutive days is recommended for beginners (47). This training frequency allows for adequate recovery between sessions (48 to 72 hr between sessions) and has proven to be effective for enhancing muscle strength and performance (47). However, trained individuals who perform more advanced programs may need more time between sessions. Factors such as training volume, training intensity, exercise selection, and nutritional intake may influence the ability to recover from and adapt to the training program. For example, trained individuals who perform a split routine may resistance train 4 times $\cdot$ wk^{-1}, but they only train each muscle group twice per week. Although an increase in training experience does not necessitate an increase in training frequency, a higher frequency does allow for greater specialization characterized by more exercises and a higher weekly training volume.

Periodization

Periodization refers to systematic variation in a resistance training program. Since it is impossible to continually improve at the same rate over long-term training, properly varying the training variables can limit training plateaus, maximize performance gains, and reduce the likelihood of overtraining. In essence, periodization is a process whereby fitness professionals regularly change the training stimulus in order to keep it effective. While the concept of periodization has been part of program design for many years, our understanding of the benefits of periodized programs compared with nonperiodized programs for long-term progression has only recently been explored in the literature (27, 47, 50).

The concept of periodization, or program variation, is not just for athletes, but for people with different levels of training experience who want to enhance their health and fitness. By periodically varying program variables such as choice of exercise, training weight (resistance), number of sets, rest intervals between sets, or any combination of these, long-term performance gains will be optimized and the risk of overuse injuries may be reduced (47). Moreover, it is reasonable to suggest that people who participate in well-designed periodized programs and continue to improve their health and fitness may be more likely to adhere to an exercise program over the long term.

For example, if an individual's lower-body routine typically consists of leg presses, leg extensions, and leg curls, performing dumbbell lunges, hip abductions, and hip adductions on alternate workout days will likely add to the effectiveness and enjoyment of the resistance training program. Further, varying the volume and intensity of training can help to prevent training plateaus, which are common after the first 2 mo of training. Many times participants can avoid a strength plateau by varying the training intensity and volume to allow for ample recovery. In the long term, program variation with adequate recovery will result in even greater gains because the body will be challenged to adapt to even greater demands. The underlying concept of periodization is based on the theory that after a certain time, adaptations to a stimulus will no longer take place unless the stimulus is altered. Periodization can promote long-term training adaptations by keeping the training stimulus effective.

Although there are many models of periodization, the general concept is to prioritize training goals and then develop a long-term plan that varies throughout the year. In general, the overall training plan is divided into specific time periods called **macrocycles** (about 1 yr), **mesocycles** (about 3 to 4 mo), and **microcycles** (about 1 to 4 wk), with each cycle having a specific goal (e.g., hypertrophy, strength, or power). The classic periodization model is referred to as a *linear model* because the volume and intensity of training gradually change over time (78). For example, at the start of a macrocycle, the training volume may be high and the training intensity may be low. As the year progresses, the volume decreases as the intensity increases.

Although the linear training model was originally designed for weightlifters and track and field athletes who wanted to peak for a specific competition, this model can be modified by fitness professionals in order to enhance health and fitness. For example, individuals who routinely perform the same combination of sets and repetitions may benefit from gradually increasing the weight and decreasing the number of repetitions as strength improves. The classic periodized model, described previously, is outlined in table 12.4. After the four-phase program is complete, individuals should be encouraged to participate in recreational activities or low-intensity resistance training to reduce the likelihood of overtraining. This period of restoration is called *active rest* and typically lasts for 1 to 3 wk. After active rest, individuals can then return to the first phase of their training program with more energy and vigor.

A second model of periodization is referred to as an *undulating (nonlinear) model* because of the daily fluctuations in training volume and intensity. For example, an individual may perform 2 sets of 10 repetitions with a moderate load on Monday, 3 sets of 6 repetitions with a heavy load on Wednesday, and 1 set of 15 repetitions with a light load on Friday. The heavy training days will maximally activate the trained musculature, while selected muscle fibers will not be maximally taxed on light and moderate training days. By alternating training intensities, the participant can minimize the risk of overtraining and maximize the potential for maintaining training-induced strength gains (33). A sample nonlinear periodized workout plan for a trained adult is presented in table 12.5. In addition, fitness professionals should consider an individual's vacation schedule or travel plans when incorporating periods of active rest into the year-long training schedule. Periods of restoration lasting from 1 to 3 wk will allow for physical and psychological recovery from the resistance training. A detailed review of periodization and specific examples of periodized programs are available elsewhere (38, 47).

Table 12.4 Sample Linear Periodized Workout for Maximizing Strength Gains in Healthy Adults

	Phase 1 General preparation	Phase 2 Hypertrophy	Phase 3 Strength	Phase 4 Peaking
Intensity	12RM-15RM	8RM-12RM	6RM-8RM	4RM-6RM
Sets	1-2	2	2-3	3
Rest period between sets	60-120 sec	60 sec	60-120 sec	120-180 sec

The workout is for major muscle group exercises performed each phase; each phase lasts about 6-8 wk. RM = repetition maximum.

Table 12.5 Sample Nonlinear Periodized Workout for a Trained Adult

	Monday	Wednesday	Friday
Intensity	8 RM -10RM	4 RM -6RM	13 RM -15RM
Sets	2	3	3
Rest period between sets and exercises	2 min	3 min	1 min

This plan is for the major muscle group exercises performed each day.

Key Point

Designing a safe and effective resistance training program involves an understanding of exercise science along with an appreciation of the art of prescribing exercise. The specific exercise, the order of exercise, the resistance used, the number of sets, the rest intervals between sets and exercises, the training velocity, and the training frequency are variables that contribute to the design of a resistance training program. Periodization is the systematic variation of program variables to optimize long-term training adaptations.

Resistance Training Models for Healthy Adults

A crucial factor to consider when designing resistance training programs is a participant's training status or training age. While any reasonable resistance training program will enhance the strength of untrained individuals, trained individuals improve at a slower rate and require more advanced programs in order to enhance muscular strength (47, 69). Thus resistance training programs designed for beginners may not be effective for trained participants who have at least 3 mo of experience with resistance training. Clearly, there is no single model of resistance exercise that will optimize training-induced adaptations in both untrained and trained individuals.

Therefore, it is reasonable for beginners to start with a general resistance training program and gradually progress to more advanced programs as performance and self-confidence in their ability to perform resistance exercise improve. However, as more advanced training programs are designed, fitness professionals must consider the additional time and effort that are required to make additional gains. For example, people with several years of training experience may need to devote a large amount of time to training in order to make relatively small gains. While athletes may be willing to make this type of commitment for small changes in performance, others may be less willing to devote a large amount of time to their resistance training.

Since long-term progression in resistance exercise requires a systematic manipulation of the program variables, fitness professionals need to make critical decisions regarding the exercise prescription. These decisions require a solid understanding of training-induced adaptations that take place in both beginners and individuals with resistance training experience. While beginners need limited variation, as the program progresses more variation and more complex training regimens are needed. General recommendations for enhancing muscular strength in beginners are summarized in the ACSM guidelines on page 200. More advanced training programs are available elsewhere (7, 38, 47).

Research Insight

Although it has been reported that individuals must resistance train at an intensity of at least 60% 1RM to induce strength gains, data regarding self-selected training intensities are scarce. Glass and Stanton (31) determined the self-selected resistance training intensity in untrained men and women. Following self-selection trials on 5 exercises, each subject's 1RM was determined. The results showed that for both genders the self-selected training intensity was 42% to 57% of the 1RM. These results suggest that untrained men and women do not self-select a training intensity sufficient to induce strength gains. In order to maximize training adaptations, fitness professionals may need to prescribe an appropriate intensity in order to maximize strength gains in untrained men and women.

Overreaching and Overtraining

Fitness professionals need to balance the demands of training with adequate recovery between workouts in order to optimize training adaptations. A resistance training program characterized by an excessive frequency, volume, or intensity of training, combined with inadequate rest and recovery, eventually results in overtraining syndrome. In essence, overtraining syndrome may occur when the training stimulus exceeds the rate of adaptation. Overtraining syndrome typically includes a plateau or decrease in performance. Other observable manifestations of overtraining include decreased body weight, decreased appetite, sleep disturbances, decreased desire to train, muscle tenderness, and an increased risk of infection (77).

Overtraining on a short-term basis has become known as *overreaching* (29). Unlike overtraining syndrome, which can last for months, recovery from overreaching can occur within a few days. In fact, overreaching is sometimes a planned part of conditioning programs as individuals train at higher volumes and intensities. Nevertheless, overreaching should be considered the first stage of overtraining and therefore warrants attention because not all people recover quickly from overreaching. Individuals may need to decrease the intensity and volume of their training program to recover from overreaching.

A downfall of many fitness programs is not allowing for adequate recovery between workouts. For example, if a person resistance trains on Monday, Wednesday, and Friday and jogs on Tuesday and Thursday, the chronic forces placed on the lower-body can injure muscles and connective tissue and decrease performance in the weight room and on the track. Overtraining can result from poor programming characterized by frequent training sessions without adequate rest and recovery between workouts. From a practical perspective, it is important to consider an individual's training age as well as all fitness activities regularly performed. Periodization can help to avoid overtraining and promote long-term gains in muscular fitness. In addition, lifestyle factors such as sensible nutrition, proper hydration, and adequate sleep can influence how people adapt to fitness training.

Key Point

Resistance training programs should be characterized by an appropriate overload and progression combined with planned periods of rest and recovery. Although beginners can make relatively large gains in performance from a general training program, individuals with resistance training experience need more advanced programs in order to progress over the long-term. Overreaching is often the first stage of the overtraining syndrome, which typically is characterized by a decrease in performance and other physical and psychological effects. Adequate rest and recovery between workouts can help to avoid overtraining syndrome.

Resistance Training Systems

Many different resistance training systems can be used to enhance muscular fitness. Some systems have been scientifically proven to be effective, whereas others are based on anecdotal evidence. The wide variety of systems illustrates the types of programs that can be developed by manipulating program variables. Five of the most common resistance training systems are the single-set system, multiple-set system, circuit training system, preexhaustion system, and assisted training system.

Single-Set System

This system of resistance training is one of the oldest and consists of performing a single set of a predetermined number of repetitions (e.g., 8-12) until volitional fatigue. More recently, the single-set approach has become known as the high-intensity training (HIT) system. This time-efficient method of resistance training is popular among some fitness professionals and has proven to be an effective method for individuals with no resistance training experience or who have not trained for several years (75). Since the acute adaptations to resistance training (i.e., 6-12 wk) are primarily due to neuromuscular adaptations (70), a single-set system can be an appropriate method of training for beginners.

Multiple-Set System

The multiple-set system is an effective training method for enhancing strength and power. This system of training became popular in the 1940s and originally consisted of 3 sets of 10 repetitions with increasing weights. For example, the classic multiple-set protocol used by Delorme in his pioneering rehabilitation work involved performing the first set of 10 repetitions at 50% of the 10RM, the second set of 10 repetitions at 75% of the 10RM, and the third set of 10 repetitions at 100% of the 10RM (18). Over the years, many multiple-set programs using different combinations of sets and repetitions have been shown to be effective. For example, the pyramid system is a multiple-set system in which the weight increases progressively over several sets so that fewer and fewer repetitions can be performed (see table 12.6). For continued progression in a resistance training program, multiple sets should be used. However, in order to reduce the risk of overtraining, the total number of sets performed per training session should gradually increase. In addition, not all exercises need to be performed for the same number of sets.

Table 12.6 Example of a Light to Heavy Pyramid Training System

Set number	Repetitions	Intensity (%1RM)
1	10	75
2	8	80
3	6	85

Circuit Training System

This system of training involves performing a series of resistance exercises in a circuit with minimal rest (about 30 sec) between exercises (see figure 12.7). Generally, moderate weights are used (about 60% of the 1RM), and 10 to 15 repetitions are performed at each exercise station. In addition to increasing muscular strength and local muscular endurance, circuit training also can improve cardiovascular fitness. However, gains in maximal oxygen consumption resulting from aerobic training are far greater than those resulting from circuit training. Starting with a 1 min rest between exercises and gradually reducing the rest to the desired range as the body adapts is recommended when an individual is beginning circuit training. A sample circuit training program is illustrated in figure 12.7

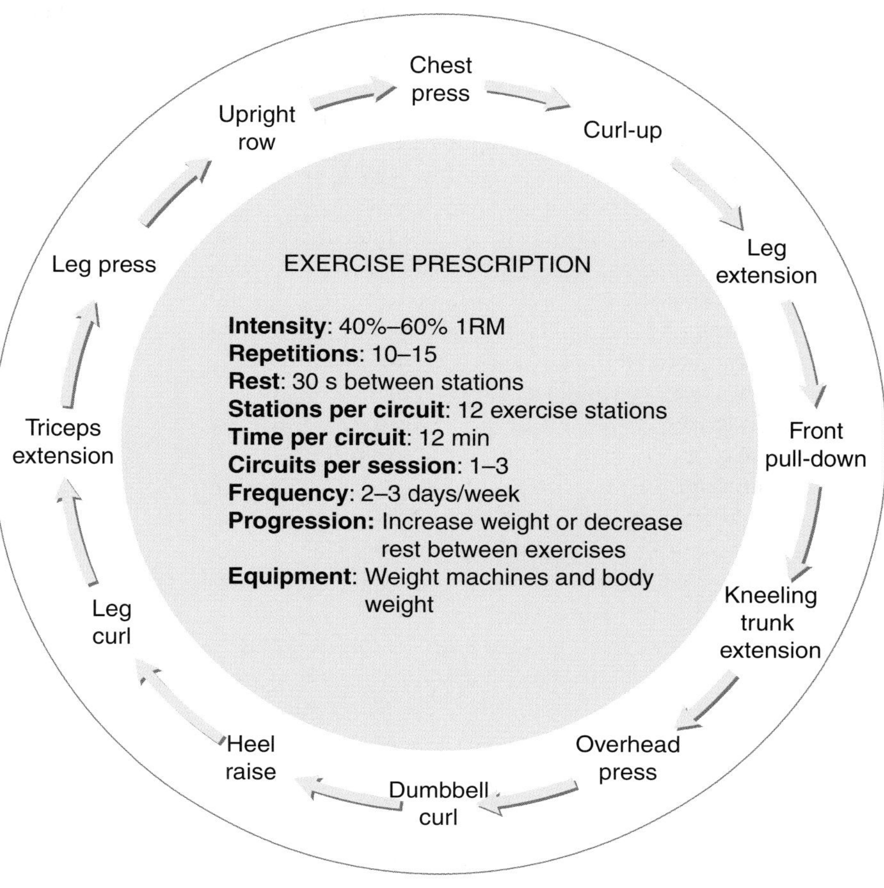

Figure 12.7 Sample program for circuit resistance training.

Adapted, by permission, from V.H. Heyward, 1991, *Advanced fitness assessment and exercise prescription* (Champaign, IL: Human Kinetics), 124.

Preexhaustion System

This training method consists of performing successive sets of two different exercises for the same target muscle or muscle group. For example, after performing one set to volitional fatigue on the bench press, the individual immediately performs a set of dumbbell flys to facilitate chest development. This type of training forces the target muscle group (e.g., pectoralis major) to work longer and harder and is often used to increase muscle hypertrophy.

Assisted Training System

As the name implies, this method of training requires the assistance of another person who, after several repetitions of an exercise are performed to volitional fatigue, can provide just enough assistance to allow the lifter to complete 3 to 5 additional repetitions. Because muscles are stronger eccentrically than concentrically, assistance may not be needed during the eccentric phase of the forced repetitions. Although this advanced training system will enhance muscular fitness, it is not recommended for beginners because it typically results in muscle soreness attributable to the reliance on heavy eccentric muscle actions. Other training systems also may result in some muscle soreness, but assisted training will increase the likelihood that soreness will result.

Key Point

Different resistance training systems can be used to enhance strength, power, and local muscular endurance. Although all training systems can be effective, the key is to match the system with the needs, goals, and abilities of each individual for long-term success. The resistance training system will influence the training-induced adaptations that take place.

Resistance Training for Special Populations

Resistance training can be a safe, effective, and beneficial method of conditioning for men and women of all ages and abilities. Although most research on resistance training has focused on trained adults, a growing body of evidence indicates that children, seniors, pregnant women, and individuals with CHD can participate safely in resistance training provided that appropriate training guidelines are followed.

Children

Despite previous concerns that children under 13 years of age would not benefit from resistance training because of inadequate levels of circulating androgens, research studies conducted over the past decade clearly demonstrate that boys and girls can benefit from resistance training. The ACSM (6), the American Academy of Pediatrics (AAP) (1), and the National Strength and Conditioning Association (23) support children's participation in resistance training provided that the program is appropriately designed and supervised. In addition to increasing muscular strength and local muscular endurance, regular participation in a resistance training program may favorably influence several measurable indexes of health, including body composition and bone mineral density (21, 22). Further, because many aspiring young athletes who enter sport programs may be ill-prepared for the demands of training and competition, participation in a preseason conditioning program that includes resistance training may decrease the risk of sport-related injuries (36).

A traditional concern associated with youth resistance training is that this type of stress may harm the developing musculoskeletal system. This myth seems to have come from an earlier report that suggested that children who performed heavy labor damaged their epiphyseal plates, which resulted in significant decreases in stature (42). However, this study did not control for other etiological factors such as poor nutrition that could be responsible for the reported growth arrest. Current observations indicate no evidence of a decrease in stature in young people who participate in resistance training in controlled environments (71). In fact, the belief that resistance training is harmful to the immature skeleton of youth weight trainers is inconsistent with current findings suggesting that childhood may be the time during which the bone-modeling process responds best to the mechanical loading of physical activities such as resistance training (9).

Another corollary of youth resistance training is its influence on body composition. As the number of overweight young people in the United States and other countries continues to increase (81), the effect of resistance training on body composition has received increased attention. Although aerobic exercise is typically prescribed for decreasing body fatness, researchers have reported that resistance training may be beneficial for treating children who are overweight (74, 79). It appears that youth who are overweight enjoy resistance training because it is not aerobically taxing and it gives all participants, regardless of body size, a chance to experience success and feel good about their performance. Further study is warranted, but the first step in encouraging these youth to exercise may be to increase their confidence in their ability to be physically active, which in turn may lead to an increase in physical activity and a decrease in body fat.

Although there is no minimum age requirement for participating in a youth resistance training program, all children who participate should have the emotional maturity to accept and follow directions and understand the benefits and risks associated with this type of training. In general, if children are ready for organized sport, then they are ready for some type of resistance training. As a point of reference, many 7- and 8-yr-old boys and girls have participated in closely supervised resistance training programs (24). Although some observers may be concerned about the stress that resistance training places on the developing musculoskeletal system, the sport-specific forces placed on the joints of children may be greater in both duration and magnitude than those resulting from moderate-intensity resistance training. Further, injury to the epiphyseal plate or growth cartilage has not been reported in any prospective study on youth resistance training. Nevertheless, fitness professionals should follow age-specific training guidelines to decrease the likelihood of an accident or injury when young people perform resistance exercises.

Research Insight

Safe and effective exercise programs are needed to treat children who are overweight. Sothern and workers (74) evaluated the effects of a multidisciplinary weight management program that included progressive resistance exercise in overweight children aged 7 to 12 yr. Weight and %BF were significantly reduced after 10 wk of training and did not increase significantly at the 1 yr follow-up. No injuries were reported and compliance to the program was 100%. These findings demonstrate that resistance training may be a valuable component of a multidisciplinary weight management program for children who are overweight.

Children should begin resistance training at a level that is commensurate with their physical abilities. No matter how big or strong a child is, adult training programs and philosophies (e.g., "No pain, no gain") should not be imposed on children. The focus of youth resistance training should be on learning proper technique for a variety of exercises. During each session, fitness professionals should listen to each child's concerns and closely monitor each child's ability to handle the prescribed training weight. Different combinations of sets and repetitions and a variety of training modes from child-sized weight machines to body weight exercises have proven to be effective. According to the ACSM, children should perform 8 to 15 repetitions of different exercises that use all the major muscle groups (6).

When working with children, remember that the goal of the program should not be limited to increasing muscle strength. Teaching children about their bodies and promoting a lifelong interest in physical activity are equally important. The following considerations for program design should be followed when developing resistance training programs for children:

- Parents or legal guardians should complete a health history questionnaire for each child.
- Qualified instructors should supervise youth fitness activities.
- The exercise area should be free of clutter and adequately ventilated.
- Children should use a light weight or wooden dowel when learning a new exercise.
- Resistance should be increased only when the child can perform the desired number of repetitions with good form.
- Two or three nonconsecutive training sessions per week are recommended.
- The resistance training program should increase motor skill and fitness level.

Seniors

The number of men and women over the age of 65 in the United States is increasing, and research studies and clinical observations indicate that seniors can benefit from resistance training (66, 72, 80, 82). Even people over the age of 90 can enhance their muscular fitness through resistance training (25). Regular participation in a resistance training program can help offset the age-related declines in bone, muscle mass, and strength that often make activities of daily life—such as climbing stairs—more difficult. Bones become more fragile with age because of a decrease in bone mineral content that results in an increase in bone porosity (65). Advancing age also is associated with a loss of muscle mass, or sarcopenia (21), which includes a proportional loss of both type I (slow-twitch) and type II (fast-twitch) fibers, with the type II fibers having the greatest loss in cross-sectional area. Evidence indicates that seniors who resistance train can improve muscle strength, muscle power, gait speed, and balance, which in turn can enhance overall function and reduce the potential for injuries caused by falls (26, 72, 80).

Seniors can adapt readily to resistance training exercises. If the training intensity is adequate, seniors can make relative gains in strength that are equal to or greater than those of younger individuals. Research studies using computerized tomography and muscle-biopsy analysis have reported evidence of muscle hypertrophy in seniors who resistance train, and others have reported that resistance training can increase the resting metabolic rate and bone mineral density of older adults who resistance train (5, 53). Although both aerobic and resistance exercise are important for seniors, only resistance training can increase muscle strength and muscle mass. These potential benefits may be particularly important for seniors who are at increased risk for osteoporotic fractures. However, adults will retain the beneficial effects of resistance training only as long as they continue their exercise program. During prolonged inactivity, adaptive changes in skeletal muscle strength and bone will return to preexercise levels (20). This is sometimes referred to as the **principle of reversibility.**

Before starting a resistance training program, seniors should undergo preparticipation health screening since many have a variety of known, coexisting medical conditions. In addition, at least during the initial phase of training, fitness professionals should provide instruction and offer assistance as needed. The ACSM recommends that older individuals begin resistance training with minimal resistance during the first 8 wk to allow for adaptations of the connective tissue (6). While the effects of high-velocity and heavy resistance training on seniors are currently being studied (34, 41), the ACSM recommends the following program design considerations for seniors who want to begin resistance training (6):

- Perform 1 set of 10 to 15 repetitions for each of 8 to 10 exercises.
- Maintain proper breathing patterns while exercising.
- Perform all exercises within a pain-free ROM.
- Perform exercises in a manner in which the momentum is controlled.
- Perform multijoint (as opposed to single-joint) exercises.
- Given a choice, use weight machines, which generally require less skill.
- Allow ample time to adjust to postural changes and balance during the transition between exercises.
- Engage in year-round resistance training.

Pregnant Women

Growing evidence suggests that regular exercise during a low-risk pregnancy poses little risk to either the mother or the fetus and improves overall maternal fitness and well-being (3,17, 64). In fact, regular exercise may play an important role in the prevention and management of gestational diabetes mellitus which is associated with long- and short-term morbidity in the offspring and mother (19). While participation in a wide range of physical activities appears safe during and after pregnancy, resistance training may be particularly beneficial because it enhances muscle strength, which allows expectant mothers to perform the activities of daily life with greater ease and possibly minimizes low-back pain, which is common during pregnancy (3, 30). Along with moderate-intensity aerobic exercise, resistance training at an appropriate intensity, duration, and frequency may offer significant health value to women with an uncomplicated pregnancy.

Exercise is not advised for all women who are pregnant, especially those who have medical complications. Thus, pregnant women should undergo a medical evaluation with their personal physician or qualified medical care provider and ask about activities that may or may not be appropriate during pregnancy. The American College of Obstetricians and Gynecologists established the following absolute contraindications for exercise during pregnancy: hemodynamically significant heart disease, restrictive lung disease, incompetent cervix or cervical cerclage, multiple gestation at risk for premature labor, persistent second- to third-trimester bleeding, placenta previa after 26 wk of gestation, premature labor during the current pregnancy, ruptured membranes, and pre-eclampsia or pregnancy-induced hypertension (3).

Limited data are available regarding resistance training for pregnant women. General guidelines for resistance training are outlined in this chapter and recommendations for exercising while pregnant are discussed in chapter 17. General exercise recommendations include maintaining adequate hydration, wearing appropriate clothing, and exercising at a comfortable intensity. Also, since pregnancy requires an additional 300 kcal · day^{-1}, pregnant women who exercise should be particularly careful to maintain adequate calories and a well-balanced diet (3, 64).

The following ACSM program design considerations are appropriate for pregnant women who perform resistance training (6):

- Avoid motionless standing, which results in venous pooling.
- Avoid ballistic exercises, which may increase susceptibility to injury.
- Practice proper breathing patterns while resistance training.
- Perform 1 set of 10 to 15 repetitions without undue fatigue (RPE 11-13).
- Avoid exercise in the supine position after the first trimester.
- Gradually increase the weight as strength improves.
- Resistance train 2 to 3 times · wk^{-1} on nonconsecutive days.
- Stop exercise in the event of any discomfort or complications such as vaginal bleeding, dyspnea before exertion, dizziness, headache, chest pain, muscle weakness, calf pain or swelling, preterm labor, decreased fetal movement, or amniotic fluid leakage.

Adults With Heart Disease

Cardiac rehabilitation programs traditionally have emphasized aerobic exercise to maintain and improve cardiorespiratory fitness. However, muscular strength and local muscular endurance are also important to prepare the patient for return to work and leisure activities (55, 61, 67). Many activities of daily living, as well as most occupational tasks, place demands on the cardiovascular system that closely resemble resistance exercise. Because many cardiac patients are deconditioned and lack the strength and confidence to perform common activities involving muscular effort, adding resistance training to an overall physical activity program provides patients with an opportunity to restore or gain optimal physiologic function. The ACSM (6), AHA (55), and the AACVPR(2) recommend resistance training as part of a comprehensive cardiac rehabilitation program.

Research indicates that medically stable cardiac patients can safely engage in resistance training provided that the program is appropriately designed and carried out within the prescribed guidelines (6, 10, 44). Regular participation in a resistance training program may favorably affect muscular strength, local muscular endurance, cardiorespiratory endurance, cardiac risk factors, and psychosocial well-being. Training-induced gains in muscular strength also can decrease the rate–pressure product (and associated myocardial demands) during daily activities such as carrying groceries and gardening (55). In general, improving physical fitness can improve a patient's quality of life and help older patients live independently (76).

Before patients begin a resistance training program, their personal physician should review their health and medical history. Although many low- to moderate-risk patients can safely participate in resistance training, the safety and appropriateness of training for patients with low fitness levels or severe left ventricular dysfunction should be decided on an individual basis. In some cases, resistance training is not advised or should be carried out only in a medically supervised environment. According to the ACSM (6), contraindications for inpatient and outpatient cardiac rehabilitations include the following: unstable angina, resting systolic BP >200 mmHg or resting diastolic BP >110 mmHg, orthostatic blood pressure drop of 20 mmHg with symptoms, critical aortic stenosis, acute systemic illness or fever, uncontrolled dysrhythmias, uncontrolled sinus tachycardia (>120 beats · min^{-1}), uncompensated congestive heart failure, third-degree AV block (without pacemaker), active pericarditis or myocarditis, recent embolism, thrombophlebitis, resting ST segment displacement (>2 mm), uncontrolled diabetes, severe orthopedic conditions, and other metabolic conditions such as thyroiditis or hypokalemia.

Recent recommendations indicate that most cardiac patients can begin resistance training 5 wk after MI or cardiac surgery provided that they participated in 4 wk of supervised endurance training in a cardiac rehabilitation program (6). Although patients can use elastic bands and light (1-5 lb, or 0.5-2 kg) weights in a progressive fashion at immediate entry into an outpatient program, consistent participation in a cardiac rehabilitation program should precede a traditional resistance training program in which patients lift weights corresponding to 50% or more of their 1RM (6).

The decision to begin a resistance training program should be based on a patient's health history and contingent on approval from the medical director or each patient's personal physician. The guidelines for designing a resistance training program for cardiac patients are the same as those for older adults. Namely, patients should start with a light weight and gradually progress as they adapt to the training program. Patients recovering from coronary artery bypass graft surgery may need to avoid exercises that cause pulling on the sternum for the first 3 mo after surgery (55).

Key Point

Resistance training can be a safe and beneficial component of a comprehensive fitness program for people of all ages and those with medical conditions provided that appropriate guidelines are followed and qualified instruction is available. Despite previous concerns, children, seniors, pregnant women, and patients with heart disease can benefit from participation in a well-designed resistance training program. Individuals should first be appropriately screened to identify those who may be contraindicated for resistance training as determined by a qualified health care provider.

Program Design Considerations for Cardiac Patients

- A physician should review each patient's health and medical history.
- Begin with a light weight and focus on slow, controlled movements.
- Perform 1 set of 10 to 15 repetitions to moderate fatigue for each of 8 to 10 different exercises.
- Perceived exertion should range from an RPE of 11 to 13.
- Train 2 to 3 times each week on nonconsecutive days.
- Avoid straining and the Valsalva maneuver.
- Avoid tight gripping of the weight handles or bar in order to prevent an excessive BP response.
- Stop exercise in the event of any warning signs or symptoms such as dizziness, abnormal shortness of breath, or chest pain.

Case Studies

You can check your answers by referring to page 472 in appendix A.

1. A 30-yr-old member at your fitness center has been resistance training for 4 mo and claims to have made significant gains in strength. He performs 1 set of 12 to 15 repetitions on 8 weight machines twice per week. However, over the past 6 wk he noticed that he isn't making the strength gains that he used to. Since his goal is to get stronger, how would you modify his training program to optimize his gains in muscular strength over the long term?
2. The director of a local assisted-living center for seniors wants to offer a new activity class at the facility, and she asks you for guidance and recommendations. In addition to a walking program that is already established, she wants you to develop a proposal for a senior resistance training program that not only enhances muscular fitness, but is safe and enjoyable for men and women over 65 yr old who have no resistance training experience. The facility does not have weight machines, but they do have several pairs of lightweight (1-5 lb, or 0.5-2 kg) dumbbells and a variety of elastic bands. Comment on program design considerations for seniors and describe a sample resistance training program using dumbbells, elastic bands, or other common household items that can be used as lightweight resistance.

APPENDIX

Selected Resistance Training Exercises for the Major Muscle Groups

Leg Press

Prime muscle movers: Quadriceps, gluteus maximus
Exercise technique: The exerciser starts in a sitting position with the knees bent at 90° and the feet placed about shoulder-width apart on the foot pad. The torso should be erect and the back should be pressed against the back of the seat. The participant extends the legs almost completely (without locking the knees) and then slowly returns to the starting position.

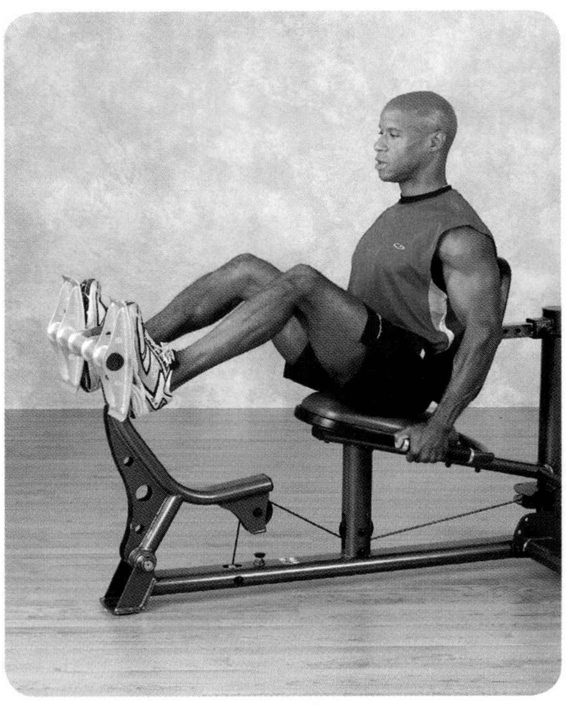

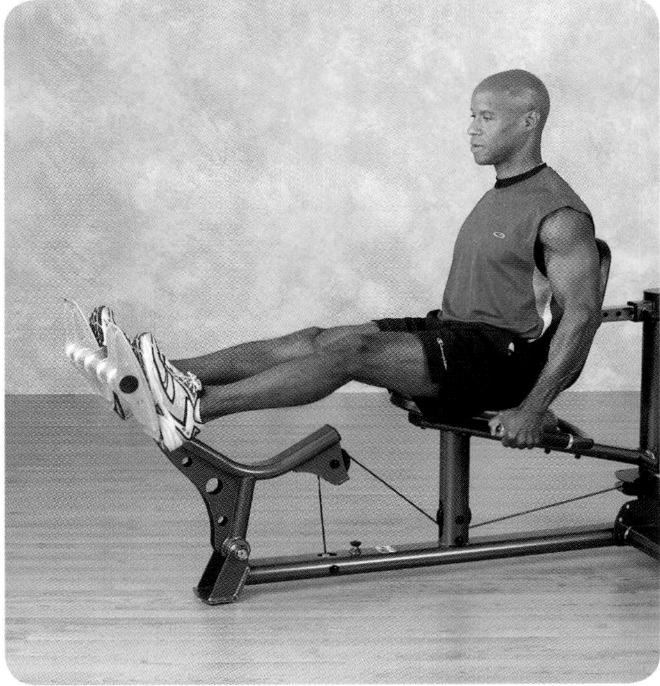

Leg Curl

Prime muscle movers: Hamstrings
Exercise technique: The participant faces the machine with one ankle in front of the pad. After grasping the handles and stabilizing the body, the participant bends the knee to lift the weight. Slowly return to the starting position and repeat the movement. Do not use momentum to complete the lift. After the desired number of repetitions, switch legs.

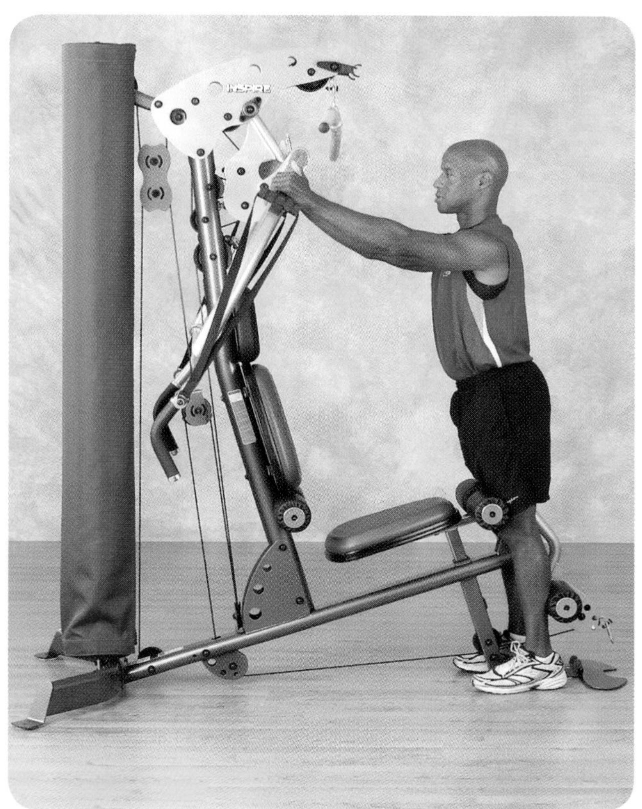

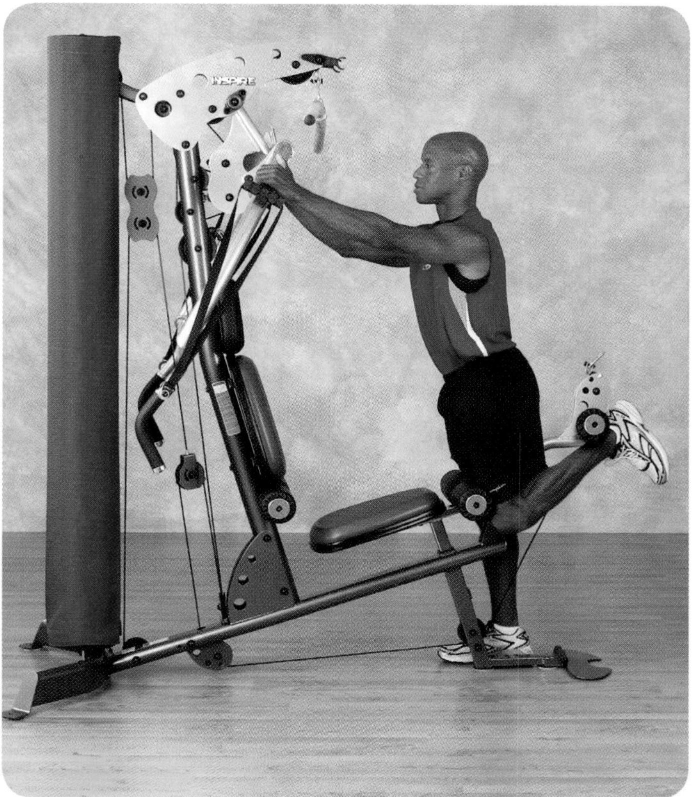

Dumbbell Heel Raise

Prime muscle movers: Gastrocnemius, soleus

Exercise technique: The participant stands with a dumbbell in the right hand hanging at arm's length and places the left hand on a wall for support. The left foot is lifted off the floor. The participant raises the heel of the right foot as high as possible and then slowly lowers it to the starting position. This exercise should be performed on both sides of the body. The participant should concentrate on keeping the torso and knees straight to avoid upper-leg involvement. To increase the ROM, a 1 to 2 in. (2.5-5.0 cm) board or weight plate can be placed under the ball of the exercising foot. If this is too difficult, the exercise can be performed with both feet on the floor or board.

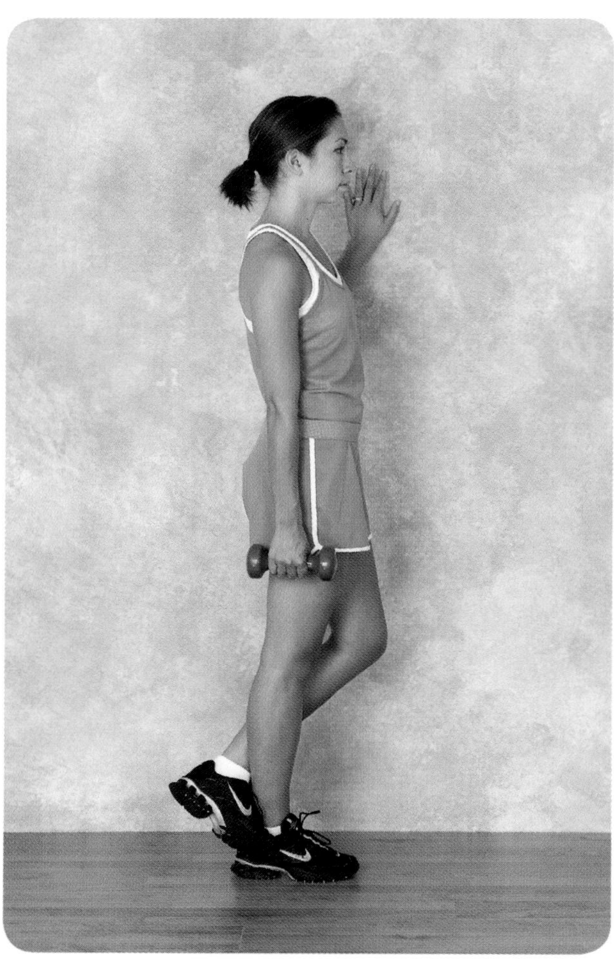

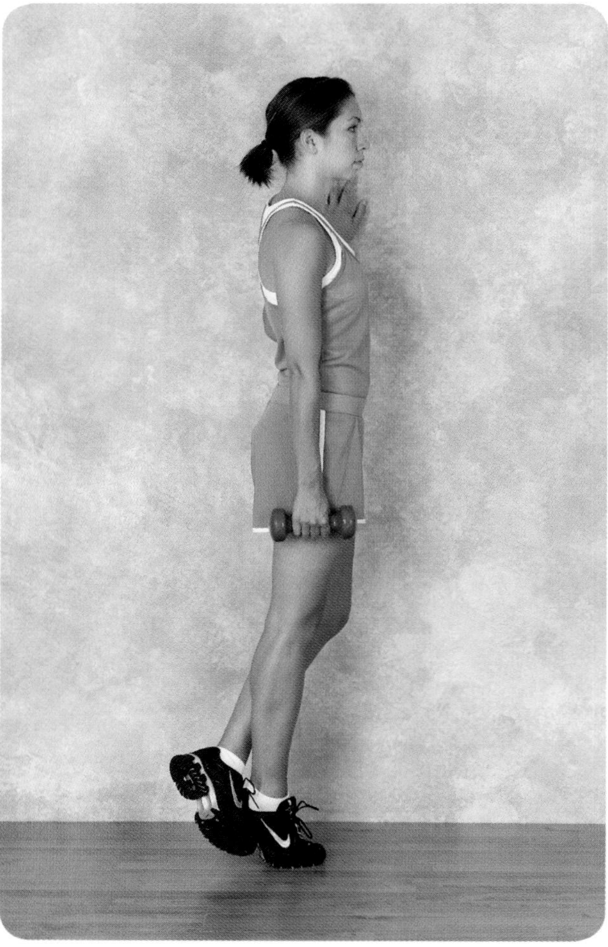

Bench Press

Prime muscle movers: Pectoralis major, anterior deltoid, triceps

Exercise technique: The participant lies flat on the bench and holds the barbell with a wider than shoulder-width grip directly above the chest, with arms straight and feet flat on the floor. The participant slowly lowers the barbell to the chest and then presses the barbell back up to the starting position. The barbell should not be bounced on the chest, and a spotter should stand by in case of a failed repetition.

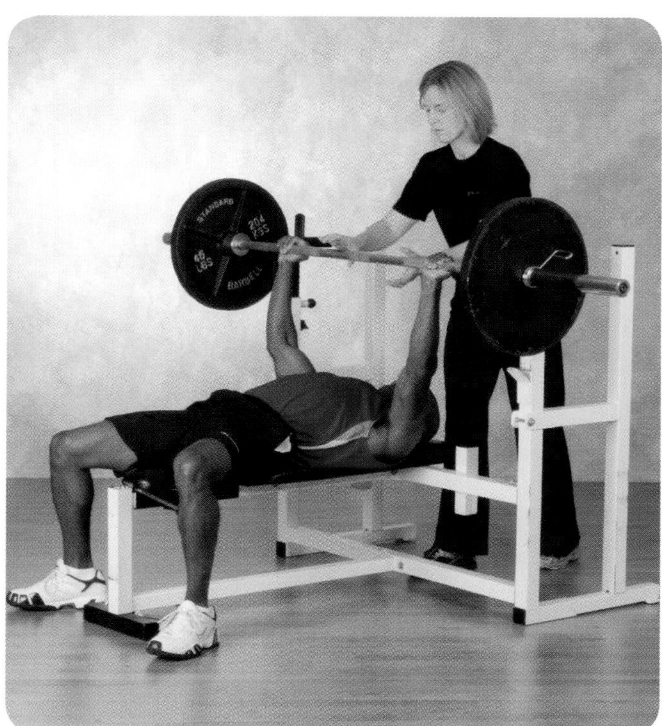

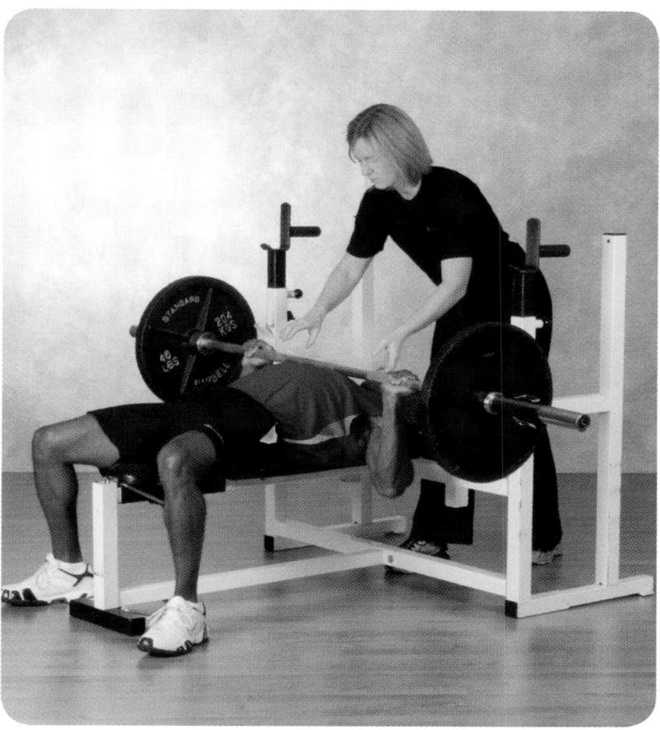

Front Pull-Down

Prime muscle movers: Latissimus dorsi, biceps
Exercise technique: The participant sits on the seat with the arms fully extended, places both knees under the exercise pad, and grips the bar underhand (palms toward the face) using a shoulder-width grip. The participant should lean slightly backward from the waist and maintain this position throughout the duration of the exercise to avoid getting hit by the bar. The bar is pulled downward just under the chin and then returned slowly until the arms are fully extended.

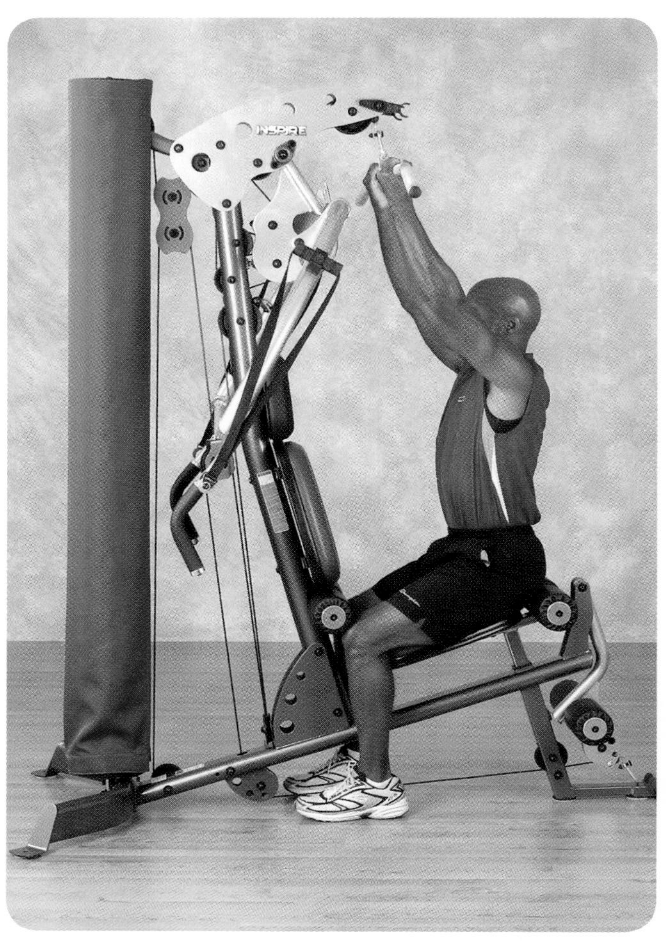

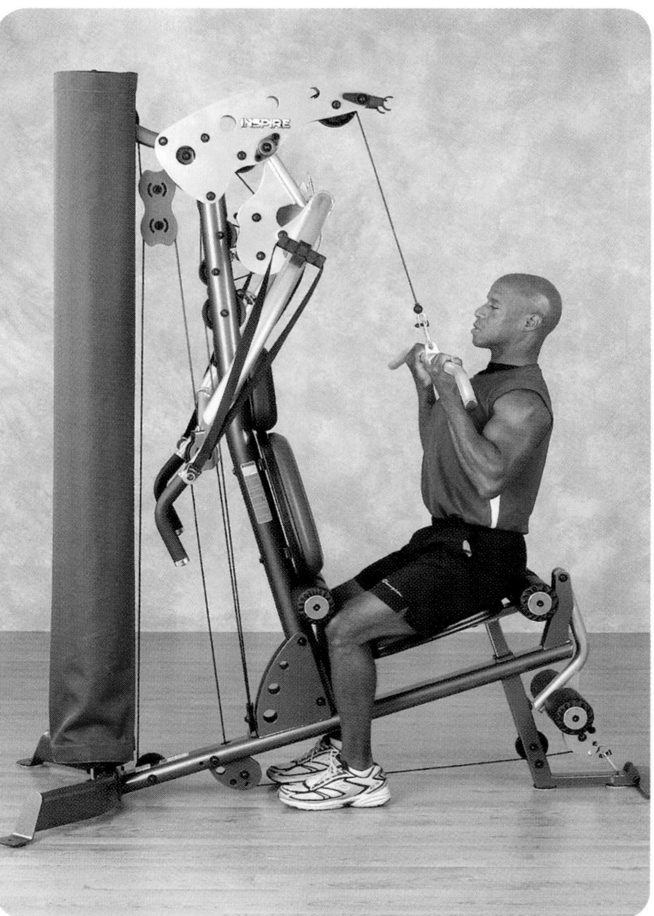

Dumbbell Overhead Press

Prime muscle movers: Deltoids, triceps
Exercise technique: In the standing position, the participant holds a dumbbell in each hand at shoulder level with palms facing forward. The participant presses the weights overhead to a straight-arm position and then slowly returns to the starting position. The participant should not bend or sway the back to complete a repetition.

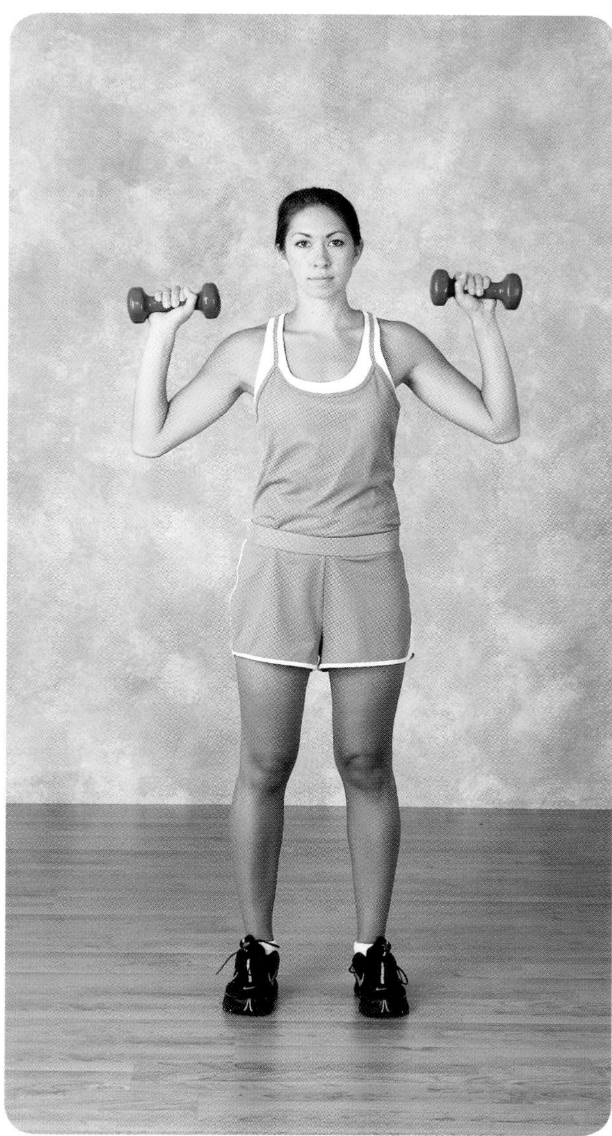

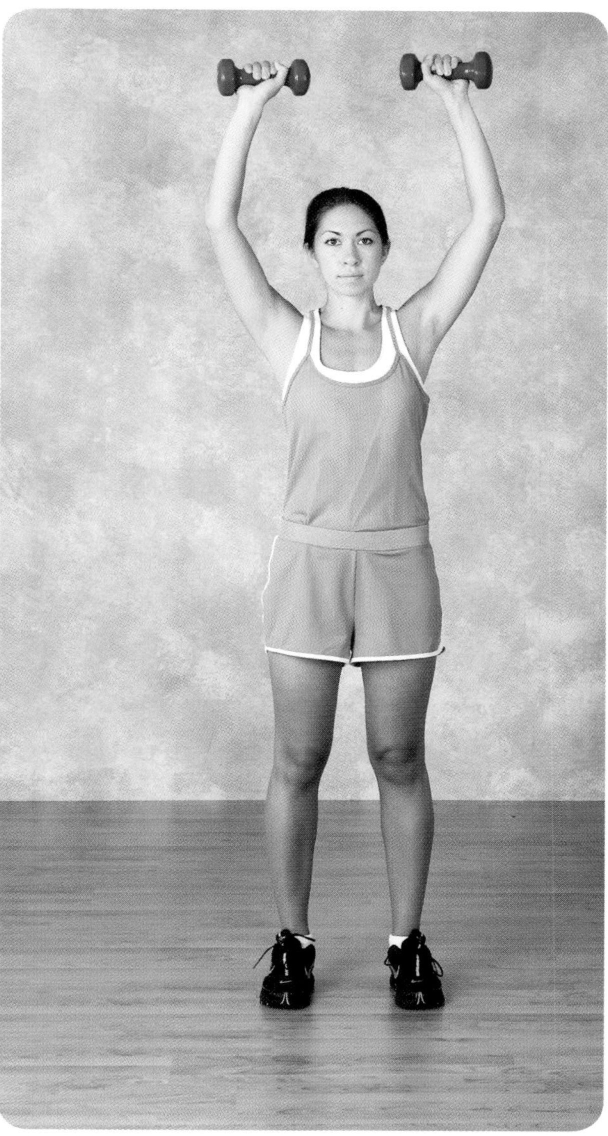

Dumbbell Curl

Prime muscle movers: Biceps
Exercise technique: The participant stands with a dumbbell in each hand (palms facing forward) and the arms at the sides of the body. The participant bends the elbows to bring the weights toward the shoulders and then slowly returns to the starting position. The back should not be bent or swayed to complete a repetition.

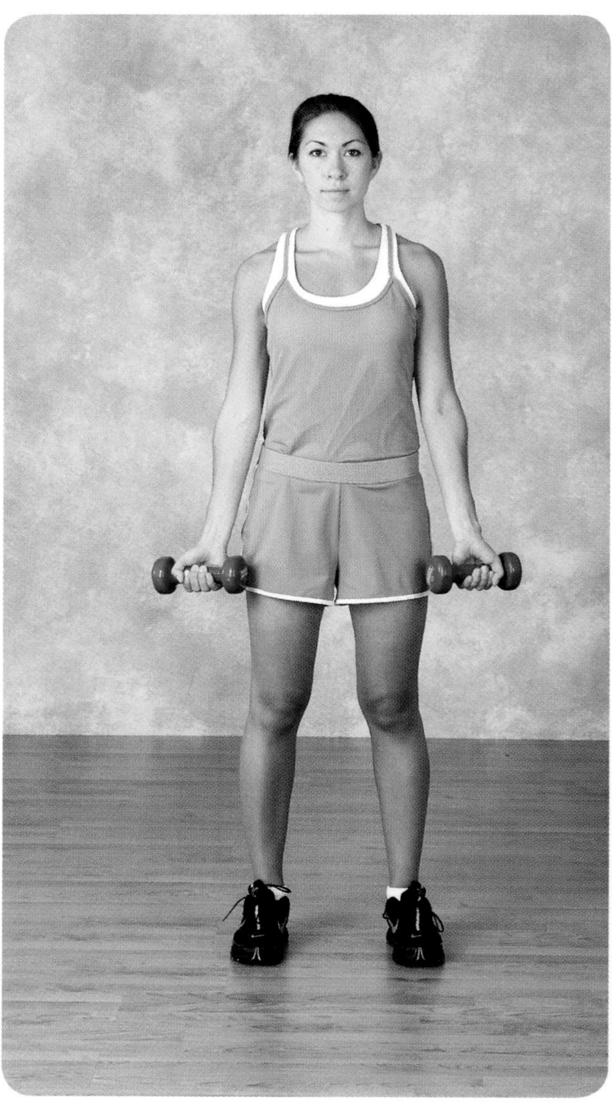

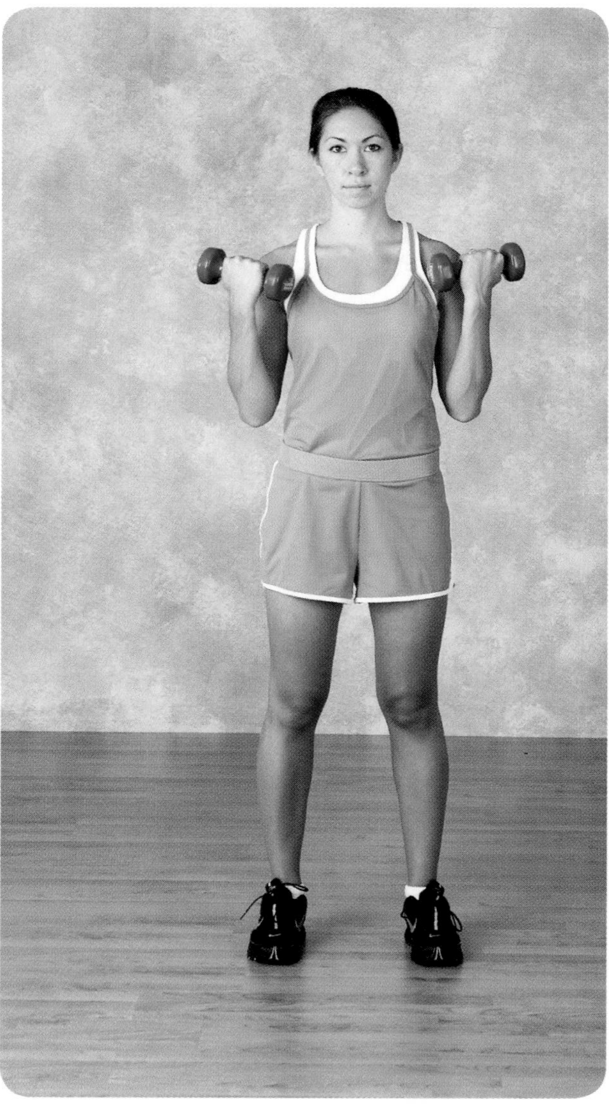

Lying Triceps Extension

Prime muscle movers: Triceps

Exercise technique: The participant lies flat on the back on an exercise bench and holds a dumbbell in each hand with arms straight over shoulders and palms facing each other. The participant lowers both dumbbells to the side of the head by bending only at the elbows and then slowly returns to the starting position. The upper arm should not be swayed to complete a repetition.

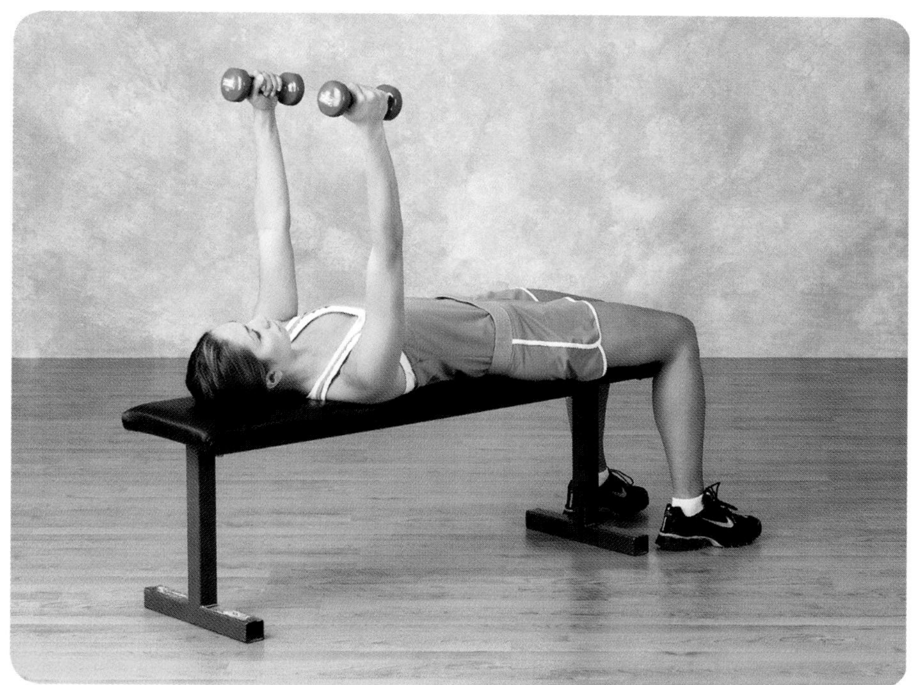

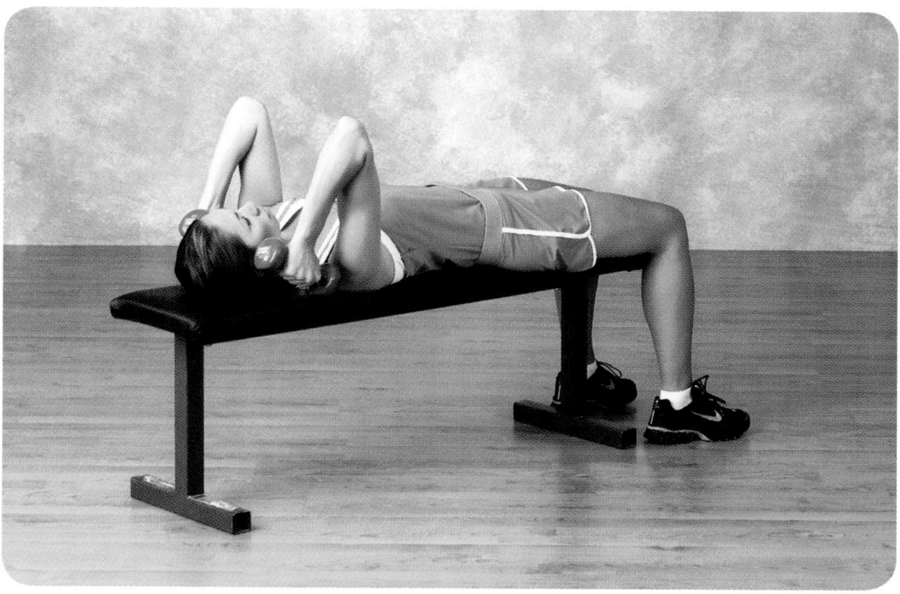

Kneeling Trunk Extension

Prime muscle mover: Erector spinae
Exercise technique: The participant kneels on the floor and supports the body on both hands and knees. The participant extends the right leg backward until it is parallel to the floor, pauses briefly, returns to the starting position, and then extends the left leg backward. To make this exercise more challenging, the participant can raise the left arm parallel to the floor while extending the right leg (and vice versa).

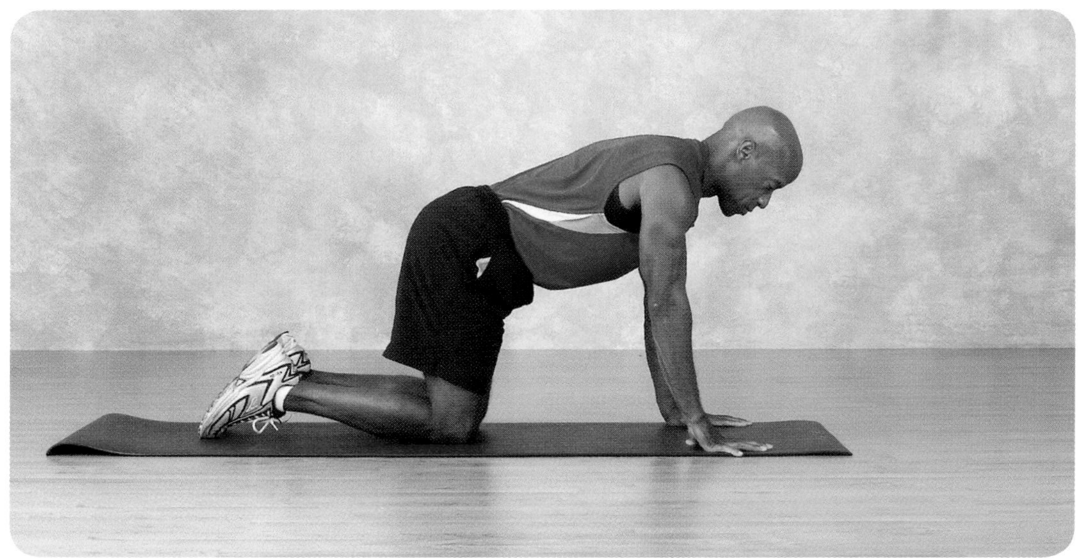

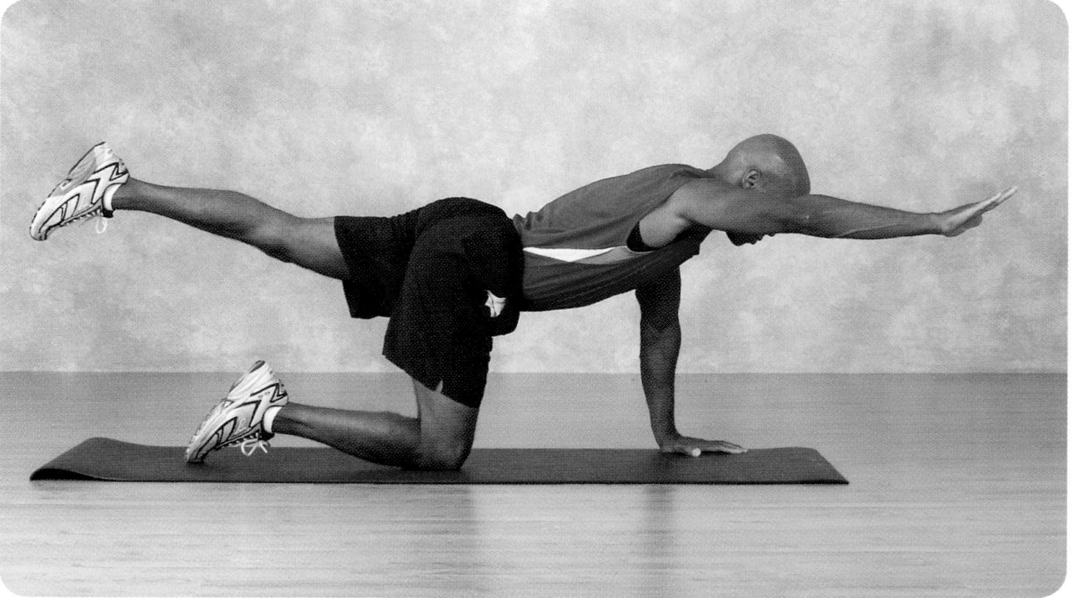

Abdominal Curl

Prime muscle mover: Rectus abdominis
Exercise technique: The participant lies flat on the back with the knees bent, feet about 12 to 15 in. (30.5-38.0 cm) from the buttocks, and hands placed on the thighs (or across the chest). Leading with the chin, the participant lifts the shoulders and upper back off the mat (about 30°-45°), moving the hands toward the knees, pauses briefly, and then returns to starting position. If the hands are placed behind the head, the participant must not pull the head forward with the hands.

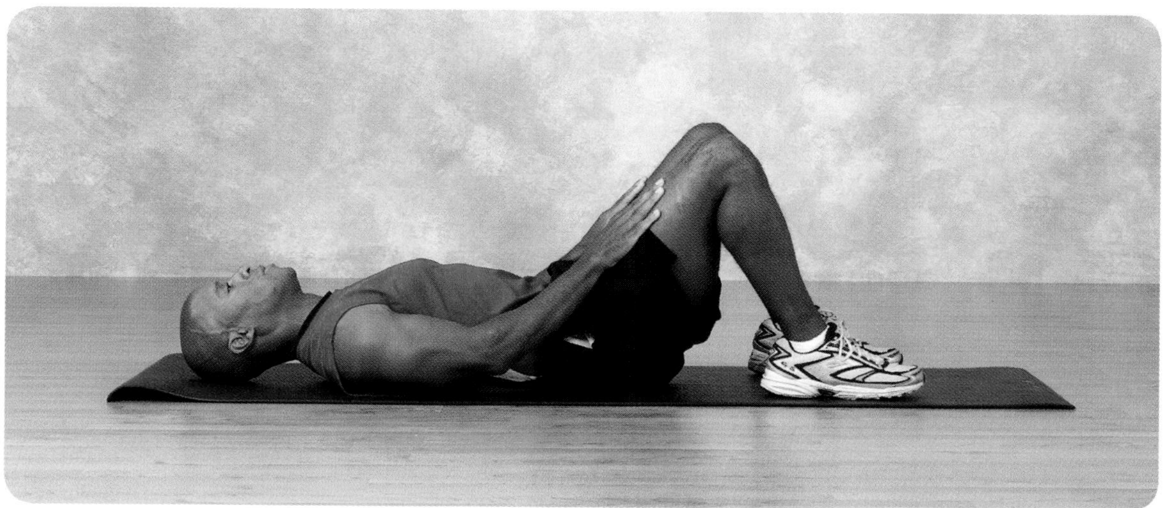

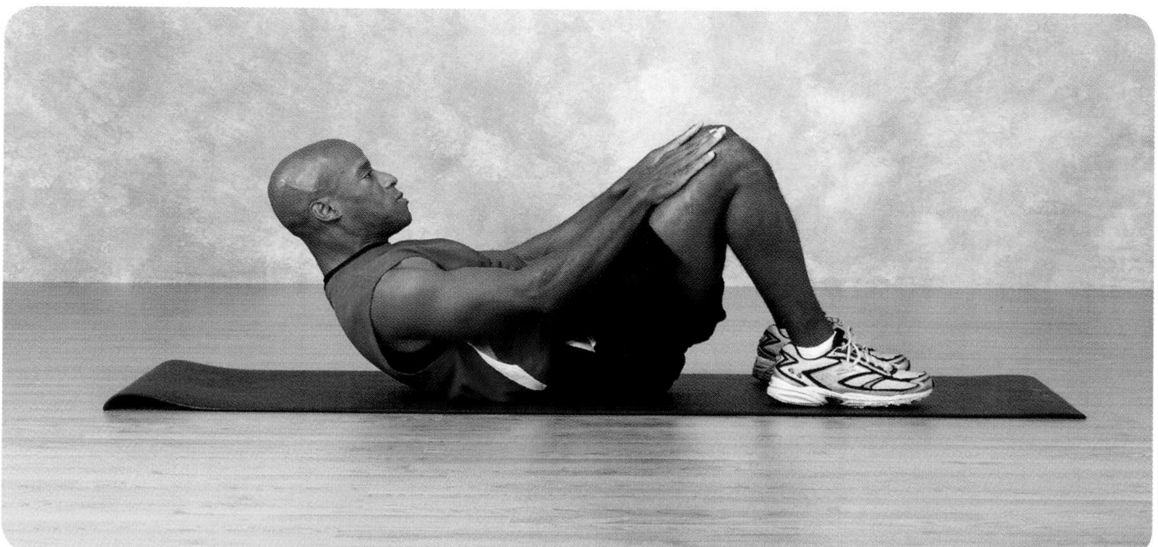

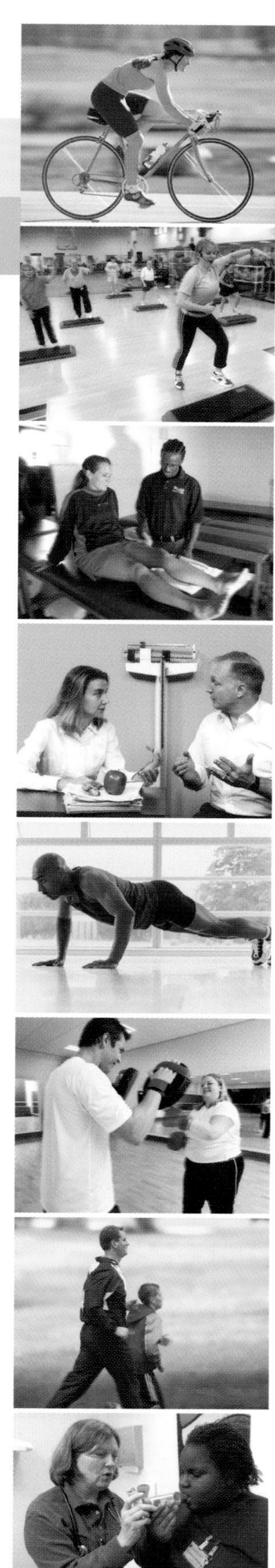

Exercise Prescription for Flexibility and Low-Back Function

Wendell Liemohn

Objectives

The reader will be able to do the following:

1. Describe motion segments and the shock absorbers of the spine, and explain the role of the facet joints.
2. Differentiate between functional and structural spinal curves and describe limitations that each may impose on exercise programs.
3. Explain why it is important that the muscles of the trunk be able to control pelvic positioning.
4. Differentiate between the low-back problems typically seen in adults and those seen in youth.

(continued)

Objectives *(continued)*

5. Describe how the anatomical limitations of ROM should be a factor as you prescribe ROM exercises.
6. Identify the components of core stability (CS).
7. Explain how the muscles of the trunk work together as a dynamic corset.
8. Describe exercises that will increase the strength and endurance of muscles that are fundamental to the development of CS.
9. Explain why CS requirements can differ for an office worker and a competitive athlete.

Low-back pain (LBP) is one of the most common complaints among adults in the United States; it accounts for more hours lost from work than any other type of occupational injury and is the most frequent cause of activity limitation in people under the age of 45. This chapter begins with a review of select anatomical and biomechanical aspects of the trunk and spine. The types of LBP seen in adults versus those seen in young people are then explored. A discussion follows on potential stresses to the spine and how they can produce symptoms related to LBP. This is followed by a discussion on core stability (CS). The last section describes exercises that can improve low-back function.

Anatomy of the Spine

The spine is depicted in figures 27.2 and 27.9. In our discussion of LBP, the emphasis is on the five lumbar vertebrae stacked on the sacrum; the latter is also the posterior wall of the pelvis. When LBP is discussed, the fundamental unit of the lumbar spine is the **motion segment,** which consists of two vertebrae and their intervening **disc** (figure 13.1). The bodies of the vertebrae and their intervening disc are sometimes referred to as the *anterior aspect* of the motion segment. The posterior aspect of the motion segment is attached to the anterior aspect by the pedicles; the latter provide the lateral boundary of the foramen (vertical passageway) for the spinal cord and its nerves. In addition to the transverse and spinous processes, the posterior elements of the vertebrae include the superior and inferior articular processes; each of their junctions is referred to as a *zygapophyseal,* or **facet joint.** In addition to assisting in supporting loads on the spine, the facet joints control the amount and the direction of vertebral movement.

A series of ligaments additionally reinforces the vertebrae of the spine. The anterior and posterior longitudinal ligaments provide stability for the anterior portion of the

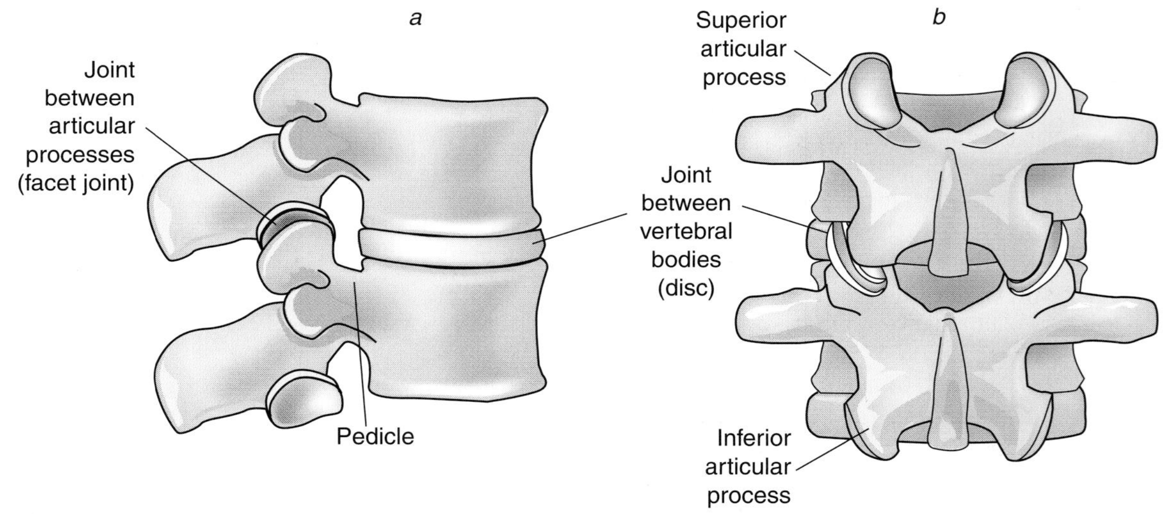

Figure 13.1 Lumbar vertebral motion segment. Note how the facet joints (i.e., the junction of the superior and inferior articular processes) are positioned to provide stability and control the amount and direction of movement. Nerves of the lumbar plexus and the sacral plexus exit the spinal cord between the pedicles.

Adapted from W. Liemohn, 2001, *Exercise prescription and the back* (New York, NY: McGraw-Hill), 8, by permission of The McGraw-Hill Companies.

motion segments; they run the length of the spine on the anterior and posterior surfaces of the bodies of the vertebrae as well as the intervertebral discs. The ligaments that support the posterior aspect of the motion segment include the ligamentum flavum, which is located immediately behind the spinal cord and serves as its posterior boundary. Also reinforcing the posterior aspect of the motion segments are the facet joint capsular ligaments that span the synovial joints formed by the superior and inferior articular processes between each vertebral pair. The posterior aspects of each motion segment are reinforced further by the interspinous and supraspinous ligaments, which are attached to the spinous processes. All of these ligaments have pain receptors; therefore, a sprain to any of them can signal a potential back problem.

The discs enable each vertebra to be more mobile (figure 13.2). Each intervertebral disc consists of a centrally placed nucleus (nucleus pulposus) surrounded by a sheath of connective tissue fibers (annulus fibrosis peripherally and vertebral end plates superiorly and inferiorly); a disc is somewhat analogous to a jelly donut (i.e., the central nucleus is the jelly and the peripheral annulus fibrosis and vertebral end plates are the bread-like parts of the donut). Intervertebral discs act as spacers and shock absorbers, and when compressive forces are placed on the spine (e.g., when a person carries a load), the nucleus of the disc exerts pressure in all directions to help absorb the force. Force absorption can also be transferred from the nucleus pulposus through the vertebral end plates into the trabeculae of adjacent vertebrae.

The disc most vulnerable to injury in the low back is the one between the fifth lumbar vertebra and the sacrum (the L5-S1 disc). Its load is greater than that of any of the other discs. The disc that is the second most often injured disc in the low back is the one between L4 and L5.[1] Except for their periphery, the discs do not have pain receptors; however, if the nucleus of a disc breaks through its normal boundaries, the disc's peripheral pain receptors will be activated. (The pain receptors in the ligaments of the spine can also quickly tell the body when something is wrong in a ligament or in an adjacent damaged disc that exceeds its normal confines.) If a disc is diseased or injured, its ability to withstand stress is adversely affected and the motion segment to which it belongs may become unstable.

The disc is avascular (i.e., without a blood supply), and its nutrition is enhanced by motion in the spine (motion enables the disc to absorb nutrients through the vertebral end plates). Long-term bed rest and smoking decrease nutrition to the disc (2). However, when we sleep, discs imbibe fluid and actually become tighter than they were at the end of the day. For this reason back injuries often occur in the morning, when these fuller discs permit less movement. Thus, slow warm-ups before strenuous exercise or work are especially important in the mornings or following sleep.

The curvatures of the spine as viewed from the side are described as **lordotic** when they are concave and **kyphotic** when they are convex; cervical and lumbar curves are normally lordotic and the thoracic curve is kyphotic. Exaggerations of these curves are not desirable. For example, an increased anterior (or forward) pelvic tilt increases the lordotic curve in the lumbar

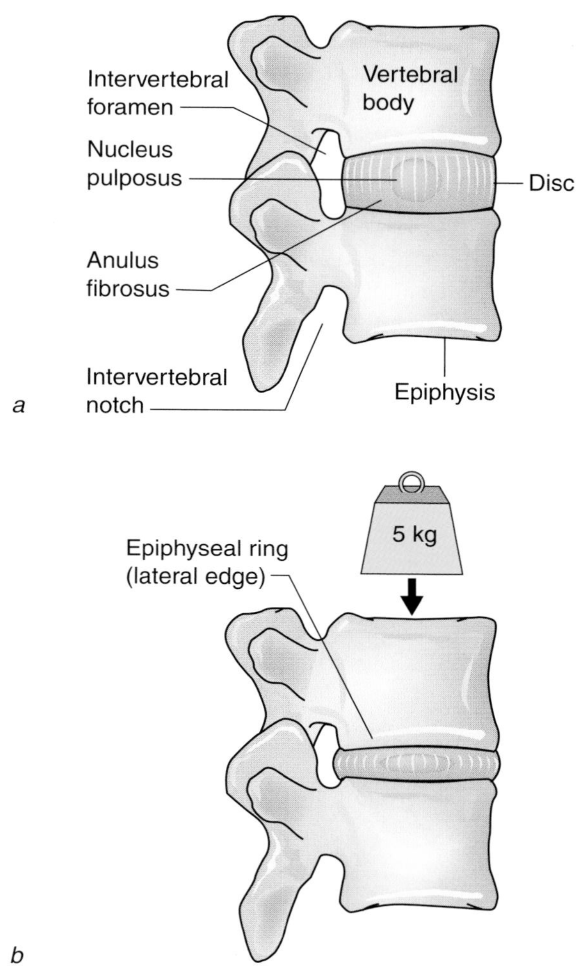

Figure 13.2 Discs allow flexibility and act as shock absorbers. *(a)* In adults, most low-back problems start in the disc. *(b)* When weight is added (in this case perpendicular to the disc), the force is absorbed in all directions; however, if the external force is applied obliquely, the pressure within the disc is away from the direction of the applied force.

Adapted from W. Liemohn, 2001, *Exercise prescription and the back* (New York, NY: McGraw-Hill).

[1] Disc pathology also occurs in the cervical spine. Poor sitting posture can contribute to this condition; however, in cervical dysfunction, a motion segment of the neck corresponding to the brachial plexus is the site of the problem.

Key Point

The fundamental unit of the spine is the motion segment, which consists of two vertebrae and their intervening disc. The spinal discs absorb shock to the vertebral column by exerting pressure in all directions. Most back problems begin in the disc; the disc most often injured is the one between L5 and S1. Natural curvatures of the spine assist the discs in cushioning compressive forces. Although the facet joints aid in supporting loads, one of their primary responsibilities is controlling the amount and direction of spinal movement such as that seen in rotation.

area; this posture increases the stresses on ligaments, discs, vertebrae, and the musculature of the spine. A small lumbar lordotic curve is natural and, along with the cervical lordosis and thoracic kyphosis, assists the discs in cushioning compressive forces occurring in the spine during activities of daily living. The neutral spine concept is based on a balance of these curves. Although some believe that an excessive lordosis is a risk factor for low-back pain, not all research supports this contention. Factors such as being overweight, wearing high heels, or lacking appropriate muscle length or strength can affect the degree of lordosis. Tightness in the hip flexors (e.g., the psoas) can increase the lordotic curve by causing an anterior pelvic tilt; conversely, tightness in the hamstrings can reduce the lordosis (see figures 9.5 and 27.10).

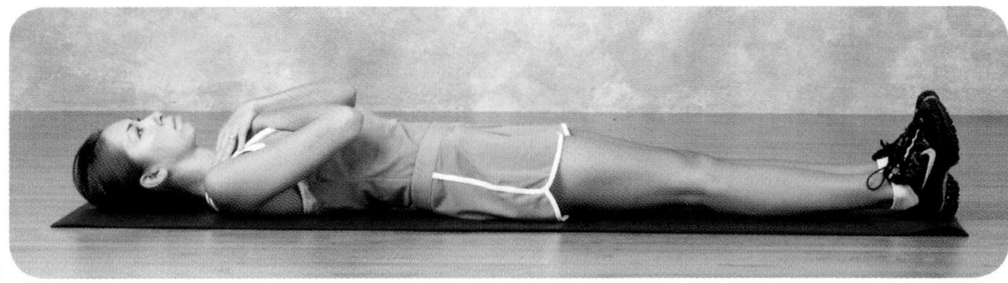

a

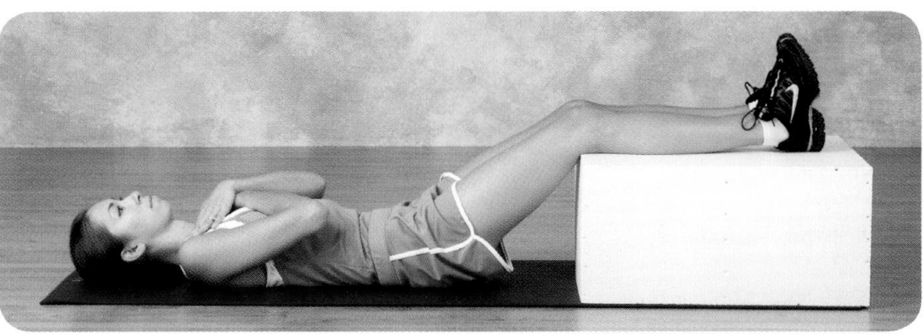

b

Figure 13.3 *(a)* When the supine posture is assumed, the pull of the psoas muscle can produce an exaggerated lordotic curve. *(b)* When the legs are supported, the psoas relaxes and the lordotic curve flattens if it is a functional curve. However, if the lordosis is a structural curve, a curve similar to that seen in *(a)* would be seen in *(b)* despite the absence of muscle tension.

Spinal Movement

Chapter 9 provides a general review of constraints on spinal movement. This section discusses flexion, spinal curvature, extension, and lateral movement.

Flexion

The flexion movements seen in curl-up exercises are discussed in chapter 27. In these exercises, each lumbar vertebra rotates from its backward tilted position to a neutral or **end-ROM** position (i.e., the lumbar spine straightens). After the lumbar spine is straightened, no further spinal flexion can take place (see figure 9.3). If the curl-up movement is continued until a full sit-up position is reached, the movement must occur at the hip joint. Then the muscles crossing this joint (e.g., psoas and iliacus) are the prime movers as the abdominal muscles contract statically; the drawbacks to this type of movement are discussed later in this chapter.

Functional and Structural Spinal Curves

Spinal curves are called **functional** if the curve can be removed by assuming a posture that takes away the force responsible for the curve. Figure 13.3 shows how leg posture affects the pull of the psoas musculature on the lumbar spine (figure 13.3*a);* when the paired psoas are relaxed (figure 13.3*b),* the lordotic curve is reduced. Habitually tight hip flexors, however, will cause an anterior tilt of the pelvis and thus reduce ROM at the hip joint; if this happens, a functional curve may become **structural.** A structural curve is not easy to straighten; such curves can result from assuming an unhealthy posture over several years. For example, if the individual in figure 13.3 had a structural lumbar lordosis, the lordotic curve would be retained even if the legs were supported.

A person with a structural lumbar lordosis would have extreme difficulty performing crunches because of lack of mobility in the **lumbosacral area.** Although this person might be able to do sit-ups by using the hip flexors while the feet are held down, this motion could exacerbate the problem. For this individual, it would be far better for the fitness professional to provide a substitute abdominal exercise such as isometric holds.

Extension

As discussed in chapter 9, spinal extension movements and postures are not used as often as spinal flexion ones in most activities of daily living; therefore, it should not be any surprise that with aging there is often a greater loss in extension ROM than in flexion ROM. For example, an individual sitting for many hours each day at a computer terminal often assumes a slumping posture for much of this time; an increase in thoracic kyphosis and rounded shoulders and a decrease in the lumbar curve might result from continuing this poor posture (see figure 9.1). If this person does not extend the spine or retract the shoulders periodically, the capability of doing these movements may be lessened and the poor posture may become structural. Sitting postures are usually more stressful on the spine than standing postures are because the lordotic curve is usually diminished; when this happens individuals may hang on their ligaments (i.e., the posterior ligaments of the lumbar spine) or use the back musculature to hold this posture. Another factor is that most people spend much more time sitting, whether at a desk, at a work station, or in a vehicle, than they do standing. The end result is that greater compressive forces are placed on intervertebral discs if the lumbar curve is not maintained. The slump posture shown in figure 9.1 is an example of a person hanging in end-ROM. Hanging in end-ROM can lengthen the ligaments and increase the compressive forces placed on intervertebral discs. Keeping the spine in a neutral position (e.g., midway between maximum flexion and extension) is much more desirable.

Lateral Flexion and Rotation

Because some of the most forceful stresses placed on the discs occur during movements that combine bending and rotation, exercises involving these movements should always be done under muscle control. In other words, exercises involving intervertebral movement should not be ballistic (e.g., movements in which momentum plays a major role). If the movement results from momentum rather than muscle control, normal end-ROM may be exceeded and connective tissue structures such as spinal ligaments or discs may be damaged.

Lateral Curvatures

When the spine is viewed from the back, ideally a straight vertical line is seen; however, minor lateral deviations are prevalent and may relate to something so nominal as hand dominance. Therapeutic exercise alone is not very effective in correcting major lateral curves (e.g., scoliosis). Moreover, inappropriate exercise prescription can worsen a scoliotic condition. Therefore, it is imperative that fitness professionals obtain advice from a physical therapist, a physiatrist, an orthopedic surgeon, or other appropriate medical personnel before prescribing exercises in an attempt to correct a scoliotic curve.

Key Point

Functional curves can be removed by assuming a posture that reduces the force that caused the curve. Structural curves usually develop over several years and are not easily removed.

In young people with a scoliosis, bracing is the mainstay of nonoperative therapy. However, because bracing is not always effective and rarely is effective for adults, internal fixation devices may be implanted surgically (5). The exercise program for patients who have a scoliosis and either external bracing or internal fixation would have to incorporate the limitations that either device places on ROM and general mobility. It is imperative that the fitness professional get advice from an appropriate medical source before prescribing exercises for someone who has a scoliosis.

Mechanics of the Spine and Hip Joint

For this discussion, refer to figures 9.3, 9.5, and 27.9. As shown in figure 9.5, the muscles crossing the hip joint can be viewed as guy-wires bracing the pelvis; if any of these guy-wires are too tight, the abdominal musculature has difficulty in controlling pelvic positioning. The individual in figure 9.5 is displaying a good neutral spine posture, in which the convex curves in the thoracic and sacral areas are balanced by the concave curves in the cervical and lumbar areas. Energy expenditure is minimal because body segments are in balance. If the convex and concave curves were not in balance, the individual in the figure would have to contract muscles more and hang on the ligaments (e.g., if head were tilted forward).

Because the sacrum (in the pelvis) is the foundation for the 24 vertebrae stacked on it, pelvic positioning is important to the integrity of the spine. Tightness in the hamstrings can severely affect the ability of the pelvis to tilt anteriorly and thus can diminish pelvic ROM.

Key Point

The pelvis serves as the foundation for the spine, so the ability of the trunk muscles to control pelvic positioning is essential for maintaining a neutral spine and a healthy back. If either the hip flexors or hip extensors are too tight, posture may be compromised.

If the body subsequently is subjected to an unplanned stress (e.g., stepping in a hole or slipping on ice), body parts are obligated to give with the resulting force. If the hamstrings cannot give, connective tissue structures of the spine may have to absorb the stress. If there is tearing or other damage to spinal ligaments, discs, or both, a step toward an acute low-back problem has been made. A shortened I-T band or a tightened piriformis also might create a problem; however, it has been contended that the piriformis syndrome is usually caused by other pathology (25). More in-depth discussions of biomechanical stresses to the spine appear elsewhere (1, 4, 10, 15, 20, 21, 23-25).

Low-Back Pain: A Repetitive Motion Injury

Even though some people might remember a specific movement that they believe caused their low-back problem, this is not generally the case. Rather, the analogy of the straw that breaks the camel's back usually better describes the occurrence of a **low-back problem.**

Low-Back Problems Seen in Adults

It has been contended that most cases of acute LBP in adults are caused by damage to the intervertebral discs (6). However, one incorrect movement seldom causes injury to a disc. LBP such as a disc injury typically is caused by a succession of inappropriate movements occurring over time; because of this, LBP often is called either a *repetitive microtrauma condition* or a *repetitive motion injury.*

If you take a paper clip and bend it once, it is still quite strong; however, its molecular makeup has been changed and it will never be the same again. The paper clip can be further bent and remain strong, but with each successive bend it becomes weaker, and with continual bending it eventually breaks. Similarly, if you use poor biomechanics to lift an object, the one poor maneuver is not apt to cause a back problem. If these poor biomechanics are repeated hundreds of times, however, connective tissue structures of the spine can weaken, like the paper clip weakens, and eventually yield to even a nominal stress (e.g., bending to the floor to pick up a paper clip). It might not be until this time that acute symptoms are noted.

Cumulative repetitive microtrauma affects the disc's homeostasis, and eventually it adversely alters the disc's pivotal responsibility as a shock absorber of the spinal unit. For example, minor tears in the periphery of the disc can be painful and can forewarn of more serious problems. Bogduk (4) relates injuries such as these as being comparable to spraining an ankle. However, if the jelly-like nucleus leaks out of its normal confines through the disc's annulus fibrosis (or the vertebral end plates), an unstable motion segment could result. This process is analogous to a radial tire losing air pressure and thus negatively affecting cornering ability. When a disc is affected, specific movements may be exceedingly painful and exceed normal ROM; the condition is apt to worsen without appropriate intervention. Thus, what started as a minor problem can evolve into a major one. The key is to never let the problem get started. Maintaining good physical fitness and strengthening the trunk musculature with appropriate exercises can help maintain a neutral spine posture and decrease the chances of having LBP.

Low-Back Problems in Youth

In young people, low-back problems are not typically seen in the disc, as in adults, but rather in the part of the vertebrae posterior to the spinal cord, including the superior and inferior articular processes (refer to figure 13.1). The part of a vertebra between the superior and inferior articular processes is called the **pars interarticularis.** Stress to this area can lead to complications such as **spondylolysis** and **spondylolisthesis.** The former condition is essentially a stress fracture in the pars interarticularis on one side; sometimes it evolves into a frank (complete) fracture on both sides of a spinous process, either because the bone does not unite properly or because it fails to withstand the stress to which it is subjected. Then the condition is called *spondylolisthesis,* and the body of the vertebra is apt to slip over the vertebra below. This injury usually occurs at the lumbosacral junction (i.e., L5 slips over S1).

Although the causes of spondylolisthesis might be genetic, stresses resulting from activities such as weightlifting or gymnastics could also be the cause. Appropriate coaching and guidance in youth athletic activities are important for avoiding unhealthy stresses on growing bones. Not all cases of spondylolysis and spondylolisthesis necessarily begin before skeletal maturity. Although the exact age of onset might be unknown, spondylolisthesis is seen in professional football players (22) and has also been cited as the most likely cause of LBP in

Key Point

LBP is often referred to as a *repetitive microtrauma* or *repetitive motion injury* because its development occurs over time as opposed to resulting from one traumatic incident. Low-back problems in adults usually originate in the disc; if low-back problems occur in young people, they usually originate in the posterior elements of the vertebrae.

patients under 26 yr of age; however, it is rarely the sole cause of LBP in people over 40 (5).

Repetitive hyperextension can also damage the facet joints. They are synovial joints and their articular cartilage can be subject to injury in this type of movement. Although this type of stress to tissue may happen in young people, damage to articular cartilage could eventually lead to arthritic problems.

Exercise Considerations: Preventive and Therapeutic

Although CS training is often used to train athletes to better perform in their particular sports, CS is also emphasized in LBP prevention and therapeutic programs. For example, stepped-up versions of therapeutic exercises often can be used as prophylactic (preventive) exercises. Ideally ROM, strength, or both should be improved before their deficiencies cause a problem.

ROM and Low-Back Function

As discussed in chapter 9, ROM deficiencies at the hip joint may be viewed as a prognostic indicator of LBP. Although lack of ROM in the spine is less apt to causally relate to LBP, a negative correlation has been seen between excessive flexibility of the spine and subsequent back injuries (16).

As displayed in figure 27.9, a limited degree of spinal mobility in the sagittal plane (e.g., flexion, extension) and the coronal plane (e.g., lateral flexion) is present in the cervical and lumbar segments. Although rotation is restricted in the lumbar and thoracic regions, a considerable amount is present in the cervical region, particularly between C1 and C2.

Spine extension is often ignored or misinterpreted in exercise programs. Although it is acknowledged that ballistic extensions (and ballistic rotations) are totally inappropriate, as discussed in chapter 9, slow and controlled extension movements are appropriate and should be included in exercise programs.

Core Stability

The trunk is sometimes referred to as the *core* of the body; the musculature of the spine and the abdominal wall is positioned to contribute to core stability (CS). CS, also called spinal stabilization, has received much attention in recent years; in addition to core strength, CS includes core coordination and endurance. CS results when the passive structures of the spinal column (i.e., vertebrae, discs, rib cage, pelvis, and all associated connective tissue) are stabilized by the active component (i.e., the musculature). In a very recent study (9), the efficacy of functionally progressive core stabilization exercises was compared with manually applied physical therapy in 160 patients with chronic low back disorder. Data were collected after the 6-month training programs and also 2 years after intervention. The CS subjects had a significantly greater reduction in both pain and dysfunction symptoms than those subjects receiving manually applied physical therapy; the latter group did, however, perform better than the 40 controls who received an educational booklet.

Having good CS can enhance performance in athletic as well as work-related activities. The CS requirements for an athlete (e.g., football player) obviously far exceed the CS requirements for a person in a sedentary job. The former needs much more strength; however, both the athlete and the office worker require coordination and endurance commensurate with the requirements of the activities in which they participate.

The large muscles of the spine that contribute to CS include the erector spinae, multifidus, and quadratus lumborum (see figure 13.4). The other trunk muscles that contribute to CS include the rectus abdominis, internal and external obliques, transversus abdominis, and quadratus lumborum. The importance of the transversus abdominis and the quadratus lumborum in CS has been emphasized in the past few years (4, 7). Again we can use the concept of guy-wires. In this case the larger muscles located more peripherally are in a position to react to greater turning moments to which the body is subjected as in contact sports or work-related activity; collectively these muscles strive to keep the spine in a relatively neutral position.

There are some extremely small muscles that are close to the spinal column; these include the intertransversarii mediales, interspinales, and rotators. Even though anatomy books present specific actions for each, their small physiologic cross-sectional area precludes any significant contribution to movement. However, Nitz and Peck (19) state that these muscles have a much richer density of muscle spindles (4.5-7.3 times) than that of the multifidus. Bogduk (4) and McGill (17) contend that these muscles can act as vertebral position sensors and play a vital role in maintaining core stability by providing feedback on the amount of contraction needed by other muscles.

Although much literature indicts weakened abdominal musculature as a prime cause of LBP, the musculature of the spine is proportionately weaker than the abdominal musculature in low-back patients, particularly in terms of endurance (3, 15). This notwithstanding, the strength of the abdominal muscles is also vital to a healthy spine; therefore, exercises that will be discussed later include strengthening exercises for all the major trunk muscles believed to be important for CS.

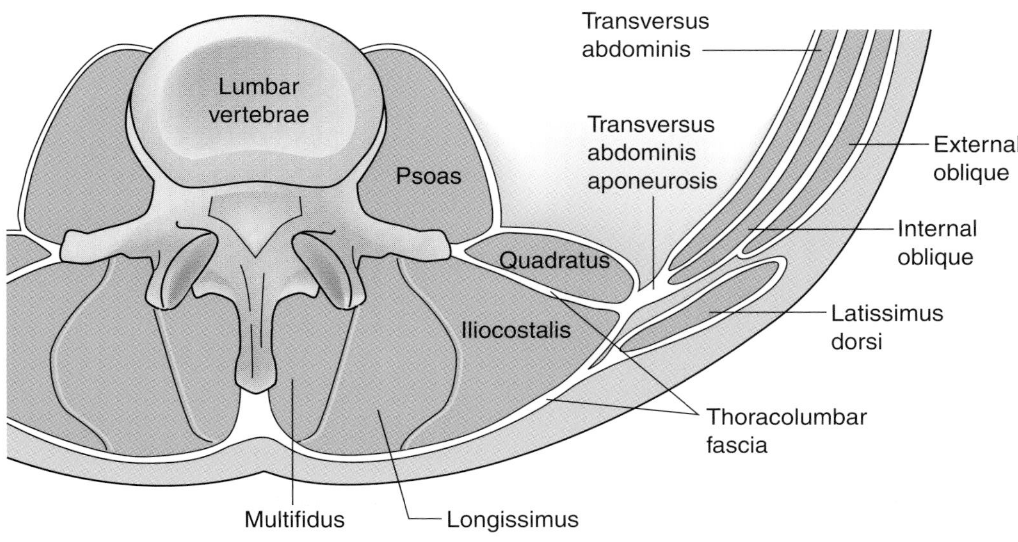

Figure 13.4 Cross-section of the major muscles of the trunk that contribute to CS. Note how the transversus abdominis (TA) attaches to the connective tissue sheath that houses the erector spinae (iliocostalis and longissimus) and multifidus; with the obliques, the TA envelopes the rectus abdominis anteriorly as its respective sides meet at the linea alba. Although the internal oblique also attaches to this sheath, its attachment is quite narrow and hence it cannot exert as much of a lateral stabilizing force (hoop tension) as the transversus abdominis exerts.

Reprinted from W. Liemohn, 2001, *Exercise prescription and the back* (New York, NY: McGraw-Hill), 21. Adapted from B. Pansky, 1996, *Review of gross anatomy* (New York, NY: McGraw-Hill). Reprinted by permission of the McGraw-Hill Companies.

Exercises Involving CS Muscles

Although muscle strength and endurance contribute to CS, specific CS exercises also require balance and coordination. One CS exercise that has gained in popularity in recent years both as a therapeutic exercise in the clinic as well as an exercise that can be used in conditioning programs is the quadruped (see appendix at the end of the chapter). Although it is not considered a challenging strength-building exercise for the back musculature, it can improve the endurance of these important muscles; moreover, the compression force that it places on the discs is only about 30% of maximum voluntary contraction (MVC) (16). If the contralateral limbs are raised, the quadruped exercise becomes more difficult and requires additional bracing; this raises the MVC of the extensors about 10%, but the contraction is unilateral (16). However, the lateral abdominal muscles are also active if the exercise is performed correctly (i.e., the trunk is virtually motionless and the hips and shoulders are kept level). This exercise, as well as many other CS exercises, can be made more challenging by performing it on a stability ball (8, 13, 14, 16). For example, performing the crunch on a stability ball will involve the lateral abdominal muscles much more than if the same exercise were done on a mat.

A muscle of the spine that once received little emphasis but now is deemed important to spine function and core stability is the quadratus lumborum (see figure 13.5). Because its origin is on the posterior part of the iliac crest and the iliolumbar ligament and its insertion are on the last rib and the transverse processes of the upper four lumbar vertebrae, it is well positioned to stabilize (i.e., control forces to which the body is subjected) the core in the frontal plane. McGill (16) contends that the contraction of the quadratus lumborum is virtually isometric. An exercise that develops not only the quadratus lumborum but also the lateral abdominal muscles is the horizontal isometric bridge (see appendix). Because this exercise involves only nominal contraction of the psoas, it does not place much

Research Insight

Because CS is greatly dependent upon coordination as well as strength and endurance, it is a difficult construct to measure. Liemohn and colleagues (11) examined core stabilization exercises used in rehabilitation research and then adapted four of these exercises so that they could be performed as a test on a stability platform with the dependent variable being subject time in balance. The ability of university students with no low-back pathology to perform CS-training exercises such as the quadruped on a stability platform was then examined. After some trial and error a measuring schedule was developed that maximized internal consistency and stability reliabilities. (For two of the four tests, stability reliability coefficients exceeded 0.90, and this is considered high.) This testing protocol provides a very good indication of CS because it integrates strength and endurance of the trunk musculature with neural control.

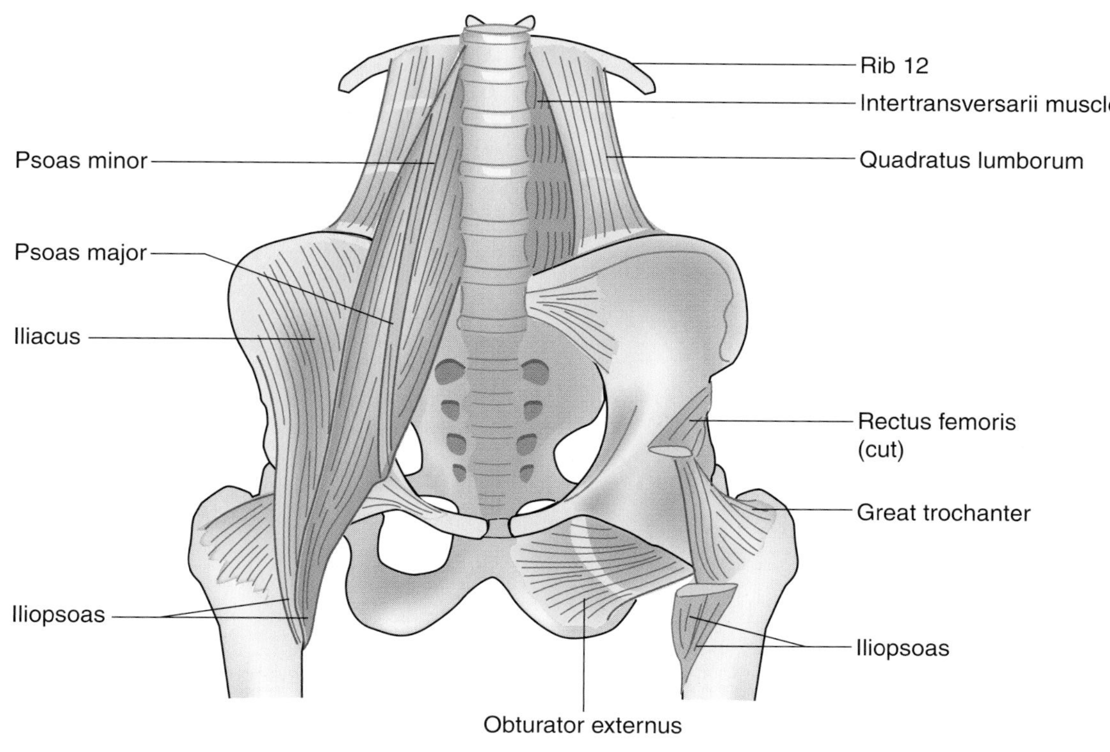

Figure 13.5 The inner fibers of the quadratus lumborum are positioned to note and control movement of the lumbar vertebrae in the frontal plane. Note also the direction of the fibers of the psoas; although the psoas is a strong flexor at the hip joint, its fibers are so aligned that this muscle exerts strong compression forces on the lumbar intervertebral discs in select abdominal strengthening exercises.

Adapted from B. Pansky, 1996, *Review of gross anatomy* (New York, NY: McGraw-Hill), 391, by permission of the McGraw-Hill Companies.

compressive pressure on the intervertebral discs of the lumbar vertebrae (1, 10). This CS exercise emphasizes both strength and endurance.

Another common exercise for developing spinal musculature is back extension on the Roman chair. In a review of research on exercise intervention for chronic LBP in which randomized, controlled trial designs were followed, only three studies were found, and each emphasized development of extensor muscles of the spine with the use of this type of equipment (12). This is a difficult exercise because it can place a compressive force on the intervertebral discs that exceeds 53% of MVC (16); however, in the studies we reviewed, each patient's exercise period was closely monitored by a physical therapist. (12). A modification of this equipment, called the *variable-angle Roman chair,* is appropriate for people who are too weak to use a regular Roman chair, have an acute LBP condition, or are recovering from surgery. A comparable back extension exercise can be done from a table or stability ball with assistance (see appendix). When undertaking trunk extension exercises to develop back extensor muscle strength, exercisers should never exceed their normal lordosis when doing the trunk raise (i.e., the exerciser should not hyperextend the spine). However, depending on the specific diagnosis of the spine malady, extension-biased exercises might be appropriate for one diagnosis and contraindicated for another.

Key Point

CS training is now emphasized in most low-back training as well as in rehabilitation programs; many CS exercises also emphasize coordination. Lack of strength and endurance in the back musculature are often seen in people with LBP. Moreover, in those individuals, the back musculature often is proportionately weaker than the abdominal musculature. In part, this might be attributable to neglecting extensor muscle strength in exercise programs. When performing dynamic extension exercises, the participant should not exceed the normal lumbar lordosis. Some of the exercises designed to improve the strength and endurance of the muscles of the spine are also good exercises for the lateral abdominal muscles.

Exercises Involving the Abdominal Wall

Even though the back musculature may be disproportionately weaker in LBP patients, it is still imperative that the abdominal muscles not be neglected. For example, the rectus abdominis is in a position to directly control the tilt of the pelvis (figure 9.5); this is an important consideration in maintaining a healthy spine. The rectus abdominis is emphasized in crunch-type activities. When performing these activities, it is only necessary to lift the shoulders off the exercise surface. It is critical, particularly for individuals who are less fit, to minimize the role of the hip flexors (e.g., the paired psoas) in any trunk flexion exercise. Many people believe that bending the knees reduces the role of the psoas muscles, but this is not so, particularly if the feet are supported. Moreover, the psoas muscles place extreme compressive forces on the discs of the lumbar motion segments of the vertebral column in activities such as sit-ups or bilateral leg lifts (1, 10).

Posterior rotation of the pelvis is often incorporated into abdominal strengthening exercises; for someone with disc disease, this is not always appropriate. Posterior rotation of the pelvis typically removes the lumbar lordosis, and such a movement can prompt the nucleus of the intervertebral disc to migrate posteriorly. If the disc is damaged, pressure can be placed on the damaged tissue and its pain receptors or even on spinal nerves. McGill (16) suggests that to rectify this potential problem, the exerciser should keep one leg extended while bending the contralateral knee and should place the palm of one hand on the exercise surface under the lumbar lordotic curve (i.e., the small of the back).

In standard crunch-type activities, the rectus abdominis does most of the work. The lateral abdominal muscles (i.e., transversus abdominis, internal and external obliques) also should be developed because they can enhance both anterior and posterior muscle groups due to their attachments both anteriorly (i.e., where they envelope the latter). Strong lateral abdominal muscles can brace and corset the trunk. In so doing they help prevent undesirable rotary motion in addition to protecting the back as heavy objects are lifted. From a biomechanical perspective, the lateral abdominal muscles are extremely important to attain and maintain a healthy low back.

Exercises that enhance the lateral musculature also include diagonal crunches and isometrics. Besides doing the diagonal curl dynamically, the participant can perform it isometrically by using challenging isometric holds (e.g., holds lasting 5-30 sec). Although isometric exercises may be considered passé for limb movements because they lack specificity of training, in reality isometrics are most specific to the stabilization of the spine (18). The horizontal isometric side bridge is also an excellent exercise. Strong lateral abdominal muscles make it much easier to stabilize and brace the spine, and people with a strong core will be much less susceptible to the repetitive microtrauma that can lead to serious cases of LBP.

Two excellent studies discussed trunk flexion exercises from a cost–benefit perspective (1, 10). In essence, these studies determined the %MVC of select muscles used in common abdominal strengthening activities. Concurrently they determined either indirectly or directly the amount of compressive force each exercise placed on intervertebral discs, which indicates psoas activity. Ideally, there should be a high percentage of MVC of the abdominal muscles; this would be a benefit. However, a high level of psoas activity would be a cost because the paired psoas can put an extreme amount of compression force on the spine and damage the discs. The strengthening exercises for trunk flexion presented in this chapter's appendix were selected because the MVC of the psoas was found to be relatively low and the MVC of one or more of the abdominal muscles was high (10). However, another consideration should be factored into exercise selection: the client's physical fitness level. Some exercises may benefit athletes in excellent condition but harm other people; thus, sometimes the quality of the movement should be considered along with the physical condition of the exerciser.

Key Point

In people with low-back problems, the back musculature often is proportionately weaker and has less endurance than the abdominal musculature has; in part, this might be attributable to neglect of extensor muscle strength in exercise programs. When trained the trunk musculature work together as a dynamic corset as the lateral abdominal muscles tie the flexors and extensors of the spine together to facilitate a strong core. Although the erector spinae, multifidus, and rectus abdominis are important trunk muscles, the lateral abdominal muscles and the quadratus lumborum warrant special attention to develop a strong core.

Prophylactic Exercises for Enhancing Low-Back Function

Even though many injuries and diseases of the low back can be treated conservatively with therapeutic exercise, the diversity and complexity of low-back problems are such that they preclude making a simple diagnosis and presenting an exercise regimen for that diagnosis. Moreover, arming a person with a set of therapeutic exercises when the person does not concurrently understand the nuances of different low-back conditions could be dangerous. Because it is beyond the scope of this chapter to discuss these countless nuances, the emphasis in this discussion is on sound exercises that enhance low-back function. Nevertheless, the exercises in the appendix are often used by physical therapists in treating low-back patients. For in-depth information on this subject, many other sources are available (1, 6, 8, 10, 12-14, 16, 17, 20, 23, 25).

Exercises to Enhance Flexibility

This chapter's appendix describes exercises recommended for low-back flexibility. The guy-wire concept discussed in chapter 9 (see figure 9.5) is helpful to consider when exploring exercises for low-back flexibility. Although the trunk musculature (e.g., the abdominal muscles and the erector spinae) is crucial to controlling pelvic positioning, the ability to control the pelvis may be reduced or negated if either the hip flexors or the hip extensors are too tight. The bottom line is that having good hip joint mobility is fundamental to having a healthy spine. Several exercises that can be used to improve ROM in joints and structures relevant to the low back are presented in this chapter's appendix.

Exercises to Develop the Trunk Musculature

Although by no means all inclusive, this chapter's appendix also describes exercises recommended for developing the musculature of the trunk. A key point to remember with spinal extension movements is that exercisers should not exceed their normal lumbar lordosis when moving into extension.

Posterior pelvic tilts and crunches are basic to many exercise programs for developing the abdominal musculature. As previously mentioned, when individuals do these exercises, the rectus abdominis often does most of the work and the lateral abdominal muscles are involved minimally.

Key Point

Maintenance of good hip joint ROM is essential for a healthy spine. An exerciser should not exceed the normal lordotic curve when doing active back extension exercises. The ROM capabilities of the trunk are quite nominal; keep this in mind when setting up exercise programs for clients. Isometric holds can nicely supplement regular crunches and diagonal crunches.

Case Studies

You can check your answers by referring to page 472 in appendix A.

1. An exercise leader is using a double-leg lowering task with a group of relatively fit adults, ostensibly to improve the strength of the abdominals. When questioned about the use of this exercise, he advises you that physical therapists have often used a similar activity to test the abdominal strength of their patients, even those who are symptomatic for LBP. Discuss the appropriateness or inappropriateness of such an exercise. For whom would it be least appropriate and possibly even contraindicated?
2. An exercise leader is using the sit-and-reach (or standing toe-touch) exercise presumably to improve hip joint flexibility. Because she is aware that ballistic stretches are usually contraindicated, the exercise leader strongly admonishes her group to perform the exercise with slow and easy stretches. Discuss the appropriateness or inappropriateness of these directions.
3. An exercise leader prescribes oblique (diagonal) curls that require the exerciser to maintain a 15 sec isometric contraction after at least one shoulder blade is raised from the exercise surface. Discuss the appropriateness or inappropriateness of this activity.

APPENDIX

Flexibility, Strength, and Endurance Exercises to Improve Low-Back Function

Flexibility Exercises to Improve ROM

In performing limb flexibility exercises, particularly for the lower extremities, the participant should first stretch to symmetry; after symmetry is achieved, the participant should work on improving flexibility in both limbs. Static stretches held for 30 to 60 sec are recommended; these can be repeated twice during the exercise session. However, for those areas in which extreme tightness is noted, ideally there should be several exercise bouts each day.

Hip Flexor Stretch (Standing)

The participant grasps the contralateral ankle and raises the leg while keeping the trunk straight *(a)*. Note incorrect technique of individual on the right *(b)*; tilting the pelvis precludes stretching the hip flexors.

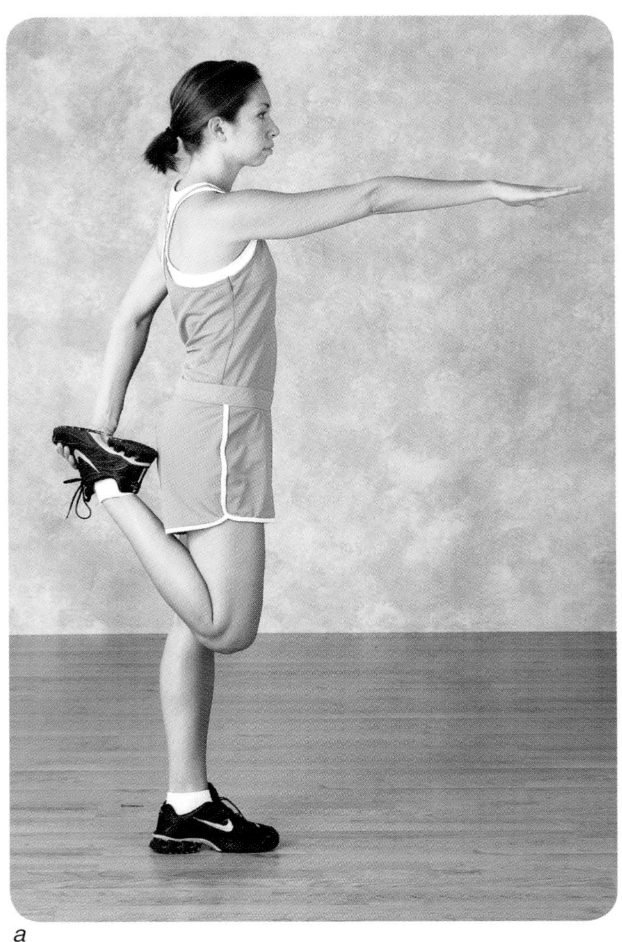

a

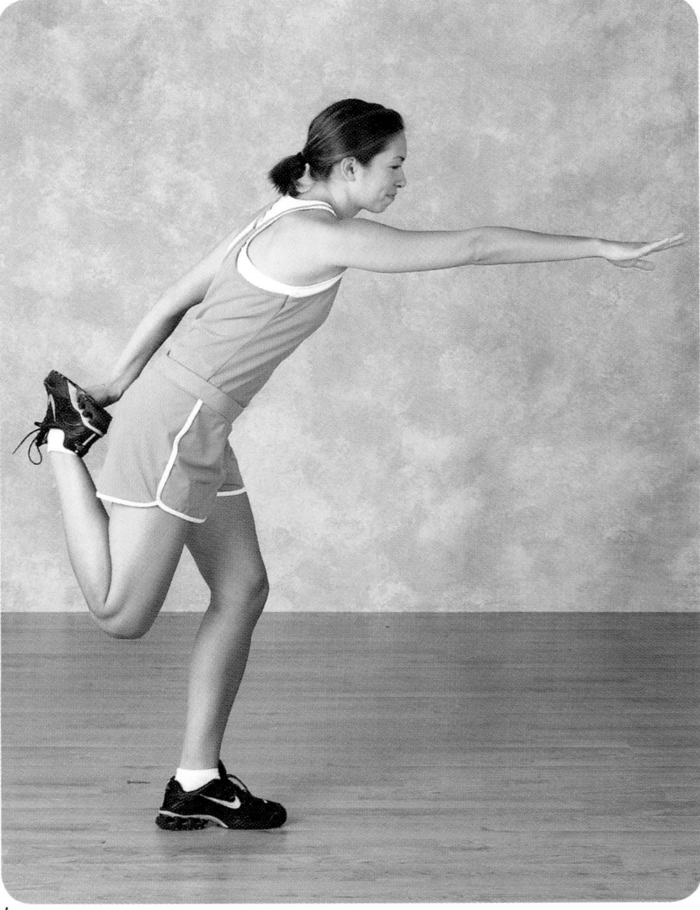

b

Hip Flexor Stretch (Supine)

The participant assumes the Thomas test position and pulls the contralateral leg back as far as possible; this posterior rotation of the pelvis can place added tension on the contralateral hip flexors.

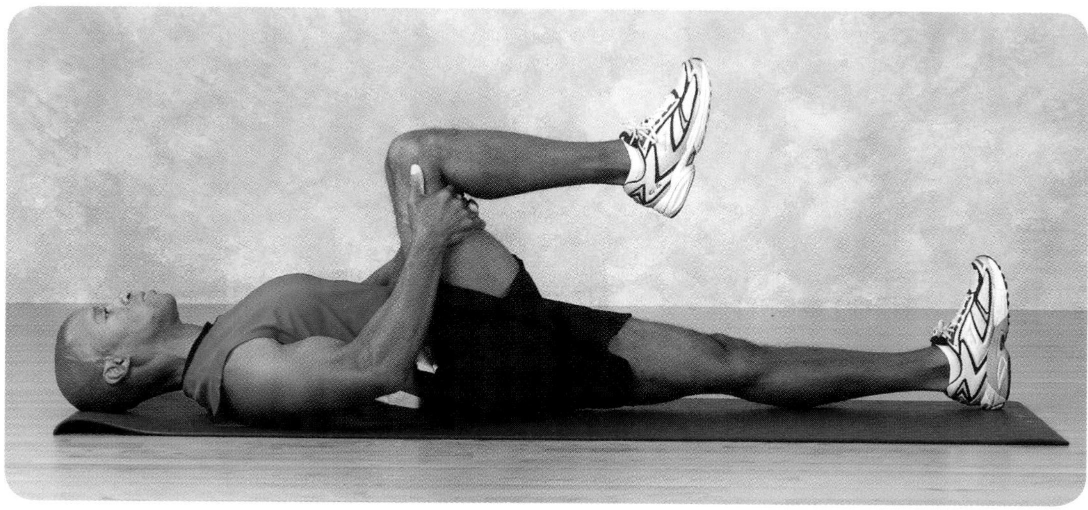

I-T Band Stretch

With hips stacked, the exerciser places the ankle of the lower leg on the lateral distal thigh; by outwardly rotating the thigh of the lower leg, the I-T band of the upper leg is stretched. (In some cases, gravity alone may be an effective stretch of the I-T band from this position.)

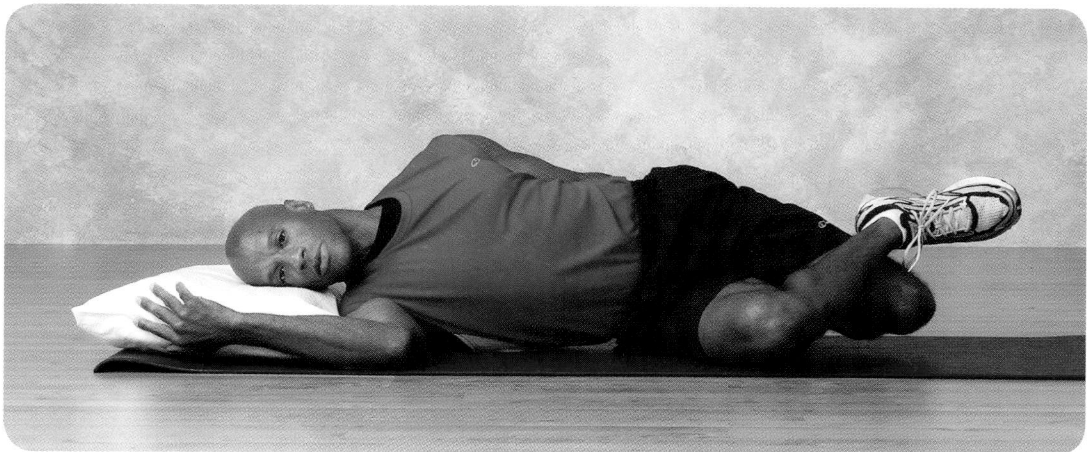

Piriformis Stretch

The piriformis of the right leg is stretched in this maneuver. This posturing is markedly similar to that achieved while sitting at a chair and placing the lateral malleolus (ankle) of one leg on the distal femur of the contralateral leg.

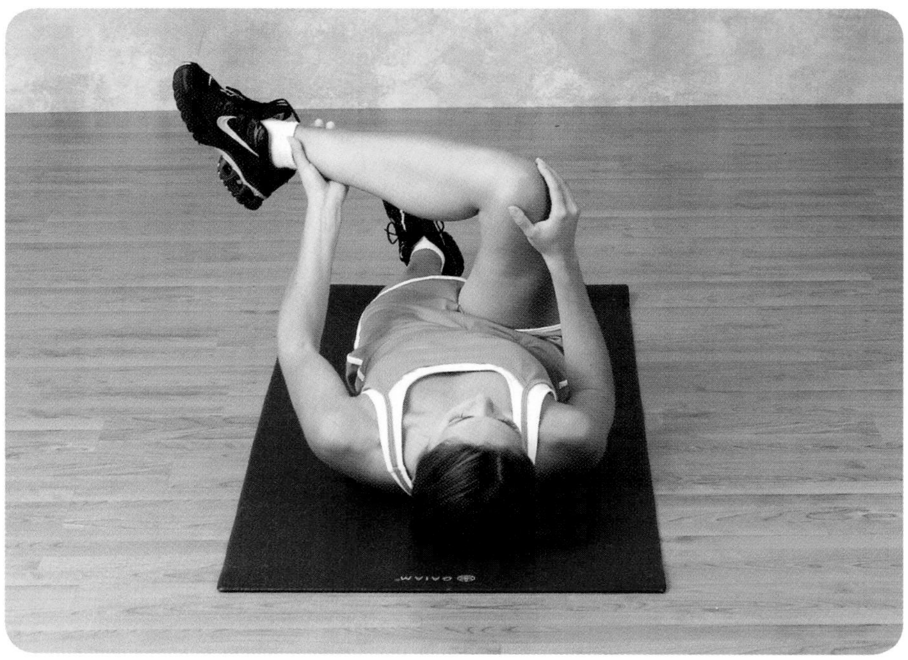

Cailliet Stretch

The exerciser should lean forward (with neutral spine) until tension is felt in the hamstrings and then hold this position. The sequence is repeated for each leg 3 to 4 times. If the hamstrings are tight (e.g., sacral angle less than 80°), stress could be placed on structures of the spine; this is not desirable. To avoid this, the back should be kept straight and the movement emphasis should be at the hip joint.

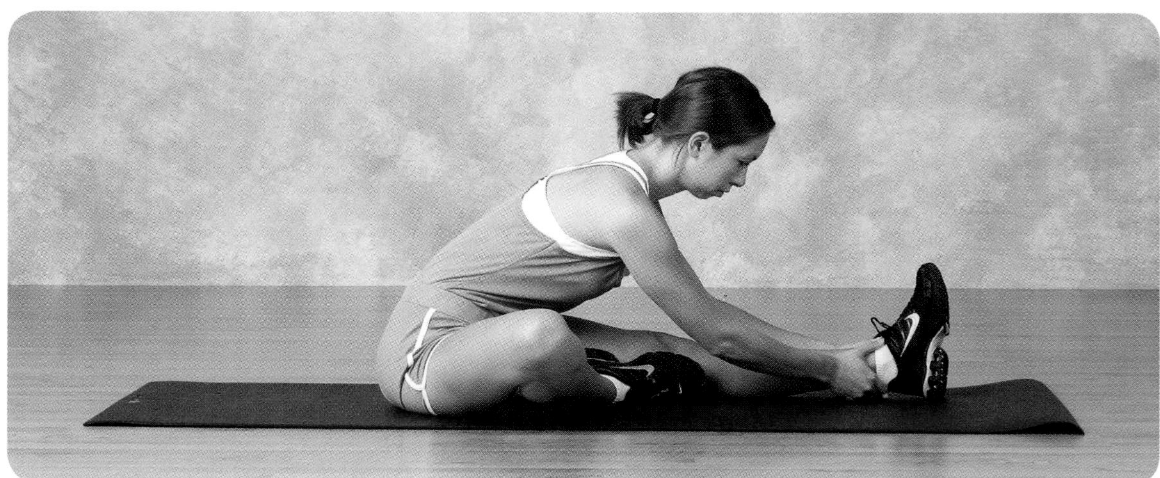

Step or Chair Stretch

The hamstrings can be isolated in the stretch if the movement is made only at the hip joint *(a)*. Although the hamstrings can also be stretched in *(b)*, the soft-tissue structures of the lower back are also stretched. This stretch can be more effective if the trunk is splinted (i.e., neutral spine/normal standing posture) so that movement only occurs at the hip joint. An appropriate stretch for the low back is presented in the next figure in the Mad Cat Stretch.

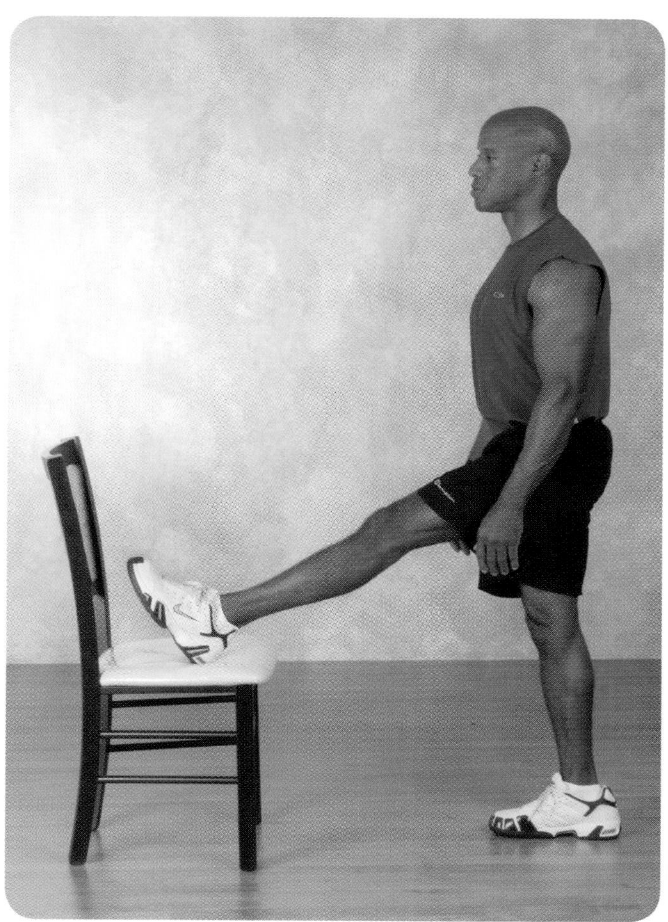

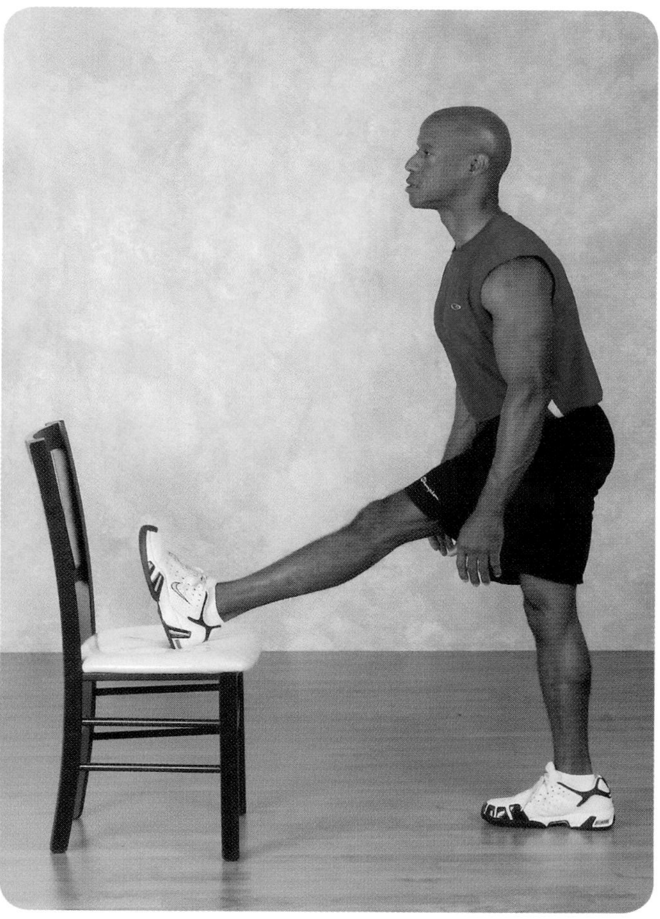

Mad Cat Stretch

The exercise involves slowly cycling through full spine flexion to full extension. This exercise is not used for increasing ROM but rather for spine mobility. Because the spinal loading is minimal, it would be a particularly appropriate morning exercise when the discs tend to be distended and tight.

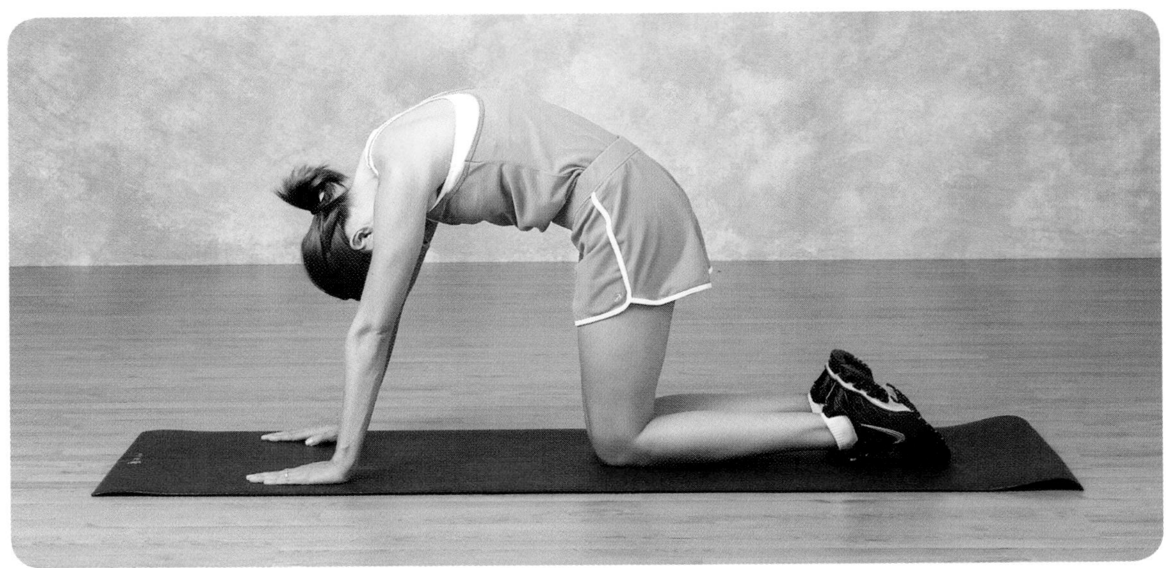

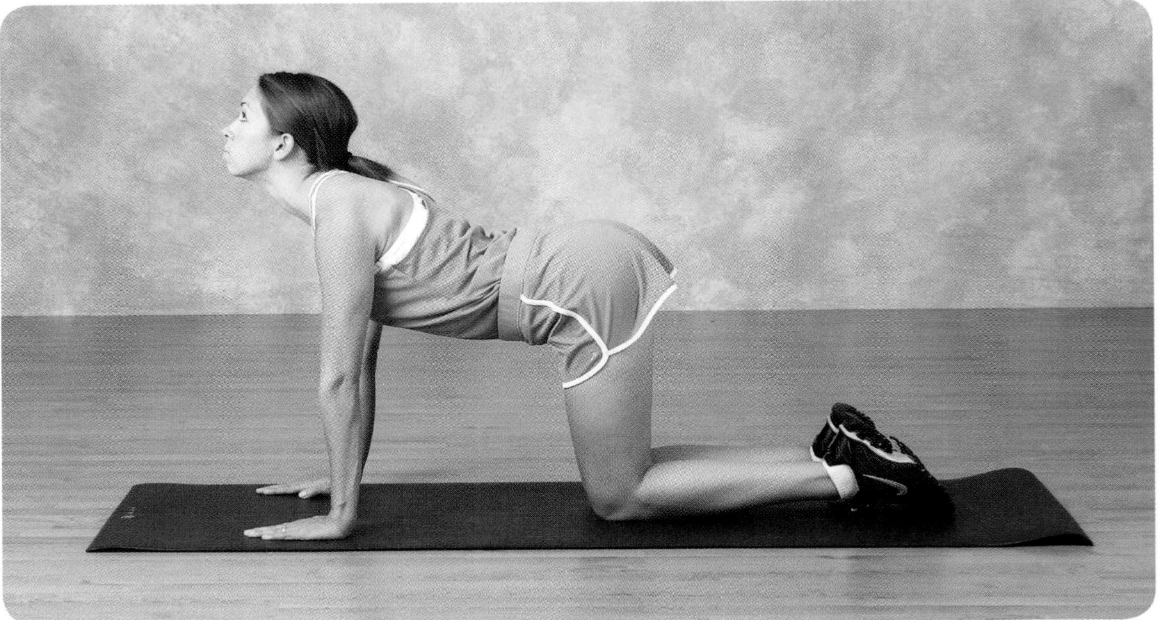

Trunk Flexion

The participant pulls one *(a)* and eventually both *(b)* knees toward the shoulders. Some disc patients might experience problems with *(b)* because in some flexion movements, the nucleus of the disc is pushed posteriorly.

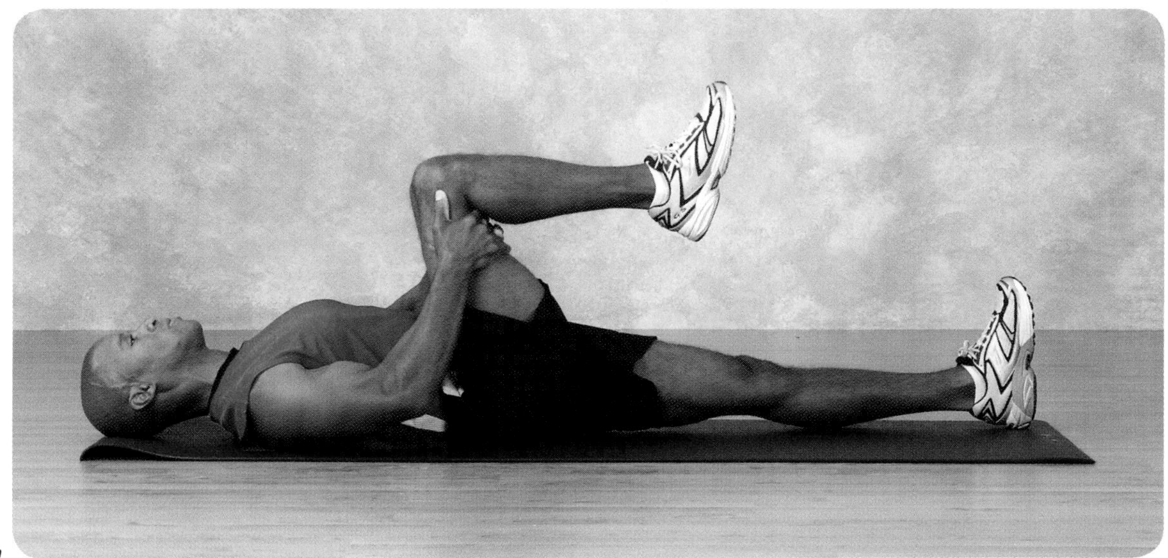

a

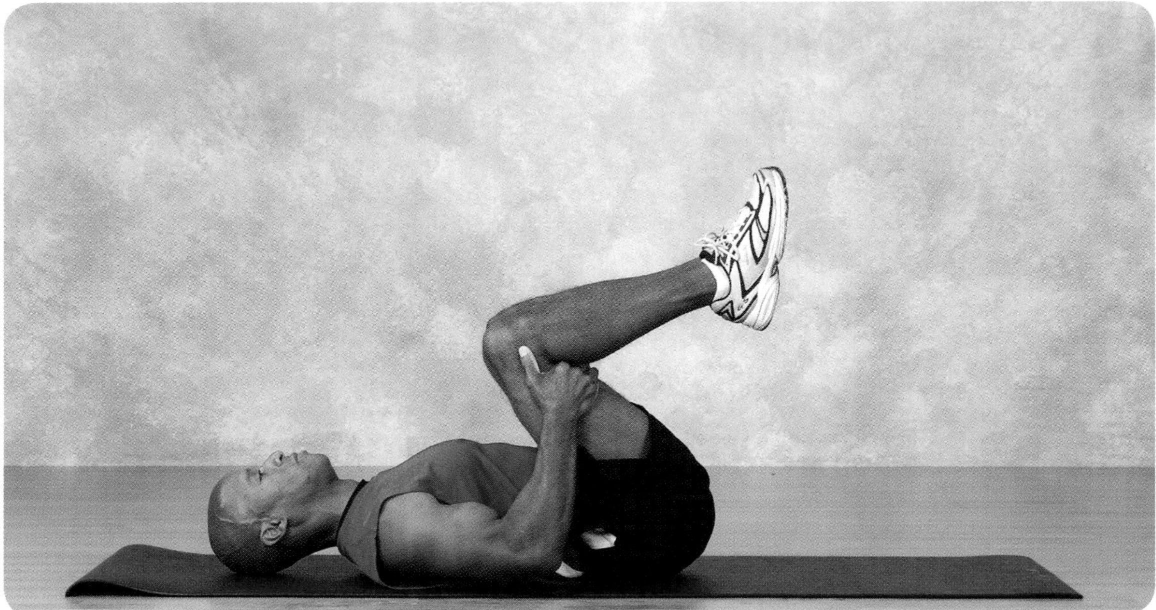

b

Trunk Extension

The exerciser places the hands under the shoulders and slowly extends the arms while keeping the pelvis in contact with the floor (back muscles are kept relaxed).

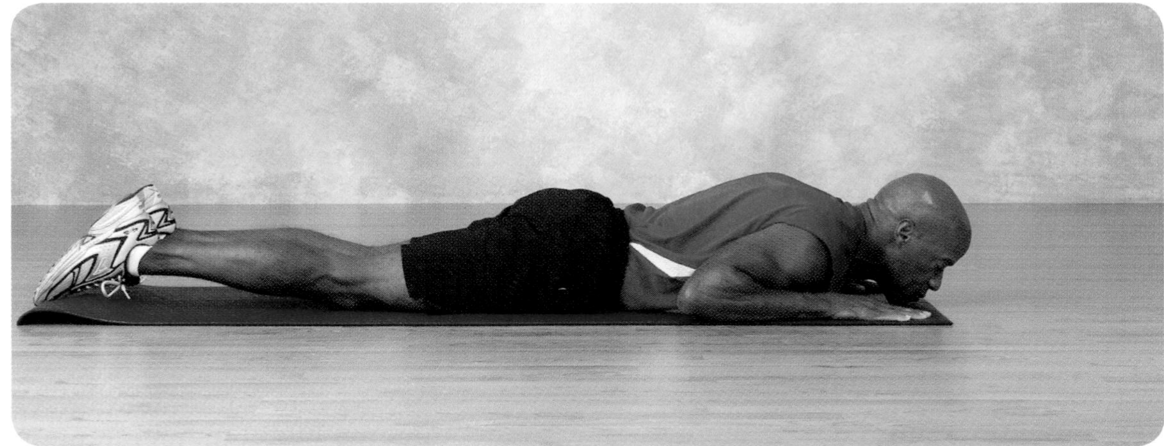

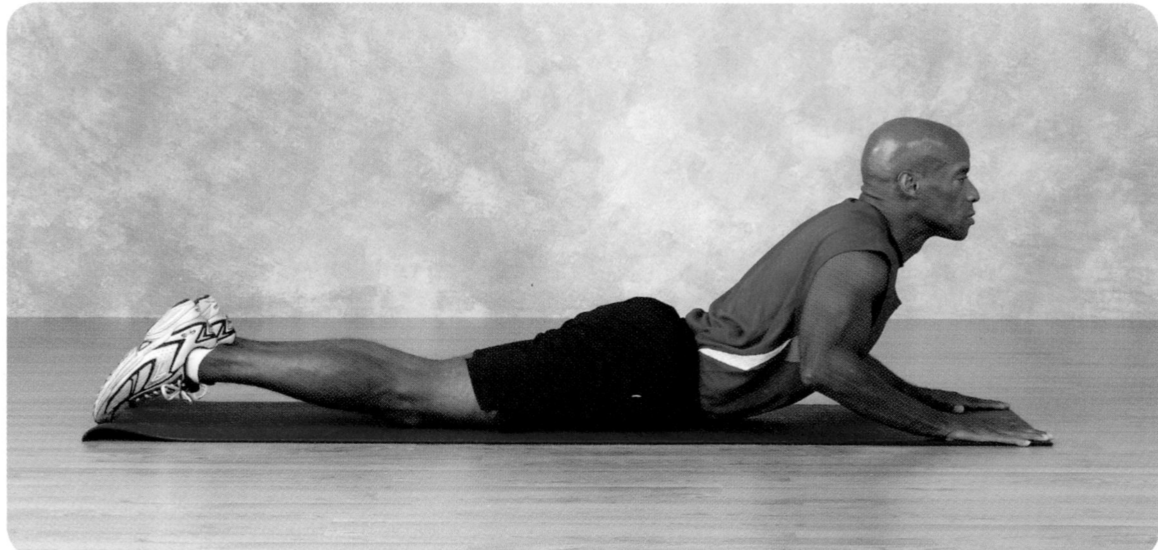

Trunk Strength and Endurance Exercises

In these, as in any other resistance training exercises, overload must be achieved. Strength can be developed by doing, for example, 10 to 15 repetitions of each exercise (or until overload is reached); however, workouts can also be varied by doing most of the exercises with 30 to 60 sec isometric holds and fewer repetitions. The latter can be advantageous for developing trunk muscle endurance, which is critical for attaining good core stability.

Quadruped

(a) Initially this exercise is done one limb at a time and then is advanced if the exerciser raises contralateral limbs; it can be done dynamically or isometrically. Abdominal bracing and core stability requirements are increased when two limbs are raised. When back patients perform this exercise, it is important that they do so in pain-free ROM and with the shoulders and hips level. There should not be any bobbing or other trunk movement during this exercise. In *(b)* the individual is performing a basic quadruped task on the stability platform as used in our research (11). It cannot be overemphasized that coordination is crucial in the development and maintenance of CS.

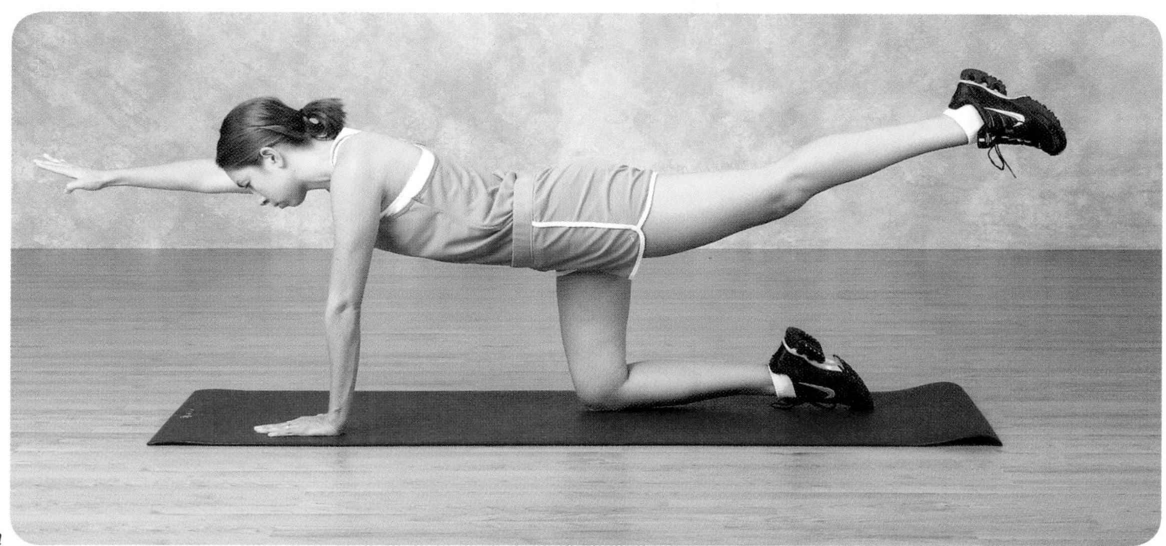

a

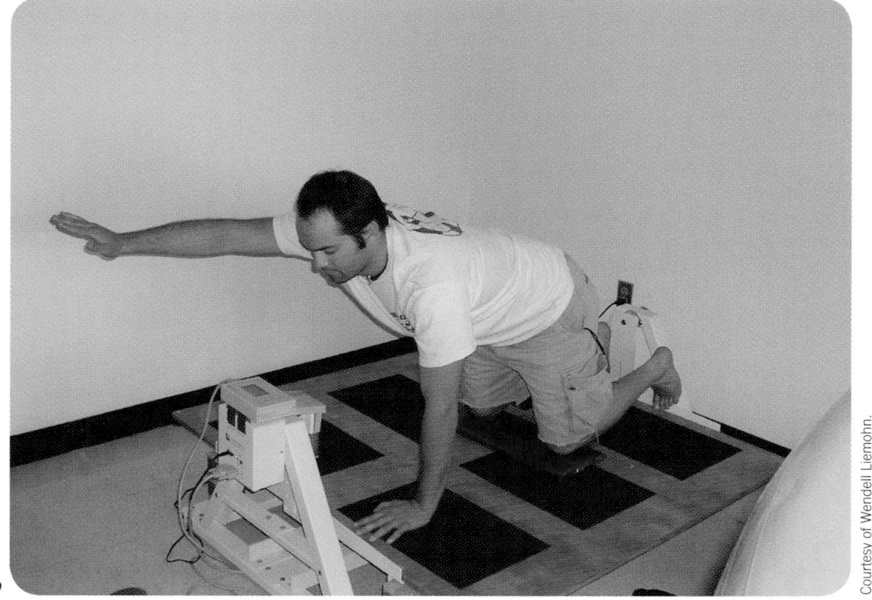

b

Courtesy of Wendell Liemohn.

Roman Chair

(a) This is an effective exercise for the lumbar erector spinae and the multifidus. For people with less strength, the activity depicted in *(b)* is more appropriate. The compressive forces on the discs are lower in *(b)* than in *(a)*; nevertheless, even the exercise depicted in *(b)* might be too difficult for some individuals.

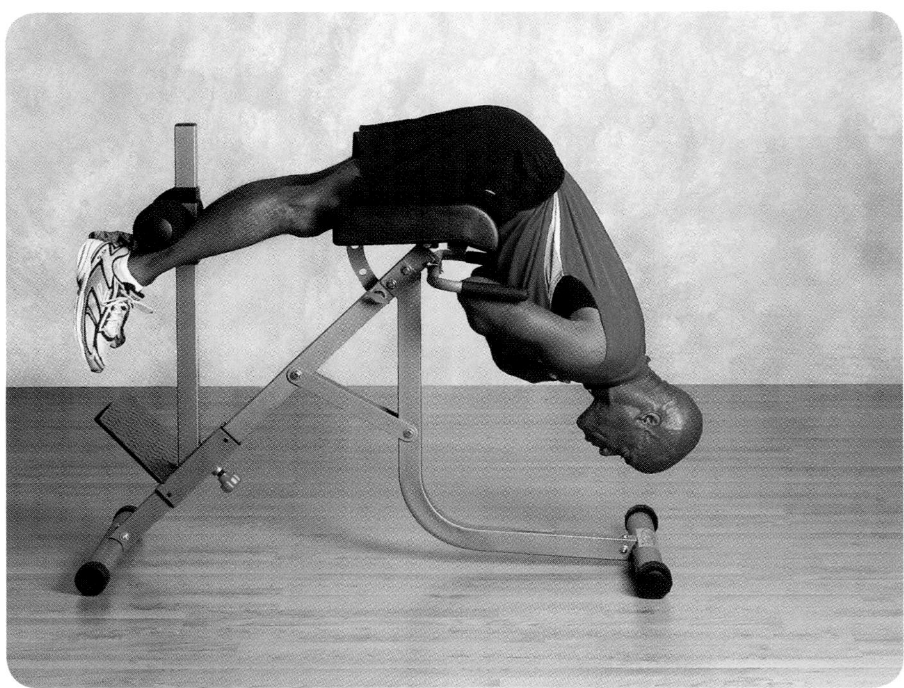

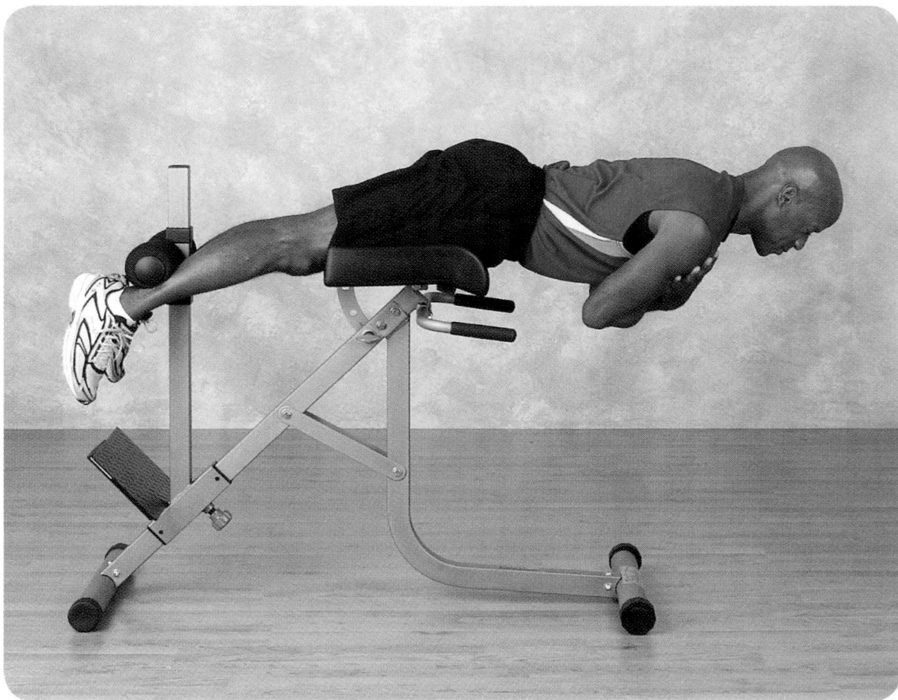

a

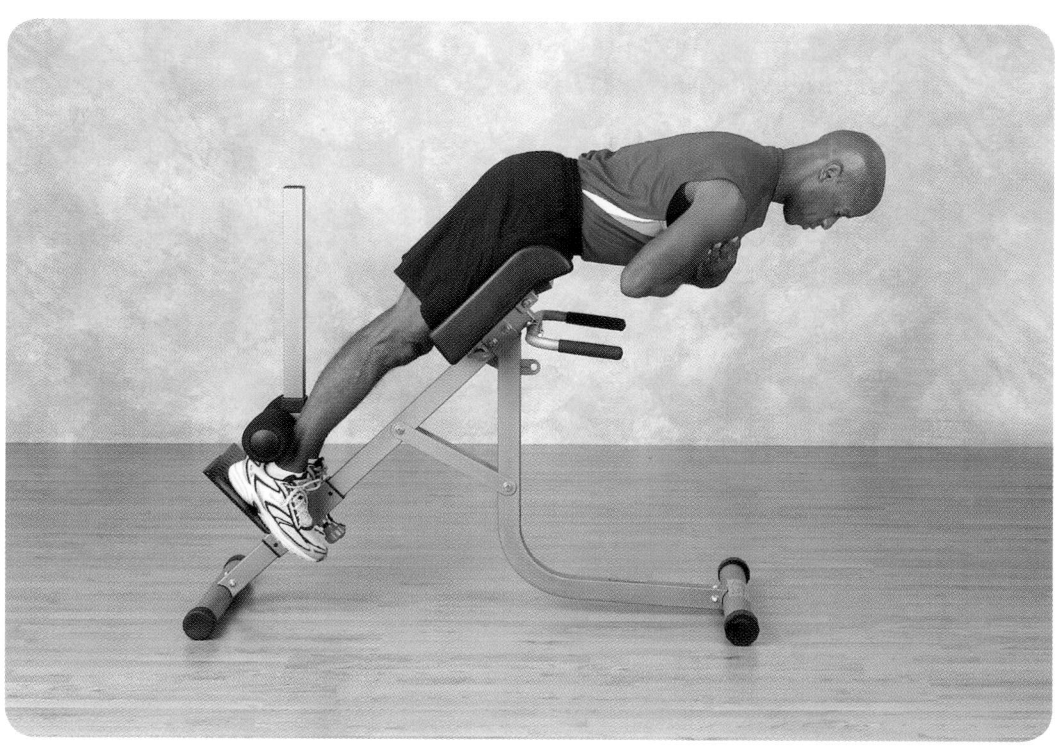

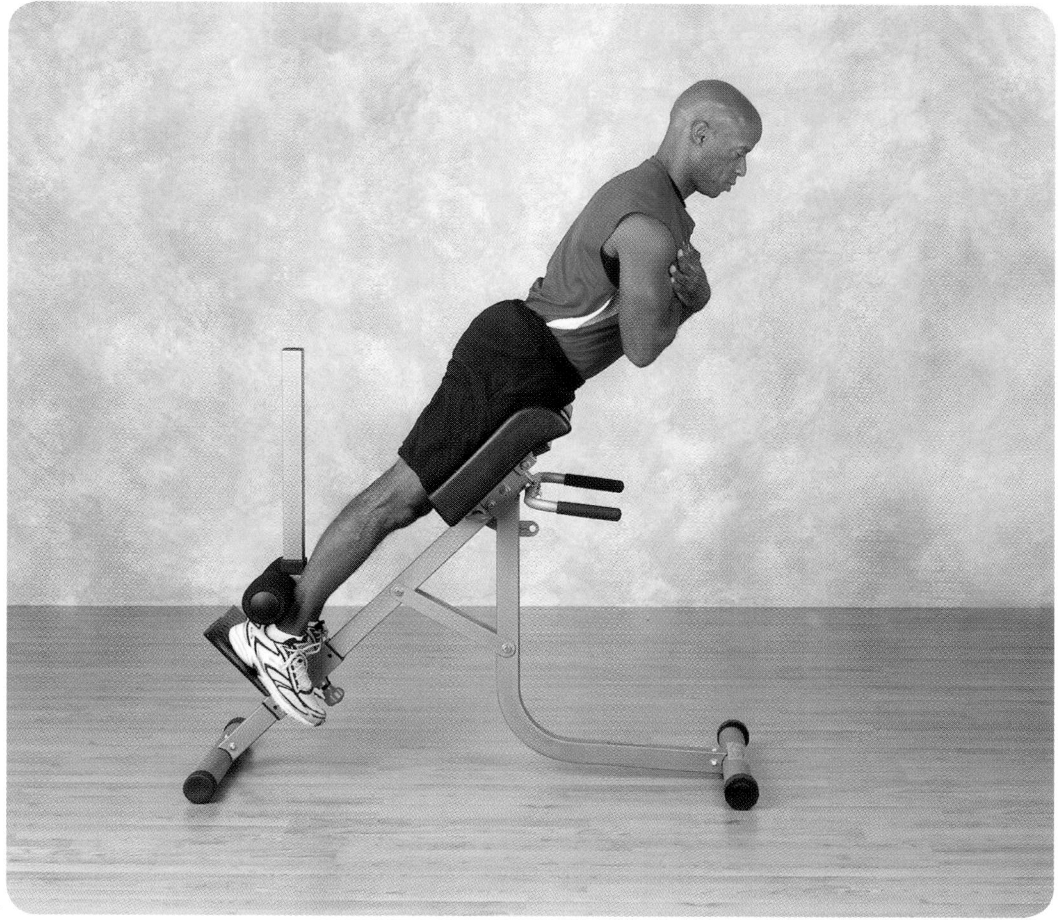

b

Posterior Pelvic Tilt

This exercise can be done by itself or as the first phase of a crunch. The participant posteriorly rotates the pelvis from starting position *(a)* until the low back is snug against the floor *(b)*. (This exercise may not be appropriate for individuals with disc pathology.)

For the following abdominal wall exercises, research is cited that indicates the degree of MVC seen for the musculature involved. As discussed previously, it is desirable to minimize psoas activity as much as possible while concurrently maximizing abdominal wall activity. The only exercises included here are those that the author thought best met these criteria. Other exercises may be appropriate for a specific population.

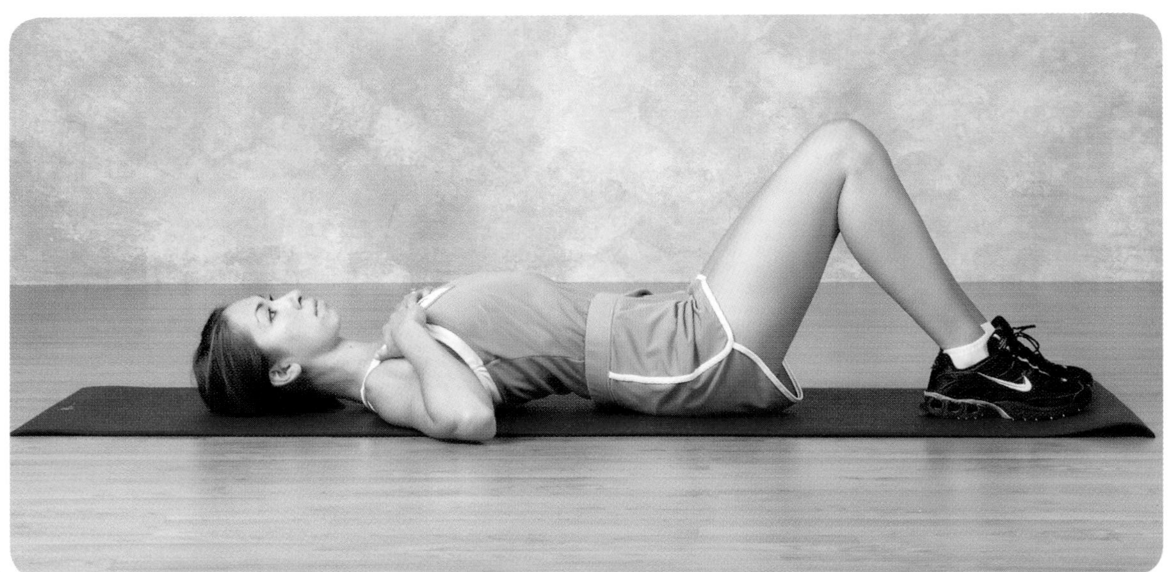

a

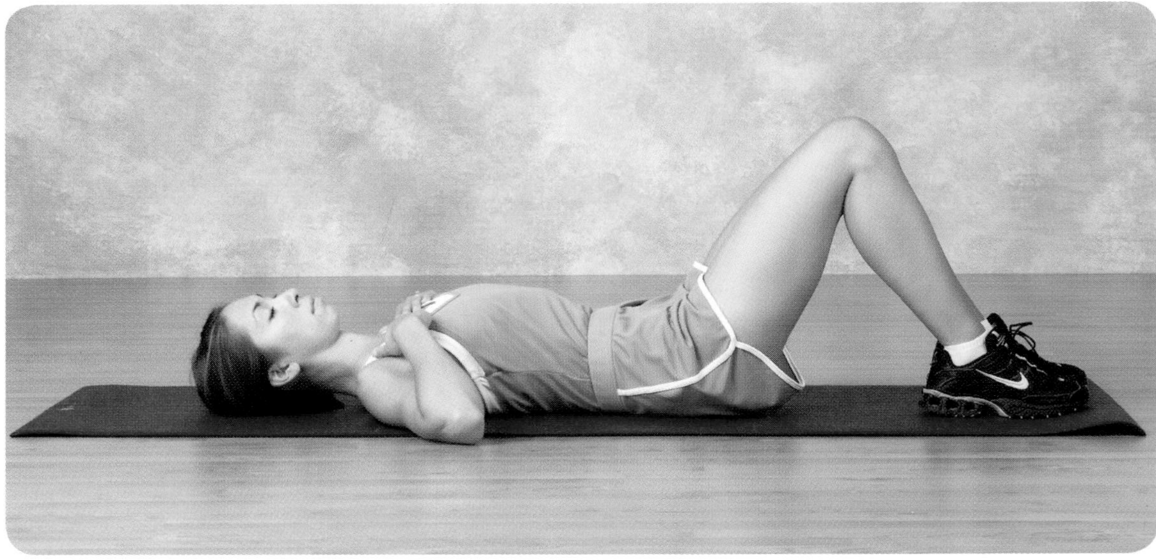

b

Crunch or Partial Curl-Up

Once the shoulders are raised from the floor, the normal lordosis has been straightened and movement should cease *(a)*. If the movement is continued, it will occur at the iliofemoral joint and the movers will be the hip flexors, because the abdominal muscles contract isometrically to stabilize the trunk. The crunch also can be performed with the thighs vertical *(b)*. A minimum of 10 to 15 repetitions should be the goal. Two or three sets may be repeated, and isometric holds of 5 sec or more can be incorporated with the up position. MVC: psoas—7% to 10%, rectus abdominis—62%, external oblique—68%, internal oblique—36%, transversus abdominis—12% (10).

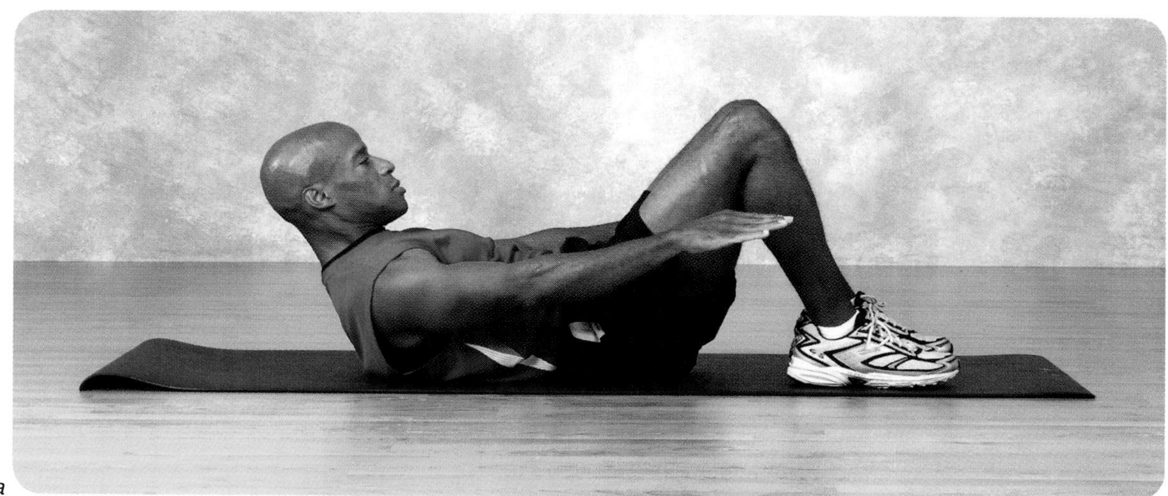

a

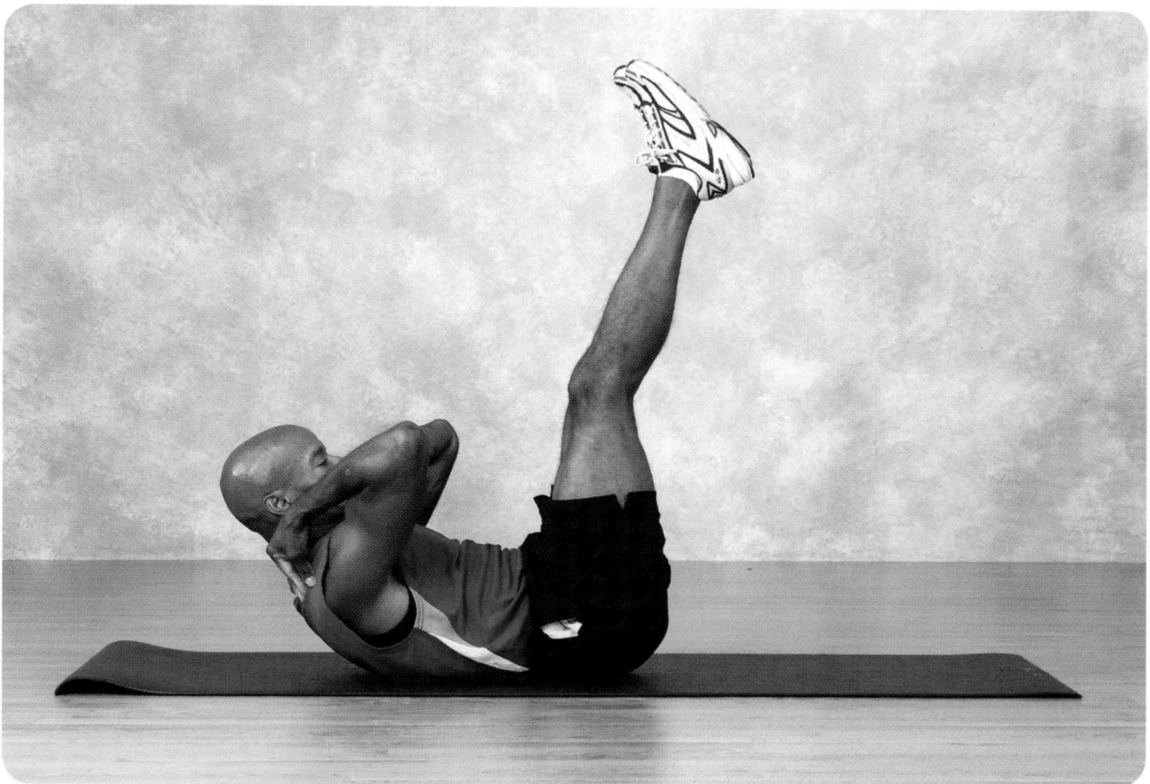

b

Cross Curl-Up

This exercise ensures greater involvement of the internal and external oblique musculature. A minimum of 10 to 15 repetitions should be the goal. Two or three sets may be repeated, and isometric holds of 5 sec or more can be incorporated with the up position. MVC: psoas—4% to 5%, rectus abdominis—62%, external oblique—68%, internal oblique—36%, transversus abdominis—12% (10).

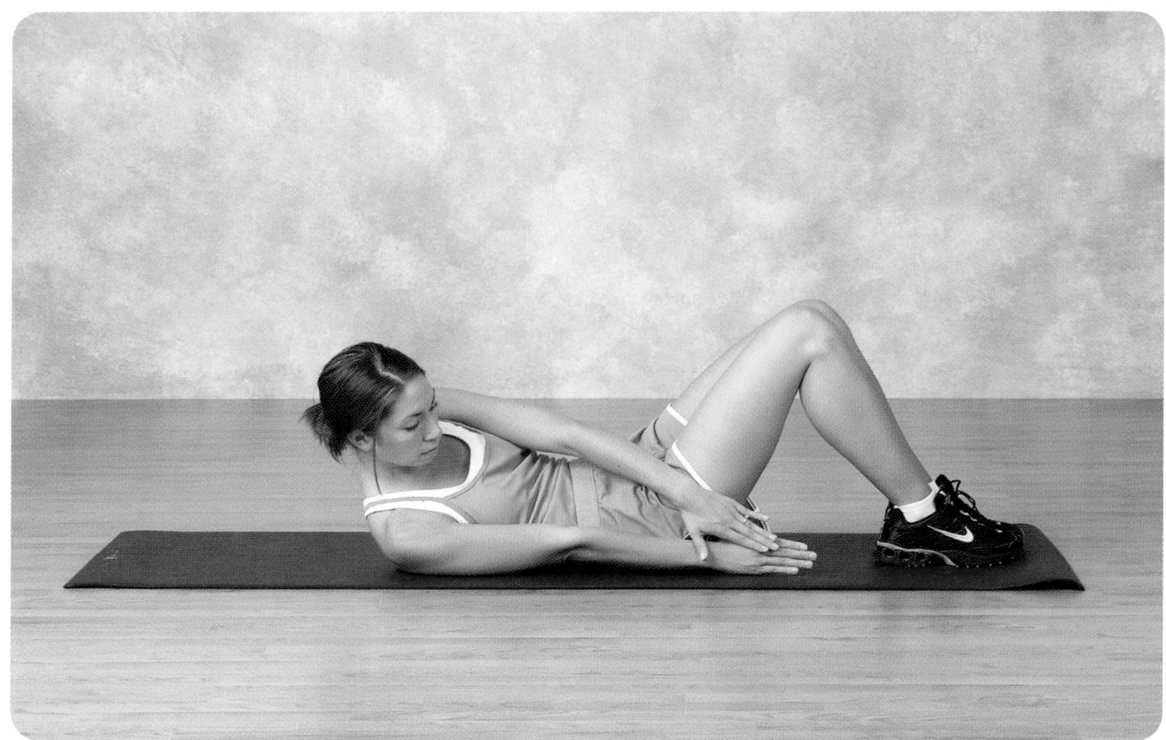

Horizontal Isometric Side Bridge

This can be done with either the knees or the feet on the floor. The latter is more difficult and increases the spine load over the figures cited. MVC: psoas—12% to 21%[2], rectus abdominis—21%, external oblique—43%, internal oblique—36%, transversus abdominis—39% (10).

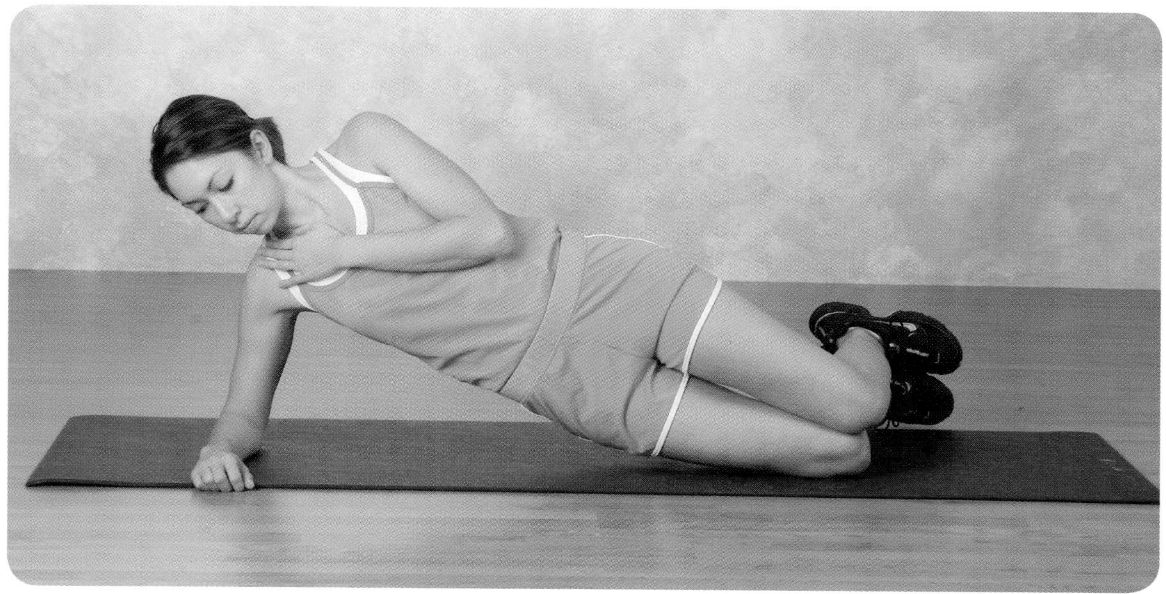

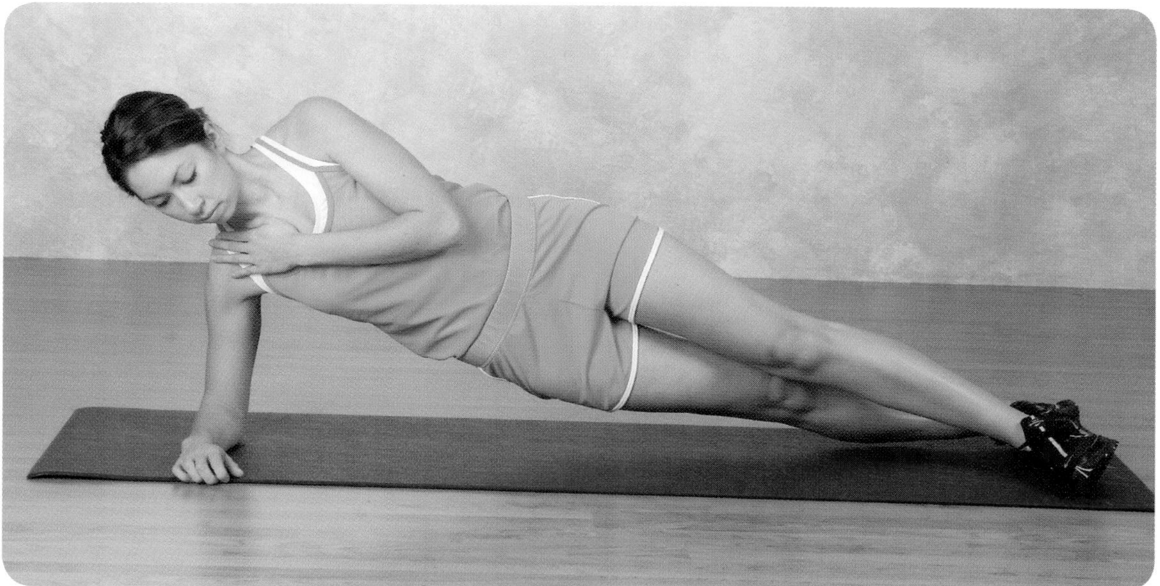

[2] Indwelling electrodes were inserted in two psoas sites.

Dynamic Side Bridge

This exercise is the horizontal isometric side bridge without the isometric hold. It can be done with the knees or the feet on the floor. The latter is more difficult and also increases the spine load over the figures cited. If this exercise is done dynamically, MVC: psoas—13% to 26%, rectus abdominis—41%, external oblique—44%, internal oblique—42%, transversus abdominis—44% (10). In the dynamic version of this bridge exercise, the hips are raised and lowered rhythmically.

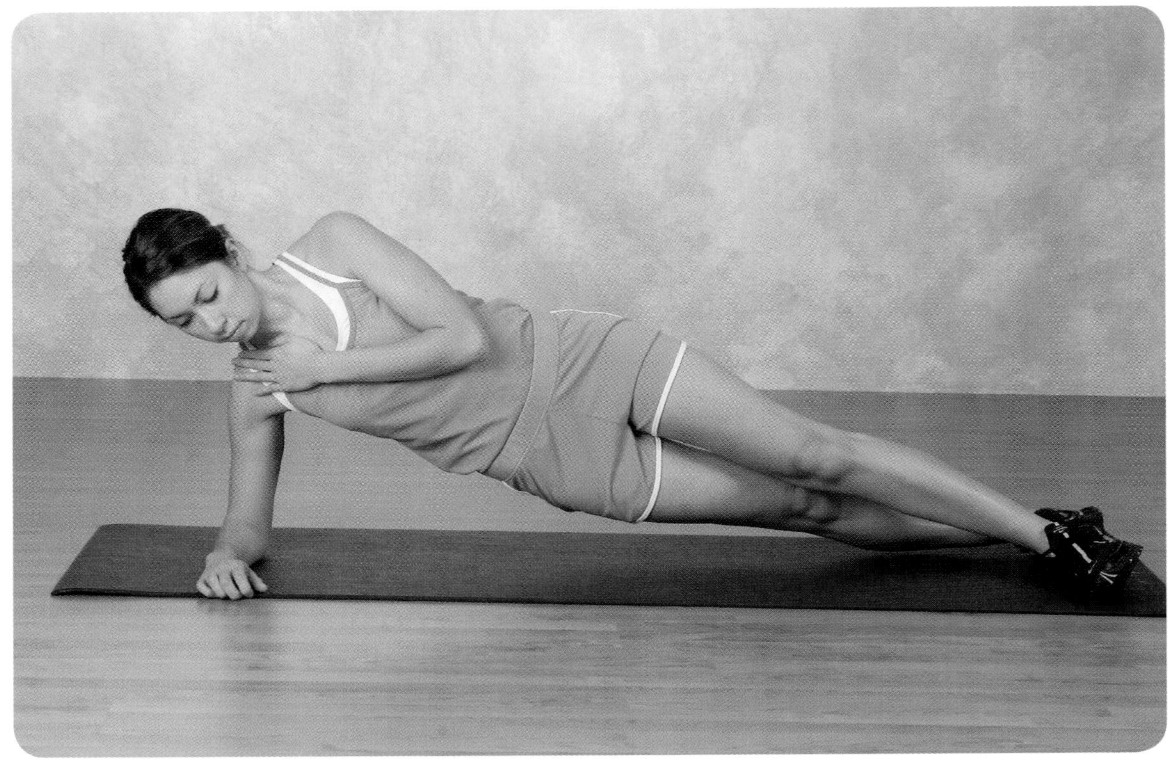

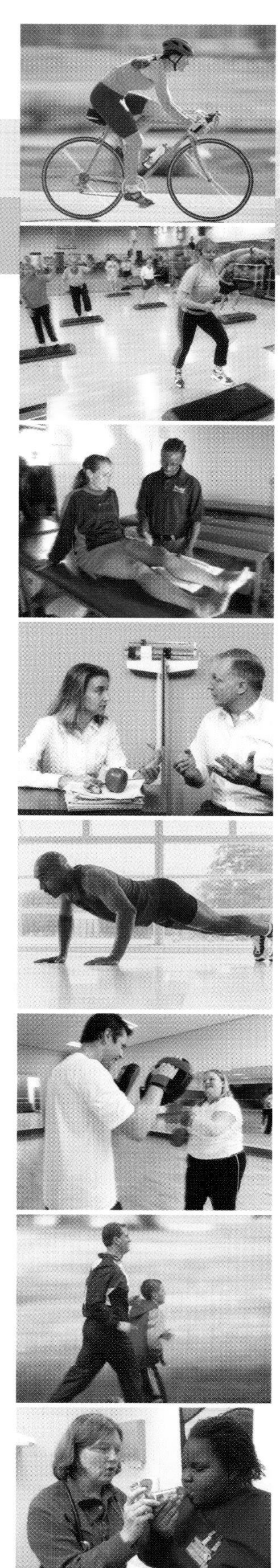

CHAPTER 14

Exercise Leadership for Health and Fitness

Objectives

The reader will be able to do the following:

1. Distinguish between moderate-intensity exercise programs recommended for everyone and systematically structured exercise programs for people interested in improving functional capacity.
2. Describe the factors related to a high and low probability of activity participation.
3. Describe the characteristics of a good exercise leader.
4. Describe safety and clothing considerations for walking and jogging programs.
5. Explain the balance between duration and intensity in a typical walking program, and list activities used in walking programs to improve enjoyment and adherence.
6. Outline appropriate walk, jog, walk intervals used at the beginning of a jogging program.
7. Describe exercise recommendations for cycling that improve cardiorespiratory fitness.
8. List the elements of games that provide effective fitness benefits.
9. Describe the activities done in a swimming pool, other than lap swimming, that can be an effective part of an aerobic exercise program.

(continued)

Objectives *(continued)*

10. Provide recommendations for beginners starting low- and high-impact dance exercise programs, and indicate the typical exercises included in such programs.
11. Recommend beginning goals for people using exercise equipment.
12. Describe a circuit training program that uses aerobic and resistance training equipment.

The purpose of a fitness program must be uppermost in the fitness professional's mind. The fitness professional is trying to help people include physical activity as a vital part of their lifestyles. This assumes that the participants understand what type of physical activity is appropriate, have sufficient skills to achieve satisfaction from the activities, and have the intrinsic motivation to continue to be active for the rest of their lives. Thus, fitness professionals help people increase their physical fitness in ways that are psychologically, mentally, and socially relevant and appealing.

Effective Leadership

Adults need 30 min of moderate-intensity physical activity daily to achieve health goals. To develop and maintain cardiorespiratory fitness, an adult should participate in aerobic exercise at least 3 days $\cdot$ wk^{-1} at an appropriate intensity and duration to expend sufficient calories consistent with that goal (see chapter 10 for details). Yet, more than 50% of American adults are not physically active at the level deemed necessary to achieve health-related goals (2). At the same time, more than half of the people who start a formal exercise program drop out within a few months (3).

Figure 14.1 summarizes the factors related to a high probability and a low probability of participation. The fitness professional must understand that a variety of factors affect people's involvement in personal or supervised exercise programs. In general, better-educated, self-motivated individuals who enjoy physical activity and believe in the health outcomes associated with physical activity are more likely to exercise regularly.

Key Point

Moderate-intensity exercise (30 min daily) is recommended for all people. Vigorous aerobic exercise should be done at least 3 days per wk to improve and maintain cardiorespiratory fitness. Unfortunately, most U.S. adults do not meet either of these recommendations.

In contrast, individuals with a high risk of CHD who also hold blue-collar jobs are less likely to participate in formal exercise. It appears that the people with the greatest need to exercise are the least likely to become involved. More than personal characteristics, however, are involved in the decision.

Support from one's spouse or partner, family, physician, and peers seems to drive participation, but this influence must be viewed against the variable of perceived convenience of facilities. People with poor time-management and goal-setting skills are less likely to be successful in meeting the exercise recommendations. What does this say about the fitness professional's role in providing exercise leadership? That exercise leadership involves much more than exercise (see chapter 22)!

Henry Kissinger once said that a leader is one who can take people from where they are to where they have not been (16). This is true for the exercise leader, who must counter the negative influences bearing down on the populations most in need of physical activity. We normally think that a fitness professional does the following:

- Screens individuals relative to health status.
- Evaluates various fitness components.
- Prescribes activities at the appropriate intensity, duration, and frequency consistent with test results and personal goals.
- Leads individuals or groups in appropriate activities.
- Monitors participants' responses within an exercise session.
- Modifies activities depending on environmental and other factors.
- Records progress and problems.
- Responds to emergencies.
- Refers problems to appropriate health professionals.

Leadership, however, means more than simply taking a class through its paces. Fitness professionals must make participants feel welcome, motivate them, and be a friend. To do all these things, the exercise leader must develop interpersonal skills. These leadership abilities are summarized on page 253.

Relationship-Oriented Abilities for Effective Leadership

- Listening skills
- Attention to individual needs
- Concern for integrating new participants
- Acceptance to group interaction
- Educational skills
- Motivational skills with participants and staff
- Rapport and empathy leading to sensitivity
- Consistency, honesty, and tactfulness
- Ability to open up communication between participants and staff

Reprinted, by permission, from N. Oldridge, 1988, Qualities of an exercise leader. In *Resource manual for guidelines for exercise testing and prescription*, edited by S.N. Blair et al. (Philadelphia, PA: Lea & Febiger), 240.

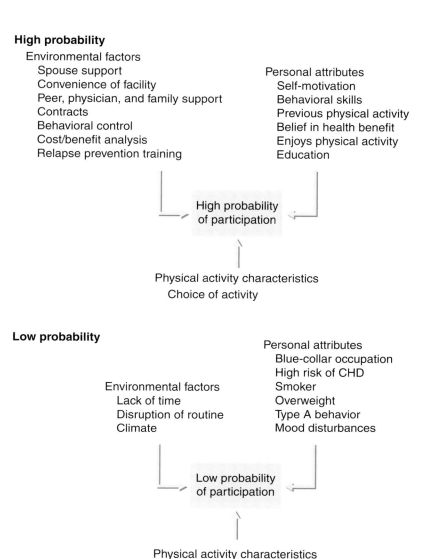

High probability

Environmental factors
Spouse support
Convenience of facility
Peer, physician, and family support
Contracts
Behavioral control
Cost/benefit analysis
Relapse prevention training

Personal attributes
Self-motivation
Behavioral skills
Previous physical activity
Belief in health benefit
Enjoys physical activity
Education

High probability of participation

Physical activity characteristics
Choice of activity

Low probability

Environmental factors
Lack of time
Disruption of routine
Climate

Personal attributes
Blue-collar occupation
High risk of CHD
Smoker
Overweight
Type A behavior
Mood disturbances

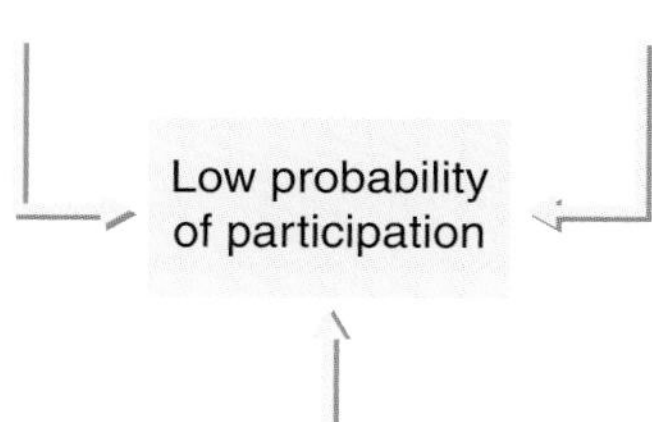

Physical activity characteristics
High-intensity activity
High perceived effort

Figure 14.1 High and low probability of participation.

Since 1980, many organizations have developed certification and education programs to promote exercise programming in preventive and rehabilitative settings. One of the earliest to do so was the ACSM (www.acsm.org). Certification requires the applicant to have a certain knowledge base and to demonstrate specific behaviors. The current ACSM certification programs include the following (1):

Personal Trainer
Health/Fitness Instructor
Exercise Specialist
Registered Clinical Exercise Physiologist

These certifications are considered the standard by many professionals in the fields of fitness and cardiac rehabilitation. However, there are a variety of other respected certification programs:

- American Council on Exercise (ACE)—Group Fitness Instructor, Personal Trainer, Lifestyle and Weight Management Consultant, and Clinical Exercise Specialist (www.acefitness.org)
- Aerobics and Fitness Association of America (AFAA)—Personal Fitness Trainer and Primary Group Exercise (www.afaa.com)
- National Strength and Conditioning Association (NSCA)—Certified Strength and Conditioning Specialist and Certified Personal Trainer (www.nsca-lift.org)

These certification programs and certifications for unique aspects of exercise leadership are presented later in this chapter. Next, the responsibilities of the fitness professional are examined in greater detail.

Be a Role Model

The fitness professional should be an inspiring role model for her clients. The idea of an overweight, out-of-shape exercise leader is one whose time has passed. A leader must plan activities, evaluate the progress of the participants, and provide incentives, but the leadership associated with many exercise programs is in the form of subtle value statements that do not require words. When the fitness professional's presence and behaviors demonstrate a healthy lifestyle, it adds much value to his words and programs.

Plan Programs

All programs must have daily, weekly, and monthly plans to provide appropriate activities, meet the needs of the participants, and reduce the possibility of boredom. This planning allows the fitness professional to judge the usefulness of the activity and encourage systematic modification from one month to the next. If the fitness professional is working with clients who exercise on their own, the need for specific exercise recommendations becomes obvious. The value of the feedback received from these individuals depends on the information they were given at the start of their program. The following considerations apply to both group and individual exercise programs.

Vary the Program

Variety should be a cornerstone of every exercise program. Some elements appear in every exercise session: a warm-up and stretching, a stimulus phase, and a cool-down. The variety comes from using different exercises in each part of a session, presenting short educational messages to the class while they are stretching or cooling down, or using games to add spice to routine exercises. The most important thing is to plan the activity sessions far enough in advance to minimize repetition and maximize variety.

Accommodate Individual Differences

A participant should be able to choose from a variety of activities. A program must address the needs, interests, and limitations of the group being served. The equipment, the activities, and the pace of the class must be considered when planning for younger or older, less fit or very fit, and skilled or unskilled participants (13). Offer people different options: 1 or 5 lb (0.5 or 2 kg) weights, low-impact or high-impact moves, or 1 mi (1.6 km) fast walks versus 3 mi (4.8 km) jogs.

Maintain Control

The exercise leader must control the exercise session. This is especially true when using games (e.g., indoor soccer), where the intensity is not as easily controlled. Control implies an ability to modify the session as needed to meet the target heart rate (THR) and total work goals of each individual. Some people will have to slow down; others may need encouragement to increase their intensity. The element of control (at a distance) for people who exercise without direct supervision can be provided through written guidelines about what to do and when to move from one stage to the next. In addition, specific information should be provided about symptoms that indicate inappropriate responses to exercise.

Monitor Progress and Keep Records

Keeping track of a participant's response to the exercise session reveals the individual's adaptation to that particular session and day-to-day changes overall. This information is important for updating exercise prescriptions and answering specific questions the participant may raise. Each exercise class should pause regularly to check HR and determine whether people are close to their THRs. Rather than keeping track of a large number of 10 sec THRs, ask each participant to indicate the number of beats over or under the 10 sec goal. This increases the participant's awareness of the THR and indicates how the intensity of the exercise should be adjusted to stay on target.

The HR response is probably the best and most objective indicator of adjustment to an exercise session, but do not stop with that. Elicit information about how the participant feels in general; ask about any new pains, aches, or strange sensations. Record keeping should include a daily attendance check, a weekly weighing, a regular BP check (if appropriate), and a column asking for comments (e.g., THR, any aches or pains). An example of such a form is the Daily Activity Form (see form 14.1). This information allows the fitness professional to make better recommendations about the participants' exercise programs and refer them to appropriate professionals if needed.

The point we have emphasized throughout this section is the need for the leader to help the participant. The behavioral strategies listed on page 256 suggest ways for fitness professionals to become better leaders.

Progression of Activities

Sedentary people who want to begin a fitness program should follow a logical sequence of activities. Moderate-intensity activities are encouraged for everyone, but a systematic program of activities helps participants increase functional capacity. The following paragraphs summarize our recommendations on how this appropriate progression of activities can be accomplished.

Phase 1: Regular Walking

The first phase for sedentary individuals is to gradually increase the moderate-intensity physical activity in their weekly patterns. Walking is the most popular activity. The major fitness goal is to increase the amount of physical activity that can be done comfortably, so no emphasis on

FORM 14.1 Daily Activity Form

Name ______________________________

Target weight ____________ Target heart rate zone ____________

Week	Day	Weight	Resting BP	Resting HR	Exercise HR	RPE	Signs, symptoms, comments
1							
2							
3							
4							

From Edward T. Howley and B. Don Franks, 2007, *Fitness Professional's Handbook,* 5th ed. (Champaign, IL: Human Kinetics).

Key Point

The effective fitness professional must develop relationship-oriented abilities, serve as a role model for others, use variety, accommodate differences, control the environment for safety, and monitor and record clients' progress. Asking for participants' HR, RPE, and any unusual responses to the exercise are ways to monitor exercise intensity during an exercise session.

intensity is necessary at this point. People in this phase start with the distance they can easily walk without pain or fatigue and then gradually increase the distance and pace until they can complete about 30 min of moderate-intensity activity (e.g., 2 mi at 4 mi · hr^{-1}, or 3.2 km at 6.4 km · hr^{-1}) each day. People with an orthopedic limitation can substitute a weight-supported activity such as cycling, rowing, or swimming for walking.

Phase 2: Recommended Work Levels for a Change in Fitness

Once phase 1 is accomplished, individuals are taught about recommended levels of work for fitness changes (see chapter 10). A work–relief interval training program is introduced—jogging is the work, and walking is the relief. The participant walks, jogs a few steps, then walks, and so forth. Gradually, jogging covers more distance than walking, until the person can jog continuously for 2 to 3 mi (3.2-4.8 km) at the THR. People interested in cycling and swimming (see later in this chapter) also can use interval training. People interested in aerobic dance should transition from the walking program to a low-intensity, low-impact class.

Phase 3: Variety of Fitness Activities

The first two phases are generally recommended for everyone (with alternative activities for people who cannot or choose not to jog, such as cycling, dancing, or

Behavioral Strategies of the Effective Exercise Leader

- Show a sincere interest in the participants. Learn why they have chosen your program and what they would like to achieve.
- Be enthusiastic in your instruction and guidance.
- Develop a personal relationship with each participant.
- Consider the various reasons why adults exercise (e.g., health, recreation, weight loss, social opportunities, personal appearance) and allow for individual differences.
- Initiate participant follow-up (i.e., postcards or telephone calls) when several unexplained absences occur in succession. Novice exercisers should be advised that an inevitable slip in attendance does not imply failure.
- Practice what you preach. Participate in the exercise sessions yourself. Good posture and grooming are essential to projecting the desired self-image. Cigarette smoking should be prohibited, and drinking soda or eating candy on the gymnasium floor also is unacceptable.
- Honor special days (e.g., birthdays) or exercise accomplishments with extrinsic rewards such as T-shirts, ribbons, or certificates.
- Attend personally to orthopedic and musculoskeletal problems. Provide alternatives to floor exercise.
- Counsel participants on proper exercise apparel.
- Avoid constantly using complicated medical or physiological terminology, but don't ignore it altogether. Concentrate on a few terms to educate participants a little at a time.
- Arrange for occasional visits by personal physicians.
- Provide newspaper or magazine articles to the participants on topics related to physical activity and other pertinent information.
- Encourage an occasional visitor or participant to lead activity.
- Designate an area for participant counseling. Avoid conversing with clients while performing another task simultaneously.
- Display your continuing education certifications and educational degrees. You are more likely to be successful at modifying behavior if you are perceived as an expert.
- Introduce first-time exercisers on the gymnasium floor or in the locker room. This orientation encourages a sense of belonging to the group.
- Reinforce participants by complimenting them on their appearance as they are exercising. Your conversation during exercise also can serve as a distracter from any unpleasant sensations that they may be experiencing.
- Consider entering city- or business-sponsored road races to pace your participants or show interest and enthusiasm by cheering clients at community fitness events.

Reprinted from B.A. Franklin et al., 1990, *On the ball* (Carmel, IN: Benchmark Press), with permission of the author, Barry A. Franklin, PhD.

running in water). Phase 3, on the other hand, is quite individualized and based on the person's interests. The purpose is to promote continued activity by having people participate in an activity they naturally enjoy. Some people prefer to continue to stretch, walk, and jog; some prefer to exercise alone; and others enjoy working out with others. Some people like cooperative and relatively low-level competitive activities, and others like the thrill of competition. Some enjoy a variety of different movement forms; others enjoy repeating similar activities. The fitness professional must provide an atmosphere where people feel free to try new things without embarrassment and allow participants to choose their fitness activities from a variety of options.

Walk, Jog, Run Programs

While walking, the participant keeps at least one foot on the ground at all times. In jogging and running, more muscular force is exerted to propel the body completely off the ground, creating a nonsupport phase. The distinction between jogging and running is not as clearly defined. Some people view the speed as being the difference, but no single criterion for speed is commonly accepted. Others distinguish between the two by the intent of the participant—a jogger is simply interested in exercise, whereas a runner trains to achieve performance goals in road races.

General Safety

A variety of safety factors common to both walking and jogging should be mentioned before we discuss how to institute walking and jogging programs.

Footwear

Any comfortable pair of well-supported shoes can be worn for a beginning walking program. Serious walkers and all joggers should invest in appropriate shoes with well-padded heels that are higher than the soles and a fitted heel cup. The shoes should be flexible enough to bend easily. The same kind of socks that will be worn while exercising should be worn during the shoe fitting to ensure a proper fit. Only the serious competitive runner needs racing shoes, which are a lighter weight and offer less cushioning.

Clothing

The weather conditions and activity intensity determine the clothing to be worn. Warm weather dictates light, preferably cotton, loose-fitting clothing. Nothing should be worn that prevents perspiration from reaching the outside air. A brimmed hat should cover the head on hot, sunny days. For the jogger, long pants are probably not needed until the temperature (windchill considered) drops below 40 °F (~4 °C).

In cold weather, walkers and joggers should dress in layers so they can remove or add clothing when necessary. Wool and polypropylene fabrics are good choices for extreme cold, but most joggers tend to overdress. A hat, preferably a wool stocking cap that can be pulled down over the forehead and ears, and gloves or mittens also should be worn. Cotton socks worn as mittens are useful not only to keep hands warm but also to act as "wipers" for the sniffling nose that often accompanies cold-weather walking and jogging.

Surface

The surface is not as crucial for walkers as it is for joggers, although some walkers (especially those with orthopedic problems) should exercise on a soft surface such as grass or a running track with a shock-absorbent surface. Many people prefer exercising off the track for visual stimulation and interest, but regular jogging on hard surfaces such as concrete or blacktop can lead to stress problems in the ankle, knee, and hip joints and in the low back. Joggers need to observe special precautions when running on the road: Jog facing traffic, assume cars at crossroads do not see joggers, and beware of cracks and curbs. Running cross country usually means running on a softer surface, but joggers must be aware of the uneven terrain and the increased potential for ankle injuries.

Safety Tips

Educate participants to practice the following tips to ensure safety when walking or jogging:

- Move toward the oncoming traffic.
- Yield the right of way to cars.
- Listen to music only while exercising on a very quiet street, and always listen for and be aware of traffic.
- Choose well-lighted streets or running tracks on school grounds.
- Walk or jog with a partner if you must exercise at night.

Key Point

Walkers and joggers should wear supportive and flexible shoes and wear clothing that accommodates weather conditions and exercise intensity. They should follow rules of the road and walk or jog in safe areas at safe times.

Walking

The advantages of walking include its convenience, practicality, and naturalness. Walking is an excellent activity, especially for people who are overweight and poorly conditioned and whose joints cannot handle the stresses of jogging.

As with all exercise programs, the participants begin with a warm-up and perhaps some static stretching. The walk should start at a slow speed and gradually increase to a pace that feels comfortable to the participant. The arms should swing freely, and the trunk should be kept erect with a slight backward pelvic tilt. The feet should point forward at all times. Many walkers have taken to malls, which provide air-conditioned comfort, safety, and a smooth surface and are usually within a short drive.

Walking programs can progress by increasing the distance or the speed. As mentioned previously, the first goal is for participants to accumulate 30 min of moderate-intensity physical activity each day. This is an important milestone and has clear health benefits (see chapter 10). Further, the 30 min can be realized in bouts of 10 min or longer. Participants should gradually increase their distance until they can easily walk 30 min at a brisk pace on a daily basis (e.g., 2 mi at 4 mi $\cdot$ hr^{-1}, or 3.2 km at 6.4 km $\cdot$ hr^{-1}). It is not appropriate to begin jogging or attempt to achieve THR in an aerobic dance class until this walking goal can be reached. The walking program on page 259 is graduated and leads to an activity level suitable for beginning a jogging program.

How do you make walking interesting for a class of 30 to 40 participants? An exercise leader must emphasize variety to keep interest high in such situations. There are several ways you might do this:

- Have participants follow the leader over hill and dale, up and down steps or slopes, with the walking speed changing from time to time.
- Have the group do line walking on a track, in which the person at the end of the line must walk faster to catch up to the front of the line, which, as a whole, moves at a steady pace. Line walking gives each person an interval-type workout.
- Add a ball to the front of the line, and have participants pass it to the side or overhead until it reaches the end of the line, at which time the last person dribbles to the front and restarts the process.
- Vary the activity used to reach the front of the line, with people skipping, jogging, and so on.
- Vary the length of the line by forming teams, and control the overall pace by balancing the teams and checking the THR.
- Plan a game of tag in a gym or field where all participants must walk, with the leader exerting control by defining the boundaries.
- Establish a distance goal for a 15 wk walking class—such as "We will walk from here to Nashville," for a total of 180 mi (290 km) walked over the 15 wk—and use a large map and stick pins to monitor each participant's progress from week to week. Award T-shirts or hold a country-western party when everyone finishes. Longer distances can be set as goals along with using the class total of miles walked to focus on group accomplishments.

Jogging

No single factor determines when a person can begin jogging. A person who can walk about 4 mi (6.4 km) briskly every other day but is unable to reach the THR range by walking should consider a jogging program to additionally improve cardiorespiratory fitness (CRF). A slow to moderate walker whose HR is within the THR zone should increase the distance or speed of walking rather than begin jogging. Also, the ability of the individual's joints to withstand the additional stresses of jogging should be considered. Remember, walking may be the first and only activity for many people; it is more important that they stay active than move to more intense activities.

Key Point

Walking programs should begin at a slow speed and gradually speed up to a comfortable pace. Distance should be increased gradually until at least 30 min (e.g., 2 mi, or 3.2 km) can be walked daily at a brisk pace. The previous list details activities that improve enjoyment and, consequently, adherence to the program.

The techniques of jogging are basically the same as those for walking. Jogging requires a greater flexion of the knee of the recovery leg, and the arms are bent more at the elbows. The arm swing is exaggerated slightly but should still be in the forward and backward direction. The heel makes the first contact with the ground; then the foot immediately rolls forward to the ball of the foot and then to the toes. As speed increases, the landing foot may contact the ground in an almost flat position. Breathing occurs through both the nose and mouth. Common faults of the beginning jogger include breathing with the mouth closed, insufficiently bending the knee during the recovery phase, and swinging the arms across the body.

Many people begin jogging at too high a speed, which results in an inability to continue long enough to accomplish the desired amount of total work; often this causes people to dislike jogging. This problem can be prevented by jogging at a speed slow enough to allow conversation and using work–relief intervals, which for beginners is slow jogging for a few seconds, then walking, then slow jogging, and so forth. Participants should be reassured that they will walk less and jog more as they become more fit. An example of such a progression is shown in the jogging program on page 260.

Key Point

Stages 1 through 5 of the jogging program are appropriate intervals to use at the beginning of a jogging program.

After a person can jog 2 or 3 mi (3.2-4.8 km) continuously within the THR zone, several approaches to a jogging program are available. A person can simply jog 3 or 4 times a week, planning only to exercise at an intensity that will elevate the HR to the training zone for a predetermined minimum length of time (or distance), with the option to go longer (or farther) on days when so desired. Other people do better with a specific program that includes progressive speed and distance goals, even if they do not plan to compete.

Walking Program

Rules

1. Start at a level that feels comfortable to you.
2. Be aware of new aches or pains.
3. Don't progress to the next level if you are not comfortable.
4. Monitor and record your HR.
5. Walk *at least* every other day.

Stage	Duration	HR	Comments
1	15 min		
2	20 min		
3	25 min		
4	30 min		
5	30 min		
6	30 min		
7	35 min		
8	40 min		
9	45 min		
10	45 min		
11	45 min		
12	50 min		
13	55 min		
14	60 min		
15	60 min		
16	60 min		
17	60 min		
18	60 min		
19	60 min		
20	60 min		

Reprinted, by permission, from B.D. Franks and E.T. Howley, 1998, *Fitness leaders' handbook*, 2nd ed. (Champaign, IL: Human Kinetics), 124 (6).

As with the walking class mentioned earlier, the fitness professional should include variety in a jogging program, and the same types of modifications cited earlier for the walking program are appropriate. In addition, in some communities jogging paths may have exercise stations at different locations to allow a person to combine walking or jogging with specific exercises for all parts of the body. Fun runs are held in many communities; the goal

Jogging Program

Rules

1. Complete the walking program before starting this program.
2. Begin each session with walking and stretching.
3. Be aware of new aches and pains.
4. Don't progress to the next level if you are not comfortable doing so.
5. Stay at the low end of your THR zone; record your HR for each session.
6. Do the program on a work-a-day, rest-a-day basis.

Stage 1 Jog 10 steps; walk 10 steps. Repeat 5 times and take your HR. Stay within THR zone by increasing or decreasing walking phase. Do 20 to 30 min of activity.

Stage 2 Jog 20 steps; walk 10 steps. Repeat 5 times and take your HR. Stay within THR zone by increasing or decreasing walking phase. Do 20 to 30 min of activity.

Stage 3 Jog 30 steps; walk 10 steps. Repeat 5 times and take your HR. Stay within THR zone by increasing or decreasing walking phase. Do 20 to 30 min of activity.

Stage 4 Jog 1 min; walk 10 steps. Repeat 3 times and take your HR. Stay within THR zone by increasing or decreasing walking phase. Do 20 to 30 min of activity.

Stage 5 Jog 2 min; walk 10 steps. Repeat 2 times and take your HR. Stay within THR zone by increasing or decreasing walking phase. Do 30 min of activity.

Stage 6 Jog 1 lap (400 m, or 440 yd) and check your HR. Adjust pace during run to stay within the THR zone. If HR is still too high, go back to stage 5. Do 6 laps with a brief walk between each.

Stage 7 Jog 2 laps and check HR. Adjust pace during run to stay within the THR zone. If HR is still too high, go back to stage 6. Do 6 laps with a brief walk between each.

Stage 8 Jog 1 mi (1.6 km) and check HR. Adjust pace during the run to stay within THR zone. Do 2 mi (3.2 km).

Stage 9 Jog 2 to 3 mi (3.2-4.8 km) continuously. Check HR at the end to ensure that you were within THR zone.

Reprinted, by permission, from B.D. Franks and E.T. Howley, 1998, *Fitness leaders' handbook*, 2nd ed. (Champaign, IL: Human Kinetics), 125 (6).

of these runs is to finish the distance, and a small prize is usually awarded.

Joggers who are not fast enough to compete successfully in road races may enjoy other competitions, such as prediction runs, in which speed does not determine the winner. The purpose of a prediction run is to see which jogger comes closest to his predicted time of finishing, which is declared before the race. A handicapped run requires joggers to declare their previous fastest times for the distance. A percentage (80%-100%) of the time difference between the fastest runner's declared time and each other runner's time is subtracted from each runner's actual finish time. For example, suppose runner A's fastest previous time is 18 min for 3 mi (4.8 km); runner B's is 19 min; and runner C's is 20 min. If 80% of the time difference is used, 48 sec (0.8 times the 60 sec difference between A and B) are subtracted from B's finish time, and 96 sec (0.8 times the 120 sec difference) are subtracted from runner C's finish time. Suppose runner A completes the race in 17:50, runner B in 18:30, and runner C in 20:10. The adjusted finish time for runner A is 17:50 (actual time), for runner B is 17:42 (18:30 – 0:48), and for runner C is 18:34 (20:10 – 0:96). Runner B is the winner. Another method of handicapping a race is to stagger the start according to each jogger's previous best time, with the slowest runner starting first and the fastest beginning last. The first runner over the finish line is the winner. Teams can be formed in which each four-member team, for example, has one runner from each of four groups classified by running speed.

Competitive Running

Almost all communities have road races sponsored by track clubs and service organizations as a means of raising funds, many for worthy purposes. Each entrant pays a registration fee, and most of the races have sex and age divisions, with prizes awarded to the top finishers, both overall and in each division. Usually every finisher receives an award such as a certificate or T-shirt. The race distances range between 1 mi (1.6 km; often called a *fun run)* and 100 mi (161 km), but the most common are the 5K (3.1 mi) and 10K (6.2 mi). Fitness participants should not be pressured to enter road races by those who enjoy them. The fitness professional should consider entering races with interested participants to help them select a starting spot and establish a pace and to provide encouragement. This may help them transition from a jogging group to an individualized jogging program.

Those who train for performance will work at the top of the THR range, 6 to 7 days each week and for more than 30 to 40 min per exercise session. Such programs are bound to result in more injuries, and the fitness professional should encourage participants pursuing such goals to have an alternative activity that they can enjoy while recovering from injuries.

Cycling

Riding a bicycle or stationary exercise cycle is another good fitness activity. Some people who have problems walking, jogging, or playing sports may be able to cycle without difficulty. The cycling program follows the guidelines for improving CRF (see chapter 10). Although bicycles and terrain vary widely, checking THR allows cyclists to adjust the speed so that they work at the appropriate intensity. Generally, a person covers 3 to 4 times the distance cycling compared with jogging; a person works up to 3 mi (4.8 km) jogging or 9 to 12 mi (14.5-19.3 km) cycling in each workout. The seat should be comfortable, and its height should be adjusted so that the knee is slightly bent at the bottom of the pedaling stroke.

Key Point

Cycling is an excellent activity, especially for those who cannot walk or jog due to joint-related issues. In general, participants should cycle 3 to 4 times the distance they would jog for an equivalent caloric expenditure and cardiorespiratory workout.

Games

One of the wonderful characteristics of children that is often lost in adulthood is playfulness. A child does not feel the need to justify spending time playing a game just for fun. One of the attributes that seems to be present in coronary-prone behavior is the inability to appreciate play for its own sake. A good fitness program can

Cycling Program

Rules

1. Adjust the seat so that it is comfortable.
2. Use either a regular bicycle or a stationary exercise cycle.
3. If you are starting at stage 1, simply get used to riding 1 or 2 mi (1.6-3.2 km). Don't be concerned about time or reaching the lower end of your THR zone.

Stage	Distance in mi (km)	THR (%HRmax)	Time (min)	Frequency (per wk)
1	1-2 (1.6-3.2)	—	—	3
2	1-2 (1.6-3.2	60	8-12	3
3	3-5 (4.8-8.0)	60	15-25	3
4	6-8 (9.7-12.9)	70	25-35	3
5	6-9 (9.7-14.5)	70	25-35	4
6	10-15 (16.1-24.1)	70	40-60	4
7	10-15 (16.1-24.1)	80	35-50	4-5

Reprinted, by permission, from B.D. Franks and E.T. Howley, 1998, *Fitness leaders' handbook*, 2nd ed. (Champaign, IL: Human Kinetics), 126 (6).

provide people with activities that increase both fitness and playfulness.

For games to be an effective part of a fitness program, certain elements must be present:

- **Competition.** Competition is not to be avoided, but little emphasis should be put on winning; the game should not be used to exclude people from participating.
- **Cooperation.** Having small groups solve problems together to accomplish fitness tasks can be enjoyable and healthy.
- **Enjoyment.** Enjoyment requires a balance of cooperation and competition, continued participation by everyone, and the chance for everyone to be a winner.
- **Inclusion.** A key ingredient for a fitness game is including everyone. This may mean modifying the rules.
- **Skill.** Some fitness games may require minimum levels of certain skills that can be taught as part of the fitness program.
- **Vigor.** The main workout should include games in which all participants are continuously active in the THR range.

Special Considerations

Participants at any fitness level can do the warm-up and cool-down activities of most games. The more vigorous games, however, usually involve high-intensity bursts, stopping, starting, and quickly changing directions. They are not recommended for the early stages of a fitness program. Some additional stretching and easy movements in different directions should be included as part of the warm-up for games. Obviously, the space, number of people, and equipment have to be considered in selecting activities. The leader must emphasize safety and should change the rules immediately when the game is not working. A variety of games should be offered so that people with different skill levels can participate. When large groups are involved in activities, the activities should change frequently to maintain interest. In addition to warm-up and cool-down activities, higher and lower intensities should be alternated to prevent undue fatigue. People should be encouraged to go at their own pace. THR should be checked periodically to ensure that people are within their ranges.

Fitness Games

Fitness games and activities are summarized below. In general, the level of control varies from that associated with circle and line activities to those with few rules, such as keep-away. Games can involve diverse muscle groups and use the body weight as resistance. Simultaneously, games develop greater balance and coordination, which are not necessarily outcomes of walking, jogging, or exercising with fixed equipment. *The Sport Ball Exercise Handbook* (5), a book written specifically to encourage games in a fitness setting, should be a part of every exercise leader's library. *The New Games Book* (14), a classic on the subject, and *Inclusive Games: Movement Fun for Everyone* (9) provide a playful and inclusive approach to games for various numbers of people. In games, as with

Fitness Games and Activities

- Skills and games with balls of various sizes. The size and type of ball can lead to innovative use—for instance, a cage ball can substitute for a basketball. Examples of other balls include tennis balls, volleyballs, playground balls, basketballs, medicine balls, handballs, softballs, mush balls, and Nerf balls.
- Activities with apparatus. Examples include hula hoops, Frisbees, paddle rackets, skip ropes, skittles, quoits, surgical tubing, culverts, and play buoys.
- Chasing games. Examples include tag, chain tag, fox and geese, and dodgeball.
- Relays with and without apparatus. Examples include running, hopping, rolling, crawling, and dribbling with hands and feet.
- Stunts and contests. Examples are dual activities such as balancing stunts, forward rolls, backward rolls, strength moves, push-ups, sit-ups, and limited combat games such as rooster fights and partner sparring.
- Lead-up games for major sport games. Examples are soccer, tennis, basketball, volleyball, handball, and football, often with rules adjusted to fit the abilities of the participants.
- Children's games. Activities include skittle ball, foursquare, and bounce ball.

Adapted, by permission, from M.D. Giese, 1988, Organization of an exercise session. In *Resource manual for guidelines for exercise testing and prescription*, edited by S.N. Blair et al. (Philadelphia, PA: Lea & Febiger), 244-247.

> **Key Point**
>
> Effective games for fitness are enjoyable, inclusive, vigorous, cooperative, competitive, and skill related.

all activities, the fitness professional needs to include people with disabilities by adapting the activities (18).

Aquatic Activities

Aquatic activities can be a major part of an exercise program or can be the needed relief from other exercises, especially during injury. The intensity of the activity can suit the needs of the least and the most fit, from the patient who's just survived an MI to the endurance athlete. HR can be checked at regular intervals to see whether THR has been reached, and a caloric expenditure goal can be achieved, given the high-energy requirement of aquatic activities. People with orthopedic problems who cannot run, dance, or play games can exercise in water. The water supports the person's body weight, minimizing problems associated with weight-bearing joints.

Target Heart Rate

One consistent finding is that the maximal HR response to a swimming test is about 18 beats · min^{-1} lower than that found in a maximal treadmill test. This suggests that for swimming, THR should be shifted downward (2 beats less for a 10 sec count) to achieve the 60% to 80% $\dot{V}O_2max$ goal associated with an endurance training effect (11).

Progression

Swimming activities can be graded not only by varying the speed of the swim but also by varying the activity. A patient who has just survived an MI and has an extremely low functional capacity will benefit from simply walking through the water. People who have had recent bypass surgery benefit from moving the arms as they walk across the pool. Following are examples of activities that can be used in aquatic exercise programs. Refer to *YMCA Water Fitness for Health* (17) for detailed information on aquatic exercise.

Side-of-Pool Activities

A variety of activities can be done while holding on to the side of the pool with one or both hands. These activities range from simply moving the legs to the side, front, or back to practicing a variety of kicks that ultimately can be used while swimming. ROM movements in the pool are a good way to warm up before undertaking the more vigorous activities of walking or jogging across the pool.

Walking and Jogging Across the Pool

A person with a low functional capacity can begin an aquatic program by simply walking across the shallow end of the pool. The water resists the movement while supporting the body weight, reducing the downward load on the ankles, knees, and hips. The arms can be involved by simulating a swimming motion; doing this increases the ROM of the arms and shoulder girdle. The speed and form of the walk can change as the person becomes accustomed to the activity. The person can take long strides with the head just above the water or sidestep across the pool. Last, the person can jog across the pool with the water at chest height. Remember to check whether THR has been achieved.

Flotation Devices

People with limited skill can use flotation devices (e.g., a life jacket or kickboard). The extra resistance of the jacket compensates for the extra buoyancy it provides. The participant should periodically determine whether THR has been reached.

Lap Swimming

Participants must be skilled to substitute swimming for running or cycling. An unskilled swimmer operates at a very high energy cost, even when moving slowly, and may become too fatigued to last the whole workout. But being unskilled at swimming doesn't mean that it should be eliminated as an option in personal fitness programs. A person can learn to swim over several months, gradually adjusting to the exercise. After learning to swim, the person can use swimming as the primary activity, even if using elementary strokes. Increasing the number of exercise activities a person can do increases the chance that the individual will remain active when something interferes with a primary activity.

Lap swimming should be approached the same way as lap running: warming up with stretching activities, starting slowly, taking frequent breaks to check the pulse rate, and gradually increasing the distance. Remember, the caloric cost of swimming compared with the cost of running the same distance is about 4:1. If jogging 1 mi (1.6 km) is a reasonable goal in a physical activity program, then swimming 400 m (0.25 mi) is equivalent in terms of energy expenditure. The swimming program on page 264 describes the stages that could be included in an endurance swimming program, beginning with walking across the pool. All steps assume that a warm-up has preceded the activity and that a cool-down follows.

Swimming Program

Rules

1. Start at a level that is comfortable for you.
2. Don't progress to the next stage if you are not comfortable with the current one.
3. Monitor and record your HR.

Stage 1 In chest-deep water, walk across the width of the pool four times and see if you are close to THR. Gradually lengthen the walk until you can do two 10 min walks at THR.

Stage 2 In chest-deep water, walk across and jog back. Repeat twice and see if you are close to THR. Gradually lengthen the jogging until you can complete four 5 min jogs at THR.

Stage 3 In chest-deep water, walk across and swim back (any stroke). Use a kickboard or flotation device if needed. Repeat this cycle twice and see if you are at THR. Keep up this pattern for 20 to 30 min of activity.

Stage 4 In chest-deep water, jog across and swim back (any stroke); repeat and check THR. Gradually shorten the jog and lengthen the swim until four widths can be completed within the THR zone. Accomplish 20 to 30 min of activity per session.

Stage 5 Slowly swim 25 yd (22.9 m); rest 20 sec. Slowly swim another 25 yd (22.9 m) and check THR. On the basis of the HR response, change the speed of the swim or the length of the rest to stay within the THR zone. Gradually increase the number of lengths you can swim (e.g., three, then four) before checking THR.

Stage 6 Increase the duration of continuous swimming until you can accomplish 20 to 30 min without a rest.

The stages in the swimming program are not discrete steps that must be followed in a particular order. Two stages can be combined or games can be introduced to make the walk-and-jog and width swims more enjoyable. The goal is to gradually increase the intensity and duration of the aquatic activities.

Key Point

Aquatic activities include upright activities (e.g., walking and jogging across the pool, using flotation devices) as well as swimming. Exercises also can be performed while holding on to the side of the pool, such as moving the legs from front to back or practicing a paddle kick.

Exercising to Music

Moving to the rhythm of music is an enjoyable way to exercise. A person can join a group at a fitness club, do individual workouts with a fitness professional, or exercise at home with videotapes or DVDs.

Advantages

Exercise to music is enjoyable for many participants, young and old, male and female. Since the mid-1970s, aerobics has evolved from the traditional high-intensity and low-impact classes to a variety of specialized classes that fit everyone's tastes and fitness levels. The inclusion of water, steps, slides, tubing, resistance balls, martial arts, and boxing provides numerous opportunities for cross-training or learning new techniques. Fortunately, certification and continuing education programs have developed in conjunction with these trends (see later in this chapter).

Getting Motivated

Working out to music is a great way to motivate people to continue exercising. The tempos and rhythms of the different songs keep the workout exciting and challenging for participants. Familiar lyrics often distract from the feeling of fatigue. Music makes routine exercises fun, and the class setting helps to promote camaraderie and regular participation.

Achieving THR

Aerobic dance programs can develop all the fitness components. The recommended frequency, intensity, and total work (see chapter 10) can be achieved when exercising to music and can increase $\dot{V}O_2$max (19). THR can be monitored easily after a music segment, but beginners need to be cautioned about doing too much too soon. One study found that THR can be achieved with either low- or high-impact routines. Although the energy cost of high-intensity, high-impact aerobic dance is higher than that of low-impact programs for the same routines and music, the activities do not differ much in caloric expenditure when multidirectional movements are included in the low-impact routines (19).

Low Skill Requirement

Movement to music can be adapted to any skill level because no competition is involved. The only rule is to keep moving at a pace needed to achieve THR. The routines can also be adapted for all ages. Most aerobics classes provide participants with an appropriate workout routine within a safe environment (assuming instructors are certified and emphasize safe exercises). Warm-ups are structured to provide low-impact movements and dynamic stretching before 30 to 40 min of cardiovascular work. Gradual progression within each session, as well as from one workout to the next, enhances enjoyment.

Fitness professionals should be familiar with the aerobic dance programs offered in their community, because some (e.g., Jazzercise) may require more knowledge of dance movements. Fitness professionals should also be aware of the programs that are appropriate for people of different ages, skill levels, and interests.

Disadvantages

Injury is always a potential risk in fitness programs, and aerobic dance is no different. One review found that about 44% of students and 76% of instructors reported injuries resulting from aerobic dance, with the injury rate being 1 injury per 100 hr of activity for students and 0.22 to 1.16 injuries per 100 hr for the instructors. The severity of the injuries, however, was such that only once in 1,092 to 4,275 hr of participation did an individual require medical attention (7). For those who want to participate in aerobic dance, a reasonable suggestion is that they do so only after they can walk 2 mi · day^{-1} at a moderate intensity, without discomfort. They should move from low-intensity, low-impact sessions to more strenuous sessions using THR as a guide. Further, introductory classes to step or other specialized forms of aerobics should be taken to develop the skills needed for participation in the regular classes.

It is not uncommon for individuals to experience muscle soreness, as well as a variety of acute soft-tissue injuries, because of regularly participating in aerobic activities. In addition, evidence shows that chronic conditions may develop because of improper form or simply from doing many repetitions of a specific exercise. These chronic conditions can include the following:

- Chronic shoulder soreness from too many overhead pulls
- Elbow or wrist pain from using handheld weights in aerobics classes
- Achilles tendinitis and plantar fasciitis from high-impact forces and improper step techniques
- Groin pulls and shin splints from improper slide technique
- Low-back problems from exercising with weak abdominals (anterior pelvic tilt) and from improperly stretching
- Knee problems from using a step that is too high

It is also common for instructors and participants to experience some hearing losses from music played too loudly. See chapter 25 for advice on how to prevent and deal with acute and chronic problems associated with exercise participation.

Here are some suggestions to minimize the risk of injury when exercising to music:

- Participants should warm up with low-impact activity and dynamic stretching and should cool down by statically stretching the following muscles: calf, anterior tibialis, quadriceps, hamstrings, hip flexors, low-back area, and shoulders.
- Participants should avoid hyperextension of the neck.
- Participants should avoid forward flexion of the spine unless supported by a bent knee balanced directly over the heel.
- Participants should practice correct standing posture (i.e., pelvis in neutral position, buttocks tight, head and chin up, shoulders back).
- Participants should avoid deep-knee bends and should not squat to where the thighs are below parallel and the knees are over the toes rather than placed properly over the middle of the foot.
- Participants should wear shoes with good cushioning and support.
- Participants should work all muscle groups evenly to achieve a balanced workout.
- Participants should not stop in the middle of a routine, because this can cause venous pooling in the lower legs.
- The leader should practice routines to ensure that movement transitions are smooth, safe, and easy to follow and should teach basic movements before using them in combination.
- The leader should monitor the class at all times and use eye contact, emphasize safe movements by making corrections while leading, and check THR or RPE regularly.

Music Selection

The music for different phases of the exercise session sets the tone for the intensity of the warm-up, aerobic, and cool-down phases (10, 12). The music can vary, depending on choice, from Top 40 hits to instrumental Muzak. The warm-up starts slowly, with a music tempo of about 100 beats · min^{-1}. The cardiorespiratory endurance phase includes increasingly intense aerobic exercises at a faster pace (no more than 160 beats · min^{-1}), whereas the muscle conditioning phase (typically including abdominal work) is set to a slower tempo (usually 118-130 beats · min^{-1}). Step classes are limited to 118 to 125 beats · min^{-1}, and slide classes are restricted to <140 beats · min^{-1}. In the final cool-down, the music tempo and volume are decreased for a relaxing conclusion.

The leader should consider purchasing music selections from one of the many aerobic music companies in the fitness market. They sell professionally mixed music selections with appropriate tempos for each class. Not only are the tapes made for specific classes (e.g., step, slide, low impact), but most companies pay the licensing fees that protect the instructor from suits related to fraud. The music should be changed periodically to provide variety.

Components

There are no set routines; the instructor can individualize the program. An exercise session should include a full-body warm-up (including low-impact and dynamic flexibility exercises); exercises for cardiorespiratory endurance using a variety of muscle groups; a recovery cool-down; exercises for muscular endurance and strength for the arms, legs, and abdominal muscles; and a final cool-down.

An easy progression for beginners includes 25 to 30 min of mostly flexibility activities, with light muscular and cardiorespiratory endurance activities. A more advanced program lasts 45 to 60 min, devoting more time to all of the fitness components. The phases of classes for exercising to music are discussed next.

Warm-Up

For a gradual progression, the program should begin with low-impact movements and dynamic stretching for the whole body. Dynamic flexibility includes exercises such as arm circles, side bends, back rolls, half-knee bends, stationary lunges, toe taps, and Achilles curls. The warm-up should continue for 5 to 10 min, gradually increasing the HR and preparing the body for the cardiorespiratory workout to come.

Cardiorespiratory Endurance

In this segment, movements concentrate on the large muscles of the legs, with arm movements adding flair and extra cardiorespiratory intensity (arm movements are optional). This segment is specific to the class. For the high-intensity, low-impact classes, marches, step touches, hops, strides, skips, knee lifts, hamstring curls, jumping jacks, step hops, crossover steps, toe–heel kicks, and so forth are used to elevate the HR to within the target zone. The instructor can individualize the style from a calisthenics workout to a funky dance routine.

If the class uses a step or slide, the leader should be trained in that form of movement to provide safe instruction. Aerobics instructors must hold a national certification and be able to lead a class with smooth transitions before leading a class on their own.

The cardiorespiratory section lasts 15 to 40 min, with THR taken about every 15 min. The intensity of this segment can be increased by using more vigorous arm movements or higher hops (power jumps), and it can be decreased by lowering the arms, slowing the pace, and walking rather than jogging through the movement. Stay within the safety guidelines for speed of music, height of step, and width of slide. This element of control will enhance the participants' safety.

Recovery Cool-Down

A 2 to 5 min active, standing cool-down should follow the cardiorespiratory segment. It should begin by lowering the intensity of the previous activities (e.g., with walking) to decrease the HR. Dynamic stretches should be repeated, followed by static stretches.

Muscular Endurance

Once the recovery cool-down is completed, muscular endurance exercises can be performed for 10 to 20 min. These activities should begin in the standing position and gradually move to the floor. Many classes end with abdominal work in the supine position.

Final Cool-Down

The final cool-down consists mainly of static stretches done lying on the floor. The stretches are held for at least 10 sec. Incorporate every muscle group, especially those specifically worked on during the class, and focus on the hamstrings and low back.

Aerobic Dance Organizations

Here are some of the many aerobic dance organizations that certify instructors as well as provide educational and professional support materials:

- Aerobics and Fitness Association of America (AFAA) (www.afaa.com)
- American Council on Exercise (ACE) (www.acefitness.org)
- Jazzercise (www.jazzercise.com)

Key Point

Beginning dance exercisers should be able to walk 2 mi · day^{-1} at a moderate intensity and without discomfort before participating in aerobic dance programs. Components of an exercise session include a full-body warm-up; exercises for cardiorespiratory endurance using a variety of muscle groups; an active recovery cool-down; exercises for muscular endurance and strength for the arms, legs, and abdominals; and a final cool-down.

Exercise Equipment

The traditional walk, jog, run, and dance programs have been supplemented in many fitness clubs by exercise equipment such as treadmills, cycle ergometers, ski machines, rowers, climbing ergometers, and stepping devices. Equipment can help a participant stay with an exercise program as well as provide feedback about the number of calories used. Participants with orthopedic limitations can choose weight-supported activities (e.g., cycle ergometers). People training for specific performance goals can do so in air-conditioned comfort, although air conditioning may be a problem for participants who plan to engage in races scheduled for hot days. The issue of acclimatization to a hot environment must be addressed for reasons of performance and safety (see chapters 10 and 25).

If a participant plans to buy exercise equipment for home use, the fitness professional can help with the decision by encouraging experimentation with all types of equipment and, within each type (e.g., rowing machines), with as many brands as possible. Equipment may appear expensive in the short term, but it may be a wise investment in the long run by reducing health care costs.

Generally, fitness clubs provide a variety of resistance training equipment that can be used as part of an overall workout or as a separate resistance training workout. Chapter 12 covered recommendations for gains in muscular strength and endurance. The emphasis at the start of a program must be endurance, low resistance, and high repetitions. As strength and interest increase, some participants may shift to high-resistance, low-repetition workouts. It is important to work all the major muscle groups evenly rather than concentrate on gaining strength in only a few muscle groups.

Key Point

Exercise equipment can add variety to a program and increase the number of muscle groups engaged in a workout. In addition, some devices (e.g., cycles) can provide relief for those who experience joint-related pain or discomfort.

Circuit Training

Circuit training can be an effective exercise program. The point is to maximize the variety of exercise, distribute the work over a larger muscle mass than can be engaged with a single form of exercise, and include exercises for all aspects of a fitness session. Circuits can include the following:

- Moving from one piece of exercise equipment to another with a brief rest accompanying each move. A person might exercise for 5 to 10 min (or 50-100 kcal) on a cycle ergometer, then on a treadmill, then on a rower, then on a bench step, and so on.
- A typical workout for muscular strength and endurance, in which one set is done on a specific machine before moving to the next, and the rotation is repeated 2 to 3 times (see chapter 12).
- A circuit set up around the perimeter of a large room with signs posted describing specific exercises that the participant should do during one trip around the circuit. The circuit could include warm-up activities, flexibility activities, strengthening exercises using body weight as a resistance, and, of course, aerobic activities. Beginning, intermediate, and advanced goals specifying the number of repetitions (or duration) can be posted at each station. Include a station to check the THR after the aerobic exercise stations.

Good examples of walk, jog, run circuits have been in place for the past decade. Many communities have set up jogging trails that have signposts along the way indicating specific exercises to do at each stop. They can be found in many cities, and they provide a break in the regular routine of steady jogging or running while adding flexibility and strengthening exercises.

Key Point

Circuit training offers variety and can include exercises in all aspects of fitness (e.g., cardiorespiratory, muscle strength and endurance, flexibility). The preceding list suggests a few circuit training possibilities.

Case Studies

You can check your answers by referring to page 473 in appendix A.

1. You are making a presentation to a group of adults who have their own neighborhood walking program. What topics should you address to emphasize safety and comfort?
2. A participant who has been involved in your walking program for the past 10 wk asks your advice on taking an aerobic dance class. What would you recommend?

PART IV

Special Populations

This section for the fifth edition of the *Fitness Professional's Handbook* is based on several interrelated factors:

- Physical activity benefits people of both sexes, all ages, and a variety of medical conditions.
- Recommendations for physical activity need to address unique factors that can have a bearing on the exercises selected for the individual (e.g., age, medical condition, etc.)
- Strategies for behavior modification need to be appropriate for different groups.
- Fitness professionals are increasingly expected to work with individuals with a variety of clinical conditions.

In chapters 15, 16, and 17 we explain special characteristics and health challenges for children, older adults, and women. In chapters 18, 19, 20, and 21, we provide

(continued)

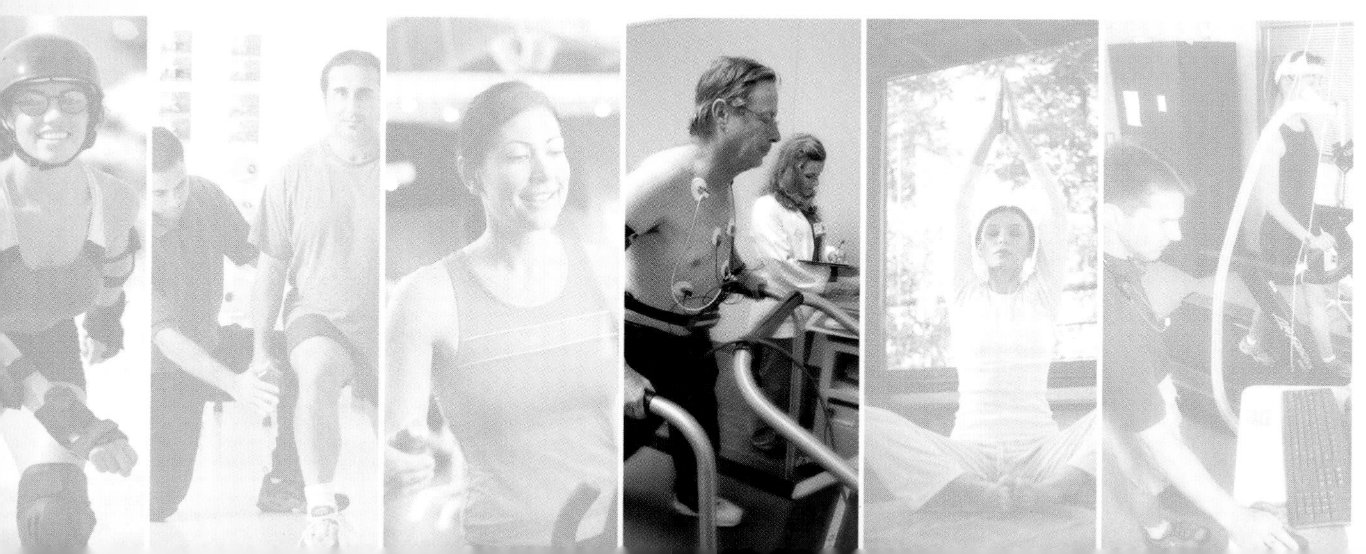

recommendations to ensure safe and effective physical activity for people experiencing some of the major health problems of today, including

- heart disease and hypertension (chapter 18);
- obesity, the new public health epidemic (chapter 19);
- diabetes (chapter 20); and
- asthma and other pulmonary problems (chapter 21).

Any one of these topics could make a complete book in and of itself. Our purpose is to help fitness professionals appreciate the importance of these populations; understand the role of physical activity in the quality of life for all people; and provide practical guidelines for special screening, testing, supervision, and activity modifications for each population.

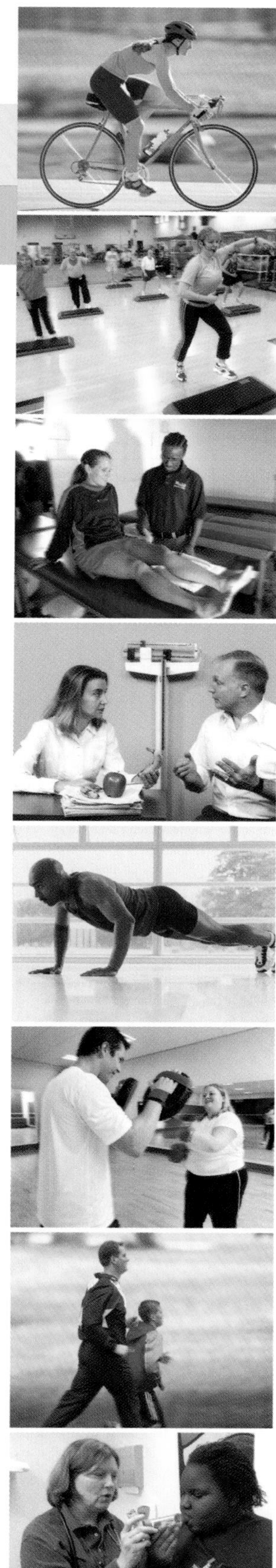

15 CHAPTER

Exercise and Children and Youth

Objectives

The reader will be able to do the following:

1. Understand why physical activity is important for children and youth.
2. Compare the responses of children, youth, and adults to acute and chronic exercise.
3. Prescribe physical activity for children and youth.
4. Describe health-related physical fitness testing for children and youth.
5. Describe special precautions for exercise and testing of children and youth.

Evidence shows that physical activity is essential for attaining the highest quality of life throughout the life span; however, most of the experimental research on how exercise affects fitness has been conducted on young adults. Most of the epidemiological research on how physical activity improves health outcomes has emphasized older adults. One of the common conclusions drawn from the research is that regular physical activity needs to be integrated with one's lifestyle. It is recommended that this active lifestyle begin early in life. Although the correlations for tracking physical activity across various ages are not very high, Malina (11) concluded, "Allowing for the different methods for estimating habitual physical activity, change associated with normal growth and maturation, and lack of control for important covariates in studies of tracking, physical activity tracks reasonably well from childhood into young adulthood" (p. 7). There is increasing evidence that physical activity also enhances the health and fitness of children and youth.

In the United States, there is increasing emphasis on motivating people of all ages to begin and continue regular physical activity (31). In addition, physical fitness testing for children and youth is a part of many physical education programs.

This chapter deals with how to implement regular physical activity programs for children and youth and the role of fitness testing in the young. We focus on school-aged children and youth. Although not covered in this chapter, physical development is vital in preschool infants and children (8, 15). The emphases of activity during the first years of life are primarily on motor development and healthy growth and are very individualized.

Key Point

Regular physical activity is essential for attaining the highest quality of life throughout the life span. Children and youth need physical activity as an integral part of their lifestyle.

Response to Exercise

This section reviews the immediate (acute) and long-term (chronic) effects of physical activity for children and youth and compares the exercise reactions of children and youth with those of adults (see chapter 28).

Acute

Zwiren (33) described in detail the differences between children and adults in terms of acute response to exercise. Adults and children are similar in

- $\dot{V}O_2max$ in $ml \cdot kg^{-1} \cdot min^{-1}$ (endurance tasks can be performed well), and
- creatine phosphate + ATP (children can deal well with very brief, intense exercise).

Children are lower in their

- capacity to generate ATP via glycolysis (children have a lower capacity to do intense activity lasting 10-90 sec),
- ability to dissipate heat via evaporation and acclimatize to heat (children have an increased potential for heat-related illness), and
- economy of walking and running (children require more oxygen to walk or run at the same speed; standard equations listed in chapter 4 for estimating energy expenditure of walking and running cannot be used for children).

Children are better in achieving a steady state in oxygen uptake (children experience a smaller oxygen deficit and faster recovery; they are well suited to intermittent activities).

Key Point

Children have similar acute responses to exercise compared with adults. They are well suited for intermittent activities and should use caution in extreme environmental conditions.

Chronic

Evidence from a recent comprehensive review of the literature on the effect of physical activity on school-aged youth (28) is summarized on page 273. Children and youth experience many of the same health and fitness benefits from regular physical activity that adults experience. An active lifestyle seems to be natural for children, and activity is a normal and essential part of the growth and development that take place during these years (8, 14). This chapter emphasizes the fitness and health aspects of activity for children and youth, but achieving fundamental motor skills (e.g., moving, throwing, catching) is also an important aspect of the active lifestyle (33).

Special Considerations

Children and youth with various medical problems need special attention (3). Young children need to be protected from overemphasizing a specific sport or activity and the

Benefits of Chronic Physical Activity: Children and Youth

Strong Evidence*

Musculoskeletal health
Cardiovascular health
Adiposity in youth who are overweight
Blood pressure in youth who are mildly hypertensive

Adequate Evidence**

Lipid and lipoprotein levels and adiposity in youth with normal weight
Blood pressure in youth with normal weight
Self-concept
Anxiety and depression symptoms
Academic performance

* >60% of studies support finding.
** >30% and <59% of studies support findings.

From W.B. Strong, R.M. Malina, C.J.R. Blimkie, S.R. Daniles., R.K. Dishman, B. Gutin, A.C. Hergenroeder, A. Must, P.A. Nixon, J.M. Pivarnik, T. Rowland, S. Trost, and F. Trudeau, 2005, "Evidenced based physical activity for school-age youth," *J. Pediatrics* 146:732-737.

Key Point

Chronically active youth not only prepare for maintaining active lifestyles as adults but also derive health and fitness benefits during their childhood and adolescence.

intense training that often accompanies it, which can lead to physical or emotional problems. Children and youth should be encouraged to choose many different activities in an enjoyable and fun atmosphere. Young children do not adapt to extreme environmental conditions; thus, more precautions need to be taken when exercising in very hot or cold conditions (1, 33).

Although exercise-related deaths are rare in children, they are most often linked to congenital heart defects (i.e., abnormalities of the heart resulting in imperfect oxygenation of the blood as manifested by cyanosis and breathlessness) or acquired myocarditis (i.e., inflammation of the myocardium). Children with these conditions should avoid intense activities. Children (as well as youth and adults) with other medical conditions (see chapters 18-21) need to modify their activities, but in almost all cases activity can still be healthful. These children and their parents should work with health care professionals to reasonably modify activities (e.g., longer warm-up and cool-down, lower intensity).

Key Point

Children and youth should be screened for cardiovascular problems that might cause exercise-related deaths. Other medical problems can be addressed by modifying activity. The fitness professional should encourage children to enjoy a variety of activities with less emphasis on intense training for competition in one specific sport.

Testing

Concern for the fitness of children and youth goes back over a century. Park's (16) historical review of the topic of fitness and fitness testing indicates that leaders of physical education from the latter part of the 19th century were convinced of the connections among exercise, fitness, and health. Not surprisingly, fitness testing was a part of physical education. Initially, testing in the United States was concerned more with anthropometry and strength, and it sometimes included a medical exam. Tests of motor ability also were developed, but it was a long time before a national test battery of fitness tests for youth became a reality.

The driving force for promoting fitness in the United States in the first half of the 20th century was war or the threat of war, attributable to the concern raised when a large number of young men could not pass a fitness exam for induction into the armed forces. In the early 1950s, a new alarm was sounded when a study showed that a large percentage of American children could not pass basic flexibility and power tests. In response to this concern, President Eisenhower established the President's Council on Youth Fitness. Soon after that, the American Association for Health, Physical Education, and Recreation (AAHPER) published its Youth Fitness Test, with fitness items such as the pull-up, sit-up, shuttle run, standing broad jump, 50 yd (45.7 m) dash, softball throw for distance, and 600 yd (548.6 m) run or walk. This test battery focused on skill-related fitness with an emphasis on muscular power (16).

In the early 1980s, the publications of *Healthy People* and of *Promoting Health/Preventing Disease: Objectives for the Nation* shifted the focus to health-related fitness. In support of this focus, the American Alliance of Health, Physical Education, Recreation and Dance (AAHPERD) published the *Health-Related Physical Fitness Test Manual* for testing fitness components related to health, including the 1 mi (1.6 km) run for cardiorespiratory fitness, skinfold measurements to evaluate body composition, and the sit and reach and the sit-up to evaluate low-back function. Following this publication, the introduction of criterion-referenced standards was advocated to focus on health-related goals rather than maximal performance (16). The criterion-reference standard for cardiorespiratory fitness is 42 ml · kg^{-1} · min^{-1} for males aged 5 to 17. For females, the standard is 40 ml · kg^{-1} · min^{-1} for ages 5 to 9, at which age the standard decreases 1 ml · kg^{-1} · min^{-1} per year until age 14, when the standard becomes 35 ml · kg^{-1} · min^{-1} (9). In short, these standards differ little from those recommended for adults.

Physical Fitness

There are two major physical fitness tests for children and youth (see table 15.1), namely, the Fitnessgram (7) and the test by the President's Council on Physical Fitness and Sports (PCPFS) (18). Both assess cardiorespiratory fitness, muscular strength and endurance, and flexibility. The Fitnessgram and the health-related part of the PCPFS test also check body composition. The PCPFS test includes a test of agility.

The Fitnessgram and the health-related portion of the PCPFS test use health criteria as standards for the tests, whereas the physical fitness portion of the PCPFS test uses percentiles (by age and sex) for its standards.

Clinical Testing

In addition to the contraindications to exercise testing for adults (see chapter 5), Zwiren (33) listed the following reasons not to test children:

- Dyspnea at rest (or forced expiratory volume <60% of predicted value)
- Acute renal disease or hepatitis
- Insulin-dependent diabetes (in subjects who do not take insulin as prescribed) or ketoacidosis
- Acute rheumatic fever with carditis
- Severe pulmonary vascular disease
- Poorly compensated heart failure
- Severe aortic or mitral stenosis
- Hypertrophic cardiomyopathy with syncope

Cardiorespiratory Fitness

Measuring $\dot{V}O_2$max in children using the cycle ergometer or the treadmill has a sound historical foundation (2, 19). The graded exercise (GXT) format is used for children, and the test (initial grade and speed on the treadmill, increments per stage) must match the child in the same way as tests are matched to adults (see chapter 5). Treadmill testing may be easier because the child's shorter attention span can interfere with a cycle protocol. In addition, local muscle fatigue may shorten a cycle ergometer test before the child reaches maximum aerobic power. If a cycle is used for young children, the handlebars, seat height, crank length, and resistance scale must be adjusted (33). Many laboratories use the Bruce protocol, with 2 min stages, or a Balke protocol in which a speed of 3 to 3.5 mi · hr^{-1} (4.8-5.6 km · hr^{-1}) for walking or 5 mi · hr^{-1} (8.1 km · hr^{-1}) for running is constant and the grade is increased 2% per stage (1). Table 15.2 lists the ACSM's recommendations for suitable cycle ergometer protocols for testing children (1).

Table 15.1 Physical Fitness Tests

Fitness component	Fitnessgram[a]	PCPFS[b] fitness	PCPFS health-related
Cardiovascular	1 mi (1.6 km) run[c]	1 mi (1.6 km) run[d]	1 mi (1.6 km) run[d]
Muscular strength and endurance	Curl-up; push-up	Curl-up; push-up[e]	Curl-up; push-up
Flexibility	Sit and reach[e]; trunk lift	Sit and reach[f]	Sit and reach
Body composition	Skinfolds or BMI	—	BMI
Agility	—	Agility run	—

PCPFS = President's Council on Physical Fitness and Sports; BMI = body mass index.
[a]Cooper Institute for Aerobic Research (7).
[b]President's Council on Physical Fitness and Sports President's Challenge (18).
[c]Or the PACER (7).
[d]Shorter distances for younger children (18).
[e]Uses one leg at a time (7).
[f]Or V-sit (18).

Table 15.2 Cycle Ergometer Test Protocols for Children

Protocol	Cadence	Body size	Initial load	Increment per stage	Stage duration (min)
McMaster	50	Height (cm)	W	W	
		<120	12.5	12.5	2
		120-140	12.5	25	2
		140-160	25	25	2
		>160	25	25 (female) 50 (male)	2
James	60-70	Body surface area (m^2)	$kgm \cdot min^{-1}$	$kgm \cdot min^{-1}$	
		<1.0	200	100	3
		1.0-1.2	200	200	3
		>1.2	200	300	3

Reprinted, by permission, from American College of Sports Medicine (ACSM), 2006, *ACSM's guidelines for exercise testing and prescription*, 7th ed. (Philadelphia, PA: Lippincott, Williams & Wilkins), 239. (1). Adapted from O. Bar-Or, 1983, *Pediatric sports medicine for the practitioner* (New York, NY: Springer-Verlag), 315-338, and F. James, S. Kaplan, C. Glueck et al., 1980, "Responses of normal children and young adults to controlled bicycle exercise," *Circulation* 61: 902-912.

Key Point

Fitness testing of children and youth is a part of many school and youth agency programs. The emphasis has usually been on field tests of health-related components of physical fitness. Children and youth can be tested on GXTs with minor modifications.

Recommendations for Physical Activity

As seen on page 273, children and youth enhance their health and well-being through regular physical activity. At a time when many adult diseases are increasingly diagnosed in children and youth, we must be concerned with health throughout the life span. Risk factors for heart disease are increasingly appearing in young people, including obesity, hypertension, and type 2 diabetes (31). The recent increase in childhood obesity is considered a public health epidemic (26, 29). Both healthy and unhealthy behaviors often begin early in life and are more difficult to acquire or change as age progresses. Thus, encouraging children and youth to incorporate physical activity into their daily life may provide the basis for a lifetime of this healthy habit (11). It is now well established that regular physical activity can reduce the risk of developing a wide variety of health problems at all ages (30, 31).

Currently, the trend is to emphasize the physical activity behavior more than the fitness test scores. The major question is, What kinds of physical activities should children do?

During childhood most motor skills (e.g., throwing, jumping, running, riding bikes, swimming) develop. Children are inherently active, and one of the most important elements adults must provide for them is an opportunity to play (8, 14). The need for children to develop motor skills must be kept in mind when attending to fitness goals (33).

Both national physical fitness testing programs (7, 18) now recognize the behavior of physical activity (through the Activitygram and the Presidential Active Lifestyle Award). This allows teachers and youth leaders to reward both the behavior of regular physical activity and the physical fitness outcomes. The Activitygram (7) provides a profile of the type, amount, and intensity of activity. It recommends at least 45 min (in three segments) for children and 30 min (in two segments) for adolescents. The Presidential Active Lifestyle Award (18) provides an award for participating in at least 60 min of activity 5 days per wk for 6 wk. Both are based on the child's self-report of activity. The Activitygram provides more information about the type of activity, although the Presidential Active Lifestyle Award is easier to use.

There are three major reasons for emphasizing an active lifestyle for children and youth:

- Enhancing health and fitness
- Beginning an active lifestyle that can be continued throughout life
- Reducing risks for health problems throughout life

Exercise Prescription for Children (Preadolescents)

The recommendations for adult physical activity can be applied to older, **postpubescent** adolescents. Children

Physical Activity Recommendations for Children Aged 5 to 12

- Avoid extended inactivity (for 2 or more hr), especially during the daytime.
- Accumulate at least 60 min and up to several hours of age-appropriate physical activity on most if not all days of the week.
- Include moderate to vigorous activities lasting 15 min or more, usually on an intermittent basis with lighter activity or rest in between.
- Choose a variety of activities.

Adapted from 8, 14, 17, 33.

(prepubescent and **pubescent)** need to be considered separately—as is often said, they are not miniature adults. The physical activity recommendations for children (6, 8, 14, 17, 33) are summarized above. The recent evidenced-based review of the effects of physical activity on youth supported each of these recommendations (28).

Cardiorespiratory Fitness

In general, the same exercise prescription for cardiorespiratory fitness (CRF) for adults (see chapter 10) can be used for children. Corbin, Pangrazi, and LaMasurier (8) recommended more physical activity for children, recognizing that activity will slightly decline with age. There is some disagreement about whether the standard prescription will increase $\dot{V}O_2max$. The prescription may increase $\dot{V}O_2max$ in pubescent and postpubescent children but may be less effective in younger children (1, 33). This suggests the focus should be on health-related benefits of aerobic exercise rather than simply $\dot{V}O_2max$. When the focus is on health-related benefits, using a variety of continuous physical activities (e.g., cycling, running, in-line skating), team sports (e.g., basketball, soccer), individual and dual sports (e.g., tennis, racquetball), and recreational activities (e.g., hiking) can contribute to energy expenditure and its associated benefits. Parents, schools, and communities must (a) provide opportunities for children to have safe places to walk, run, and cycle; (b) provide organized programs for children to learn and play sports; and (c) focus on personal achievement rather than on winning at all costs.

Key Point

Children should focus on health-related physical activity with a variety of endurance activities appropriate for their age. Long durations of inactivity should be avoided.

Strength

Children can improve muscular strength and endurance by participating in formal resistance training programs. Safety precautions must be taken, however, because children are anatomically, physiologically, and psychologically immature (4, 21, 33). Chapter 12 discusses resistance training programs, including those for children. We will simply highlight some of the more important considerations for children:

- Have the parent or legal guardian complete a health history for each child.
- Ensure that trained personnel supervise each session.
- Adapt equipment to children.
- Teach proper lifting techniques.
- Have children perform 1 or 2 sets of 8 to 10 different exercises (with 8-15 repetitions per set) and include major muscle groups.
- Increase resistance only when the child can perform the desired number of repetitions in good form.
- Do 2 or 3 nonconsecutive sessions each week.
- Encourage other activities.

Key Point

Children can benefit from resistance training. Such training should emphasize safety, supervision for proper form, and muscular endurance (i.e., less resistance and more repetitions).

Exercise Prescription for Youth (Pubescent and Postpubescent)

Rowland (20) pointed out that the motivation for activity shifts from a biological one in children to a more psychosocial one in adolescence. Many of the adolescent psychosocial factors negatively influence physical activity, resulting in the well-known decline in physical activity, especially among females. Although the recommendations for physical activity are essentially the same as those for adults (25), the strategy for enhancing motivation must target these adolescent psychosocial factors (22). Youth sport can fill the need for appropriate motivation. An increasing number of females are participating in sport (27), from fewer than 300,000 in 1971 to more than 2 million in 1995; however, that number is still only 63% of the number of male participants. Both Bunker (5) and Weiss (32) emphasized a wide variety of accessible activities that promote self-esteem and can be done in an enjoyable atmosphere.

As Morrow and Jackson (13) indicated, physical education helps promote physical activity for children and adolescents. A number of programs, such as Coordinated School Health (12), SPARK (23), and PATH (10), have shown that physical education programs can have a positive effect on both children (23) and youth (10). In addition, the increased time spent on physical education does not diminish achievement in other subject areas (24). Finally, a principal recommendation from the evidenced-based review of physical activity and youth was to restore daily physical education programs and after-school intramural programs to address the lack of physical activity in adolescents (28). In the United States, we must invest in our children when we can influence their physical activity—when they are at school. If we don't invest the money now, we will pay interest in the form of disease-related costs in the years ahead.

Key Point

Young people can benefit from adult exercise prescription; however, motivation for physical activity shifts toward peer influence.

Case Studies

You can check your answers by referring to page 473 in appendix A.

1. A parent has read that for major strength gains, the weightlifter should use a resistance that can be lifted for only 3 to 6 repetitions. He knows that strength is important for some of the sports his 9-yr-old son wants to play, so he asks for your advice. What would you tell him?
2. A parent's group is recommending that additional reading and math be included in the schools by reducing time for physical education and recess. The school board has asked you to respond to this recommendation. How would you respond?

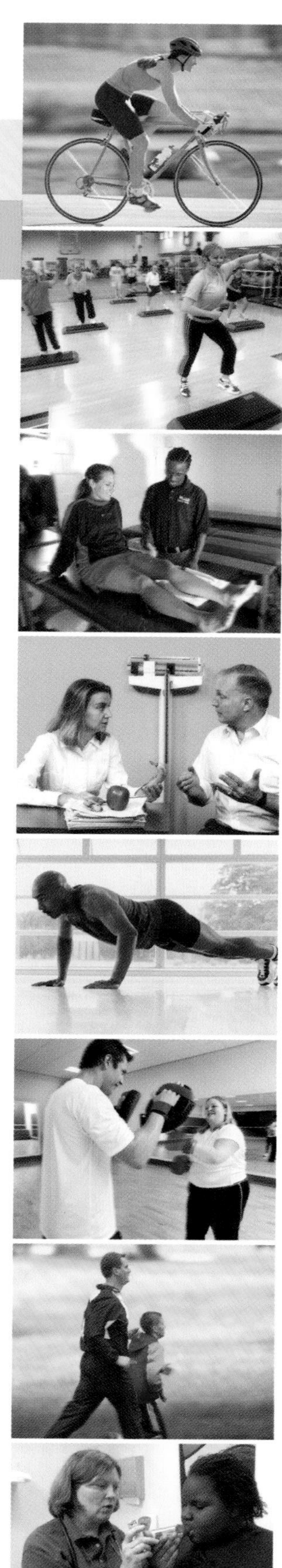

16 CHAPTER

Exercise and Older Adults

Objectives

The reader will be able to do the following:

1. Describe the changes in the number of people older than 65 yr that will take place during the first three decades of the 21st century, and provide a brief profile of the older population, indicating factors that affect the delivery of fitness-related programs.
2. Describe the typical changes in $\dot{V}O_2max$, strength, body composition, and flexibility that occur with age and the effect of exercise training on each.
3. Describe modifications to exercise tests to accommodate typical limitations seen in the older population.
4. Describe functional tests used to evaluate the different components of fitness.
5. Explain why it is necessary to address individual differences in the older population regarding exercise prescription.
6. Provide general guidelines for exercise prescription for cardiorespiratory fitness, muscular fitness, and flexibility for the older population.

A constant theme throughout this text is the importance of physical activity and exercise in leading a healthy life. This message is especially important for older people, the fastest growing segment of the population. The baby boom generation (those born between 1946 and 1960) was a spike in the birth rate in the United States after World War II; these individuals are now coming to full maturity. Figure 16.1 shows the changes in the number of persons over age 65, projected to the year 2030 (26). The number actually doubles between 2000 and 2030 because of the baby boom generation. In addition, because of advances in hygiene and medicine over the past century, life expectancy has increased in general and with it the numbers of individuals living to advanced ages. Shephard (21) described age classifications and characteristics of those aged 40 to 85 and older:

- Middle age—40 to 65 yr; 10% to 30% loss of biological functions.
- Old age—also called young old age; 65 to 75 yr; further loss of function.
- Very old age—75 to 85 yr; substantial impairment in function but can still lead an independent life.
- Oldest old age—over 85 yr; institutional or nursing care typically is needed.

Currently, there are 16 times more persons in the 75 to 84 age group and 38 times more persons in the 85+ age group than there were in 1900 (26). These latter age groups already have had a major effect on health delivery systems, financing of health care, family issues in caring for parents and grandparents, and general concerns about quality of life for those contemplating retirement. These changes also affect the role of the fitness professional in providing appropriate physical activity and exercise programs to increase and maintain health and fitness in older individuals. Are fitness clubs ready to welcome older participants when the focus has been on younger, healthier age groups? Are the personnel trained to serve the special needs of the older age groups? This chapter summarizes important health and fitness information related to this age group. We recommend consulting the following references to gain a more complete understanding: *Physical Dimensions of Aging* (23), *Aging, Physical Activity, and Health* (21), the ACSM's "Exercise and Physical Activity for Older Adults" (1), and Holloszy and Kohrt's review on aging and exercise in the *Handbook of Physiology* (13).

Overview

A variety of demographic and physiological characteristics of the older population (>65 yr of age) affect the planning of fitness facilities, the programming options available, and the kinds of emergencies to anticipate. The following, from *A Profile of Older Americans: 2003* (26), provides some insights into the population as a whole:

- There are four times as many widows (8.9 million) as widowers (2 million) in this age group.
- The majority live in a family setting; however, as the population ages, the number living alone or in an institution increases.

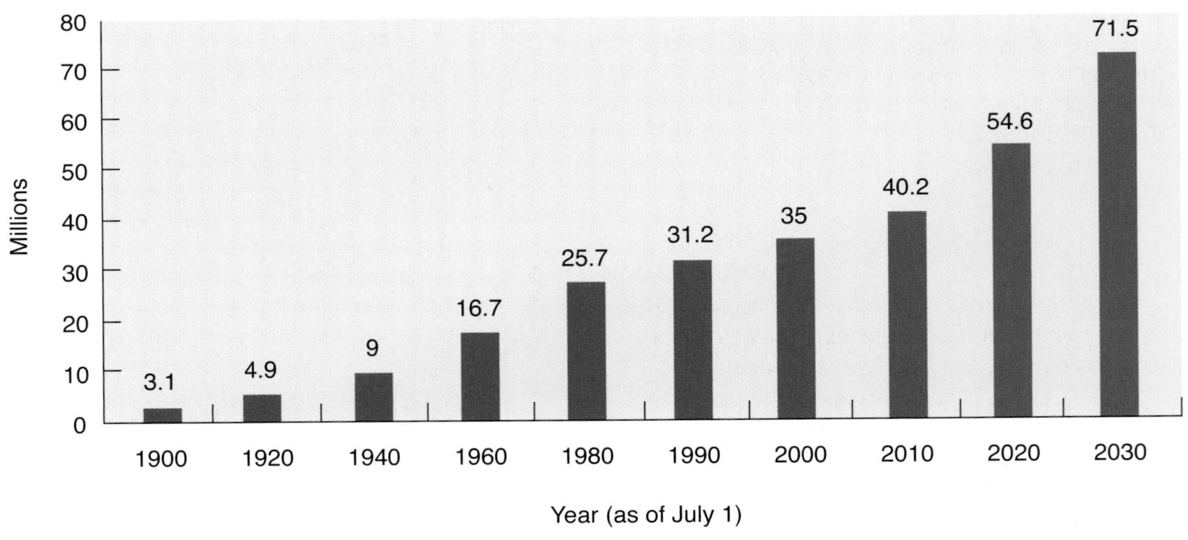

Figure 16.1 Number of persons aged 65 yr and older, from 1900 to 2030. Increments in years are uneven.
From U.S. Department of Health and Human Services, 2003, *A profile of older Americans: 2003* (Washington, DC: Author).

- In 2003, 75.4% of older White Americans rated their health as excellent or very good, versus 57.7% of African Americans and 60.5% of Hispanics.
- Physical activity limitations increase with age. More than half (54.4%) of those over 65 yr report one disability, and a third (37.7%) report a severe disability. The disabilities interfered with their capacity to carry out activities of daily living (ADLs) and instrumental activities of daily living (IADLs), that is, preparing meals, shopping, and doing housework.
- Most older persons have at least one chronic condition and many have several. These include hypertension (49%), arthritis (36%), heart disease (31%), any cancer (20%), and diabetes (15%).

This brief demographic profile indicates that fitness programs must address health-screening issues, the need for socialization, joint-protective activities, prevention or treatment of chronic diseases, and pragmatic goals to maintain independent living (21). However, these characteristics (i.e., type and severity of disease, physical limitations, fitness) are not uniformly distributed across the older population and we must attend to individual differences. We address this issue in the sections dealing with exercise prescription.

Key Point

The number of older individuals in the United States is increasing as the baby boom generation comes to full maturity. Older participants present special challenges to fitness professionals because of chronic disease conditions and physical activity limitations. Programs must address prevention and reduction of the progression of chronic diseases as well as increasing or maintaining fitness to allow for independent living.

Effects of Aging on Fitness

There is no question that physiological function decreases with age; however, some functions age faster than others. Further compounding the problem, each person displays a unique rate of aging that is influenced by genetic and environmental (e.g., education, health care, economic status, nutrition, exercise) factors (23). Consequently, it is not uncommon to find a person who is intellectually young but physically old or a 70-yr-old who has the physiological capacity of a 50-yr-old.

In general, the common chronic diseases that contribute to morbidity in older adults respond to exercise interventions in a manner similar to that of younger adults. Endurance training

- improves blood lipids (linked more to a reduction in body fatness rather than exercise),
- lowers BP to the same degree as shown for younger individuals with hypertension, and
- improves glucose tolerance and insulin sensitivity (1).

As described earlier in the text, the primary fitness components (cardiorespiratory fitness, muscular fitness, body composition, and flexibility) affect our ability to perform work and engage in recreational pursuits at any age. Although natural changes in these fitness components occur with age, the evidence is overwhelming that regular exercise maintains fitness at considerably better levels than does a sedentary lifestyle. The following sections address each fitness component.

Cardiorespiratory Fitness

Figure 16.2 shows that maximal aerobic power ($\dot{V}O_2max$) decreases at the rate of about 1% per year in healthy men and women after the age of 20 (13). This decrease is due to both inactivity and weight gain as well as to aging. Some studies show that this rate of decline is reduced by half in men who maintain a vigorous exercise program, but not without exception (2, 13). Women show a 10% decline per decade independent of activity status (7); however, trained women, as expected, have a higher $\dot{V}O_2max$ at any age compared with their sedentary counterparts (9). It should be no surprise that the decrease in $\dot{V}O_2max$

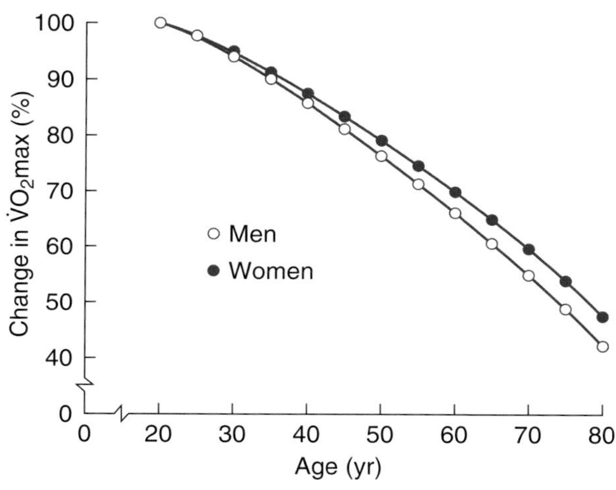

Figure 16.2 Percent change in $\dot{V}O_2max$ with age in men and women.

Adapted, by permission, from J.O. Holloszy and W.M. Kohrt, 1995, Exercise. In *Handbook of Physiology, Section II: Aging*, edited by E.J. Mason (Bethesda, MD: American Physiological Society), 633-666, figure 24.2.

affects endurance performance. Average running speed in distance races decreases about 1% per year, suggesting a link between the decrease in $\dot{V}O_2max$ and performance in distance running. However, a variety of other factors (e.g., running economy, lactate threshold, joint trauma) also might affect running performance (13).

The fact that all people experience a decline in $\dot{V}O_2max$ with age means that by the time of retirement, the ability to engage in routine physical activities has been compromised. This reduced capacity for work can further reduce physical activity, setting up a vicious cycle leading to lower and lower levels of cardiorespiratory fitness. This may result in the inability to perform ADLs, which would affect quality of life and independence (23).

Maximal oxygen uptake (see chapter 28) equals the product of maximal cardiac output (maximal HR · maximal stroke volume) and maximal oxygen extraction (systemic arteriovenous oxygen difference). There is no question that maximal HR decreases with age (e.g., 220 – age) and is the major contributor to the age-related decrease in maximal cardiac output. The Frank-Starling mechanism (greater stretch of the ventricle due to higher venous return) appears to compensate for the lower maximal HR in middle age and so reduces the magnitude of change in maximal cardiac output, but this mechanism is less effective in old age (1, 13). Maximal oxygen extraction is also lower in the elderly compared with younger sedentary adults, but this decrease is probably attributable more to their level of inactivity than to a true aging effect. Endurance training increases $\dot{V}O_2max$ about 10% to 30% in older individuals, an increase similar to that of young adults (1, 13). The increase in $\dot{V}O_2max$ is due to an increase in both maximal cardiac output and oxygen extraction in older men but is due almost entirely to an increase in oxygen extraction in older women. This may be related to the observation that older women show little or no increase in left ventricle mass, end diastolic volume, or maximal stroke volume after endurance training. The increase in oxygen extraction is due to increases in capillary number and mitochondrial enzymes, just as in younger adults (13).

Key Point

$\dot{V}O_2max$ decreases about 1% per year in sedentary men and women because of a decrease in both maximal cardiac output and maximal oxygen extraction. Endurance training increases $\dot{V}O_2max$ in older adults as it does in younger adults. The greater $\dot{V}O_2max$ results from gains in both maximal cardiac output and oxygen extraction in men but is due solely to an increase in oxygen extraction in women.

Muscular Strength and Endurance

Muscular strength begins to decline at about age 30, but the majority of the decrease occurs after age 50, when it falls at the rate of 15% per decade, with a more rapid decline of 30% per decade after age 70 (15, 20). The loss of strength relates directly to a loss of muscle mass (sarcopenia), with the latter attributable primarily to a loss of muscle fibers (motor units) and secondarily to an atrophy of those muscle fibers (primarily type II) that remain (see figure 16.3). However, the distribution of fiber types is maintained across age, as is strength per cross-sectional area of muscle (1, 13, 15, 20).

Maintaining muscle mass is important, not only for preserving the ability to carry out daily activities but also for its link to resting metabolic rate (see chapter 11) and the risks of type 2 diabetes and hypertension (2, 20). Considerable evidence shows that an intense (~80% 1RM) resistance training program increases both muscle mass

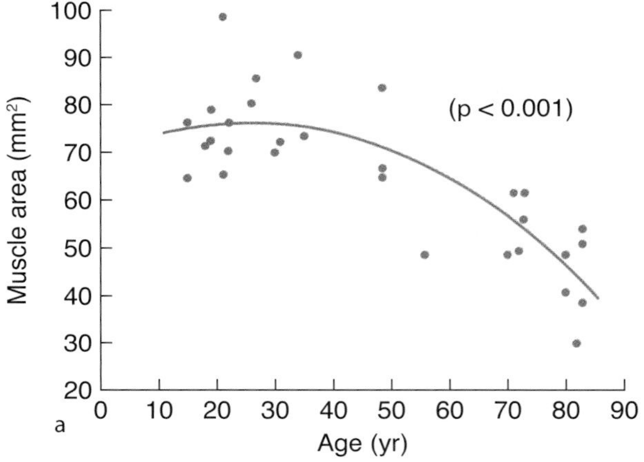

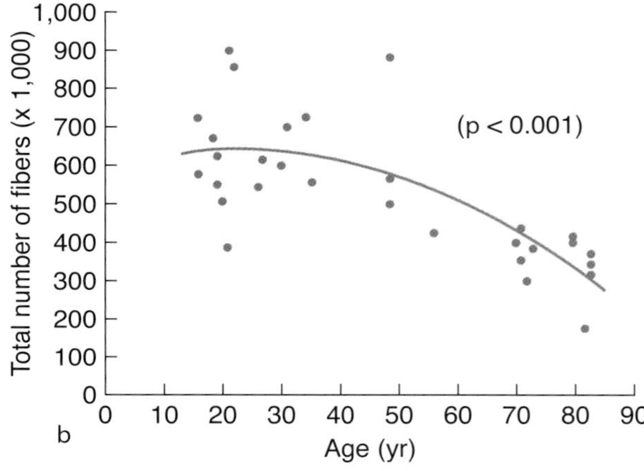

Figure 16.3 *(a)* Relationship between age and muscle area of whole vastus lateralis muscle cross sections. *(b)* Relationship between total number of fibers and age in whole vastus lateralis muscle.

Adapted, by permission, from M.A. Rigers and W.J. Evans, 1993, "Changes in skeletal muscle with aging: Effects of exercise training," *Exercise and Sport Sciences Reviews* 21: 65-102.

Key Point

Muscular strength decreases with age because of a loss of motor units (muscle mass) as well as a reduction in the size of the muscle fibers that remain. Intense resistance training (~80% 1RM) causes large (>100%) increases in strength, attributable primarily to neural factors, because muscle fiber size increases only 10% to 30%.

and strength in 60- to 96-yr-old individuals (8, 12). These training programs resulted in modest increases in muscle fiber area (10%-30%) but very large increases (>100%) in 1RM strength. The disproportionate increase in strength is similar to what is observed when young adults participate in intense resistance training programs (see chapter 12) and is ascribed to neural adaptations. There is also evidence that resistance training can increase $\dot{V}O_2max$ in this population (11). For the elderly who are frail, it is even recommended that resistance training should precede aerobic conditioning because they must be able to rise from a chair and maintain balance and posture in order to walk (1).

Body Composition

Chapters 6 and 11 provided details about health risks, measurement issues, and fitness programs for body composition. In general, body fatness increases from about 16% (males) and 25% (females) in 25-yr-olds to 28% (males) and 41% (females) in 75-yr-olds. This amounts to a gain of about 10 kg of fat for both groups during that time. Fat-free mass is stable until about age 40 but decreases 3% (males) and 4% (females) per decade between age 40 and 60 and 6% (males) and 10% (females) per decade from age 60 to 80 (13).

Evidence indicates that the increase in body fat relates to a sedentary lifestyle rather than to an increase in food intake or an aging effect. Cross-sectional and longitudinal studies on older male and female athletes suggest that regular vigorous exercise is associated with maintaining a stable weight during aging (13). However, observations of highly trained athletes indicate that body fatness still increases about 2% per decade. Consequently, vigorous exercise attenuates, but does not prevent, the increase in body fatness that accompanies age. However, when body composition in older adults changes due to exercise, most of the body fat is lost from central stores, which reduces the risk of metabolic and cardiovascular diseases (13). Exercise is also important in dealing with the loss of bone mineral density with age, but there is more to that story (see Bone).

Key Point

An increase in body fat with age is attributed more to a decrease in physical activity than to an increase in caloric intake. Vigorous exercise is associated with maintaining a stable body weight with increasing age, and exercise intervention results in the loss of body fat from central stores, which is associated with reduced risk of cardiovascular and metabolic diseases.

Bone

Bone mineral density (BMD), a measure of bone mass, decreases with age at about the same rate as the fat-free mass; however, in women bone loss accelerates after menopause (13). Accelerated bone loss is a major concern because the risk of fractures increases as BMD decreases. A general recommendation is to maximize BMD through adequate calcium intake and physical activity before age 30 and then to reduce the rate of loss from that point in time (3, 5). Hormone levels (estrogen and testosterone), calcium intake, and physical activity affect the rate of loss of BMD. The higher rate of loss of BMD after menopause can be prevented by hormone replacement therapy. Vigorous exercise and calcium intake are important in maintaining BMD but cannot substitute for hormone replacement therapy. Older individuals need additional calcium (see chapter 7) to help maintain BMD and possibly to realize the full benefits of increased physical activity. The most effective exercise programs for bone health in older women include activities that

- involve a wide variety of muscle groups and movement directions,
- are weight bearing (e.g., walking, jogging),
- strengthen most muscle groups, and
- generally exceed 75% of maximal capacity for both strength and endurance.

However, in older adults with severe osteoporosis, impact-producing and forward spinal flexion exercises should be avoided (5).

Flexibility

The ability to move a joint through its normal ROM is an important factor related to the ability to carry out daily activities and to the risk of low-back pain (see chapter 9). Joint motion is influenced by the condition of the muscle, connective, and cartilage tissues associated with the joint. In general, the increase in collagen cross-linkages in tendons and ligaments and a degradation of articular cartilage contribute to decrease joint ROM with age (1). However, in evaluating the health of a joint it is difficult to separate aging effects from those associated with chronic inactivity.

Because of the variability in the number of subjects, the types of research design, and the methods of assessment in studies investigating the effect of training on flexibility, it is difficult to provide a general profile of the training effect as was done for $\dot{V}O_2$max and strength (1, 18, 23). However, general programs of physical activity as well as special ROM exercise programs have been shown to improve flexibility in people who are very old (21). Clearly, additional research is needed in this area.

Key Point

Possessing adequate flexibility throughout old age contributes to the ability to perform ADLs and maintain independence. Flexibility can be improved through general programs of physical activity and special ROM exercises.

Special Considerations Regarding Exercise Testing

Age is a risk factor because the likelihood of developing serious conditions increases with age. The passage of time allows the consequences of poor health behaviors (e.g., smoking, high-fat diet, inactivity) to add up and manifest themselves as a major medical problem (e.g., lung cancer, atherosclerosis, glucose intolerance). Consequently, fitness professionals must follow the ACSM risk stratification guidelines (3) closely when working with the elderly (1).

Risk stratification provides clear guidance for test selection and personnel requirements. Clearly, with the higher incidence of CVD in the older age groups, diagnostic exercise testing may be used as part of a medical exam. However, standard submaximal CRF tests (see chapter 5) may be used as part of a fitness assessment. Independent of the reason for testing, modifications may be necessary to address certain limitations (3, 7, 22):

Instrumentation

- A cycle ergometer may be a better choice for those with arthritis of the knee or hip or those with balance problems.
- Tracking cadence may be a problem unless an electronic cycle ergometer is available.
- If a treadmill is used, additional practice may be needed, with emphasis on slow walking speeds.

Intensity and Progression

- As mentioned in chapter 5, for deconditioned persons with low $\dot{V}O_2$max values, the initial intensity of a GXT should be low, increments per stage should be small, and perhaps the time (3 versus 2 min) per stage should be longer so the person can achieve a steady state.

Exercise Prescription

The Surgeon General's report on physical activity and health (25) documented that many adults do not participate in any leisure-time physical activity. The problem gets worse with age; 27% of persons aged 65 to 74 report that they engage in regular leisure-time physical activity, compared with only 17% of those aged 75 or older (26). Clearly, the general recommendation that adults should participate in moderate physical activity on most, preferably all, days of the week is an essential message for all ages, but especially for older individuals who are positioned to gain substantially from an increase in physical activity (17). However, an activity that might constitute moderate work for a younger, fitter adult may be classified as very heavy for an older adult (see figure 10.8) (14).

The only thing two 65-yr-old men in your fitness class may have in common is their age! They may differ substantially in their health risk (chronic diseases), cardiorespiratory fitness ($\dot{V}O_2$max), and experience with exercise. Scientists and clinicians (10, 19, 23) have developed a variety of classification schemes to deal with this reality; Rimmer's (19) classification scheme is representative of these:

Level I *Healthy:* No major medical problems; in relatively good condition for age; has exercised the past 5 yr.

Level II *Ambulatory, nonactive:* No major medical problems; has never participated in a structured exercise program.

Level III *Ambulatory, disease failure:* Diagnosed as having severe CAD, arthritis, diabetes, or chronic obstructive pulmonary disease.

Level IV *Frail elderly:* Relies on partial assistance from professional staff for ADLs; can stand or walk short distances, usually less than 100 ft (30.5 m) with an assistive device; spends most of the day sitting.

Level V *Wheelchair dependent:* Relies on total assistance from professional staff for ADLs; cannot stand or walk.

These classifications of abilities and problems should be viewed as a continuum rather than discrete categories. As a person moves across the continuum, the following occurs:

Risk of Disease Increases

- Need for supervision by medical personnel is greater.
- Use of medication increases.
- Testing moves from fitness to diagnostic to functional (see Functional Testing).

Fitness Level Decreases

- Range of suitable fitness activities decreases.
- Fitness professionals must be creative and adapt conventional activities to the limitations of the individual.
- Fitness professionals must incorporate socialization as part of the activity.

Personnel Needs Change

- Personnel need more education in gerontology, pathophysiology, and pharmacology.
- Staff mix may include fitness, nursing, physical therapy, and therapeutic recreation personnel.

Cardiorespiratory Fitness

A formal program of activities aimed at improving CRF should be built on a base of moderate-intensity activities that are tied to an individual's lifestyle (1). Like any workout, it should begin with a formal warm-up and end with a cool-down, during which flexibility exercises can be done. It is crucial to adapt the activities to the abilities of the people in the group. Those at the high end of the fitness continuum can participate in a wide variety of activities similar to those used for younger adults. Those who have the $\dot{V}O_2$max of cardiac patients (5-7 METs) can follow an exercise routine that would not be too different from those used in a cardiac rehabilitation program (see chapter 18). However, prescribing activities for those at the low end of the functional continuum, in whom $\dot{V}O_2$max may be only 2 to 4 METs, demands special creativity and attention to safety. Exercises can be done standing with support, seated on a chair, or in the

Functional Testing

A common method to evaluate the capabilities of older adults involves a series of performance tests that are linked to underlying fitness components. The Senior Fitness Test, developed by Rikli and Jones (18), uses the following tests to evaluate the different fitness components:

Chair stand—Number of times within 30 sec a person can stand from a seated position with arms folded across the chest (assesses lower-body strength).

Arm curl—Number of curls that can be completed in 30 sec with a 5 lb (2.3 kg; women) or 8 lb (3.6 kg; men) dumbbell while participant is seated (assesses upper-body strength).

6 min walk—Number of yards the participant can walk in 6 min around a 50 yd (46 m) course (assesses aerobic endurance).

2 min step—Number of full steps the participant can complete in 2 min, raising knee to midway between knee and hip while standing in place. This is an alternative to the 6 min walk.

Chair sit and reach—Number of inches between extended fingertips and tips of toes when the participant is sitting in a chair with legs extended and hands reaching toward toes (assesses lower-body flexibility).

Back scratch—Number of inches between the extended middle fingers when the participant reaches with one hand over the shoulder and the other hand up the back (assesses upper-body flexibility).

8 ft up and go—Number of seconds required to get up from a seated position, walk 8 ft (2.4 m), turn, and return to the seated position (assesses agility and dynamic balance).

Height and weight—Used to calculate BMI.

These tests have been shown to be valid and reliable, and normative data are provided for men and women aged 60 to 94 yr (18). These practical and easy tests can be used to track progress over the course of a training program or to document loss of function that might necessitate additional medical attention.

water (4, 18). Because of the prevalence of joint-related problems, exercise modes should be chosen that do not aggravate the problem. The need for additional assistance with balance and attention to safety regarding the risk of a fall should be incorporated into the routine (see Balance and Falls).

Balance and Falls

Loss of balance can lead to a fall, with dire consequences. The lower bone density in elderly people predisposes them to fractures, and about half are unable to return to regular walking after a fracture (23).The ability to maintain balance is influenced by a variety of factors, such as strength, vision, proprioception, medications, illnesses, flexibility, and environmental hazards (23). Considerable information shows that exercise programs improve balance and reduce falls, but not without exception (1, 21). The general recommendation is to include activities for balance training, resistance exercise, walking, and weight transfer (1). However, medications, environmental hazards, and vision also must be addressed to reduce the risk of falls (23).

The general exercise prescription for older adults is similar to what was described in chapter 10 for the typically sedentary individual (2, 3):

- Intensity: THR can be used to set the exercise intensity, but measured maximal HR is preferred to predicted maximal HR. Intensity guidelines are similar to those for younger adults, but the low end of the THR zone should be emphasized at the beginning of the program, and RPE also should be used to determine whether the intensity is suitable.
- Duration: If the client is extremely deconditioned, the exercise sessions should be divided into segments (5-10 min) that can be done throughout the day (or within the context of a single class period). Some participants may not be able exercise continuously for 30 min.
- Frequency: Moderate activity daily. Formal exercise sessions should be done 3 times each week, with a rest day between the exercise days.

Muscular Strength and Endurance

The exercise prescription for increasing strength is described in chapter 12. It is highlighted here (3):

- Instruct participants on safety, proper lifting technique, and breathing.
- Begin with minimal resistance for the first 8 wk to allow for adaptations of the connective tissue.
- Participants should perform 8 to 10 exercises that use the major muscle groups.
- Participants should stay within the pain-free ROM.
- Participants should not exercise if an arthritic joint is painful or inflamed (see Osteoarthritis).
- Each set should involve 10 to 15 repetitions that elicit an RPE of about 12 to 13 (e.g., somewhat hard).
- Participants should perform the workout at least twice a week, with 48 hr between sessions.

Osteoarthritis

Osteoarthritis, a common problem in many older adults, is a degenerative joint disease associated with damage to the articular cartilage that lines joint structures. The swelling and pain associated with osteoarthritis affect joint ROM and may prevent an individual from participating in physical activity. A variety of over-the-counter and prescription medications can reduce pain and inflammation and allow participation in physical activity. Activity programs should not excessively load the involved joint (e.g., participants with a knee or hip problem should perform stationary cycling or pool work instead of jogging or stair-climbing). Select the modes that provide the least discomfort. Gradual warm-up and flexibility exercises should be included, and the intensity and duration of the endurance exercise program should be at the low end of the spectrum. Resistance training should begin with only 2 to 3 reps and gradually progress to 10 to 12 reps, using pain threshold as a guide (3, 16).

Flexibility

A flexibility program should involve all joints with the goal to maintain their normal ROM. Tai chi and yoga programs can be used to achieve and maintain flexibility goals. However, for most people, flexibility goals can be achieved within the context of a regular exercise class. Elements of the program include the following (3):

- Slow movements through pain-free ROM, with static stretches held for 15 to 30 sec
- Two to four repetitions per muscle group

- Movements performed as a regular part of the warm-up and cool-down, as for younger individuals; whole sessions could focus on flexibility for the most deconditioned participants

Key Point

The exercise prescription for older adults is similar to that for younger adults, with additional attention to risk stratification, level of CRF, and limitations related to chronic or degenerative (e.g., osteoarthritis) diseases. Exercises should be selected to minimize joint trauma, provide an additional measure of safety against falling, and accomplish fitness goals in a socially supportive environment.

Psychological and Social Functioning

This chapter focused on the fact that regular participation in physical activity is associated with better health (lower risk of chronic diseases) and fitness (cardiovascular function, strength, body composition, and flexibility) during aging. However, regular participation in physical activity also has been shown to improve both psychological and social functioning (1, 6, 24, 27). This is a good example of how regular physical activity affects the whole person, leading to a more active and fulfilling life. The World Health Organization (27) has summarized the immediate and long-term benefits of physical activity on psychological and social functioning:

Immediate Benefits Attributable to Current Exercise Session

- Enhanced relaxation
- Reduced stress and anxiety
- Enhanced mood state
- Empowerment to be more independent and self-sufficient
- Enhanced social and cultural integration, especially from small-group programs

Long-Term Benefits Attributable to Regular Participation Over Time

- Improved general well-being
- Improved mental health
- Improved cognitive function: better central nervous system processing speed and reaction time
- Improved motor control and performance for both fine and gross motor skills
- Increased skill acquisition; new skills can be learned
- Enhanced integration; less likely to withdraw from society
- Formation of new friendships, particularly in small groups and other social environments
- Widened social and cultural networks
- Role maintenance and new role acquisition (the person remains active in society)
- Enhanced intergenerational activity (diminishes stereotypic perceptions about aging and the elderly)

Case Studies

You can check your answers by referring to page 473 in appendix A.

1. A 67-yr-old male who has been actively involved in jogging and tennis most of his life has developed arthritis in his left knee. The problem has caused him to reduce his jogging, and his lack of fitness, as he calls it, is affecting his tennis game, which he is determined to continue. He comes to your health club for testing and advice about what he can do to increase and maintain his fitness. How would you address his concerns?

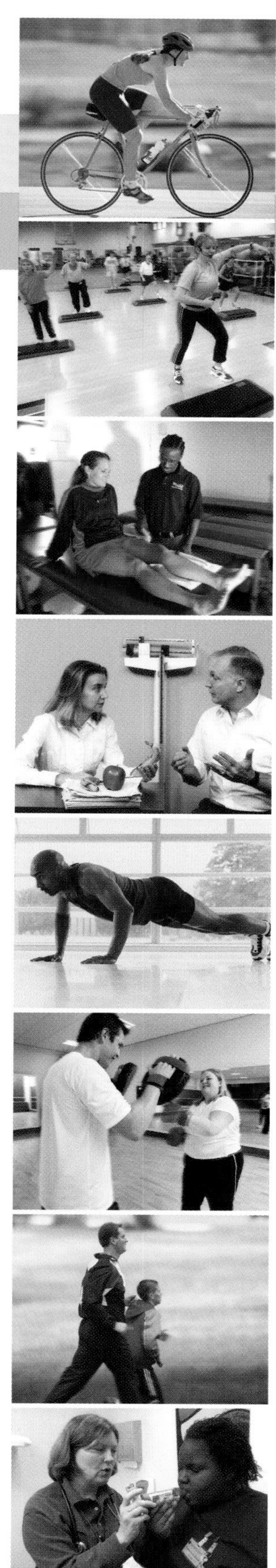

17
CHAPTER

Exercise and Women's Health

Dixie L. Thompson

Objectives

The reader will be able to do the following:

1. Describe the risks and benefits of exercising during pregnancy, and suggest ways to alter exercise to make it more comfortable and safe for pregnant women.
2. Define osteoporosis and risk factors for this disease, and prescribe exercise to promote bone health.
3. Define the female athlete triad.

Women and men share many of the obstacles to good health (e.g., cardiovascular disease, type 2 diabetes, obesity). Likewise, the benefits of exercise that combat these diseases are similar for men and women, as are exercise guidelines. However, some conditions are faced exclusively, or primarily, by women. In this chapter, we examine three of these: pregnancy, osteoporosis, and the female athlete triad.

Pregnancy and Exercise

Pregnancy places enormous demands on a woman's body. Justified concern about the safety of the fetus and the mother leads to questions about whether exercise is wise during pregnancy. Fortunately, there is substantial evidence that for healthy pregnant women, exercise is safe and beneficial during this critical time (4). Although difficult to document, proposed benefits of exercise during pregnancy include greater psychological well-being, less fatigue, and shorter and easier delivery (6, 18). However, some conditions require that exercise be approached cautiously. Pregnant women with cardiovascular, pulmonary, or metabolic disease as well as those with severe obesity or who are considerably underweight should seek physician guidance concerning exercise (9). The contraindications for exercise during pregnancy as determined by the American College of Obstetricians and Gynecologists (ACOG) (5) are shown below. The Canadian Society for Exercise Physiology (CSEP) has prepared a Physical Activity Readiness Examination for Pregnancy. This tool screens for potential medical problems and assists with exercise prescription and can be found on the CSEP Web site (www.csep.ca/forms.asp).

Potential Problems of Exercising During Pregnancy

Concerns about exercise during pregnancy target four crucial areas: heat dissipation, oxygen delivery, nutrition supply, and premature delivery. During the first trimester, the fetus is particularly vulnerable to developmental defects caused by excessive heat. Although the body's core temperature can increase with exercise, there are no known links between a greater prevalence of birth defects and exercise. An increase in the woman's blood volume provides adequate blood for heat dissipation, exercise, and nourishment of the fetus. Increases in ventilation and skin blood flow also help protect against excessive changes in body temperature (18). Additionally, the temperature at which sweating begins decreases as pregnancy progresses, providing an additional protective mechanism against higher core temperatures (9).

Concern that vigorous exercise could compromise uterine blood flow is also unsubstantiated. The increase in maternal blood volume coupled with a decrease in systemic vascular resistance results in an increase in cardiac output and provides adequate blood flow, and therefore oxygen, to the fetus (6, 18). The fact that fetal HR is only modestly, if at all, affected by exercise provides evidence that this type of physical activity does not significantly

Contraindications for Exercise During Pregnancy

Absolute Contraindications

- Hemodynamically significant heart disease
- Restrictive lung disease
- Incompetent cervix or cerclage
- Multiple gestation at risk for premature labor
- Persistent second or third trimester bleeding
- Placenta previa after 26 wk of gestation
- Premature labor during current pregnancy
- Ruptured membranes
- Preeclampsia or pregnancy-induced hypertension

Relative Contraindications

- Severe anemia
- Unevaluated maternal cardiac arrhythmia
- Chronic bronchitis
- Poorly controlled type 1 diabetes
- Extreme morbid obesity
- Extreme underweight (BMI < $12\ kg \cdot m^{-2}$)
- History of extremely sedentary lifestyle
- Intrauterine growth restriction
- Poorly controlled hypertension
- Orthopedic limitations
- Poorly controlled seizure disorder
- Poorly controlled hyperthyroidism
- Heavy smoker

Adapted, by permission, from American College of Obstetricians and Gynecologists, 2003, "Exercise during pregnancy and the postpartum period," *Clinical Obstetrics and Gynecology* 46(2): 497.

distress the fetus (6, 18). Because of the nutritional demands of pregnancy, greater caloric consumption is needed. The nutritional demands of exercise and fetal development must be adequately met by the exercising woman. For most women, the energy demands of pregnancy are approximately 300 kcal · day^{-1} (4). Evidence that exercise does not compromise the nutritional needs of the developing fetus comes from studies showing very little difference between the weights of newborns from exercising and nonexercising mothers (6, 18).

Another major concern is that exercise may cause premature delivery. For normal pregnancies, there is no evidence that gestational length is affected by exercise (6, 18). Care should be taken, however, to avoid activities (i.e., contact sports) in which injury could lead to fetal injury or premature delivery (5).

Exercise Testing and Prescription During Pregnancy

Maximal exercise testing should be avoided, unless under the direction of a physician, and submaximal exercise testing, if needed, should be stopped at <75% HRR (4). Moderate and even vigorous exercise can be performed safely by previously active pregnant women. The type, intensity, frequency, and duration of activity should conform to the woman's health and comfort. Encourage regular (at least 3 days per wk) rather than intermittent exercise. Unless there are medical complications, 30 min or more of moderate-intensity activity on most, if not all, days of the week are recommended (4). Intensity can be gauged with RPE, with a recommended range of 11 to 13 (4). It is suggested that women who were sedentary before becoming pregnant receive physician approval and initially engage in low-intensity (20%-39% HRR) programs if they begin an exercise program while pregnant (4).

The mode of exercise depends on comfort and convenience. Some women find that non-weight-bearing exercises such as swimming and stationary cycling are more comfortable, especially as pregnancy advances. During the postpartum stage, the return to activity should be gradual and based on individual response. A pregnant client should take the following precautions when exercising (4, 5).

- Avoid exercise in a supine position after the first trimester. The enlarged uterus can apply pressure to the surrounding blood vessels and limit venous return.
- Take steps to avoid heat injury. To prevent hyperthermia, avoid exercising in hot and humid environments, ensure adequate hydration (before, during, and after exercise), and dress appropriately for the heat.
- Limit exposure to falling and impact injury. Although completely eliminating the risk is impossible, do not participate in competitive contact sports (e.g., soccer, boxing) and activities where trauma risk is great (e.g., skydiving, water skiing). As pregnancy advances, center of gravity and balance change; therefore, exercise that requires rapid changes in direction may be more problematic than it was before pregnancy.
- Be aware that joint laxity increases during pregnancy. The release of relaxin allows the pelvis to undergo the changes needed during pregnancy and delivery. However, this hormone also leads to greater laxity in other joints. Follow the precautions in the previous point on this list to help prevent joint injury.
- Resistance training can be used during pregnancy, but observe the following precautions: (a) Avoid the Valsalva maneuver during lifting, (b) keep the programs at low to moderate intensity (resistance should be low enough that at least 12 repetitions can be completed without fatigue), and (c) use slow and steady rather than ballistic movement patterns. For more information on resistance training during pregnancy, see chapter 12.
- Avoid exercise in which extremes in air pressure occur. Scuba diving should be avoided because it puts the fetus at risk for decompression sickness. Exercise at altitudes over 6,000 ft (1,829 m) could be potentially dangerous and should be performed with caution.
- Be aware of the body's warning signs (5). Each woman should closely monitor her body for signs or symptoms that something may be wrong. If any of the following occur, stop exercise and consult a physician:

  Vaginal bleeding
  Dyspnea before exertion
  Dizziness
  Headache
  Chest pain
  Muscle weakness
  Calf pain or swelling
  Preterm labor
  Decreased fetal movement
  Amniotic fluid leakage

Key Point

Exercising during pregnancy is safe and beneficial for most women. Protecting against traumatic impact, heat injury, musculoskeletal injury, and overexertion is the key to planning safe exercise programs for pregnant women.

Osteoporosis

Osteoporosis is a disease characterized by fragile bones. Approximately 10 million Americans over age 50 have osteoporosis and another 34 million have low bone mass **(osteopenia)** and are at risk for developing osteoporosis (17). Annually, osteoporosis accounts for $12 to $18 billion in direct medical costs (17). The most common sites for osteoporotic fractures are the hip, vertebrae, and wrist. Bone strength is determined by **bone mineral density (BMD)** and the structural integrity of the bone. BMD is measured by dual-energy X-ray absorptiometry (DXA; see chapter 6) and reflects the amount of bone mineral per unit area ($g \cdot cm^{-2}$). BMD, accounting for about 70% of bone strength, is highly correlated with a bone's resistance to fracture (14). Structural integrity is determined by the microarchitecture of the bone and is much more difficult to assess, requiring invasive testing of bone (1). Because of the low risk, the ease, and the availability of DXA, it has become the preferred method for diagnosing osteoporosis. According to WHO guidelines, osteoporosis is defined as a BMD that is 2.5 standard deviations below the mean for young white women. When BMD is in the osteoporotic range, fracture risk is high. Common pharmaceutical treatments for osteoporosis are selective estrogen receptor modulators, hormone replacement therapy (for women), and bisphosphonates. These drug interventions slow bone loss and some even increase BMD. More information can be found on osteoporosis and its treatment at the Web site of the National Institute of Arthritis and Musculoskeletal and Skin Diseases (www.niams.nih.gov).

Risk Factors for Osteoporosis

Osteoporosis can affect both males and females across all ages and ethnicities. However, older women, particularly of Caucasian and Asian descent, are especially at risk. Bone accumulates during childhood and generally peaks in early adult life (12). Although BMD declines somewhat during the middle adult years, the most rapid loss in women occurs in the years surrounding menopause (7, 12). The decline in estrogen levels around the time of menopause is the reason for the rapid bone loss, which can be as great as 3% to 5% of bone mass each year. In men, bone loss is typically slow but steady from the time of peak accumulation until death. In general, men are less likely than women to experience osteoporotic fractures because their peak BMD is higher than women's. However, men are not completely protected from osteoporosis. Some estimate that 1 in 4 men over age 50 will experience an osteoporotic fracture (15). In addition to sex, race is a factor in determining peak bone mass. Peak BMD is generally higher in individuals of African descent when compared with those of European and Asian ancestry (14).

Sometimes osteoporosis accompanies another medical condition. Examples of conditions that can lead to osteoporosis are endocrine disorders, gastrointestinal diseases, nutritional deficiencies, and the long-term use of glucocorticoid medications. Because of the many factors that may lead to low bone density, people of all ages, including children, can develop osteoporosis. Low intake of calcium and vitamin D can limit the accumulation of bone during childhood, and it is estimated that only 25% of boys and 10% of girls achieve the recommended levels for calcium intake (14). Attaining a peak bone density that is lower than expected increases the risk of osteoporosis in later life. The International Osteoporosis Foundation has developed a screening tool to assess risk for osteoporosis. This simple 10-question test, designed to help identify people at particularly high risk for osteoporosis, is found on page 293.

Risk Factors for Osteoporosis

Female
Older age
Estrogen deficiency
Caucasian or Asian race
Low weight or BMI
Diet low in calcium
Alcohol abuse
Inactivity
Muscle weakness
Family history of osteoporosis
Smoking
History of fracture

Exercise in Prevention and Treatment of Osteoporosis

One of the primary means for preventing osteoporosis is maximizing bone accumulation during childhood and adolescence. In addition to adequate calcium and vitamin D intake, physical activity is important for developing strong bones. Studies demonstrate that children who exercise regularly have higher bone mineral levels than their sedentary peers, and this increase in bone carries over into adulthood (3). The primary goal for children is to participate in activities that maximize bone accrual.

The research examining exercise as a tool to increase bone density among adults has produced mixed results. Although some studies have demonstrated gains in bone

Millennium One-Minute Osteoporosis Risk Test

1. Have either of your parents broken a hip after a minor bump or fall? Yes _____ No _____
2. Have you broken a bone after a minor bump or fall? Yes _____ No _____
3. Have you taken corticosteroid tablets (cortisone, prednisone) for more than 3 mo? Yes _____ No _____
4. Have you lost more than 3 cm (just over 1 in.) in height? Yes _____ No _____
5. Do you regularly drink heavily (in excess of safe drinking limits)? Yes _____ No _____
6. Do you smoke more than 20 cigarettes a day? Yes _____ No _____
7. Do you frequently have diarrhea (caused by problems such as celiac disease or Crohn's disease)? Yes _____ No _____

For Women:

8. Did you undergo menopause before the age of 45? Yes _____ No _____
9. Have your periods stopped for 12 mo or more (other than because of pregnancy)? Yes _____ No _____

For Men:

10. Have you ever had impotence, lack of libido, or other symptoms related to low testosterone levels? Yes _____ No _____

If you answered yes to one or more of these questions, it is possible that you are at increased risk for osteoporosis, and consultation with your physician is recommended.

Reprinted from the International Osteoporosis Foundation, *Millennium One-Minute Osteoporosis Risk Test* [Online]. Available: www.osteofound.org.

density with exercise, others have shown that exercise has little effect. The wide variety among research protocols is one reason for the mixed results. Some common elements among studies that yielded the most profound effect on adult bone health are moderate to vigorous activity, adequate calcium intake in conjunction with exercise (1,000-1,500 mg · day^{-1}), and movements that involve either impact loading or resistance training. For older adults, exercise alone may not be adequate to prevent age-related bone loss; however, exercise is essential in slowing this potentially devastating condition. Older adults with osteoporosis should be encouraged to engage in exercises designed to lower the risk of falling (e.g., balance and resistance training) in order to help protect against osteoporotic fractures.

Exercise Prescription for Bone Health

Exercise for children and adolescents helps maximize bone density. Regular participation in high-intensity loading activities should be encouraged. The ACSM recommends the following (3):

- Mode: activities and sports that involve weight bearing and jumping (e.g., volleyball, gymnastics) and moderate resistance training
- Intensity: high-loading forces in jumping, moderate (<60% 1RM) resistance training
- Frequency: at least 3 days per wk
- Duration: 10 to 20 min

For nonosteoporotic adults, loading exercises and muscle-building activities promote bone health. An excellent example of this type of program is described by Metcalfe and colleagues (13). Using the evidence available, the ACSM recommends the following approach to preserve bone during adulthood (3):

- Mode: weight-bearing aerobic exercise, jumping activities (e.g., basketball), and resistance exercise
- Intensity: moderate to high
- Frequency: weight-bearing endurance exercise 3 or 4 times · wk^{-1}; resistance exercise 2 or 3 times per wk
- Duration: 30 to 60 min

Exercise Testing and Prescription for Osteoporotic Individuals

For individuals with osteoporosis, precautions should be taken with both exercise testing and prescription. The benefits versus the risks of exercise testing must be weighed, and physician approval for exercise testing is recommended (4). For individuals with severe kyphosis that limits forward vision or balance, stationary cycling may be a better choice than treadmill walking (4). Testing muscular strength can be important in designing programs

Key Point

Osteoporosis, a disease characterized by fragile bones, affects millions of Americans. Although males and females of all ages can develop osteoporosis, it is most commonly seen in postmenopausal women. Healthy eating practices and an active lifestyle are keys to promoting bone health. Exercises that involve either impact loading or resistance training appear most beneficial for promoting bone development. Special care should be taken when testing and prescribing exercise for osteoporotic clients.

for osteoporotic clients; however, exercises that involve significant spinal flexion should be avoided because of the risk of compression fractures. Tests of balance and functionality can be useful in designing programs to reduce the risk of falling. Improving functional muscle strength and balance is key to reducing the risk of falls (7). Exercise prescription for the osteoporotic client must be individualized and based on the severity of disease and the presence of other conditions. In general, exercise prescription should focus on aerobic activity, exercises that strengthen muscle, and activities that improve balance. This combination incorporates three major components: cardiovascular health, bone health, and reduced risk of falling. For more details on exercise testing and prescription for osteoporotic clients, see Bloomfield and Smith (7).

Female Athlete Triad

The female athlete triad (figure 17.1) includes three major components: disordered eating, amenorrhea, and osteoporosis (2). This condition, if left untreated, can produce significant health consequences including glycogen depletion, anemia, and electrolyte imbalances (2). The precipitating factor in this triad is disordered eating. Anorexia nervosa and bulimia nervosa are two eating disorders commonly associated with the female athlete triad. Among athletes who develop the female athlete triad, the range of unhealthy eating practices varies. Some athletes clearly present with eating disorders, whereas others limit calories without meeting the strict clinical definitions of an eating disorder (10). The unhealthy eating pattern with insufficient calories and nutritional density leads to amenorrhea. The estrogen deficiency seen in amenorrhea leads to osteopenia and potentially even osteoporosis. This loss of bone puts the athlete at great risk for stress fractures and for osteoporotic compression fractures.

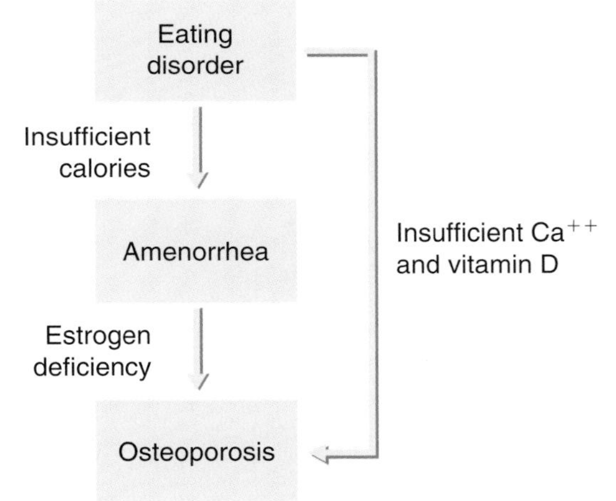

Figure 17.1 Female athlete triad.

In the general adult population, anorexia nervosa occurs at a rate of 0.5% to 1% and bulimia nervosa occurs at a rate of 2% to 4% (11). Although it is difficult to determine the percentage of athletes struggling with unhealthy eating practices, the prevalence of these eating disorders among them seems at least as high as that for the general population (2). A meta-analysis found that some athletes are at particular risk for eating disorders (elite athletes, dancers, athletes in sports that emphasize thinness), whereas others (nonelite status, athletes in sports that do not emphasize thinness) may actually have some protection from unhealthy eating (16). When left untreated, eating disorders can lead to seriously deteriorating health and potentially even death (see chapter 11).

Amenorrhea, or lack of menses, is clinically divided into two categories. **Primary amenorrhea** is characterized by the absence of menarche (i.e., first menses) in girls aged 16 or older. When there is a lack of menses for 3 or more consecutive months in females after menarche, it is classified as **secondary amenorrhea.** The cause of amenorrhea can be difficult to establish and involves a complex interaction among the hypothalamus, pituitary gland, and ovaries. Because of inadequate stimulation, the ovaries do not function normally, resulting in lower than normal estrogen and progesterone levels. The high prevalence of irregular menstruation has been observed in athletic women for a number of years, but the consequences on bone largely were ignored until Drinkwater and colleagues' landmark study (8) in which the bones of young amenorrheic athletes were found to be comparable in density to those of postmenopausal women. To help protect against bone loss, many physicians now treat amenorrheic athletes by replacing the missing endogenous estrogen with oral contraceptives (10).

Recognizing the signs of disordered eating (see chapter 11) is necessary before successful intervention. Often coaches and athletes are ill informed about the female athlete triad. Therefore, education is an important first step in battling this condition. Successful intervention for the female athlete triad requires a multidisciplinary approach that includes input from medical, nutritional, and psychological professionals (2, 10).

Key Point

The female athlete triad is characterized by disordered eating, amenorrhea, and osteoporosis. Anorexia nervosa and bulimia nervosa are eating disorders frequently seen in the female athlete triad and can lead to significant health impairment, even death, if left untreated. Intervention for the female athlete triad should be multidisciplinary and should include psychological counseling.

Case Studies

You can check your answers by referring to page 473 in appendix A.

1. A sedentary 52-yr-old woman with a family history of osteoporosis comes to your facility for information on exercise to promote bone health. Her doctor says she is in generally good health and does not have osteoporosis, but there are signs that her bones are weaker than when she was younger (i.e., osteopenia). What type of exercise would you recommend?

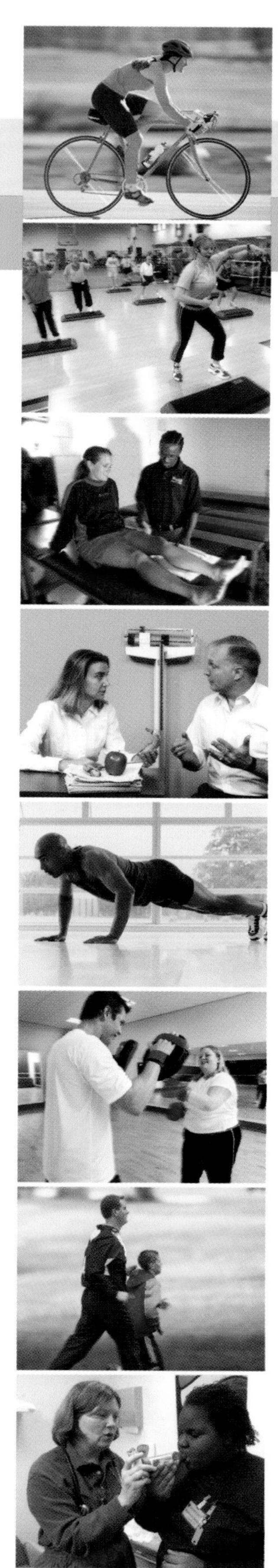

CHAPTER 18

Exercise and Coronary Heart Disease

David R. Bassett Jr.

Objectives

The reader will be able to do the following:

1. Describe the atherosclerotic process and the resulting outcome if blood flow becomes obstructed in the arteries of the heart, brain, or periphery.
2. Quantify the magnitude of cardiovascular disease as a health problem in the United States and list the various subcategories of cardiovascular disease.
3. Identify the various patient populations found in cardiac rehabilitation programs.
4. Describe the physiological and mental health benefits of exercise for individuals with cardiovascular disease.
5. Define what is meant by secondary prevention of CHD.
6. Describe special tests that can help diagnose the presence or absence of CHD, including those that use exercise and nonexercise challenges to stress the heart.
7. Describe how to prescribe aerobic exercise (frequency, intensity, and duration) in cardiac rehabilitation programs.
8. Discuss special considerations in prescribing exercise intensity for individuals who are taking beta-blocker medications.

Coronary heart disease (CHD) is a major problem in the United States and in other industrialized nations. This chapter provides the fitness professional with a basic understanding of the development of CHD, the types of patients found in cardiac rehabilitation programs, the benefits of exercise for a cardiac population, and the special considerations for exercise prescription in this group. It is not a comprehensive guide to exercise in cardiac rehabilitation; a number of excellent texts provide more complete information on the topic (3, 5, 12).

Atherosclerosis

Atherosclerosis refers to an accumulation of lipid deposits in the large and medium-sized arteries (figure 18.1), a process that provokes fibrosis and calcification. The atherosclerotic process begins early in life, as evidenced by studies of soldiers killed in the Korean War. Approximately three fourths of the 300 soldiers examined (mean age 22.1 yr) had some degree of blockage in their coronary arteries (7). It is believed that the atherosclerotic process begins when the **endothelial cells** lining the artery become damaged because of smoking, toxic agents, or high blood pressure (see Hypertension on page 299). When lipoproteins are deposited at the damaged site, plaque formation (or atherosclerosis) occurs. Eventually, these deposits impede blood flow in the affected arteries, sometimes to the point of complete occlusion (18).

Consequences of Atherosclerosis

Atherosclerosis can occur in various arteries throughout the body, with different results. Blockages in the coronary arteries will lead to **myocardial ischemia** (reduced blood flow to the heart) and in severe cases to **myocardial infarction (MI).** If the blood vessels in the brain become occluded, a **stroke** will result. Blockages in the peripheral leg vessels can result in **claudication,** or intermittent muscle pain that occurs with exertion (17).

Cardiovascular Disease

In the United States, cardiovascular disease (CVD) is the leading cause of death, with 433,825 males and 493,623 females dying from CVD in 1998. CHD accounts for 53% of these deaths, with stroke (18%), hypertensive disease (5%), and congestive heart failure (6%) making up most of the other leading causes (4). (CVD refers to any disease of the heart and the blood vessels or circulation, while CHD is a more specific condition resulting from reduced blood flow in the coronary arteries.) The death rate attributable to coronary artery disease has declined in recent decades, but it remains a problem of huge proportions. According to the AHA, approximately 1,100,000 Americans will have a coronary attack this year. About 650,000 of these will be first heart attacks, and the rest are recurrent attacks. Of those

Key Point

Atherosclerosis is a disease that starts early in life and leads to blockages in the arteries of the heart, brain, or peripheral muscles. If a blockage occurs in a coronary artery, myocardial ischemia or infarction results. There is a high prevalence of such health problems in the United States.

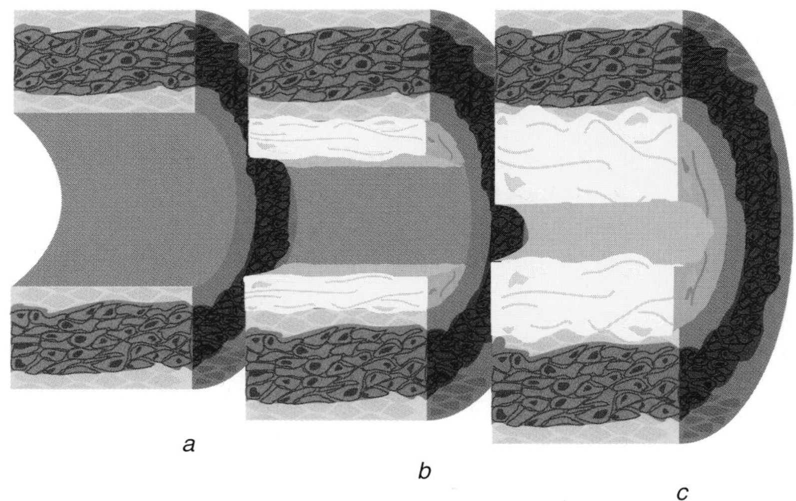

Figure 18.1 Stages of atherosclerosis: *(a)* normal artery, *(b)* partially blocked artery, and *(c)* significantly blocked artery.

Hypertension

Hypertension, or high BP, greatly increases a person's risk of developing cardiovascular disease. It usually is defined as an SBP of 140 mmHg or a DBP of 90 mmHg. It is estimated that 65 million people in the United States have hypertension (4). Typically, hypertension is controlled through medication (see chapter 24), particularly if the patient's BP is very high (e.g., BP of 160 mmHg systolic or 95 mmHg diastolic). For those who have only moderate hypertension, a variety of nonpharmacological approaches to reducing BP are recommended. Dietary change includes reducing sodium intake, which has been shown to independently lower SBP and DBP by 5 and 3 mmHg, respectively (11, 13). Obesity is linked to hypertension, and research shows that a loss of 1 kg of body weight decreases SBP and DBP by 1.6 and 1.3 mmHg, respectively (11, 13). Last, participating in an endurance exercise program has been shown to decrease SBP and DBP by 7 and 6 mmHg, respectively, in hypertensive individuals (1).

The standard ACSM exercise prescription for improving $\dot{V}O_2$max (see chapter 10) also reduces BP in previously hypertensive individuals (1, 11). In addition, endurance exercise at moderate intensities (40%-60% $\dot{V}O_2$max) has been shown to reduce BP. Moderate-intensity exercise should be done frequently and for durations long enough to expend a large number of calories. Furthermore, for those with higher BPs who are taking medication, such an exercise program along with changes in diet, smoking, and body weight can lower BP. In these cases, BP should be checked frequently so medications can be reduced as needed. Gradually establishing appropriate diet and exercise habits improves the chance that a person will maintain an appropriate BP once it has been normalized.

experiencing a heart attack, 60% will survive, and some of these individuals will be referred to cardiac rehabilitation programs (4).

Populations in Cardiac Rehabilitation Programs

Cardiac rehabilitation programs include persons who have experienced angina pectoris, MI, **coronary artery bypass graft** (CABG), and angioplasty (8, 9). **Angina pectoris** refers to the chest pain attributable to ischemia of the ventricle resulting from an occlusion of one or more of the coronary arteries. The pain appears when the oxygen requirement of the heart (estimated by the double product SBP · HR) exceeds a value that coronary blood flow cannot meet. The ischemia can be transient and may subside once the oxygen demand of the heart returns to normal.

MI patients have actual heart damage (death of ventricular muscle fibers) caused by the occlusion of one or more of the coronary arteries. The degree to which left ventricular function is affected depends on the mass of the ventricle permanently damaged. Individuals who have experienced an MI usually take medications (betablockers) to reduce the work of the heart and control the irritability of the heart tissue so that dangerous arrhythmias (irregular heartbeats) do not occur. Generally, these individuals experience a training effect similar to that of people who did not have an MI.

CABG patients have had surgery to bypass one or more blocked coronary arteries. In this procedure, a blood vessel is sewn into existing coronary arteries above and below the blockage in order to reroute the blood flow (see figure 18.2). People with chronic angina pectoris before CABG find a relief of symptoms, with 50% to 70% experiencing no more pain. Generally, with an increased blood flow to the ventricle, left ventricular function and the capacity for work improve (20). These patients benefit from systematic exercise training because most are deconditioned before surgery as a result of activity restrictions related to chest pain.

Some CHD patients undergo a special procedure, **percutaneous transluminal coronary angioplasty (PTCA),** to open occluded arteries. In this procedure, the chest is not opened; instead, a balloon-tipped catheter (a long slender tube) is inserted into the coronary artery, where the balloon is inflated to push the plaque back toward the arterial wall (see figure 18.3). These patients tend not to have as severe CHD as those who undergo CABG. For these patients, PTCA has some advantages, including being less invasive, requiring a shorter hospital stay (1-2 days instead of 6-9 days), and costing less (9). However, with PTCA the coronary artery becomes reoccluded in approximately one third to one half of patients within 6 mo of the procedure (10).

To help prevent reocclusion, **intracoronary stents** are often used to help keep the lumen of the coronary artery open. Stents are composed of a metal mesh that is inserted into the artery on a balloon catheter and positioned in the area of obstruction. The balloon is first inflated to increase the lumen size, and then it is deflated and pulled back while the stent remains embedded in the artery. The main disadvantage of metal stents is that they increase the risk of blood clots; hence, anticoagulation therapy is needed to reduce this risk (5).

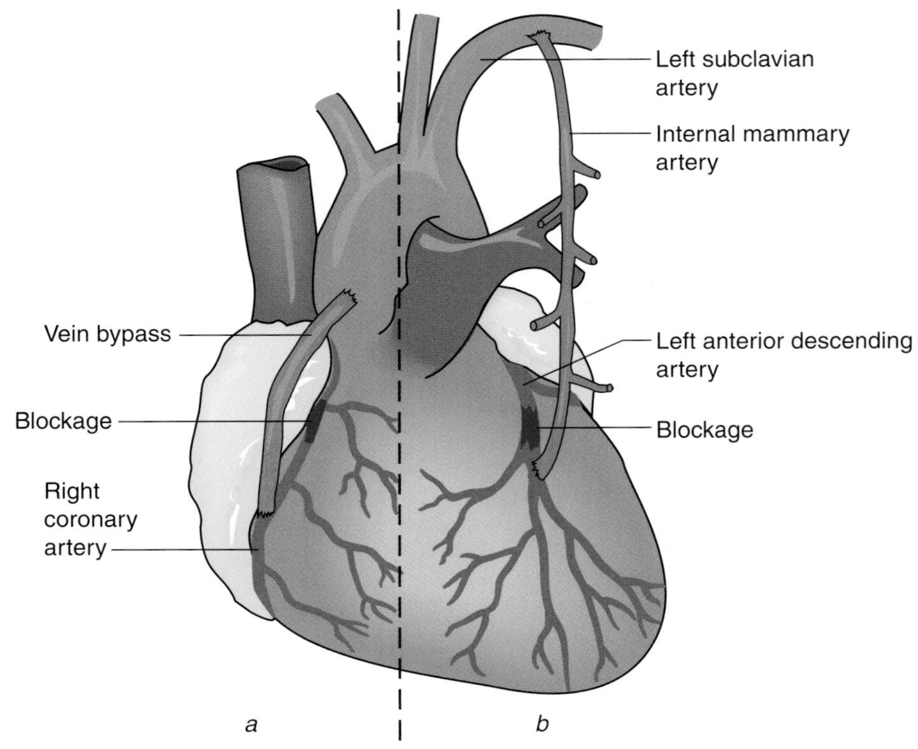

Figure 18.2 Coronary artery bypass surgery. *(a)* Coronary artery bypass graft using saphenous vein, and *(b)* coronary artery bypass graft using mammary artery. Blood flow is rerouted around the site of obstruction by taking a blood vessel from another part of the body and sewing it to the affected coronary artery, distal to the site of the obstruction. Blood vessels typically used in the procedure are the saphenous (leg) vein and the mammary artery.

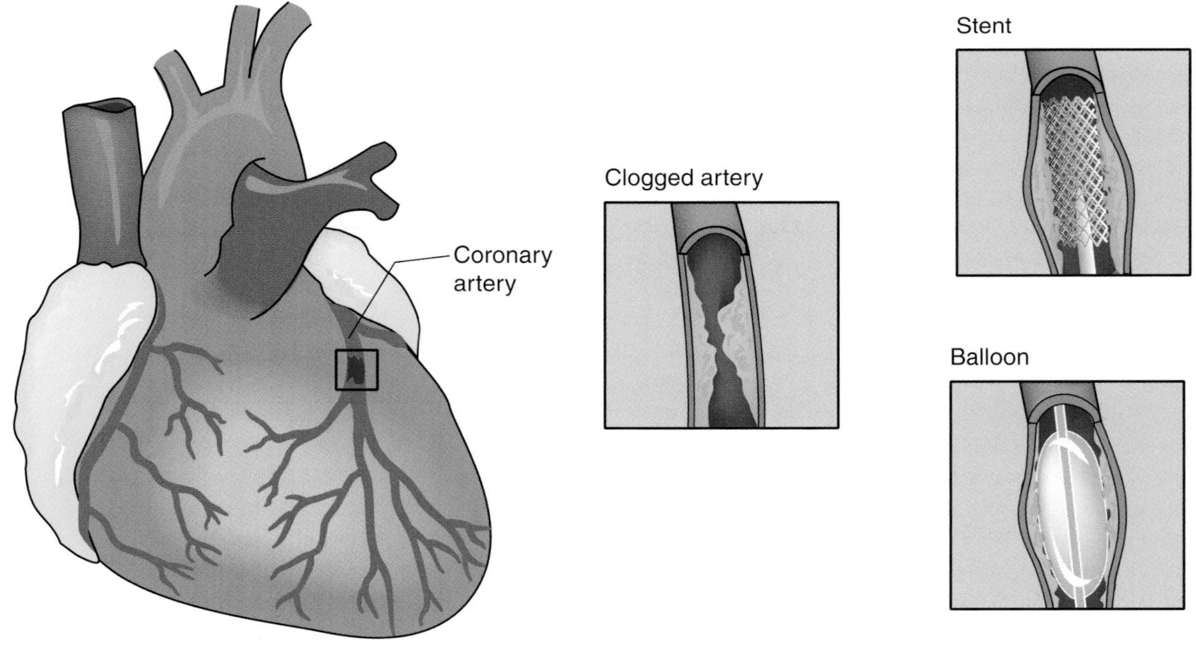

Figure 18.3 Percutaneous transluminal coronary angioplasty. A guide wire is used to position the balloon catheter at the site of obstruction inside the coronary artery. The balloon is inflated, increasing the lumen size and capacity for blood flow. The catheter is then deflated and removed. In some cases, a metal stent is placed inside the artery to keep it open.

Key Point

CHD is treated by CABG, angioplasty, or intracoronary stent. Patients who have undergone these procedures are candidates for a hospital-based cardiac rehabilitation program.

Evidence for Exercise Training

Fifty years ago, the most common advice given to patients who had experienced an MI was to take several weeks of complete bed rest (3). Today, however, exercise training is an ordinary part of treatment for people with CHD. Cardiac rehabilitation programs use a multidisciplinary approach of education and exercise to help clients with heart disease return to normal function, within the limits of their disease (12).

There is no question that patients with CHD have improved cardiovascular function as a result of exercising. This is evidenced by higher $\dot{V}O_2$max values, higher work rates achieved without ischemia (as shown by angina pectoris or S-T segment changes), and an increased capacity for prolonged submaximal work (6, 16, 19). Moderate reductions in body fat, blood pressure, total cholesterol, serum triglycerides, and LDL-C have been shown to occur with regular exercise, along with increases in HDL-C. The improved lipid profile is a function of more than the exercise alone, given that weight loss and the saturated fat content of the diet can modify these variables.

A major focus of cardiac rehabilitation programs is to reduce the occurrence of subsequent MIs (3). This is referred to as **secondary prevention** of CHD. The Framingham Heart Study has shown that people who have experienced one heart attack are at increased risk of a second heart attack. Further, the likelihood of recurrence clearly is associated with many of the same risk factors that caused atherosclerosis in the first place. Thus, cardiac rehabilitation personnel must monitor blood pressure, blood cholesterol levels, and smoking in their patients. In general, research studies have shown that a cardiac rehabilitation program involving exercise results in a 20% to 25% reduction in all-cause and cardiovascular mortality after an MI. This is good news, because it indicates that such patients derive a substantial benefit from participating in cardiac rehabilitation. In addition, patients gain an improved sense of well-being (12).

One of the most exciting developments in cardiac rehabilitation in recent years is the demonstration that lifestyle modification can reverse coronary artery disease. Ornish and colleagues (14) conducted a series of studies in which they showed that a program consisting of a strict vegetarian diet, yoga, meditation, smoking cessation, and physical activity reversed the atherosclerotic process. Patients in this study showed actual reversal of blockages in their coronary arteries, lending credibility to the idea that this condition can, in some cases, be treated with nonsurgical interventions.

Key Point

Cardiac rehabilitation programs help people with heart disease regain their fitness and return to normal, everyday activities. The benefits of such programs include increased work capacity and reduced cardiovascular risk factors. Cardiac rehabilitation programs generally lower the risk of a second heart attack.

Special Diagnostic Tests to Detect CHD

Testing a patient with CHD is much more involved than testing the apparently healthy person. There are some classes of patients with CHD for whom exercise or exercise testing is inappropriate and dangerous (2). In other persons, however, the benefits of a **graded exercise test (GXT)** outweigh the risks. Diagnostic exercise testing is nearly always performed in a hospital environment, with a physician present. A 12-lead electrocardiogram (ECG) is monitored at discrete intervals during the GXT, and three leads are displayed continuously on an oscilloscope. Blood pressure, rating of perceived exertion (RPE), and various signs and symptoms also are noted. Emergency equipment includes a defibrillator, supplemental oxygen, and emergency medications. Personnel trained and certified in advanced cardiac life support are on hand to provide assistance if needed.

Treadmill tests commonly used in diagnostic exercise testing are the Naughton, Balke, Bruce, and Ellestad protocols, named after their developers (2). These protocols are all GXTs that increase speed or grade at regular intervals to increase the exercise intensity. For those who are unable to perform treadmill exercise, a cycle test or arm ergometer test may be used. The criteria for terminating the GXT focus on various pathological signs (e.g., S-T segment depression on the ECG) or symptoms (e.g., angina pectoris) rather than on achieving some percentage of age-adjusted maximal heart rate. A subjective angina scale may be used to assess the severity of the symptoms (see table 18.1).

• Table 18.1 Angina Rating Scale •

1	Mild, barely noticeable
2	Moderate, bothersome
3	Moderately severe, very uncomfortable
4	Most severe or most intense pain ever experienced

This scale is used in rating the subjective pain associated with myocardial insufficiency.

Adapted, by permission, from American College of Sports Medicine (ACSM), 2006, *ACSM's guidelines for exercise testing and prescription*, 7th ed. (Philadelphia, PA: Lippincott, Williams & Wilkins), 107. (2).

Other tests of heart function include radionuclide procedures, typically administered in conjunction with either exercise or pharmacological (nonexercise) stress tests (5, 15). In the latter case, the pharmacologic agents provoke myocardial ischemia through either increased myocardial oxygen demand or coronary vasodilation. For instance, thallium-201 (a radioactive substance) can be injected intravenously to assess myocardial perfusion. Thallium is taken up by well-perfused myocardium similarly to the way potassium is taken up. Ischemic myocardium tends not to take up the thallium, thus identifying areas of the heart with poor blood flow. Another technique involves a radioisotope that binds to the red blood cells (technetium-99m), which is useful for cardiac blood pool imaging. This allows the end-systolic volume (ESV) and end-diastolic volume (EDV) to be measured, and the ejection fraction then can be computed as follows: ejection fraction = (EDV – ESV) ÷ EDV. Ventricular wall motion abnormalities also can be identified (15).

The most definitive tests for CHD are **coronary angiography** and **positron emission tomography (PET)** scans. In angiography, a cardiac catheter is inserted into the femoral artery and pushed all the way up the aorta until it reaches the entrance to a coronary artery, where the curved tip of the catheter guide allows it to be inserted into the artery. A contrast dye is injected through the catheter into the coronary artery. By viewing an image of the coronary arteries on a screen, the cardiologist can measure the degree of occlusion (narrowing) that exists (see figure 18.4). PET scans use [^{18}F]-deoxyglucose or [^{13}N]-ammonia. These substances allow the level of myocardial cell metabolism to be assessed. Metabolically active areas, indicative of good perfusion, can be distinguished from underperfused areas by color.

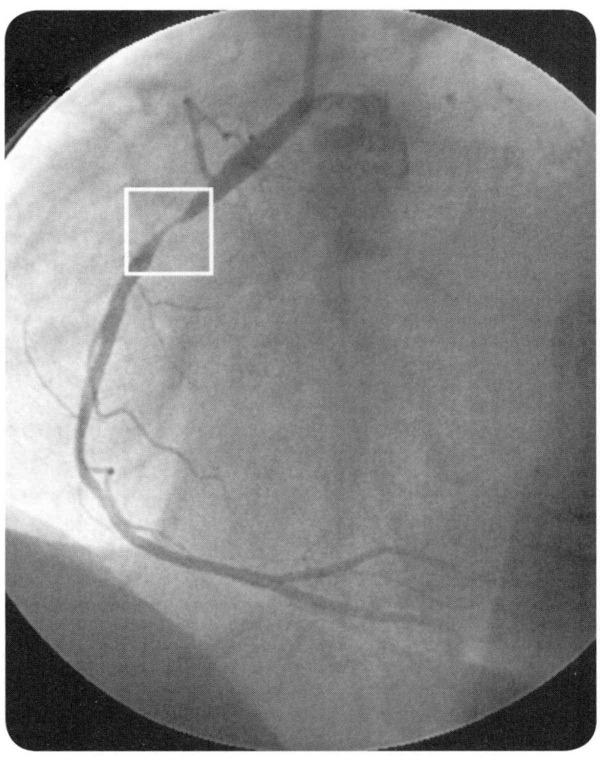

Figure 18.4 Coronary angiogram showing occlusion (narrowing) of a coronary artery. A catheter has been inserted into a coronary artery and radiographic contrast dye injected to allow the artery to be seen.
Courtesy of David R. Bassett Jr.

Key Point

Special types of diagnostic tests can determine whether a patient has CHD. Using GXTs on the treadmill (with close monitoring of the ECG and blood pressure) is a common method of detecting signs and symptoms of heart disease. Radionuclide tests can more definitively confirm the presence or absence of heart disease.

Typical Exercise Prescription

The details of how to design and implement cardiac rehabilitation programs, from the first steps taken after patients are confined to bed to the time that they return to work and beyond, are provided in the American Association for Cardiovascular and Pulmonary Rehabilitation guidelines (3). This section briefly introduces these programs.

Cardiac rehabilitation programs are organized in progressive phases of programming to meet the needs of clients and their families. Phase I (the acute phase) begins when a patient arrives in the hospital step-down unit, after leaving the intensive or coronary care unit (12). Within 1 to 3 days of the MI or revascularization procedure, the patient has already begun the rehabilitation process. Patients are exposed to orthostatic or gravitation stress by intermittently sitting and standing. Later, bedside activities and slow ambulation (i.e., walking) in the hallways are recommended (3).

Phases II and III refer to outpatient exercise programs conducted in a hospital environment. Rhythmic activities using large muscle groups are recommended for physical conditioning; these activities include treadmill exercise, cycle ergometry, combined arm and leg exercise, rowing, and stair-climbing. Light to moderate resistance training is accomplished with free weights (dumbbells) and elastic tubing (Thera-Band). Special care must be taken when prescribing upper-body exercises to clients who have undergone CABG procedures, because of limitations related to the chest incision. See chapter 12 for more details on resistance training in cardiac populations.

Recommendations for aerobic exercise programming in outpatient cardiac rehabilitation (phases II and III) are as follows (8, 9):

- Frequency: 3 to 4 days per wk
- Intensity: 40% to 75% of $\dot{V}O_2$max or HRR
- Duration: 20 to 40 min per session
- 5 to 10 min of warm-up and cool-down exercises

Fitness professionals who work in cardiac rehabilitation must have knowledge of cardiovascular medications (for a description of these, see chapter 24). Patients who are on beta-blockers require special consideration, because the Karvonen formula for computing THR range is invalid if the client was not on beta-blockers at the time of testing. For these individuals, a THR is sometimes computed by adding 20 to 30 beats $\cdot$ min^{-1} to the client's standing, resting HR. However, in view of the wide differences in physiological responses to beta-blockade, another approach is to use RPE ratings around somewhat hard, which correspond to 11 to 14 on the original Borg RPE scale (3).

In phase II, clients are monitored carefully for vital signs (HR, BP, ventilation), and the ECG is monitored at a central observation station via telemetry (radio signals). A single-channel recording of 6 to 10 patients can be monitored simultaneously on a computer screen, and in the event of arrhythmias or S-T segment changes, a rhythm strip is printed out. Phase II programs typically last about 12 wk and are covered by insurance reimbursement.

Phase III programs are hospital-based programs in which clients are encouraged to continue their exercise regimens and are provided access to continuing health care and patient education. In these cases, the client's ECG usually is not monitored by telemetry but clients continue to follow an individualized exercise prescription and continue to attend patient education classes. Eventually, clients may enter the maintenance phase and move to a phase IV program in a nonhospital setting.

Key Point

Cardiac rehabilitation programs are divided into four phases. Phase I is the acute phase, performed while the patient is still in the hospital. Phases II and III are conducted on an outpatient basis, and phase IV is the maintenance phase. Cardiac patients can benefit from aerobic and resistance training, but working with this population requires special knowledge of their medical conditions.

Case Studies

You can check your answers by referring to page 473 in appendix A.

1. John is a 46-yr-old male. He is an insurance executive who is married with two children. John is active in his church and plays golf on the weekends. He went to see his cardiologist because he experienced recent fatigue with chest pain on exertion. He has never smoked but he consumes 1 to 2 alcoholic drinks per day. His medical history reveals a blood cholesterol level of 263 mg · dl^{-1}, a triglyceride level of 195 mg · dl^{-1}, and an HDL-C value of 45 mg · dl^{-1}. Considering his sex, age, symptoms, and risk factors, what do you think is the likelihood he has CHD? What would be a reasonable next step to diagnose the presence or absence of CHD?
2. Jane is a 61-yr-old retired female. She recently underwent a left heart catheterization, which revealed significant occlusion in the left anterior descending artery and the circumflex artery. Therefore, a balloon angioplasty procedure was performed. Approximately 2 wk later, she performed a GXT with the following results:

   Protocol: Balke (3.3 mi · hr^{-1}, or 5.3 km · hr^{-1})

   Resting: HR = 72 beats · min^{-1}, BP = 130/72 mmHg

   End point: stage 3 for 1 min (approximately 7 METs)

   HR = 126 beats · min^{-1}, BP = 160/90 mmHg

   Reason for termination: Fatigue

   No S-T segment depression, no reported symptoms

   Jane was taking atenolol (a beta-blocker) at the time of her test, and her physician instructed her to continue taking this medication. She was referred to the cardiac rehabilitation center for supervised exercise and risk factor modification. List some types of exercise that would be appropriate for her.

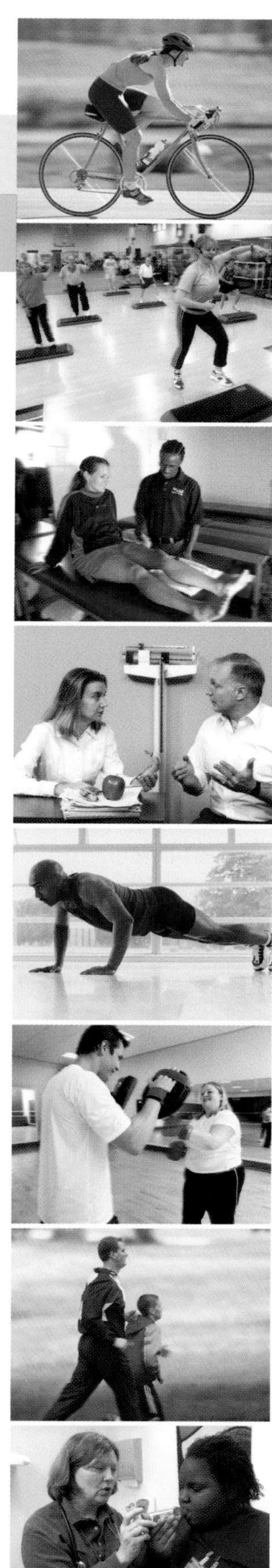

19 CHAPTER

Exercise and Obesity

Dixie L. Thompson

Objectives

The reader will be able to do the following:

1. Define obesity and describe health risks of obesity.
2. Describe the role that exercise plays in preventing and treating obesity.
3. Explain the modifications to standard testing procedures necessary for clients who are obese.
4. Write an exercise prescription for someone who is obese.

Obesity is characterized by excessive adiposity. Obesity can be documented by examining the relationship between height and weight (e.g., BMI) or by evaluating percent body fat (%BF). Because BMI requires simple measurements and, for the majority of adults, closely relates to body fatness, it has become the clinically preferred method of assessing obesity (see chapter 6). Generally accepted guidelines classify a BMI of 30 kg · m^{-2} or higher as obese (8). The following are subclasses of obesity:

- Class I obesity—30.0 to 34.9 kg · m^{-2}
- Class II obesity—35.0 to 39.9 kg · m^{-2}
- Class III (extreme) obesity—40 kg · m^{-2} or higher

Although there are no universally agreed on standards for classifying obesity from %BF, a %BF of >38% for females or >25% for males generally is considered in the obese range (19, 22). Another tool used to screen for obesity is waist circumference (see chapter 6 for more details). Adiposity located in the abdominal region is strongly linked with chronic disease risk; therefore, a waist circumference of ≥102 cm in men or ≥88 cm in women is used to classify individuals with abdominal obesity (8).

Potential Causes

Although consuming calories in excess of daily caloric need is an easily identified culprit in the etiology of obesity, this condition is much more complex than suggested by that simple explanation. Both biological (e.g., genetic predisposition attributable to lower than normal metabolic rate) and psychological (e.g., poor body image) factors can contribute to obesity and can pose significant obstacles when a person attempts to lose weight (13). Some studies show that genetics contribute around 25% to 40% of the variation in body composition (6), but others argue that genetics are responsible for 50% to 70% of this variation (5). Many biological factors have been identified as possible mechanisms that predispose a person to obesity. These factors include the protein leptin, sympathetic nervous system activity, several neuropeptides, and some hormones (27). Suggested pathways through which these factors work include lowering resting metabolic rate, influencing eating behaviors, or slowing the rate of fat oxidation. Because of the attention recently focused on the genetic roots of obesity, individuals who are obese can become discouraged from attempting to lose weight. Although biological factors clearly contribute to obesity, the imbalance between energy intake and expenditure ultimately leads to fat accumulation. Educating clients on the role of good nutrition and appropriate exercise in maintaining a healthy weight is an important aspect of the fitness professional's responsibilities.

The prevalence of obesity in the United States and in many countries around the world is increasing (20). The U.S. prevalence of obesity rose from 13.4% in the early 1960s to 30.9% in 2000 (9). Figure 19.1 shows the increase in BMI and waist circumference in recent decades. Recent national surveys reveal that 65.1% of American adults now have a BMI of 25 kg · m^{-2} or higher and thus are classified as overweight or obese (15). Minority women (i.e., non-Hispanic Blacks and Mexican Americans) appear particularly at risk for overweight and obesity, with over 70% having a BMI ≥25 kg · m^{-2} (15). According to criteria for waist circumference, 38.3% of men and 59.9% of women have abdominal obesity (25). Another disturbing trend is the increasing rate of obesity among children (29). Current estimates are that 31% of children are at or above the 85th percentile for BMI (the standard used to indicate excessive weight for height) (15). Some researchers have linked the rising prevalence of childhood obesity to an increase in inactive leisure pursuits such as television viewing (12, 26). The rapid increase in obesity in the United States over the last four decades supports the contention that lifestyle choices (i.e., diet and physical activity), not genetics, are primarily responsible for the increasing prevalence of obesity.

The increasing prevalence of obesity is important because of the negative health complications that accompany it. Obesity is linked with increased mortality and morbidity rates. Diseases and conditions associated with obesity include coronary heart disease (CHD), conges-

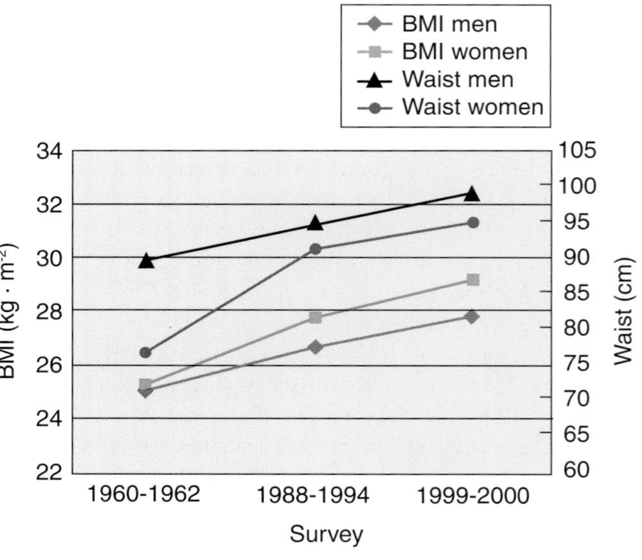

Figure 19.1 Changes in BMI and waist circumference for men and women (9, 25).

tive heart failure, stroke, type 2 diabetes, hypertension, dyslipidemia, gallbladder disease, osteoarthritis, some cancers (e.g., breast, colon), sleep apnea, and respiratory problems (24). Women who are obese are more likely to experience menstrual irregularities and complications with pregnancy (24). Estimates of annual U.S. deaths attributable to obesity range from 112,000 (10) to 300,000 (3). The direct cost of obesity in 1995 was approximately $51 billion, with the total economic cost near $100 billion (24). In 2000, the total economic cost of obesity increased to approximately $117 billion (32). Clearly, obesity results in major personal as well as financial strains. The serious effects of overweight and obesity are reflected by the issuance of *The Surgeon General's Call to Action to Prevent and Decrease Overweight and Obesity* (32). This report outlines the problem of overweight and obesity and calls for both public and private commitments to address this health concern.

Key Point

Obesity is a complex condition with biological and lifestyle links. Nearly one third of U.S. adults are classified as obese, and the prevalence is rising. Comorbidities of obesity include type 2 diabetes, CHD, stroke, and some cancers. In the United States the economic cost of obesity is more than $100 billion per year.

Physical Activity in Prevention and Treatment of Obesity

The rapid increase in obesity prevalence appears linked to both low physical activity and excessive energy intake (31). This suggests that increasing physical activity and reducing caloric intake will lower rates of obesity. Although the evidence is indirect, an overview of cross-sectional and prospective studies suggests that active people are less likely to be obese, and those who maintain an active lifestyle are least likely to become obese over time (7, 18). A recent international consensus meeting concluded that 45 to 60 min of daily moderate activity is needed to prevent obesity (28). However, estimating energy intake and expenditure on a population level is crude, the studies do not always agree, and much additional research is needed to clarify these issues. Despite the need for more research, there is general agreement in the medical (30) and public health (32) communities that both exercise and dietary modification should be used in treating patients who are obese.

A number of studies have used exercise as a means for treating obesity. Most of these trials were short term, and many had design flaws that limit the conclusions that can be drawn. In general, well-controlled, randomized control trials typically have found modest weight reduction when exercise is used to treat obesity (14, 35). Slightly greater weight loss typically is seen when caloric restriction is combined with exercise. There is also evidence that a combination of dietary restriction and exercise is better at helping maintain weight loss than is either method alone (14, 35). The data from the National Weight Control Registry (NWCR) suggest that regular aerobic exercise is common among those who successfully maintain significant weight loss (36). See the following Research Insight for more information on the characteristics of people who are successful at maintaining weight loss. Exercise recommendations for individuals who are obese can be found later in this chapter.

Research Insight

The NWCR was established in 1994 to provide insight into ways that people successfully lose weight and then maintain weight loss. Currently, more than 3,000 people participate in the NWCR, with an average weight loss of 30 kg maintained for 5.5 yr. About half of these participants used commercial weight loss programs, whereas the others lost weight without formal guidance. Several interesting facts have been gathered from these successful losers: (1) 89% report using both caloric restriction and exercise in their weight loss programs, (2) the most common dietary approach involved choosing a diet low in total calories and low in fat (~24% of calories from fat), (3) most participants weighed themselves frequently to provide feedback on the success of their behaviors, (4) a typical exercise routine was 1 hr · day^{-1} of moderate physical activity, and (5) walking was the most frequently reported exercise (77% of participants), while about 20% used resistance training. For more information on the NWCR, see Wing and Hill (36).

Key Point

Active people are less likely to be overweight or obese. Exercise can be an important part of a weight loss program and is a key to maintaining weight loss.

Special Medical Screening

Several conditions frequently coexist with obesity (e.g., type 2 diabetes, hypertension) (8). The high prevalence of these comorbidities requires that fitness professionals carefully screen individuals who are obese before performing exercise testing. Health histories and pretesting screenings should be designed to identify any comorbidities (see chapter 3). These conditions as well as the individual's overall physical condition will determine the types of exercise testing needed before exercise programming. Once the initial health history screening process is completed, the ACSM risk stratification (2) can be used to decide on the need for medical clearance and physician supervision of exercise tests.

Medications

Like all clients, a person who is obese should provide documentation of medications. Because of the wide-ranging comorbidities that can exist with obesity, a variety of medications may be prescribed. It is common to find clients who are obese and who take several medications, including those for hypertension and glucose control. Before exercise testing and prescription, fitness professionals should consider the possible effect of these medications.

Prescription medications for weight loss or weight control are available for individuals under a physician's care (21, 30). Two commonly prescribed drugs used to treat obesity are orlistat (i.e., Xenical) and sibutramine (i.e., Meridia). Orlistat interferes with the absorption of fat in the digestive system and commonly results in weight loss and improved blood lipid profile. Although an increase in BP occasionally is reported with using orlistat, more common side effects are oily discharge and fecal urgency. Sibutramine works through the brain neurotransmitters serotonin and norepinephrine. It increases metabolic rate, creates a sense of fullness, and elevates energy levels. Potential cardiovascular side effects include increased HR and BP. Over-the-counter weight loss aids and herbal supplements are also taken frequently by people desiring weight loss. In 2004, the U.S. Food and Drug Administration banned ephedrine alkaloids (ephedra) in over-the-counter weight loss products because of the reported occurrence of tachycardia, hypertension, strokes, and heart attacks. It is beyond the scope of this chapter to review all products used to promote weight loss. Fitness professionals should encourage clients to be wise consumers of such products by learning about all the potential side effects and discussing these substances with their physicians.

Exercise Testing

Typically, standard testing modes and protocols can be used when testing persons who are obese; however, the initial intensity as well as the incremental increases should reflect the individual's fitness and activity level (see chapter 5). This is particularly important because of the severe deconditioning that often exists with obesity. With severe obesity or when ambulation is problematic, it may be preferable to use cycle or arm ergometry for testing. However, when walking is the exercise of choice for programming, treadmill testing provides useful insight into the velocity that the client can maintain during walking. This can be helpful information when designing a workout with a targeted caloric expenditure.

The physiological response to exercise typically is similar in people who are obese and people who are normal weight, except that excessive weight often reduces cardiorespiratory function. However, comorbidities, especially hypertension and type 2 diabetes, can alter the exercise or postexercise response. For more information on testing clients who are obese, refer to the review by Wallace (33).

Key Point

The large number of comorbidities that accompany obesity necessitates careful screening of clients who are obese. Exercise testing of these clients should be individualized, taking into account any special needs.

Surgical Procedures for Weight Loss

For individuals with extreme obesity (BMI $\geq$40 kg · m^{-2}) who have been unsuccessful in previous weight loss attempts and who have serious comorbid conditions, **bariatric surgery** may be an option (23, 30). There are a variety of surgical options, but all modify the gastrointestinal system so that food intake is restricted and nutrient uptake is diminished. These procedures often lead to significant weight loss, but they also have a number of serious side effects (23). These surgeries require major modifications in eating patterns. Once individuals recover from surgery, exercise programming is recommended. The dietary planning and exercise programming for these patients should be overseen by medical professionals.

Exercise Prescription

Weight loss, greater fitness, and improved chronic disease risk factors are the focus of exercise programs for individuals who are obese. ACSM guidelines state that all adults, including those who are obese, should exercise on most, if not all, days of the week for a minimum of 150 min · wk^{-1} in order to protect against chronic disease (1, 2). However, evidence indicates that an even greater caloric expenditure (i.e., 200-300 min · wk^{-1}) may be most beneficial for long-term weight control (1, 2). Some groups advocate 45 to 60 min of daily moderate activity to prevent weight gain and 60 to 90 min for individuals who were previously obese to prevent weight regain (11, 28). When first beginning an exercise program, participants may be unable to exercise this long, so an initial focus of programming is to build enough endurance to sustain aerobic activity to reach these duration goals. Accumulating activity in shorter bouts throughout the day should be considered as an option. The ACSM recommends the following approach to exercise for weight loss (2):

- Frequency: 5 to 7 days per wk
- Intensity: initially moderate (40%-60% HRR), with progression to higher intensity (50%-75% HRR)
- Duration: progress from short, easily tolerated bouts to 45 to 60 min daily

Designing exercise programs for individuals who are obese requires some special considerations. One of the primary aims of any exercise program should be safety. For individuals who are obese, avoiding orthopedic injuries is a particular concern because of the additional loading to joints. Therefore, low-impact activities (water exercise, cycling, and walking) are preferable when individuals who are obese begin to exercise regularly. After some weight loss and conditioning occur, they may participate in higher impact sports and activities. Another safety concern is thermoregulation (33). Because of excessive body fatness and the increased energy demands of activity, keeping the body cool during exercise can be problematic for people with a lot of body fat. They should be encouraged to exercise at cool times of the day or in temperature-controlled environments. These exercisers should maintain hydration by drinking adequate amounts of water.

Resistance training also may be an important component of the overall exercise program. Although resistance training typically does not burn off a large number of calories, it can serve important functions in weight loss (1). During weight loss, both lean and fat tissues typically diminish. However, lean tissue may be maintained, or at least muscle loss can be minimized, by using resistance training during caloric restriction. Maintaining muscle mass benefits both functional capacity and metabolic rate. Compared with fat, muscle is a metabolically active tissue, so maintaining lean mass helps minimize decreases in metabolic rate.

Rarely will individuals who are obese begin exercise without also setting goals related to weight loss (although exercise provides benefits even in the absence of weight loss; see Exercise Without Weight Loss on page 310). Fitness professionals should assist the client in developing healthy weight loss goals. Appropriate weight loss goals are 0.5 to 1 kg · wk^{-1}. For example, reducing caloric intake by 500 kcal · day^{-1} and expending an additional 300 kcal · day^{-1} creates a caloric deficit that approximates a 0.7 kg loss in 1 wk (7 [500 + 300] = 5,600 kcal · wk^{-1}). Typically, diets with fewer than 1,200 kcal · day^{-1} are not recommended without physician supervision. A well-planned, low-fat diet with a caloric deficit of 500 to 1,000 kcal · day^{-1} gradually reduces weight without sacrificing nutritional needs (1). An appropriate distribution of macronutrients along with the necessary amounts of vitamins and minerals should be included in the dietary planning (see chapter 7). Diets that are low in fat, particularly saturated fat, not only are effective for weight loss but also are associated with long-term weight maintenance. See chapter 11 for additional information on weight loss and weight management strategies. Individuals who are overweight and obese should reduce body weight by at least 5% to gain health benefits such as lower BP and a more favorable blood lipid profile. For some individuals, an even greater reduction in body weight may optimize health improvement (1).

Long-term adherence to exercise is problematic for people who were previously sedentary and are obese. Fitness professionals should help clients overcome perceived barriers to living an active lifestyle. Commonly reported barriers are feeling too fat to exercise, believing that their health is too poor for exercise, and believing that an injury or disability precludes participation in exercise (4). Fitness professionals should provide education about the risks of leading an inactive life, the health benefits of regular exercise, and the variety of exercise options available. A dialogue between the fitness professional and client determines program needs, client likes and dislikes, and level of support needed to increase adherence. These discussions can lead to decisions about the specific nature of the exercise routine (e.g., structured versus lifestyle, intermittent versus continuous) (16, 17). Look for opportunities to increase energy expenditure through structured exercise (e.g., taking brisk 30 min walks) and lifestyle activity (e.g., substituting active for sedentary leisure pursuits). When it comes to long-term adherence, finding an approach that fits the needs of the client is critical.

Key Point

Prudent weight loss goals for clients who are overweight and obese range from 0.5 to 1.0 kg · wk^{-1}. Daily, or near daily, moderate aerobic activity is suggested. While 30 min · day^{-1} of moderate-intensity exercise is a minimum goal, better success is seen with 45 to 90 min. People who are obese can use both aerobic exercise and resistance training. For weight loss, exercise programs should be combined with a low-fat, reduced-calorie diet. When prescribing exercise, emphasize avoiding musculoskeletal injuries and heat injury as well as finding ways to improve adherence.

Exercise Without Weight Loss

Even without weight loss, exercise benefits people who are overweight. These benefits (e.g., an improved blood lipid profile, lower BP, and better stress management) are much the same as those seen in people who are normal weight. Although both reducing weight and improving fitness optimize health benefits, participation in regular exercise significantly protects against disease even when the individuals remain overweight. Data from the Cooper Clinic in Dallas have demonstrated that fitness protects against early death in persons who are overweight (34). Because of these findings, it is important to emphasize an active lifestyle, even if weight loss is not an outcome.

Case Studies

You can check your answers by referring to page 474 in appendix A.

1. Marsha is a 51-yr-old female who comes to your fitness facility and expresses interest in purchasing a membership. She is responding to a series of advertisements that your facility is using to attract people interested in weight loss. Your screening reveals the following:
   - Her height is 5 ft 5 in. (1.65 m) and her weight is 240 lb (109 kg).
   - Her blood pressure is 152/88 mmHg.
   - She has never exercised regularly, has a desk job, and has no active leisure pursuits.
   - It has been more than 3 yr since she had a medical examination.
   - There is a history of heart disease on her father's side of the family, and her mother developed type 2 diabetes after menopause.
     a. What, if any, medical screening would you recommend before this client enrolls in your facility's programs?
     b. What fitness testing would you suggest for her?
     c. Assuming that no medical conditions are revealed with the screening and initial testing, describe a diet and exercise program that Marsha could use to achieve her weight loss and fitness goals.

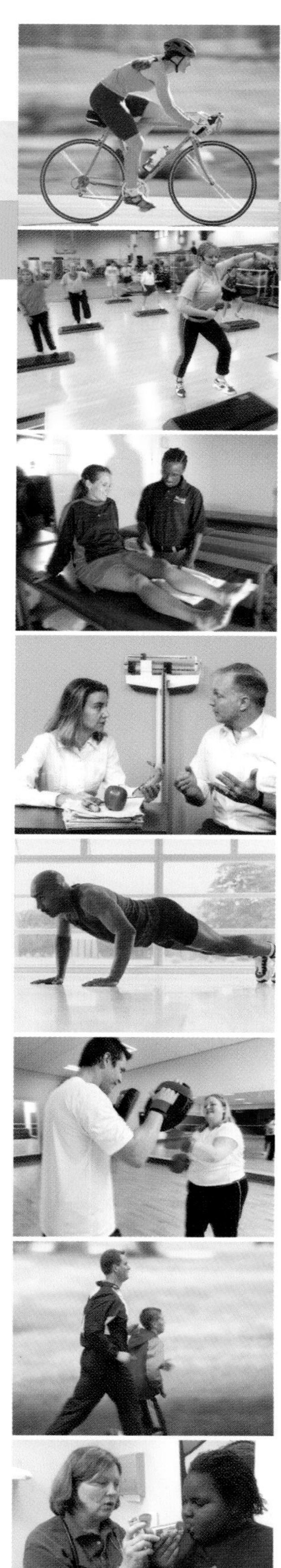

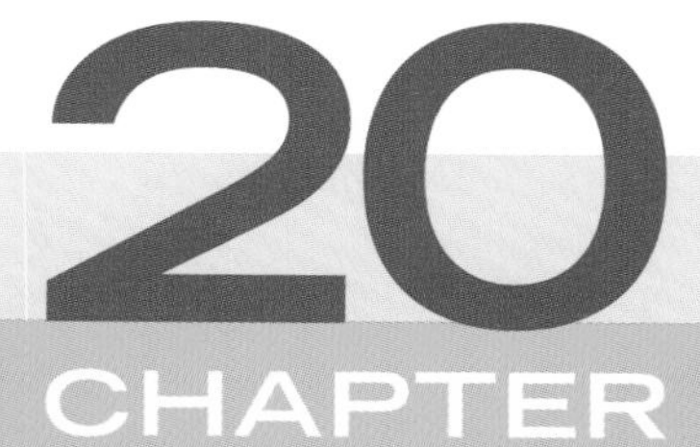

20 CHAPTER

Exercise and Diabetes

Dixie L. Thompson

Objectives

The reader will be able to do the following:

1. Define diabetes mellitus and describe the characteristics of type 1 and type 2 diabetes.
2. Describe the role that exercise plays in the prevention and treatment of type 2 diabetes.
3. Describe special considerations in exercise testing for clients with diabetes.
4. Describe special considerations in exercise prescription for clients with diabetes.

Diabetes mellitus refers to metabolic diseases characterized by **hyperglycemia** (i.e., elevated plasma glucose). The following blood glucose levels are used to identify a person with diabetes mellitus. The cause of hyperglycemia varies depending on the form of diabetes present, with the most common forms being type 1 and type 2 diabetes. **Type 1 diabetes** is characterized by a deficiency of insulin often attributable to an autoimmune destruction of the insulin-producing beta cells of the pancreas. In **type 2 diabetes,** the insulin receptors become insensitive or resistant to insulin and, because glucose cannot move readily into the cells, hyperglycemia results. Although there are other forms of diabetes mellitus (e.g., gestational diabetes), type 1 and type 2 account for the vast majority of cases. Regardless of the type, a number of complications may result from diabetes. These complications typically affect the blood vessels and nerves and include vision impairment, kidney disease, peripheral vascular disease, atherosclerosis, and hypertension (5). The estimated economic burden (direct and indirect costs) of diabetes is $132 billion each year (3).

It is estimated that more than 20 million Americans have diabetes; approximately 90% of the cases are type 2 diabetes. This form of diabetes has both lifestyle and genetic roots. Many people with type 2 diabetes are relatively inactive and overweight or obese, particularly with excessive abdominal fat. Other risk factors include a family history of type 2 diabetes, older age, and belonging to an ethnic minority (prevalence is higher among Hispanic, Native Americans, and African Americans compared with Caucasians). Type 2 diabetes frequently coexists with other conditions such as hypertension and dyslipidemia. Although type 2 diabetes can appear at any age, the highest rates are seen among people aged 60 yr and older (14). However, there is an increasing prevalence of type 2 diabetes among children, and this trend seems to be linked to increasing obesity rates (14).

Comparison of Type 1 and Type 2 Diabetes

Type 1 diabetes results from a lack of insulin. The most common cause is autoimmune destruction of the insulin-producing beta cells of the pancreas, leading to lack of insulin. Without insulin, the body's cells are unable to take in glucose. Unlike type 2 diabetes, type 1 diabetes often appears early in life and is more closely linked to genetic than lifestyle factors. People with type 1 diabetes require insulin injections. There are many types of insulin, and they vary by how rapidly they begin working, their peak time of action, and how long they continue to work. Insulins used to treat diabetes are listed in table 20.1. Some people with type 2 diabetes also require insulin injections. More often, however, they take other types of prescription medications to lower blood glucose. Many types of medications are used for this purpose (see table 20.2). For more information on medications used to treat diabetes mellitus, see the Web sites of the American Diabetes Association (www.diabetes.org) and the National Institute of Diabetes and Digestive and Kidney Diseases (www.niddk.nih.gov).

Type 2 diabetes is characterized by **insulin resistance,** a condition in which the body's insulin receptors no longer respond normally to insulin. Thus glucose entry into cells is impaired and hyperglycemia results. Plasma insulin levels of people with type 2 diabetes may be normal, suppressed, or elevated depending on the individual. Regardless, type 2 diabetes is considered a disease of relative insulin deficiency because the insulin available is inadequate to maintain normal glucose concentrations. Although some people with type 2 diabetes can control their disease through exercise and weight loss, others require medications such as oral hypoglycemic agents and possibly even insulin injections (see table 20.2).

Diagnosing Diabetes Mellitus (5)

For a diagnosis of diabetes, one of the following criteria must exist:

- Fasting plasma glucose of $\geq$126 mg · dl^{-1} (7.0 mM; fasting means no food intake within the past 8 or more hours)
- Symptoms of diabetes (e.g., unusual thirst, frequent urination, unexplained weight loss) and a casual plasma glucose of $\geq$200 mg · dl^{-1} (11.1 mM; casual means that time of last food ingestion before testing was not controlled)
- A glucose value of $\geq$200 mg · dl^{-1} 2 hr after the ingestion of 75 g of carbohydrate (oral glucose tolerance test)

Normal fasting plasma glucose concentration is <100 mg · dl^{-1} (5.6 mM). Fasting plasma glucose concentration of 100 to 125 mg · dl^{-1} classifies the individual as having impaired fasting glucose.

• Table 20.1 Forms of Insulin Used to Control Diabetes Mellitus •

Type of insulin	Onset of action	Peak	Duration
Rapid acting	5-20 min	45 min-3 hr	3-5 hr
Short acting	30 min	2-5 hr	5-8 hr
Intermediate acting	1-3 hr	6-12 hr	16-24 hr
Long acting	4-6 hr	8-20 hr	24-28 hr
Very long acting	1 hr	Lowers evenly for 24 hr	24 hr
Premixed (intermediate + short acting)	30 min	7-12 hr	16-24 hr

• Table 20.2 Medications to Control Type 2 Diabetes •

Class of medication	Example	Mode of action
Sulfonylureas	Glynase PresTab	Stimulates insulin production
Biguanides	Glucophage	Reduces glucose release from liver
α-Glucosidase inhibitors	Precose	Slows the absorption of carbohydrates
Thiazolidinediones	Avandia	Increases insulin sensitivity
Meglitinides	Prandin	Stimulates insulin production
D-phenylalanine derivatives	Starlix	Increases the rate of insulin production

Type 2 diabetes usually develops over time, first appearing as **impaired fasting glucose** (100-125 mg · dl^{-1}) or **impaired glucose tolerance (IGT).** Impaired glucose tolerance is a condition in which the increase in blood glucose after ingestion of carbohydrate is higher than normal and remains elevated longer than normal. A glucose level of 140 to 199 mg · dl^{-1} 2 hr after an oral glucose tolerance test indicates impaired glucose tolerance. Examples of normal and abnormal blood glucose responses are shown in figure 20.1. A person with either impaired fasting glucose or impaired glucose tolerance is classified as having **prediabetes.** Without intervention, prediabetes generally evolves into type 2 diabetes. It is estimated that 41 million Americans have prediabetes.

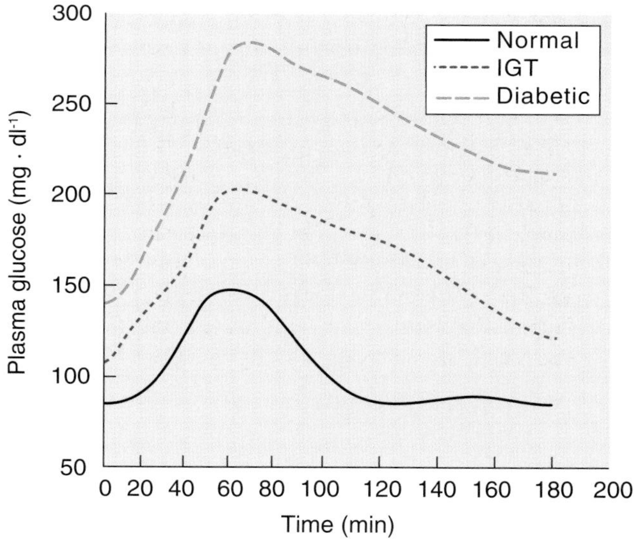

Figure 20.1 Comparison of glucose response to carbohydrate ingestion.

Key Point

Diabetes mellitus is characterized by hyperglycemia. More than 20 million Americans have diabetes mellitus, and the economic cost is approximately $132 billion each year. Type 1 diabetes results from a lack of insulin production. Type 2 diabetes, the most common form of diabetes, is characterized by the cells becoming insensitive to insulin. Risk factors for type 2 diabetes include older age, a family history of type 2 diabetes, excess weight, and inactivity.

Exercise for Clients With Diabetes

Exercise can provide many benefits to individuals with either type 1 or type 2 diabetes. This is particularly true because of the strong link between diabetes and cardiovascular disease and the role that exercise plays in reducing cardiovascular disease risk. Although exercise will not prevent or cure type 1 diabetes, exercise should be encouraged in this population for a number of reasons (4). Exercise improves insulin sensitivity and reduces disease risk for people with diabetes, much like in the population without diabetes. Because of the high rate of cardiovascular disease among people with diabetes, exercise can help promote overall well-being. Exercise protects against coronary artery disease, dyslipidemia, hypertension, and obesity. Increased physical activity and improved physical fitness also promote psychological health and quality of life.

Exercise helps prevent and treat type 2 diabetes. Inactivity and obesity are common characteristics of persons with type 2 diabetes. Research has shown that individuals who are regularly active are 30% to 50% less likely to develop type 2 diabetes than are their inactive counterparts (6). Additionally, people who have impaired glucose tolerance are less likely to develop type 2 diabetes if they begin to exercise regularly (1, 12). Evidence is mounting that people with type 2 diabetes experience better glucose tolerance and improved insulin sensitivity through regular exercise (1, 7). There are a number of reasons why exercise can benefit the treatment of type 2 diabetes (11, 15), including the following:

- Lower fasting blood glucose concentrations
- Better glucose tolerance (less of a spike in glucose after eating)
- Improved insulin sensitivity (more glucose uptake with a given amount of insulin)
- Weight control (increased lean mass and reduced fat mass)
- Improved lipid profiles
- Reduction in blood pressure for those with hypertension
- Lower risk of cardiovascular disease
- Stress management (stress can affect glucose control via increased levels of catecholamines)

Key Point

Exercise has been shown to be effective in preventing and treating type 2 diabetes. Regardless of the type of diabetes, exercise benefits people with diabetes in a number of ways.

Screening and Testing Clients With Diabetes

Medical clearance should be required of all clients with diabetes mellitus to ensure that they can safely perform exercise (2). Individuals should discuss with their physicians how to modify their insulin dosage with exercise. Because exercise increases glucose uptake from peripheral tissues regardless of insulin levels, hypoglycemia may result if insulin intake is not adjusted (see next section for tips on avoiding hypoglycemia). Diabetes is a primary risk factor for the development of cardiovascular disease, so clients with diabetes should be screened carefully for signs and symptoms of disease (chapter 3). The ADA recommends that individuals undergo a full medical screening with particular attention to diabetes-related complications (e.g., CAD, retinopathy, nephropathy) before beginning an exercise program (5).

People with type 2 diabetes frequently are overweight and hypertensive and have a poor blood lipid profile; therefore, they may be taking a number of medications that can influence the exercise response. For people who have had diabetes for a number of years, peripheral neuropathy may be a problem. Damage to the sensory nerves in the feet can lead to ulcerations, and if there is damage to blood vessels, healing can be slow. Because of these and other issues, conducting a thorough medical history is particularly important with these clients.

The type of testing performed before exercise programming depends on the person. Diagnostic exercise stress testing, under the supervision of a physician, may be necessary for individuals with numerous risk factors. The protocol will depend on the client's age and functional ability. Submaximal exercise testing can be used to estimate aerobic power (see chapter 5). However, autonomic neuropathy can cause unusual HR and BP responses during exercise.

The decision of whether to perform exercise testing for clients with diabetes should be made in consultation with the client's physician. Generally, before the client begins a moderate or vigorous exercise program, exercise testing with CAD screening is recommended (13). It is also recommended that high-risk patients be tested before any program (see Guidelines for Clients With Diabetes on page 315). Some low-risk participants will be able to begin low-intensity programs (<39% HRR) without stress testing. For additional information on testing clients who have diabetes, see *ACSM's Resource Manual for Guidelines for Exercise Testing and Prescription* (13) and

Key Point

Because of the increased risks for exercise-related complications associated with diabetes mellitus, physician clearance should be obtained before exercise testing. The type of tests will depend on the client's needs.

Guidelines for Clients With Diabetes

High-risk individuals who meet one of the following criteria should undergo diagnostic exercise tests before beginning any exercise programming:

- Previously sedentary and aged 35 yr or older, or sedentary and has had diabetes >10 yr (whatever the current age)
- Has had type 1 diabetes >15 yr or type 2 diabetes >10 yr
- Has additional major CAD risk factors
- Has peripheral vascular disease, kidney disease, microvascular disease, cardiomegaly, or congestive heart failure
- Has advanced autonomic, renal, or cerebrovascular disease
- Has known CAD

Low-risk individuals who meet the following criteria may begin a low-intensity (≤39% HRR) exercise program without diagnostic exercise testing:

- Anticipated exercise level roughly equivalent to ordinary walking pace
- Under 35 yr old
- Has no other major CAD risk factors
- Shows no other risk factors for sudden death
- Has a normal resting ECG

Adapted, by permission, from American College of Sports Medicine (ACSM), 2005, *ACSM's resource manual for guidelines for exercise testing and prescription*, 5th ed. (Philadelphia, PA: Lippincott, Williams & Wilkins), 246-247. (13).

ACSM's Exercise Management for Persons with Chronic Diseases and Disabilities (11).

Exercise Prescription

The goals of exercise programming for clients with diabetes (e.g., increasing aerobic power, reducing disease risk, increasing flexibility, increasing muscular strength and endurance) are similar to those for clients who do not have diabetes, with the exception of increased attention to improving glucose control. The basic elements of exercise prescription should be applied for clients with diabetes, but with special considerations as outlined in the following sections.

Type 1 Diabetes

A person with type 1 diabetes must carefully consider modifying insulin dosage and carbohydrate ingestion before beginning an exercise program. Increasing the intake of carbohydrate or reducing insulin dosage is often necessary to maintain proper glucose control and to avoid hypoglycemia that can result from exercise. The adjustment in carbohydrate intake and insulin dosage depends on the intensity and duration of activity. Glucose should be measured before initiating an exercise session. If glucose is <100 mg · dl^{-1}, carbohydrate (20-30 g) should be ingested before beginning exercise. If glucose is >300 mg · dl^{-1} or >250 mg · dl^{-1} with urinary ketones, exercise should be delayed (2).

For the client with type 1 diabetes who was previously inactive, progression should be slow, with careful monitoring of blood glucose and symptoms of cardiovascular and metabolic distress. Initially, supervised exercise is recommended. After the person is able to maintain glucose control with exercise, unsupervised exercise is acceptable. However, it is always preferable that clients with diabetes do not exercise alone because of the need to have someone nearby in case of a hypoglycemic event. Symptoms of hypoglycemia include dizziness, nausea, headache, confusion, and irritability (2). The following precautions should be observed for avoiding exercise-induced hypoglycemia:

- Measure blood glucose immediately before and 15 min after exercise (also during exercise if the exercise lasts longer than 30 min).
- Consume carbohydrate if glucose is <100 mg · dl^{-1}.
- Delay exercise if glucose is >250 mg · dl^{-1} with ketone bodies or >300 mg · dl^{-1} without ketones.
- Avoid exercising during times of peak insulin action.

- Reduce insulin dose (and inject into inactive areas) on days of planned exercise.
- Consume carbohydrate after exercise. Hypoglycemia can appear several hours after exercise, so monitoring after exercise is crucial.
- Avoid exercise late at night because hypoglycemia could occur while sleeping.
- Extend the warm-up and cool-down if needed.

Regular (3 or more times a week) aerobic exercise is recommended to maximize blood glucose control. The intensity of the exercise should match the characteristics of the client. Although moderate-intensity resistance exercise is safe for most people with diabetes, those with advanced complications (e.g., kidney disease, vision impairment) should avoid heavy lifting, where extreme BP elevation is possible. The American Diabetes Association provides specific examples of recommended and discouraged exercises depending on the severity of the disease (4).

Because peripheral neuropathy can lead to ulcerations of the feet, good foot care is essential. Properly fitting and supportive shoes are particularly important for clients with diabetes who are engaging in weight-bearing exercise. For more information, Neil Gordon's book, *Diabetes: Your Complete Exercise Guide,* provides guidelines for foot care that may be useful (9). For those with advanced peripheral neuropathy, low-impact and potentially non-weight-bearing exercises are more appropriate (4).

Type 2 Diabetes

The ACSM recommends that individuals with type 2 diabetes engage in both endurance and resistance training, unless significant complications or limitations exist (1). At least 1,000 kcal $\cdot$ wk^{-1} should be expended in aerobic activity. For those who are overweight or obese, aerobic activity should focus on caloric expenditure and weight control. Although at least 3 nonconsecutive days of exercise per week are recommended, individuals may choose to engage in daily physical activity to maximize glucose control and caloric expenditure.

Moderate-intensity exercise is generally recommended (2), although the participant's characteristics should be considered when determining intensity. Activity at higher intensity is acceptable for those who are conditioned and choose more vigorous exercise. Because of the possibility of autonomic neuropathy, using HR to monitor exercise intensity may be problematic. Therefore, RPE may be a better choice for individuals to self-monitor exercise intensity (see chapter 5). Exercise intensity and duration should be balanced to achieve goals for caloric expenditure. Typically, exercise sessions lasting at least 10 to 15 min are suggested, with physical activity accumulating to 30 to 60 min each day. The mode of aerobic exercise should fit the client's needs and abilities. Walking is the mode of choice for many, but for those with peripheral nerve damage, other modes (e.g., swimming, nonimpact exercise equipment) may be preferable.

Resistance training also is suggested for many people with type 2 diabetes (1, 2). Resistance training maintains or even increases muscle mass and assists with glucose tolerance and insulin sensitivity. The program should focus on major muscle groups (8-10 exercises) and consist of at least 1 set of 10 to 15 repetitions (see chapter 12). This routine should be performed at least 2 day $\cdot$ wk^{-1}. People without advanced complications can follow more aggressive programs. However, for those with eye or kidney damage resulting from diabetes, particular caution should be taken to avoid extreme BP elevations (4).

Because many clients with type 2 diabetes have a history of being relatively inactive and are often overweight, beginning and then maintaining an active lifestyle presents particular challenges. Creating a supportive environment is critical to the success of these clients. Early in the exercise program, it is particularly important to provide information on the benefits of a lifetime commitment to exercise. The program should progress slowly, be based on realistic goals, and incorporate the client's needs and desires. Additional information on increasing adherence to exercise can be found in chapter 22 and in the ACSM position stand on exercise and type 2 diabetes (1).

Key Point

Exercise prescription for the client with diabetes must take into account special needs caused by the disease. Careful monitoring of blood glucose levels is needed to help avoid hypoglycemic events. For individuals with type 2 diabetes, the ACSM recommends an exercise program that burns at least 1,000 kcal $\cdot$ wk^{-1}. Resistance training can be used with clients who have diabetes as long as the client avoids damage to already weakened blood vessels.

Metabolic Syndrome

Metabolic syndrome (also called *syndrome X)* is a condition in which a number of CAD risk factors exist together. People with metabolic syndrome have a much higher risk for atherosclerotic cardiovascular disease. In order to be diagnosed with metabolic syndrome, a person must have at least three of the following (10):

- Abdominal obesity: waist circumference ≥102 cm (men) or ≥88 cm (women)
- High triglycerides: ≥150 mg · dl^{-1}, or drug treatment
- Low HDL-C: <40 mg · dl^{-1} (men) or <50 mg · dl^{-1} (women), or drug treatment
- Elevated blood pressure: ≥130/≥85 mmHg, or drug treatment
- Elevated fasting glucose: ≥100 mg · dl^{-1}, or drug treatment

A recent study found that approximately 29% of American adults have metabolic syndrome (8). Without intervention, chronic disease risk (e.g., CVD, diabetes) is much higher for these individuals. The approach to control metabolic syndrome depends on the symptoms that are present. Since abdominal obesity is common, weight loss is frequently suggested (7%-10% weight loss the first year and then continued reduction to reach a BMI of <25 kg · m^{-2}) (10). Physical activity is also commonly recommended because of the effect of regular exercise on all characteristics of metabolic syndrome. See chapter 19 for recommendations about physical activity for clients who are obese.

Case Studies

You can check your answers by referring to page 474 in appendix A.

1. Mr. Conner is a 40-yr-old man who, in response to doctor's orders, appears at your medical wellness facility for exercise programming. He recently sought the care of his physician after experiencing fatigue and headaches. Mr. Conner's physician ordered a series of tests, including a diagnostic exercise stress test. Here are Mr. Conner's test results:

   Weight = 265 lb(120 kg)

   Cholesterol = 270 mg · dl^{-1}

   Fasting glucose = 132 mg · dl^{-1}

   Height = 5 ft 9.5 in. (1.77 m)

   LDL-C = 190 mg · dl^{-1}

   Blood pressure = 148/94 mmHg

   No smoking

   HDL-C = 32 mg · dl^{-1}

   $\dot{V}O_2max$ = 22 ml · kg^{-1} · min^{-1}

   High stress

   Previously inactive

   No ischemia with GXT

   Mr. Conner was diagnosed with type 2 diabetes, placed on medication to lower his cholesterol, and placed on a diuretic to lower his blood pressure. He was told to begin to exercise and lose weight in an attempt to lower his blood glucose. Mr. Conner will enroll in a 3 mo weight loss and supervised exercise program at your facility. Determine a reasonable 3 mo weight loss goal for Mr. Conner and determine a caloric intake and exercise plan to help him realize this goal.

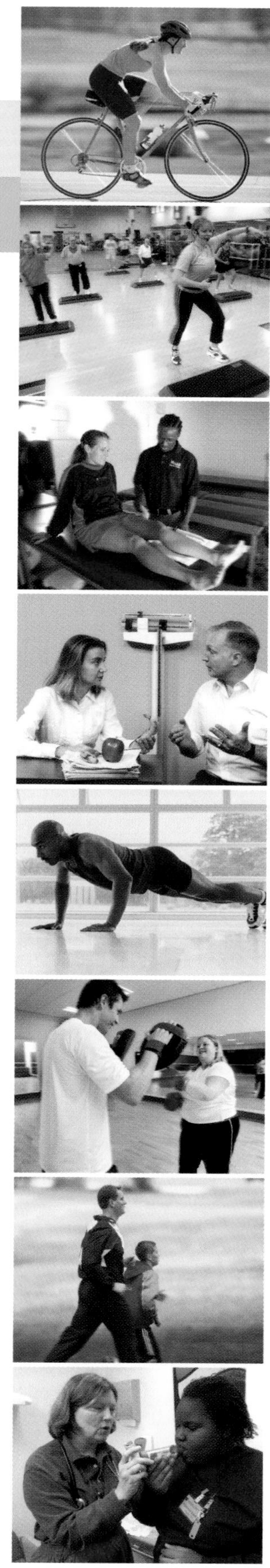

21
CHAPTER

Exercise, Asthma, and Pulmonary Disease

David R. Bassett Jr.

Objectives

The reader will be able to do the following:

1. Describe the differences between chronic obstructive lung diseases and restrictive lung diseases.
2. Define the underlying physiological problems associated with asthma, emphysema, bronchitis, and cystic fibrosis.
3. List physiological and mental health benefits of exercise for individuals with pulmonary disease.
4. Describe how pulmonary function testing can be used to diagnose chronic obstructive lung diseases versus restrictive lung diseases.
5. Describe how signs (e.g., dyspnea) and symptoms (e.g., hypoxemia) of pulmonary disease typically are monitored during a GXT.
6. Describe how to prescribe aerobic exercise (frequency, intensity, and duration) in pulmonary rehabilitation programs.
7. Identify the benefits of upper-body training in pulmonary rehabilitation.

(continued)

8. Discuss the use of supplemental oxygen therapy and pursed-lip breathing for individuals with chronic obstructive pulmonary disease.
9. List the common categories of medications used to treat pulmonary disease and examples of each category and discuss the probable effect of these medications on exercise performance.

Pulmonary diseases can be subdivided into two major categories. In **chronic obstructive pulmonary diseases** (COPDs), the airflow into and out of the lungs is impeded. In restrictive lung diseases, the expansion of the lungs is reduced because of conditions involving the chest cavity or parenchyma (lung tissue). Some pulmonary diseases are genetically inherited (e.g., cystic fibrosis), but in other cases a history of cigarette smoking, environmental pollutants, or occupational exposure to silica, coal dust, or asbestos is the primary contributing factor. All pulmonary diseases show a disruption in the exchange of gases between the ambient air and the pulmonary capillary blood. As a result, $\dot{V}O_2max$ is reduced, the work of breathing is increased, and the ability to perform exercise is limited.

Chronic Obstructive Pulmonary Diseases

COPDs cause a reduction in airflow that can dramatically affect a person's ability to perform daily activities. Characteristics of COPDs include expiratory flow obstruction and shortness of breath on exertion. These diseases include chronic bronchitis, emphysema, and bronchial asthma. Each of these diseases obstructs airflow, but the underlying reason for obstruction differs for each (4):

- Bronchial asthma is caused by bronchial smooth muscle contraction and increased airway reactivity.
- Chronic bronchitis results from persistent production of sputum attributable to a thickened bronchial wall with excess secretions.
- Emphysema is caused by loss of elastic recoil of alveoli and bronchioles and enlargement of those pulmonary structures.

According to 1994 data from the U.S. National Center for Health Statistics, 14 million Americans have chronic bronchitis and 2.2 million Americans have emphysema (15). Unfortunately, the mortality rates associated with COPDs have increased over the past two decades. Chronic bronchitis and emphysema are not reversible. The patient with COPD perceives an inability to perform normal activities without dyspnea, but, tragically, by the time this occurs the disease is well advanced (4, 18).

Asthma

An estimated 14.6 million people in the United States have asthma (15); 36% are children under the age of 18 (6). It is a condition that can reverse itself and varies from wheezing and slight breathlessness to severe attacks that may result in suffocation. Causes of asthma include allergic reactions to antigens such as dust, pollen, smoke, and air pollution. Nonspecific factors such as emotional stress and exercise as well as viral infections of the bronchi, sinuses, or tonsils can also result in asthma. People with exercise-induced asthma may have normal resting pulmonary function but experience bronchospasms during exercise. In some cases, no specific cause of the asthma can be identified (18). Treatment involves bronchodilators (often administered by inhalers) and other drugs that thin the mucous secretions and help eject them (expectorants) (7).

Exercise-induced asthma is a reactive airway disease affecting between 4% and 20% of the U.S. population (19). With this condition, exercise tends to cause the bronchioles to constrict. One method of diagnosing exercise-induced asthma is to have a patient run for 6 to 8 min on the treadmill at 85% to 90% of maximal heart rate (2). The forced expiratory volume in 1 sec (FEV_1) is measured before exercise and 3 to 9 min after exercise. A positive test occurs when the postexercise FEV_1 is 15% below the pretest value (2).

People with exercise-induced asthma can usually engage in exercise training (16). In fact, some notable Olympians like Jackie Joyner-Kersee (gold medalist in heptathlon, 1988 and 1992) and Amy Van Dyken (gold medalist in four swimming events, 1996) have had this condition. Oral inhalers, such as Ventolin and Flovent, are helpful for managing exercise-induced asthma. Other strategies to improve exercise tolerance include exercising in warm, moist environments rather than in cold, dry ones. Many people with asthma tolerate swimming better than running. In addition, a long warm-up can lessen the airway constriction that is more likely to occur with sudden, strenuous exercise (2, 19).

Cystic Fibrosis

Cystic fibrosis, another type of COPD, is a recessively inherited genetic disorder. It is a fatal disease. Three decades ago, most cystic fibrosis patients died in childhood, but better treatments have prolonged life expectancy by 20 yr (12). In Caucasian children, 1 in 2,500 is born with the condition, although the disease is rare in Asians and African Americans (12). Thick mucous secretions by the exocrine glands affect many systems in the body. In fact, clinical diagnosis is based on excessive chloride concentration in the sweat. In the lungs, the mucous secretions plug the airways and cause inflammation of the airways and chronic bacterial infections. Treatment for cystic fibrosis consists of having patients lie with the head facing downhill while percussion is used to enhance mucous drainage. In addition, aerobic exercise has been shown to help clear the lungs and prevent bacterial infections. The increased use of antibiotics is yet another reason that survival of cystic fibrosis patients has increased dramatically in recent years (13).

Key Point

COPDs reduce the capacity for airflow during respiration. Bronchitis and emphysema are irreversible. Bronchial asthma is an intermittent condition caused by restriction of airways; it can be relieved with medications. Cystic fibrosis is a fatal disease that results from a genetic defect.

Restrictive Lung Diseases

Restrictive lung diseases have many causes, including diseases of the rib cage and spine such as kyphoscoliosis and pectus excavatum (sunken chest). Other causes include pulmonary edema, pulmonary embolism, exposure to toxic substances (coal workers' pneumoconiosis, silicosis, asbestosis), chemotherapy, and radiation therapy. Often, these inflame the interstitium and fibrotic tissue develops. Various types of neuromuscular diseases (spinal cord injury, amyotrophic lateral sclerosis or Lou Gehrig's disease, Guillain-Barré syndrome, tetanus, and myasthenia gravis) can also cause restrictive lung disease. Obesity and pregnancy can restrict lung expansion because of the abdomen pushing up into the thoracic cavity. In general, people with restrictive lung diseases have reduced residual volume (RV), inspiratory reserve volume (IRV), expiratory reserve volume (ERV), forced vital capacity (FVC), and maximal tidal volume (TV) (see figure 21.1). Breathing is more difficult because the respiratory muscles must work harder to inflate the lungs (9, 18).

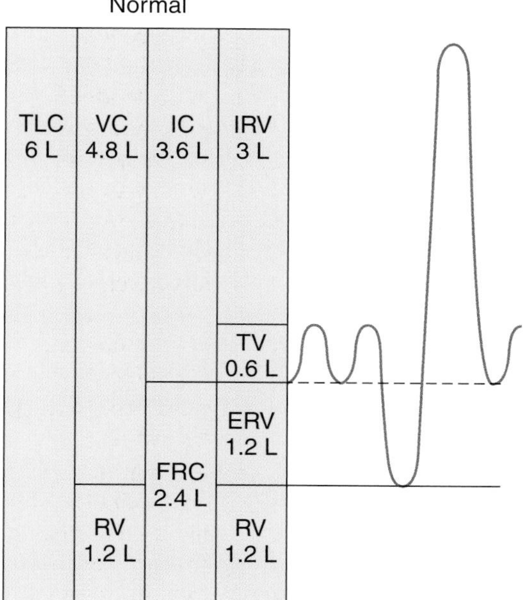

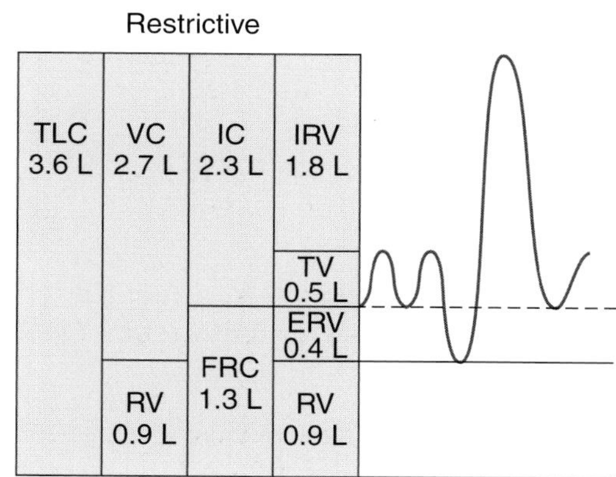

Figure 21.1 Lung volumes in a person with restrictive lung disease versus a person with normal pulmonary function. Lung volumes are total lung capacity (TLC), vital capacity (VC), inspiratory capacity (IC), inspiratory reserve volume (IRV), tidal volume (TV), functional residual capacity (FRC), expiratory reserve volume (ERV), and residual volume (RV).

Reprinted from *Essentials of cardiopulmonary physical therapy*, 2nd ed., edited by E.A. Hillegass and H.S. Sadowsky, p. 186, Copyright 2001, with permission from Elsevier.

Key Point

Restrictive lung diseases have numerous causes, but all are characterized by the reduced capacity to expand the lungs. Thus, smaller lung volumes, assessed through pulmonary function testing, typically are seen in people with these diseases.

Evidence for Exercise

Pulmonary rehabilitation programs are often found alongside cardiac rehabilitation programs in many hospitals. Most pulmonary rehabilitation programs focus on people with COPD, although people with other types of pulmonary disease may also benefit from exercise (3, 8). Support for pulmonary rehabilitation programs is limited by the fact that patients typically show little or no improvement in $\dot{V}O_2$max, tests of lung function, and mortality rates. As a result, many insurance providers are reluctant to pay for pulmonary rehabilitation because they view it as medical management rather than a way to restore the patient to normal function (as much as possible).

However, most pulmonary rehabilitation patients do improve in functional outcomes, including symptom-limited GXT, symptoms of dyspnea, quality of life, and frequency of hospitalization (3). Thus, pulmonary rehabilitation should be viewed as a desirable part of the patient's medical treatment (10). The overall goals are to improve the patient's general health, to optimize oxygen saturation, to make activities of daily living more easily accomplished, and to improve self-efficacy (3).

Key Point

Patients with lung diseases can benefit from a pulmonary rehabilitation program. Although patients usually demonstrate little improvement in $\dot{V}O_2$max and pulmonary function tests, they do improve in their ability to carry out tasks and in other measures of quality of life.

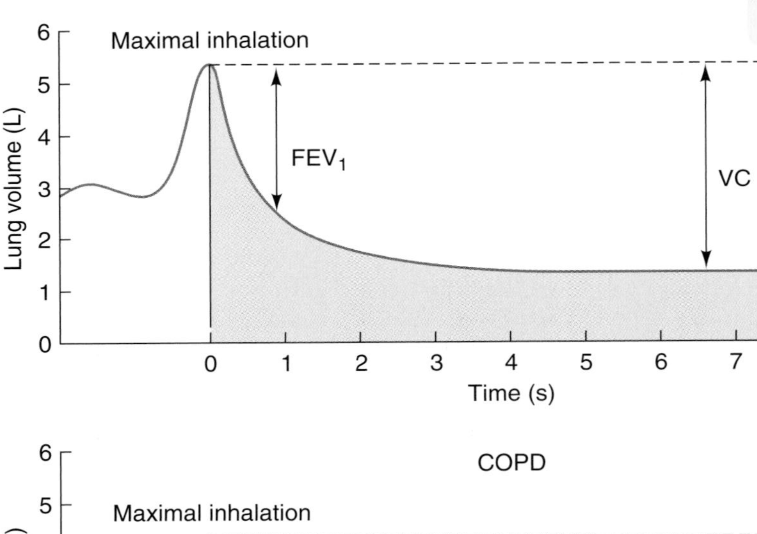

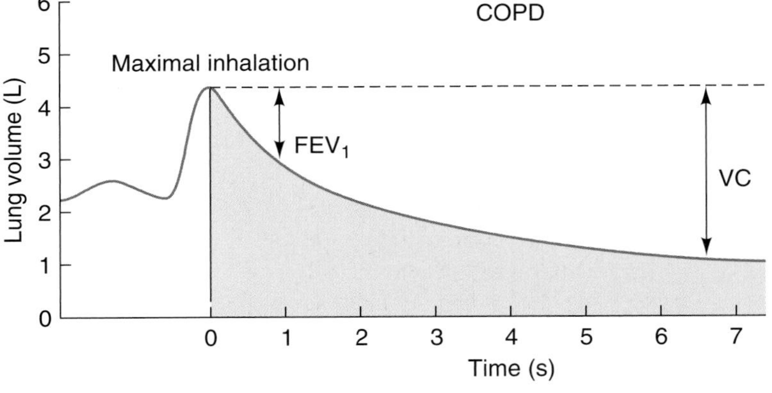

Figure 21.2 Pulmonary function test showing the volume versus time curves in a normal person and a person with obstructive lung disease. FEV_1 = forced expiratory volume in the first second of exhalation; VC = vital capacity.

Testing and Evaluation

In most instances, **pulmonary function testing** is carried out for diagnostic purposes and to assess the severity of the disease (14). Computerized spirometry systems measure lung volumes and flow parameters. In COPD, the principal measure is **forced expiratory volume (FEV_1)**, which reflects the maximum volume of air that can be moved in 1 sec (see figure 21.2). Sometimes forced expiratory volume is expressed as FEV_1/VC, where **VC (vital capacity)** is the volume of air that can be breathed out when going from maximal inhalation to maximal exhalation. Because of airway obstruction, individuals with COPD have a decreased ability to exhale quickly; if the FEV_1 is below 80% of the expected value, the test is considered abnormal (6). In restrictive lung disease, the lung volumes (e.g., RV, IRV, ERV, FVC, and maximal TV) are smaller than normal because lung expansion is limited. People with restrictive lung disease compensate by taking faster, smaller breaths, which reduces the work that the respiratory muscles must perform to inflate the lung.

Exercise tests are often administered to assess the patient's ability to exercise. The test may be a standard graded exercise test (GXT) on a treadmill or cycle ergometer or a simple 6 or 12 min walk test on a flat surface. In a pulmonary patient, exercise capacity is limited more by the lungs than the cardiovascular system. As a result, these patients typically experience **hypoxemia** (low arterial oxygen content) and **dyspnea** (shortness of breath). Measurements of maximal ventilation rates ($\dot{V}_E$max), obtained during the final minute of an exercise test, are also clinically useful. $\dot{V}_E$max is typically 60% to 70% of the maximal voluntary ventilation (MVV), although in COPD patients it may approach 80% to 100%. MVV can be measured via a special spirometry test, or it can be predicted from the following formula: MVV = $FEV_1 \cdot 40$.

A **pulse oximeter** is used to assess the percent saturation of hemoglobin in the arterial blood (S_aO_2) of pulmonary patients. This noninvasive device shines a light beam through the finger or earlobe to assess the color of the arterial blood (figure 21.3). Values for S_aO_2 below 90% indicate that the client needs supplemental oxygen to increase the driving force for diffusion of oxygen into the lungs. Frequently, a dyspnea rating scale is used to evaluate symptoms during exercise testing (5, 17). Cardiovascular, pulmonary, metabolic, and power output measurements are obtained and used to evaluate the severity of disability (table 21.1).

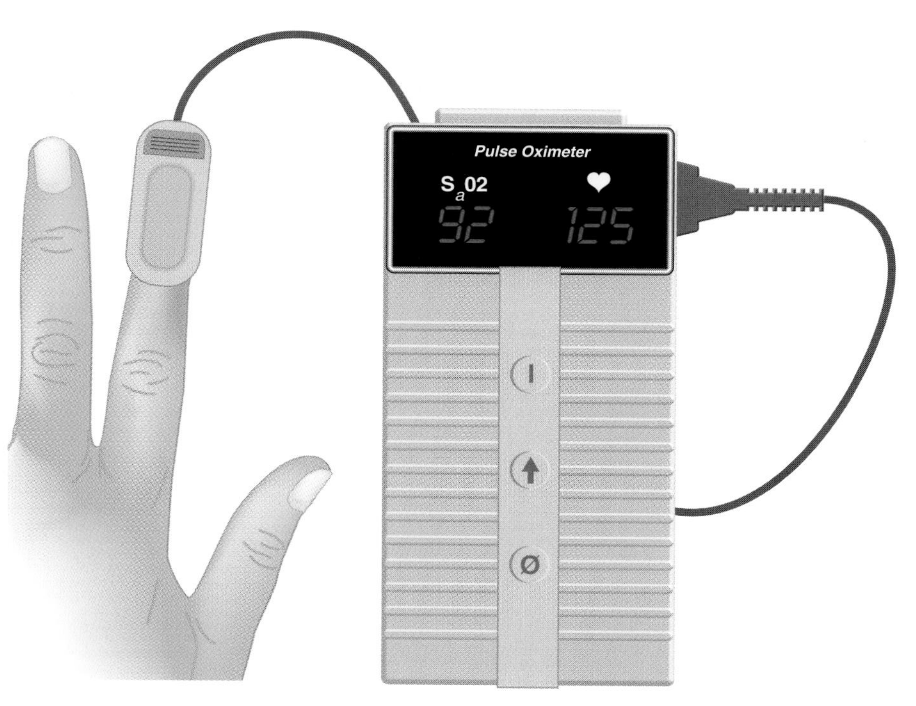

Figure 21.3 Portable pulse oximeter used to assess a pulmonary patient's arterial oxygenation. The number on the left of the display shows the percent saturation of hemoglobin in arterial blood (S_aO_2), whereas the number on the right shows the heart rate.

Key Point

One of the main pulmonary function tests for COPD is the FEV_1. COPD patients demonstrate a reduced ability to exhale quickly because of obstruction of the airways. In restrictive lung diseases, lung volumes are often reduced because the ability to expand the lungs is compromised. Exercise testing of patients with lung diseases, with appropriate monitoring of signs (hypoxemia) and symptoms (dyspnea) to assess the severity of the patient's condition, is beneficial.

Typical Exercise Prescription

The goal of a typical pulmonary rehabilitation program is the client's self-care, and to achieve that goal, physicians, nurses, respiratory therapists, exercise specialists, nutritionists, and psychologists are recruited to deal with the various manifestations of the disease (3). The pulmonary patient receives education about the ways to deal with the disease, including breathing exercises, ways to approach the activities of daily living at home, and ways to handle work-related problems. The emphasis in most pulmonary rehabilitation programs is on the COPD patient, although patients with restrictive lung disease often participate as well (3, 19). The AACVPR published a detailed description of exercise testing and prescription in its *Guidelines for Pulmonary Rehabilitation Programs* (1).

Aerobic training is usually accomplished with rhythmic, dynamic exercise that uses large muscle groups. As with healthy individuals and other clinical populations, the frequency is typically 3 to 5 times a week, with each session lasting at least 30 min. However, assigning appropriate exercise intensities poses a particular problem. Pulmonary patients usually cannot achieve the same peak HRs as healthy individuals of the same age achieve. Thus, computing a target heart rate (THR) from a typical percentage of age-predicted HRmax often results in target intensities that are too high. On the other hand, using THR values computed from a typical percentage of measured HRmax underestimates the appropriate training intensity (1, 6).

Table 21.1 Guide to Grading Chronic Obstructive Pulmonary Disease

Grade	Cause of dyspnea	FEV_1 (% predicted)	$\dot{V}O_2max$ ($ml \cdot kg^{-1} \cdot min^{-1}$)	Exercise $\dot{V}O_2max$ ($L \cdot min^{-1}$)	Blood gasses
1	Fast walking and stair-climbing	>60	>25	Not limiting	Normal P_aCO_2, S_aO_2
2	Walking at normal pace	<60	<25	>50	Normal P_aCO_2, S_aO_2 above 90% at rest and with exercise
3	Slow walking	<40	<15	<50	Normal P_aCO_2, S_aO_2 below 90% with exercise
4	Walking less than one block	<40	<7	<30	Elevated P_aCO_2, S_aO_2 below 90% at rest and with exercise

Table is based on a 40-yr-old man.

Reprinted, by permission, from N.L. Jones et al., 1987, Chronic obstructive respiratory disorders. In *Exercise testing and exercise prescription for special cases*, edited by J.S. Skinner (Baltimore: Lea & Febiger), 175-187.

Various methods can be used to estimate the appropriate exercise intensity for pulmonary patients. Generally, the method of assigning exercise intensity varies with the level of the disability. In patients with mild or moderate impairment, setting the intensity at the anaerobic threshold or the point where the person became noticeably dyspneic is appropriate. In clients with more severe disability, it is often necessary to let symptoms of dyspnea be the guiding factors (6). Intermittent exercise, interspersed with rest, may be all that the client can tolerate. If the impairment is severe, supplemental oxygen will be needed to maintain S_aO_2 above 90% (11).

Individuals with emphysema should be instructed in pursed-lip breathing, which involves pressing the lips together and exhaling through a small opening in the center of the mouth. Doing this slows the rate of respiration and prevents collapse of small airways, resulting in better oxygenation (3, 18). In some instances, a resistive breathing device may be recommended to specifically train the respiratory muscles at rest.

Upper-body exercise is recommended for pulmonary patients. This exercise can be achieved through using exercise modalities that require both arm and leg muscles, such as the Schwinn Airdyne or the rowing ergometer. Additionally, resistance training can be accomplished with dumbbells, machines, or elastic bands. Increasing arm strength and endurance improves the client's ability to perform functional activities and decreases local muscle fatigue (3, 6).

Key Point

Pulmonary rehabilitation programs involve many different types of health professionals. The primary goals are to educate patients about dealing with their disease and help them improve their exercise capacity. A health professional in pulmonary rehabilitation must understand the client's medical conditions and physiological limitations. Sensations of dyspnea and pulse oximeter readings are frequently used to determine the appropriate exercise intensity.

Medications for Pulmonary Diseases

Bronchodilators relax smooth muscle surrounding airways in the lungs and relieve the symptoms of asthma, bronchitis, and related lung disorders (7). These medications can be taken orally or from an inhaler. The inhalers are generally used for acute asthma episodes, whereas long-term bronchodilation usually is obtained orally. Most of these drugs stimulate the $beta_2$ receptors that relax bronchial smooth muscle and increase the airway lumen. Because of their beta-adrenergic stimulating effect, these medications can increase HR and BP, although they mostly focus on the smooth muscle found in airways. Some of the inhaler brand names include Brethaire Inhaler, Alupent, and Maxair. A second class of drugs comprises the methylxanthines, which include Theobid, Aminophyllin, Theo-Dur, and many others. Side effects of this class include tachycardia, arrhythmias, central nervous system stimulation, and risk of seizures. Anticholinergics (Atrovent) make up a third class of bronchodilators.

Additional medicines are used to treat common respiratory disorders. These include **decongestants** to dry out the mucous membranes, **antihistamines** to relieve symptoms of seasonal allergies (e.g., hay fever), anti-inflammatory agents, expectorants, and cough medications. Antibiotics are often given to fight off infections

(7), which tend to occur if mucous secretions block off the airways.

Diuretics are important in treating cor pulmonale, a condition that occurs in about half of pulmonary patients with severe disease. Cor pulmonale is defined as pulmonary hypertension with right ventricular hypertrophy. Because failure of the right ventricle often follows, diuretics may be needed to enhance fluid excretion (10). There are three different types of diuretics: thiazide diuretics (e.g., Esidrix), potassium-sparing diuretics (e.g., Aldactone), and loop diuretics (e.g., Lasix) (7).

Key Point

Bronchodilators are the most common medications for patients with COPD. Decongestants, antihistamines, anti-inflammatory agents, and antibiotics are often prescribed to treat respiratory disorders. Diuretics are sometimes needed for patients with severe pulmonary disease who also develop heart failure.

Case Studies

You can check your answers by referring to pages 474 and 475 in appendix A.

1. A 38-yr-old woman with asthma would like to enter your fitness program. What kinds of questions would you ask her during your screening interview?
2. A 50-yr-old man with a history of smoking a pack of cigarettes a day for the past 25 yr enters a hospital complaining of dyspnea. A chest X ray shows that his lungs are hyperinflated, and spirometry tests show that his FEV_1 is only half of the normal value. What type of pulmonary disease does he have, and what is the logical course of treatment?
3. A middle-aged patient with severe kyphoscoliosis is referred to a pulmonary rehabilitation program. He has restrictive pulmonary disease, demonstrating a vital capacity of only 1.5 L (compared with the normal value of 5.0 L). During a 6 min walk test, he manages to cover 865 ft (264 m), stopping once because of shortness of breath. His S_aO_2 at the end of the test has fallen to 87%. What type of exercise training would you recommend? What types of other therapies might assist this person in completing his exercise sessions?

PART V

Exercise Programming

The previous parts of this handbook covered assessment and exercise prescription for components of physical fitness for people with a variety of characteristics and health conditions. This section includes other elements needed for a comprehensive and effective fitness program. In chapter 22, we go over ways to help motivate individuals to adopt and maintain a healthy lifestyle. In chapter 23, we provide an overview of mind-body (mindful) exercises (e.g., yoga, Pilates, etc.). In chapter 24, we review analysis of the electrocardiogram and current medications for cardiovascular problems. We summarize the prevention and treatment of injuries in chapter 25. Finally, in chapter 26 we describe program administration and management.

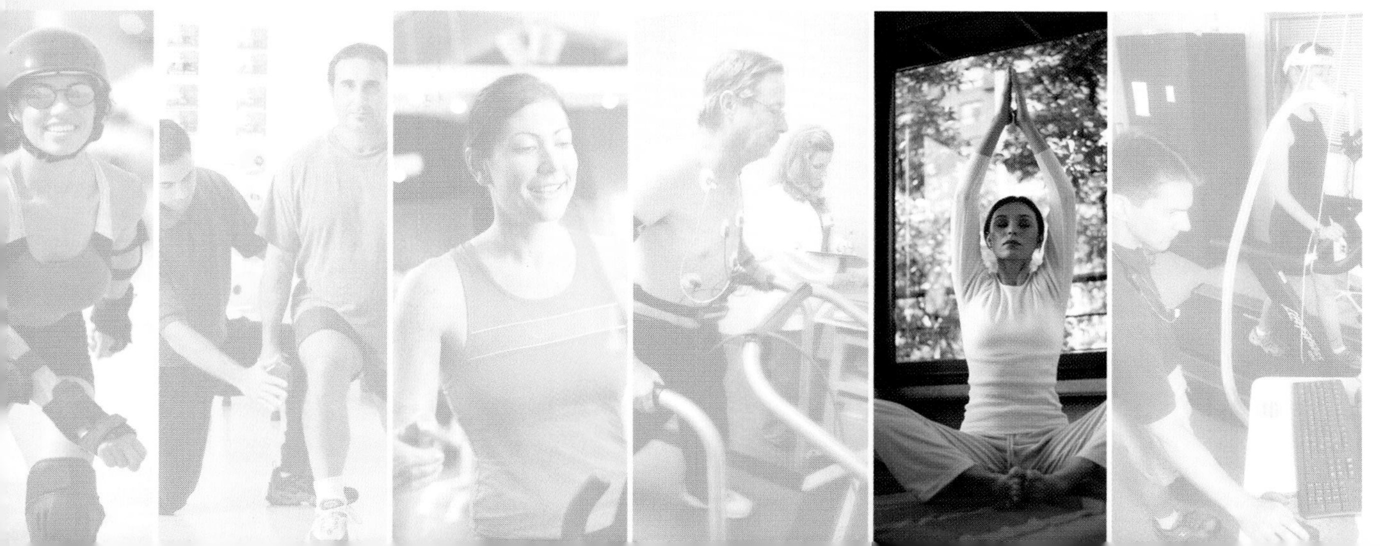

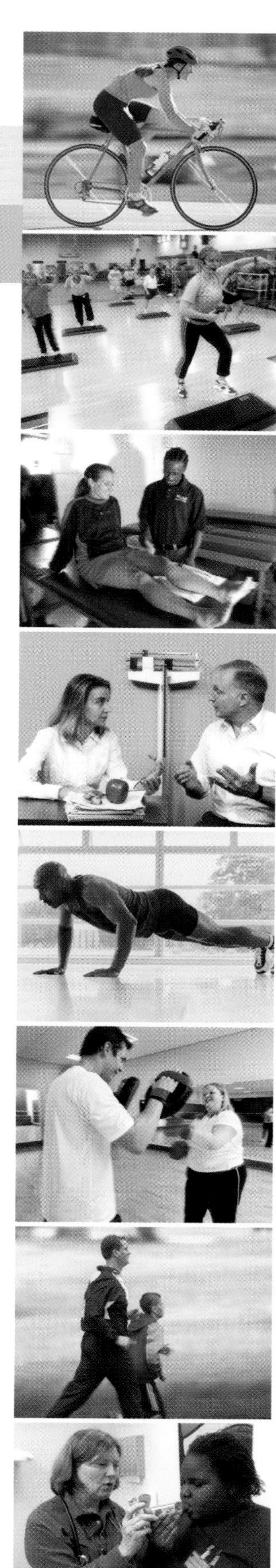

Behavior Modification

Janet Buckworth

Objectives

The reader will be able to do the following:

1. Describe the transtheoretical model and stages involved in healthy behavior change.
2. Discuss the role of motivation in exercise adoption and adherence and identify behavioral strategies for enhancing motivation.
3. List and describe six strategies that fitness professionals can use to monitor and support behavior change.
4. Describe ways to apply relapse prevention to exercise behavior.
5. Identify effective communication skills useful in motivating and fostering healthy behavior change.

Translating the desire to change a health-related behavior into action is a challenge for most people. They may wish to be more active or to eat a healthier diet but may not have the knowledge, skills, or sufficient motivation to make the necessary behavior modifications and stick to them. To help people adopt and maintain a healthier lifestyle, the fitness professional should understand basic principles of behavior change and develop the skills to put those principles into practice.

This chapter begins with a brief description of theoretical models for explaining and predicting human behavior, in particular the transtheoretical model of behavior change (also known as the *stages of change model).* Methods and strategies are presented in the context of behavior change as a process, with suggestions for use based on stages of motivational readiness. For an excellent review of the transtheoretical model applied to exercise, refer to Prochaska and Marcus (21). Factors for fitness professionals to consider as they help participants move through each stage of the model are discussed along with specific strategies for encouraging adoption of and adherence to exercise and other healthy behaviors. Additional strategies and suggestions for interventions can be found in Annesi's (2) text on enhancing motivation to exercise, in the chapter by Southard and Southard (24) in the ACSM resource manual, and in *Motivating People to Be Physically Active* by Marcus and Forsyth (16). The last section in this chapter examines communication skills that fitness professionals should possess in order to motivate participants and foster healthy behavior change.

Transtheoretical Model of Behavior Change

Several theories guide strategies for changing exercise behavior, such as behavior modification, social cognitive theory, and the transtheoretical model of behavior change (3). Behavior modification theory is based on the assumption that behavior is learned and can be changed by modifying the antecedents (cues) and consequences (rewards, punishments). A cue could be a flyer listing the benefits of walking during lunch, and a reward could be a certificate presented to the aerobics participant with the best attendance. Social cognitive theory offers the view that behavior is influenced by the dynamic relationships among the person's characteristics, the environment, and the behavior itself. Someone training for a marathon would be more motivated than a novice fitness walker to exercise outside in the rain, but even the most dedicated marathoner would not run in a lightning storm. Although effective strategies for behavior change have been developed with these and other theories, most theories of behavior treat change as an all-or-none event. In other words, participants go from being sedentary to being regularly active in response to an intervention.

The transtheoretical model presents change as a dynamic process whereby attitudes, decisions, and actions evolve through different stages over time. In the late 1970s and early 1980s, Prochaska and DiClemente (20) developed the transtheoretical model of behavior change by observing smokers trying to quit without professional intervention. They discovered that self-changers used specific strategies that varied over time as they tried to decrease or eliminate their high-risk behavior and that the self-changers progressed through distinct stages. Although the model was developed to explain how people stop high-risk behaviors, it has been applied to promoting exercise with some success (1). The rest of the chapter describes the transtheoretical, or stages of change, model and ways this model can be used to help people think about, decide to begin, and continue an active lifestyle.

Concepts

The **transtheoretical model** is a model of intentional behavior modification. Behavior change is a dynamic process that occurs through a series of interrelated stages that are mostly stable but open to change (22). This model emphasizes the individual's motivation, readiness to change, and personal history regarding the target behavior. For example, people who exercised successfully in the past would have more confidence in their ability to exercise again than would people who have been sedentary most of their lives. The problem with most interventions is that they are for people who are prepared to take action (21). According to the transtheoretical model, traditional strategies for participant recruitment will not affect people who are not ready to change. Different strategies must be used to persuade people to consider change and then motivate them to take action. Other approaches will be more effective in supporting adherence to the new behavior.

Dimensions

The transtheoretical model has three dimensions (22): (1) stages of change, (2) attitudes, beliefs, and skills for behavior change, and (3) level of change (context for change). By evaluating the participant in respect to these factors, the fitness professional can design individually tailored and stage-specific interventions.

Dimension 1: Stages of Change

1. *Precontemplation:* In this stage, the individual is not seriously thinking about changing an unhealthy behavior in the next 6 mo or is denying the need to change.

2. *Contemplation:* The individual is seriously thinking about changing an unhealthy behavior within the next 6 mo.
3. *Preparation:* This is a transitional stage in which the individual intends to take action within the next month. Some plans have been made, and the individual tries to determine what to do next.
4. *Action:* This stage is the 6 mo following the overt modification of an unhealthy behavior. Motivation and investment in behavior change are sufficient in this stage, but it is the least stable and busiest stage and has the highest risk of relapse.
5. *Maintenance:* Maintenance begins after the individual has successfully adhered to the healthy behavior for 6 mo. The longer someone stays in maintenance, the less risk of relapse.

Dimension 2: Attitudes, Beliefs, and Behavioral Skills Hypothesized to Influence Behavior Change

- *Self-efficacy* is confidence in one's ability to engage in a positive behavior or abstain from an undesired behavior. This expectation of success is an important factor in making the decision to change and in maintaining the new behavior.
- *Decisional balance* refers to evaluating and monitoring potential gains (pros) and losses (cons) arising from any decision. Perceived gains increase and perceived losses decrease in respect to the target behavior as the person moves through the stages of change described in dimension 1.
- *Processes of change* are strategies used to change behavior. Experiential or cognitive processes are strategies that involve thoughts, attitudes, and awareness. Behavioral processes involve taking specific actions directed toward yourself or the environment. For example, seeking out information about the best exercise for losing weight is a cognitive process, and creating reminders to register for a water aerobics class is a behavioral process.

Dimension 3: Level of Change (Context for Change)

Identifying the context in which the problem behavior occurs helps the fitness professional determine what factors people must change to be successful. The root of the problem can be situational barriers, maladaptive cognitions, current interpersonal or family conflicts, or intrapersonal conflicts. For example, one person may want to exercise but does not have access to facilities (situational barrier), and another person may think she does not have the willpower to stick with a program (maladaptive cognitions). The first person would be helped with a home exercise program, whereas the second would benefit from social support and rethinking discouraging thoughts.

Applying the Transtheoretical Model to Exercise

The transtheoretical model is applied to exercise by matching the appropriate intervention strategy to a person according to his physical activity history and readiness for change (22) (see figure 22.1). For example, the goal in working with people in the precontemplation stage is to get them to begin thinking about changing their level of physical activity. Discussing information from a fitness test or health risk appraisal followed by education about personal benefits of physical activity is an appropriate strategy for participants in the precontemplation stage. The goal with people in the contemplation stage is to help them prepare to take action. They would benefit from accurate, easy-to-understand information about how they can start an exercise program or begin to be more active. Someone in the preparation stage is doing some

Maintenance: Encourage new activities with others, reinforce self-regulatory skills, review and revise goals, introduce cross-training, conduct periodic fitness testing

Action: Identify social support for maintaining exercise, set up stimulus control, teach self-reinforcement, implement self-efficacy enhancement strategies, set goals, teach self-monitoring, employ relapse prevention

Preparation: Conduct psychosocial and fitness assessments, evaluate supports/benefits and barriers/costs, design personalized exercise prescription, set goals, develop behavioral contracts, teach time management skills

Contemplation: Market benefits of exercise, foster self- and environmental reevaluation, provide clear and specific guidelines for starting an exercise program, be a positive role model, identify social support for exercise

Precontemplation: Implement an exercise promotion media campaign, education about personal benefits of exercise, foster values clarification, conduct health risk appraisals and fitness testing

Figure 22.1 Intervention strategies for the various stages of change.

exercise but realizes that it is not enough and needs help to set up a personalized exercise program. She is aware of the benefits of exercise, but there are still barriers that must be resolved. While participants in the contemplation stage may not be ready to set goals, those in the preparation stage are ready to set goals and get a personalized exercise prescription.

Participants in the action stage are at a high risk of relapsing into a more familiar, inactive lifestyle. They are participating in regular activity, but exercise is not a habit. Relapse prevention, which is discussed later, can help move them on to the maintenance stage. Movement from the action stage to the maintenance stage follows a decrease in the risk of relapse and an increase in self-efficacy. Helpful strategies include periodic reevaluations of goals and plans for coping with life events such as travel, inclement weather, or medical events that can disrupt regular exercise.

Key Point

The transtheoretical model addresses the dynamic nature of behavior change. Practitioners apply this model by selecting interventions based on characteristics of the individual, environment, and stage of change. Interventions should match the stage the individual is in and the context in which the problem behavior occurs (see figure 22.1).

Promoting Exercise: Targeting Precontemplators and Contemplators

Understanding the knowledge, attitudes, and behavioral skills that foster adoption of a regular exercise program is important in helping people in the early stages of exercise behavior change. People in precontemplation are sedentary and have no plans to start exercising. They may be in this stage because they lack information about the long-term personal consequences of physical inactivity. They also may be demoralized from previous unsuccessful attempts to stick with an exercise program and may have low self-efficacy for exercise. People in the precontemplation stage may feel defensive about their lifestyle because of social pressures to be physically active. They have no personally compelling reasons to change, and the costs of exercising seem to outweigh the benefits. Given these attitudes and beliefs, your clients' perceptions about the benefits of exercise should be strengthened and the costs reduced. Activities to help people develop a personal value for exercise and information about the role of exercise in a healthy lifestyle are useful in moving someone to the next stage (16).

Sedentary individuals move to the contemplation stage because of information that is convincing, personal, and timely (17). Contemplators are planning to become more physically active, but they are still ambivalent about changing. For them, the costs of starting to exercise balance out the perceived benefits. Things that support the contemplator's desire and motivation to exercise and counter perceived costs and barriers can initiate the move to preparation. Role models, perceived barriers and benefits, and psychosocial variables such as self-efficacy for exercise are other factors that will influence exercise adoption. The cognitive processes of change, such as increasing knowledge about the health benefits of regular exercise and being aware of how one's inactivity affects others, are critical in these early stages of change.

Specific factors related to the adoption of regular exercise are presented next, followed by a review of strategies to market exercise and increase motivation.

Influencing Exercise Adoption: Successful Planning for the Preparation Stage

Identifying individual, social, and environmental factors related to exercise adoption can help the fitness professional select more effective interventions for behavior change. Working with a participant who is in the preparation stage must include a thorough assessment and a specific plan for change. Behavioral strategies come into play more as someone moves from the preparation stage, where he is doing some exercise, to the action stage and regular exercise. Assessment (both fitness and psychosocial), evaluation of supports and benefits and barriers and costs, goal setting, behavioral contracts, and time management training are practical strategies to use with participants in the preparation stage.

Individual Influences

Individual characteristics that influence the initiation of exercise include demographics, activity history, past experiences, perception of health status, perception of access to facilities, time, enjoyment of exercise, aptitudes, beliefs, self-motivation, and self-efficacy (25). Higher education, higher income, gender (male), and younger age are positively associated with exercise (25). Exercise history is an important factor in current level of physical activity. Past participation is linked with physical activity in supervised exercise programs and in treatment programs for patients with CHD and obesity (6). Past exercise experience also can influence expectations about exercise and self-efficacy, and high exercise self-efficacy is associated with increased exercise participation.

Motivation is another individual variable influencing exercise adoption. Motivation depends on expectations for future benefits or outcomes from exercise, such as good health, improved appearance, social outlets, stress management, enjoyment, and opportunities for competition (18). Self-motivation for exercise is the ability to continue an exercise program without the benefit of external reinforcement. Participants high in self-motivation are probably good at goal setting, monitoring exercise progress, and self-reinforcement (23). People with little self-motivation may need more external reinforcement and encouragement (e.g., group activities and social support) to adopt and adhere to exercise.

Perceived behavioral control has been found to be significantly correlated with the intention to exercise (10). If participants believe they have more control over the exercise and have choices about when and how to exercise, they are more likely to begin a program. It follows that participants who set their own goals will have a greater chance of success than if goals are assigned to them (15).

Social Influences

Social support involves comfort, assistance, and information provided by individuals or groups. While practical help, such as providing a ride to the fitness facility or problem-solving tips, can result in tangible benefits to the participant, emotional support, too, plays a key role. For example, emotional support (encouragement and expressions of care, concern, and sympathy) could be helpful when a participant is emotionally stressed. Other types of emotional support include esteem support (reassurance of worth, expressions of liking or confidence in the other person), network support (expressions of connection and belonging), and even informational support (information and advice).

Research Insight

Social support plays a big role in exercise adherence, and most research has assumed that other people will have a positive influence on behavior. Gabriele, Walker, Gill, Harber, and Fisher (9) asked 244 young adults about social influence (encouragement *and* constraint), exercise motivation, and exercise behavior. Encouraging social influence was related to exercise behavior through influencing motivation, but social constraint, which involves expectations or norms that create a sense of obligation or intrusion, was not. It seems that we cannot assume that all social influence is helpful for the adoption and maintenance of exercise.

Social support for exercise from family, friends, and physicians is usually associated with physical activity (25). Spouses appear to provide a consistent, positive influence on exercise participation; in one study, individuals who joined a fitness center with their spouse had better adherence and lower dropout than married individuals who joined without a spouse (26). Group factors may be particularly important for older adults and people who are motivated to exercise primarily for social reinforcement.

Environmental Influences

Research has shown that environmental prompts, social support, and convenience are factors in exercise adoption (4). Environments that have cues for exercise, easily accessible facilities, and few real or perceived barriers make exercise maintenance easier. Posters, e-mails, self-sticking notes, visibly located exercise equipment, and bike and walking paths are examples of environmental cues.

The convenience of exercise is influenced by the sequence, or chain, of behaviors that must be completed for the person to exercise. The longer and more complicated the behavior chain, the more barriers there are to exercise. For example, there is a greater potential for a break in the link if a person must leave work, drive home, gather up exercise clothes, drive to a facility, park, sign in, and change clothes to walk on a treadmill than if the person walks first thing in the morning in her neighborhood. For many people, exercising in the morning may be easier to stick with than exercising during the day when numerous demands compete for time.

The primary reason given for not exercising is lack of time (4). Time can be a true determinant, a perceived determinant, an indication of poor time management, or a rationalization for the lack of motivation to be active. Flexibility in an exercise program (e.g., classes offered at many different times of day and evening, a lunch-hour walking group) can help with actual time problems. Accumulating several shorter bouts of exercise throughout the day may be another effective strategy. The fitness professional can help identify how time is a barrier and then choose appropriate interventions, such as modification of an exercise schedule or referral to a time management class.

Researchers and practitioners recognize that the physical environment powerfully influences the level of physical activity in communities (7). For example, accessible, attractive, and safe places to walk, bike, or run can make physical activity more appealing and convenient. Certainly, workout facilities that are clean, are well ventilated, and have a good selection of equipment and adequate parking will be more enticing to novice exercisers than poorly maintained or managed fitness centers.

Research Insight

Loops and lollipops is not a new snack treat, but rather a description of road patterns in neighborhoods characterized by urban sprawl. There is a growing concern that car-friendly environments indicative of sprawl are not good for public health. Ewing, Schmid, Killingsworth, Zlot, and Raudenbush (8) looked at the relationship among sprawl, level of physical activity, and obesity. Using county and metropolitan sprawl indexes and controlling for variables known to influence exercise and obesity, such as age, education, and fruit and vegetable consumption, Ewing and colleagues found small but significant associations between the county sprawl index and minutes walked, obesity, BMI, and hypertension. Greater sprawl in metropolitan areas was also associated with fewer minutes walked.

Marketing and Motivational Strategies for Inactive Stages of Change

Your goal as a fitness professional may be to help people who have not yet considered exercise to begin thinking about starting a fitness program (i.e., precontemplation stage). For example, the primary goal of a media campaign may be to capture the attention of inactive people and motivate them to contemplate beginning an exercise program or another healthy behavior. This might involve putting informational prompts at the point of decision to act, such as hanging catchy posters next to elevators encouraging people to take the stairs (13). Bulletin boards, pamphlets, flyers, and handouts with upbeat information about the benefits of exercise and practical suggestions for increasing physical activity can also catch the attention of potential exercisers. Handing out passes at local restaurants for an aerobics class is a proactive form of recruitment. Fun runs and walks supporting a local or national charity may motivate people who primarily want to help the organization to begin thinking about exercise for its own sake. Wellness fairs, health risk appraisals, and fitness testing can also prompt contemplation and enhance motivation to become more active.

To increase participation in the early stages of behavior change, the fitness professional's role is to provide education about why people should be more active, to describe how to exercise sensibly, and to offer encouragement to follow through with a personal exercise program. Specific strategies to increase adoption and early adherence are recommended (4, 16, 17):

- Ask participants about their exercise history. They may need proper information to dispel myths (e.g., the myth of no pain, no gain) and to develop positive attitudes about exercise.
- Explore ways exercise can benefit them personally. Find out what they think they will get out of being physically active and provide information and resources about additional benefits.
- Help participants develop knowledge, attitudes, and skills to support the behavior change. In addition to providing information and training in self-management skills, the fitness professional may use cognitive restructuring to identify discouraging thoughts and replace them with positive statements (see Cognitive Restructuring: Reframe Negative Statements Into Positive Statements).

Cognitive Restructuring: Reframe Negative Statements Into Positive Statements

Negative Statements

- I'm never going to get in shape.
- I'm fatter than everyone else in the class.
- I've tried to stay with exercise and each time I fail.
- It's just impossible to find time to exercise with my schedule.

Positive Statements

- Change takes time. I didn't get out of shape overnight, and I am making progress bit by bit.
- Everyone has to start somewhere. Other people have worked long and hard to get where they are.
- Every time I begin a new exercise program, I get closer to sticking with it for good.
- I can take a little time for myself to exercise every day because I deserve it. I'm the one in control.

- Bolster the participant's exercise self-efficacy with success-producing learning experiences. Strategies for enhancing self-efficacy include the following:

  Mastery experiences. These experiences include behavioral rehearsal with proper supervision and positive feedback. The fitness professional can make sure participants have chosen activities that are appropriate for their fitness and skill level. Practical feedback will also help participants be successful and thus feel more confident. In addition, an increased sense of competency is motivating.

Verbal persuasion or self-persuasion. The fitness professional can provide verbal encouragement and can teach participants positive self-talk.

Modeling. Modeling has been effective in increasing self-efficacy. The fitness professional can set up situations in which participants see someone like themselves succeed (e.g., post a newspaper story about seniors who now exercise regularly) or watch a peer who has trouble with the task succeed (e.g., point out to a new participant that "Lynette also had difficulty jogging 3 mi when she first started the program, but after months of hard work, she has now reached her goal!").

Interpretations of physiological and emotional responses. The typical increased HR, respiration, and muscle tension that occur during exercise may make novices feel anxious or uncomfortable. The fitness professional can make sure that participants have information about the normal physiological responses to exercise and know how to interpret these responses.

- Clarify expectations and make sure they are reasonable and realistic. Use guidelines for goal setting to ensure initial successes.
- Identify potential barriers to behavior change and brainstorm with the participant about ways to overcome these barriers. Barriers can be personal (low exercise self-efficacy), physical (past injuries), interpersonal (peer pressure from sedentary friends to engage in sedentary behaviors instead of exercising), or environmental (inclement weather or lack of transportation to an exercise facility).
- Foster motivation to adopt and maintain an exercise program. Set up incentives to exercise. Incentives can be tangible (e.g., T-shirts, certificates, water bottles, recognition on a bulletin board) or intangible (e.g., sense of competence, enjoyment). Tangible incentives are useful early in a program. Offer a variety of incentives and foster intrinsic motivation, like a sense of accomplishment or avoidance of obesity, for long-term adherence. Strategies to increase motivation are listed in Motivational Strategies.

Motivational Strategies

- Provide positive behavioral feedback.
- Encourage group participation and group support to offer the opportunity for social reinforcement, camaraderie, and commitment.
- Recruit spouse and peers to support the behavioral change.
- Use upbeat, positive music. Make the program enjoyable.
- Provide a flexible routine to decrease boredom and increase enjoyment. Consider alternatives to traditional exercise modes, such as games and backpacking, to provide a variety of exercise options.
- Provide periodic exercise testing to show progress toward goals and offer an opportunity for positive reinforcement.
- Use strategies for behavioral change, such as personal goal setting, contracting, and self-management, to foster personal control and perceived competency.
- Chart progress on record cards, graphs, or computer programs. Note and record progress daily to give immediate, positive feedback.
- Recognize goal achievement in newsletters and bulletin boards. Individual effort increases when that effort is identifiable.
- Set up group or individual competitions.
- Offer lotteries based on individual or group accomplishment of a specific goal. Everyone can contribute money; set a winning criterion (such as the first person to walk 15 mi · wk^{-1} for 5 wk wins) for which the winner gets all the money. An alternative is to set a criterion (e.g., attending 20 of 24 aerobic classes) for participation in a random drawing.
- Organize teams to train for a charity-sponsored fun run and walk or road race.

Key Point

Individual, social, and environmental factors motivate people to move from precontemplation to contemplation of an exercise program and then to actually set up a plan to begin. A variety of strategies can be used, from mass media campaigns to fitness testing, to motivate people to move from contemplation into the preparation and action stages. Six strategies to facilitate adopting and maintaining exercise are 1) ask participants about exercise history and use what you learn to set up a personalized plan; 2) help participants develop knowledge, attitudes, and skills to support behavior change; 3) bolster self-efficacy; 4) set clear and realistic goals; 5) identify and resolve barriers to change; and 6) foster motivation.

Enhancing Adherence: Methods of Behavior Change for Participants in the Action and Maintenance Stages

Various strategies have been discussed to illustrate principles of behavior change and to describe ways to market and motivate exercise. Once a participant has started an exercise program (action stage), the fitness professional plays an important role in monitoring and supporting the establishment and maintenance of behavior change. For example, together, the fitness professional and the participant should set goals that are consistent with capabilities, values, resources, and needs. Exercise self-efficacy predicts adoption and maintenance; it can be increased with mastery experiences. Thus, initial goals should be set that are challenging but are certain to be met, which will foster increased exercise self-efficacy. The fitness professional and participant also should evaluate environmental and social supports and barriers and use this information to determine ways that barriers can be modified to promote the new behavior.

Assessment

Regardless of the intervention, comprehensive fitness and psychosocial assessments are necessary to select and carry out the appropriate strategies of behavior change for participants in the preparation and early action stages. Reassessment should be conducted periodically to evaluate the effectiveness of the plan.

First, the problem must be identified and defined in behavioral terms. For example, being overweight is not the problem but rather the result of overeating and underexercising. The fitness professional can also help the participant decide what can be realistically changed and what cannot.

Next, examine past attempts at behavior change. Find out what worked, what did not, and why. This information will be useful in goal setting and identifying high-risk situations (see Relapse Prevention on page 339).

Also find out if initiation of the behavior change is voluntary or recommended by someone else. This will give you a sense of motivation and commitment to change. Participants who are there because a doctor prescribed exercise may need help finding personal reasons for exercising. There are many different reasons for beginning an exercise program (e.g., health, weight loss, anxiety reduction), but the initial motivation may not be why someone continues to exercise. Ask these participants what they expect to get out of exercise and be prepared to pique their interest by presenting additional short- and long-term benefits.

Another useful assessment tool is the decisional balance sheet. The participant lists all short- and long-term consequences, positive and negative, of both changing and not changing the behavior. The participant and the fitness professional then brainstorm ways to avoid or cope with the projected negative consequences of behavior change.

Self-Monitoring

Part of the assessment process can be accomplished by self-monitoring, in which the participant records information about the target behavior and also indicates thoughts, feelings, and situations before, during, and after the behavior. The participant can identify the internal and external cues and behavioral consequences that inhibit and prompt exercise. Barriers and supports also become evident with self-monitoring. The fitness professional can help the participant develop strategies to cope with the barriers and use the supports. The chain of behaviors encompassing exercise can also be evaluated and weak links identified. For example, if the participant discovers she always skips her 5:30 p.m. aerobics class when she oversleeps and doesn't have time to pack her workout clothes before she leaves for work, you can suggest that she pack her workout bag the night before. Immediate benefits and reinforcements tailored to individual preferences can also be established at critical links in the chain (e.g., if she packs her workout bag the night before, she can push the snooze button for an extra 10 min of sleep the next morning). Electronic notebooks, computer programs, calendars, graphs, and charts can be used for self-monitoring as part of the initial assessment and as a way to record progress.

Research Insight

Achieving the CDC's recommendation for 30 min of moderate physical activity each day can be accomplished through the widely advertised 10,000 steps a day walking program (11). A popular tool for monitoring steps is the pedometer. This device has been used in several studies to effectively increase the number of steps walked and to help participants become more aware of when and how they can fit physical activity into their day. For example, Croteau (5) used goal setting, pedometers, self-monitoring, and weekly e-mail reminders in a lifestyle intervention to increase walking. After 8 wk, the participants significantly increased daily steps to more than 10,000. Gains were greatest for participants who were obese and for those starting with fewer than 6,000 daily steps.

Goal Setting

The purpose of **goal setting** is to accomplish a specific task in a specific time frame. Goals can be as simple and time limited as making a sandwich for lunch to the complicated and encompassing aim of earning an advanced degree. Goal setting provides a plan of action that focuses and directs activity and emphasizes a clear link between behavior and outcome.

Effective goal setting has several characteristics. Goals should be behavioral, specific, and measurable. Plans are easier to make if the goal is stated in behavioral terms. For example, a goal of walking 4 days $\cdot$ wk^{-1} for 30 to 45 min is easier to implement than a goal to get in shape. Specific, measurable goals make it easier to monitor progress, make adjustments, and know when the goal has been accomplished. Goals also must be reasonable and realistic. A goal might be achievable, but personal and situational constraints can make it unrealistic. Losing 2 lb $\cdot$ wk^{-1} (0.9 kg $\cdot$ wk^{-1}) through diet and exercise is reasonable for many people, but it may be almost impossible for the working mother of three who has minimal time for exercise and cooking. Unrealistic goals set the participant up to fail, which can damage self-efficacy and adherence to the program for behavior change.

By using information from the assessment and self-monitoring, the fitness professional can help participants set positive, realistic behavioral goals based on their age, sex, fitness, health, interests, exercise history, skills, and schedule. Both short-term and long-term goals should be included. Short-term goals mobilize effort and direct present actions, but both short- and long-term goals lead to a more effective plan of action (15) (see Characteristics of Effective Goals).

Reinforcement

Social **reinforcement** and self-reinforcement are crucial in the action phase, especially because the longer someone has been inactive, the longer it takes until exercise itself becomes reinforcing. Immediate consequences of exercise can be pain and fatigue, so external, immediate, positive rewards are necessary for beginners. Monitoring progress is rewarding and can involve charting miles walked after each session or asking for feedback from instructors after a difficult exercise class. Positive reinforcement from others can enhance self-esteem, especially when feedback comes from people who are important to the participant. Praise is more effective if it is immediate and behaviorally specific (12). "You worked hard in class last week" is not as effective as, "Sally, you did a great job getting through all the leg lifts today," especially if Sally has been struggling with leg lifts.

Self-reinforcement should involve rewards that are important to the participant. Using special spa soaps and creams only after an aerobic workout and getting tickets to the big game after logging a certain number of miles are rewards that are personalized and self-administered.

Social support can be verbal or tangible, such as transportation to exercise class. It can come from the class instructor, exercise partners, and family members. Significant others must be involved in the exercise plan and educated about the differences between support and nagging. Constructive verbal feedback, praise, encouragement, and positive attention will help a family member stick with exercise, whereas punishing comments, jokes about the person's efforts, or discouraging social comparisons can hinder adherence. Support focuses on what has been accomplished ("You're being consistent in your walking to lose weight. I'm proud of you."), whereas nagging harps on what has not been accomplished ("You should walk faster to lose weight. Why can't you pick up the pace?").

Friends in an exercise program can provide both social support and cues to exercise. They can be positive role models and part of a buddy system to support the exercise effort. Some participants are more likely to stick with a program if they know someone else is counting on them to be there to work out.

Behavioral Contracts

Behavioral contracts are written, signed, public agreements to engage in specific goal-directed behaviors, and they have been used effectively to increase exercise adherence (6). Contracts should include clear, realistic

Characteristics of Effective Goals

- Behavioral (Aim for actions, such as lifting weights, rather than outcomes, like losing weight.)
- Flexible (For example, jog or cycle 4-5 times each week.)
- Specific (For example, walk 3 mi without stopping.)
- Measurable (Can you quantify your goal in miles, minutes, reps, etc?)
- Reasonable (Is it possible?)
- Realistic (Does it stand a good chance of happening?)
- Challenging (Is it challenging but also realistic?)
- Meaningful (Is it important to the participant?)
- Reward for specific accomplishments (For example, buy a new CD after completing a yoga course.)
- Have a time frame (Establish a time frame for short- and long-term goals.)

objectives and deadlines. Developing a contract engages the participant in a way that is motivating, challenging, and public. The public nature of contracts is especially important because public goals are more likely to be met than private or semiprivate goals (15).

Contracts can be set by individuals or groups. The benefits of a group contract are the feeling it gives participants about not wanting to let others down and the desire to be part of a group. Individual contracts, however, can be tailored to the participant's specific situation and goals.

Consequences of meeting and not meeting the contracted goals should be clear and relevant to the participant. Contingency reinforcement can be set up so that the participant agrees to do a low-preference activity (e.g., squats) before a high-preference activity (e.g., sauna). Material and extrinsic reinforcers are good initially but should become limited as natural reinforcers, such as social reinforcement, are developed. Inherent benefits of exercise, such as enjoyment and a sense of accomplishment, can foster more intrinsic motivation and better adherence. A sample behavioral contract for a middle-aged man starting a walking program is shown below.

Key Point

Assessment is an important first step in the action stage of behavior change. Self-monitoring is useful in determining the antecedents and consequences of the target behavior as well as the potential costs of and barriers to behavior change.

Strategies such as goal setting and behavioral contracts must be tailored to the individual and should be reevaluated regularly during the maintenance stage. Some of the variables that influence exercise maintenance are enjoyment, motivation, convenience, exercise intensity, program flexibility, social support, incentives, rewards, and skills like self-regulation and self-reinforcement.

Behavioral Contract

Goal: To walk 3 mi without stopping **Time frame:** By May 15
Benefits of meeting goal: Improve my blood pressure, feel better, manage stress, lose weight, keep up with son's Boy Scout troop on weekend camping trips

To reach my goal, I will do the following:

1. Monitor my speed at the high school track during two walks on the weekend.
2. Walk at least 3 days per wk during my lunch hour with Bob or Mary.

Goal-supporting activities

1. Keep a spare pair of walking shoes and my MP3 player at work.
2. Watch sports on Saturday and Sunday only after I have completed my walks.
3. Reward myself with 30 min on the Internet each time I walk at least 30 min during my lunch hour.
4. Let my wife know about my plan and have her encourage me to walk on the weekends.
5. Purchase a new computer monitor when I reach my overall goal.

Barriers and countermeasures

1. Luncheon meetings: I will walk for 30 min before I leave work on days I have a meeting during lunch.
2. Rain: I will walk the stairs for at least 30 min during lunch when it rains.

Signed ______________________________ Date __________

Fitness professional ______________________________ Date __________

This contract will be evaluated every 2 wk:

Date __________ Revisions ______________________________

Date __________ Revisions ______________________________

Reprinted, by permission, from E.T. Howley and B.D. Franks, 2003, *Health fitness instructor's handbook*, 4th ed. (Champaign, IL: Human Kinetics), 357.

Relapse Prevention

The relapse prevention model is based on relapses in alcohol abuse, smoking, and drug abuse; the goal is to decrease a high-frequency, undesired behavior. This model is best applied to voluntary behavior. Although exercise is voluntary, the goal is to increase a low-frequency, desired behavior. Even so, the concepts and techniques of relapse prevention can be used with exercise adherence (14).

Relapse occurs when people who have been exercising regularly or engaging in other positive health behaviors stop the healthy behavior and go back to the old, unhealthy behavior. It is important to understand the concept of relapse as it applies to exercise, because relapse is likely for many people. The fitness professional must help participants understand that relapse does not mean failure; together, they can devise strategies to cope with temporary setbacks in the program for behavior change.

Defining High-Risk Situations

Relapse begins with a **high-risk situation** that challenges an individual's perceived ability to maintain the desired behavioral change. A wedding reception with all her favorite foods can be a high-risk situation for a dieter, and weekend guests can challenge a jogger's motivation to keep up with his afternoon runs. Individuals are predisposed to high-risk situations if they have a lifestyle imbalance in which shoulds exceed wants. This imbalance leads to feelings of deprivation and desires for indulgence. Rationalization, denial, and apparently irrelevant decisions can then occur (14).

Successful coping in a high-risk situation leads to increased self-efficacy and decreased probability of relapse. Not coping or inadequate coping leads to decreased self-efficacy and positive expectations about not maintaining the behavior change (e.g., being able to eat like "normal people," having more time to spend with friends). If this leads to an actual slip, the abstinence violation effect (or for exercise, the adherence violation effect) occurs in which participants perceive that they have failed. All-or-none thinking, such as the belief that you cannot skip a weekend of jogging and still be a jogger, makes the participant more susceptible to this effect. Feelings of failure lead to self-blame, lowered self-esteem, guilt, perceived loss of control, increased probability of relapse, and possibly giving up (14).

Fostering Coping Strategies for Exercise

Relapse prevention, as described by Marlatt and Gordon (19), is a method used to identify and deal with high-risk situations. The strategy begins by educating participants about the relapse process and enlisting their help as active participants in preventing a relapse. The next step is determining specific strategies to prevent exercise relapse:

- Identify situations with a high risk of relapse. High-risk situations are those that involve behaviors that are incompatible with exercise, such as eating, drinking, overworking, or smoking. High-risk situations can also involve relocation, medical events, travel, and inclement weather. Personal high-risk situations can be determined from information gathered during assessment and self-monitoring. The fitness professional should help the participant recognize aspects of the exercise behavior itself, such as time of day, place, people, moods, thoughts, and particular situations that can threaten exercise adherence.
- Revise plans in order to avoid or cope with high-risk situations. Flexible, short-term goals can be adapted to uncontrollable situational demands. Resetting goals temporarily can decrease the sense of noncompliance and increase a sense of control (e.g., "While my weekend guests are here, I will jog one day in the morning before they get up instead of trying to jog on both Saturday and Sunday afternoons").
- Improve coping responses by referring participants to classes covering techniques related to time management, relaxation, assertiveness, stress management, confidence building, and so on.
- Provide realistic expectations of potential outcomes from not exercising so the behavioral consequences of relapse are placed in proper perspective.
- Encourage participants to expect and plan for relapse. They should plan for some alternate modes of exercise, times of day, places, and so forth. If an individual is likely to skip a day of exercise when all the treadmills are in use, suggest the cycle or stair-climber on those days.
- Minimize the tendency to interpret a lapse (missing one class, not exercising during a business trip) as inevitably leading to a relapse, and then defining a relapse as a total failure. Use cognitive restructuring to change the definition of a missed exercise class from "the end of my exercise program" to "a temporary lapse that most people who exercise experience."
- Correct a lifestyle imbalance in which shoulds outweigh wants. Make exercise something participants want to do instead of something they feel they should do. Use positive reinforcement and other strategies to make exercise fun.

Key Point

Because missing regular exercise is inevitable for many people, the fitness professional must be prepared to help participants prevent lapses in an exercise routine from ending the exercise program. Strategies such as being flexible in setting and revising goals, realizing that the occasional lapse is just temporary, and building self-confidence can help participants deal successfully with a potential relapse.

Health and Fitness Counseling

The fitness professional is called on to provide counseling during assessment, exercise prescription, and ongoing monitoring of exercise programs. Good communication skills are the foundation of effective counseling. Developing good communications skills takes time and focus, so patience is critical to listening and understanding. For additional information, see the excellent chapter on health counseling skills by Southard and Southard in the ACSM resource manual (24).

Communication Skills

To be able to communicate well, the fitness professional must be able to listen effectively and respond empathetically. Listening involves being able to accurately discriminate the feeling and meaning of the speaker's message. Listening is more complicated than simply hearing words. **Communication** occurs at different levels, and thus we should not always assume that what people say is what they mean. The message includes the actual, objective meaning of the words, or the content of the message; however, tone of voice, loudness or softness of speech, speed, and nonverbal behavior can change the meaning of a statement. A participant who smiles, looks you in the eyes, and says, "My program is going really well," is not saying the same thing as a person who mumbles the same words and looks away. To enhance our understanding of the message, we must be able to attend to the verbal and nonverbal as well as overt and covert messages. The fitness professional should pay attention to facial expressions, body language, and tone of voice in addition to listening to the actual words.

The context of the message, determined by the social and cultural implications of the situation, can create noise that will interfere with sending and receiving the message. Noise is also created by the ideas, experiences, expectations, and prejudices of the speaker and listener. Barriers to communication occur not only in the context of the message but also in the way a listener responds. Ordering or commanding, threatening, criticizing, interpreting, interrupting, interrogating, and diverting (often by humor) are responses that shut off understanding and make the speaker feel you do not care. Looking over your shoulder and checking your watch are other obvious ways to shut down communications. If you don't have time to talk, be honest about it, but make sure you arrange another time when you won't be distracted and can give the participant the attention she needs and deserves.

Do not automatically assume you understand what a person is saying. We react to a communicated message according to our own perceptions of the nature of the message. Use responsive listening to clarify communication and confirm with the speaker that you comprehend his message. Reflect back what you have heard, and then ask questions and make statements that respond to the feeling and meaning of the message. Responsive listening lets people know you understand what they have expressed, helps build a relationship with them, encourages them to keep talking, and clarifies what they mean. Responsive listening is illustrated in the following exchange:

Participant: I'm the only one in this class who can't get the new step routines. (The fitness professional should observe the tone of voice, eye contact, and posture.)

Fitness professional: You think the other members of the class catch on before you do. That must be really frustrating. (The fitness professional paraphrased the participant's statement and interpreted probable underlying feelings. Other feelings could be discouragement or a sense of futility or failure. Responding with an offer to teach the participant the steps might not have addressed an underlying lack of confidence. Responsive listening keeps the communications open so the participant can express what kind of help she wants.)

Participant: Yes, I wonder if I can even do aerobics. The steps change faster than I can follow them. (The participant has low self-efficacy for this step aerobics class. The fitness professional now has more information about the problem and can offer a better solution.)

Fitness professional: You doubt this is for you because it is so fast-paced, but did you know that many of the people in this class started with Jenny's class? Jenny teaches all the basic routines at a slower pace and focuses on helping everyone learn the steps. (The fitness professional acknowledged the participant's beliefs and provided more information to put her perceptions in a different context. A beginners' class could provide mastery experiences to increase the participant's self-efficacy.)

Participant: I've always felt I didn't fit in, but I thought it was just me. Maybe I could try Jenny's step class. (The fitness professional should observe what the participant said and how she said it to see if the information met the underlying need.)

Fitness professional: This class was not the right one for you. Jenny's class can be a good way for you to learn the steps. We can check the schedule and I can introduce you to Jenny. (The fitness professional paraphrased the participant's statement and offered help rather than telling her what to do. This acknowledges the participant's ability to make choices when the fitness professional provides useful information.)

Characteristics of an Effective Helper

The role of the fitness professional as counselor is to help clients achieve their health-related goals. It is easier to provide this help when the fitness professional responds to the client with empathy, respect, concreteness, genuineness, and confrontation:

- **Empathy** is an expression of understanding of the personal meaning of events and experiences to the participant. It is different from sympathy, which is an attempt to experience another person's feelings. Empathy is also not the same as knowing what the problem is. You may know that John has 28% body fat because he eats fast food every day and does not exercise. Empathy means you have a sense of what it must be like for him to be overweight and inactive, and you are able to communicate your understanding in a nonjudgmental manner. Even if you are not sure you are being empathetic, when the participant perceives that you are trying to understand, he will be encouraged to communicate more about the problem. The additional information will help you empathize more and give you clues to the underlying nature of the problem and how to come up with a more realistic intervention plan. Your effort to understand also communicates to the participant that you value him as an individual.
- **Respect** is a feeling of positive regard for the participant. You display warm acceptance of the participant's experiences and place no conditions on your acceptance and warmth. This means not making judgments. It is often hard for the fitness professional to respect a person whose behavior (smoking, sedentary lifestyle, high-fat diet) shows a lack of self-respect for her body. We must prize the person but not necessarily the behavior. When we respect another person, we help that person develop self-respect.
- **Concreteness** is the ability to help the participant be specific about feelings and goals he is trying to communicate. Reflective listening enables the participant to become more precise in communicating what he experiences and wants to accomplish, which aids in setting goals.

Qualities of an Effective Healthy Behavior Counselor

- Knowledgeable
- Supportive
- Model of healthy behavior
- Trustworthy
- Enthusiastic
- Innovative
- Patient
- Sensitive
- Flexible
- Self-aware
- Able to access material resources and services
- Able to generate expectations of success
- Committed to providing timely, specific feedback
- Capable of providing clear, reasonable instructions and plans
- Aware of personal limitations

- **Genuineness** is being authentic and sincere in a relationship with another person. In a helpful relationship, the counselor is honest and open with the client. Some self-disclosure is appropriate and can help develop trust, but the goal of the relationship is to help the client, not deal with the fitness professional's personal issues.
- **Confrontation** involves telling the other person that you see things differently from how they are being presented to you. You point out incongruities that are observable facts about which the participant may not be consciously aware. Confrontation should be used only after you have an established relationship, and it should be directed toward the behavior, not the person.

Other qualities important in effective health counseling are listed in Qualities of an Effective Healthy Behavior Counselor.

Ethical Considerations

There is an ethical dilemma in promoting healthy behavior change in people who don't want to change. The fitness professional must weigh the importance of persuading people to behave in ways conducive to good health versus the clients' right to do as they please with their own health as long as it does not impinge on the rights of others. Informed consent theoretically gives participants a free choice after they have been given all the information needed to make a decision. If an unhealthy lifestyle is based on ignorance or incorrect information, we should provide the necessary information for an informed choice, not aggravate feelings of guilt or failure. But if an individual has chosen an unhealthy lifestyle as a matter of free will, we must accept this informed refusal, although fitness professionals often have difficulty doing this. Thus, an awareness of our own value preferences is essential in helping others set goals. We must consider whose values are to be served by the intervention, the clients' or ours, and we must respect their choices even if we disagree with them.

Confidentiality is another ethical concern for the fitness professional. In addition to client information that is clearly confidential, such as medical records, the fitness professional may become aware of other information the participant wants to keep private. Trustworthiness is an important characteristic of an effective helper and reflects an ethical stand. Participants will trust someone who keeps information confidential, treats them with respect, and keeps the relationship professional.

Also, recognize your limitations and know when to refer your client to a professional therapist. It is the role of the fitness professional to help people change unhealthy behavior, but marital problems, eating disorders, and affective disorders such as depression are a few of the areas that should be handled by someone trained to work with these issues. We must know our limits and help connect participants with the best resources for handling their unique problems.

Key Point

Listening to the actual words and the nonverbal message in context is the foundation of good communication skills. To communicate effectively, the fitness professional should practice reflective listening and empathetic responding. Characteristics of an effective helper include empathy, respect, concreteness, genuineness, and confrontation.

Case Studies

You can check your answers by referring to page 475 in appendix A.

1. Dana was given a 3 mo membership to your facility by her boyfriend, Mike, who attends aerobics classes regularly. They are going on a backpacking trip to Colorado this summer, and Mike thought you could help get her ready for the physical strain of the trip. She is a self-proclaimed couch potato. Dana started aerobics classes with Mike last year but got so sore that she stopped after 1 wk. Yesterday, you completed her fitness assessment; Dana is in good health, has 20% body fat, and is slightly below average in aerobic fitness. She said her goal is to be prepared for the trip, and she wants to try aerobics again. However, she confides she is afraid she will disappoint Mike because she is "really out of shape" and doesn't enjoy aerobics. What stage of behavior change is she in, and what strategies could you use to help her?
2. Jack is a middle-aged college English professor who joined the walking club in your facility after you conducted his fitness and psychosocial assessment 3 mo ago. His long-term goal was to walk around the world (in terms of total miles walked), and his progress has been marked on the walkers' promotional map at the front entrance. His office is two blocks from your facility, and Jack usually walks on your indoor track before he goes home for the day. You notice his mileage has decreased over the past 2 wk, and another walker tells you that Jack said, "I won't make it out of the state thanks to term papers and final exams." What stage of behavior change is he in, and what strategies could you use to help him?

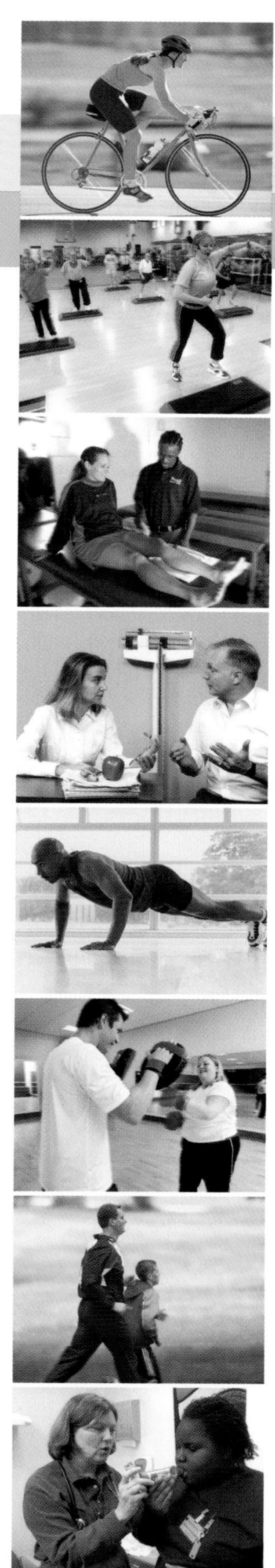

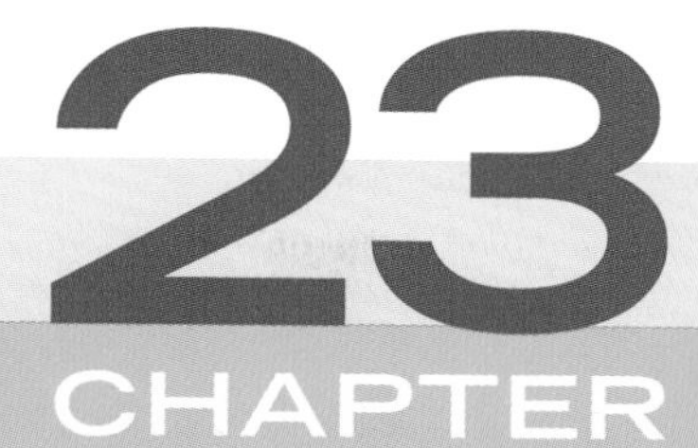

Mindful Exercise for Fitness Professionals

Ralph La Forge

Objectives

The reader will be able to do the following:

1. Understand the historical origins of two classical mindful exercise traditions and their relevance to contemporary mindful exercise programming.
2. Describe the essential components common to most mindful exercise programs.
3. Understand the essential tenets of classical and contemporary mindful exercise modalities and list potential benefits of each.
4. List psychobiological mechanisms responsible for the benefits of mindful exercise and yogic breathing.
5. Know key resources for further information on both classical and contemporary mindful exercise.

Mindful exercise (sometimes referred to as *mind–body exercise)* in its most simple form is low-to-moderate physical activity performed with a meditative, proprioceptive, or sensory awareness component. Although not universally defined, mindful exercise can also be described simply as physical exercise executed with a profound inward focus. The physical activity can be executed with a specific choreographic movement pattern such as in tai chi or can be a free-form pattern as seen in ethnic spiritual dancing (e.g., Native American spiritual dancing). The cognitive component is characteristically nonjudgmental and meditative. The descriptor *mindful* is used here in contrast to the more nebulous *mind–body* because *mindful* more appropriately defines the cognitive process involved. *Mindful* may be described as self-help knowledge to answer questions on self-control and understanding, awareness without judgment of what is via direct experience, and awareness of the moment.

The inward attention in mindful exercise is performed with specific focus on breathing and proprioception, or muscle sense. Any physical activity can integrate an inner attentiveness or a cognitive component; however, inner attentiveness is the key process in mindful exercise. Mindful exercise combines low-to-moderate muscular activity with a sensory awareness of the physical movement or posture—a self-monitoring of perceived effort. Classical mindful exercises such as Hatha yoga and tai chi are attentive to the present moment and are process oriented. This process contrasts with most conventional exercise, in which there is a relative disconnect between the mind and the kinesthesis of the physical activity, or in which the mind may disassociate from the present moment. This disconnect does not necessarily disadvantage conventional aerobic exercise; it may be a distraction from life stress or the physical exertion itself.

Mindful programs can be readily executed at low-to-moderate exercise intensities and are adaptable to a wide range of functional capacities. For example, Iyengar yoga (restorative yoga) with skillful instruction can be customized for nearly any age, level of fitness, body type, or chronic disease state. Several blankets under the upper torso during a savasana pose can provide initial support for the lower back when preparing the lower back for a bridge pose (back bend; see figure 23.1). This is one example of how including props (e.g., blankets) can prepare an older adult for a more difficult pose. For someone who is unfamiliar with Hatha yoga, the popular triangle pose may appear to be nothing more than a lateral side stretch. However, the yogi's cognition is deeply entrained on the simple kinesthesis of the pose and on breath centering. Many will find these attributes beneficial in managing musculoskeletal health concerns, in reducing anxiety and stress-related symptoms, and, perhaps most importantly, in improving self-awareness and peace of mind.

This chapter is an overview of both classical and contemporary mindful exercise. Yoga, tai chi, and qigong are addressed in more depth, as they have a much longer heritage and larger research foundation. The information in this chapter is not intended to instruct fitness professionals on how to teach yoga, Pilates, or tai chi, as each requires hundreds of hours of personal exploration and objective feedback in order for the teacher to attain sufficient instructive skill and knowledge of its tradition. The chapter objective is to introduce these forms of contemplative exercise and provide helpful resources.

Origins

The Asian yoga and tai chi disciplines are at the root of most contemporary mindful exercise programs taught today. These two ancient forms integrate mind and body along with an overt sense of spirituality and grounding in nature. At the heart of all meditative practice in Asia is what Indians call *yoga.* Yoga is a complex system

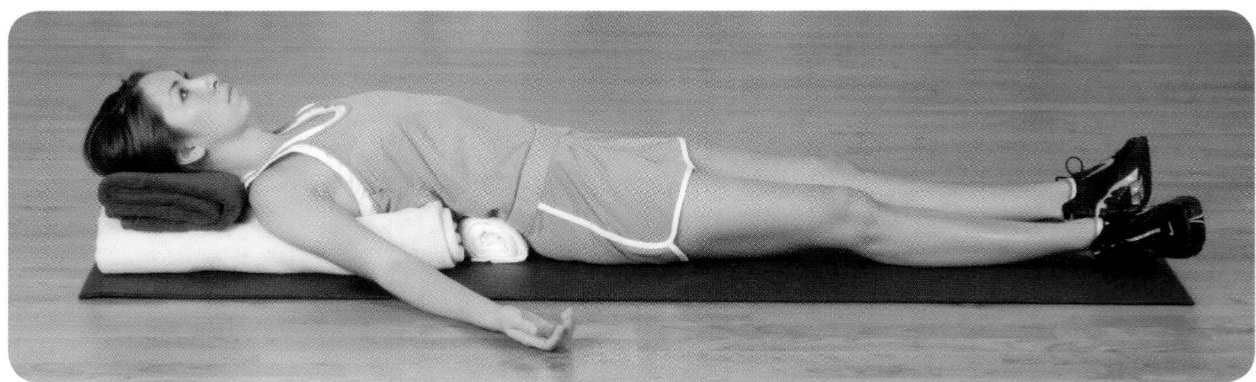

Figure 23.1 Supported corpse pose using towels and blankets for back support.

of physical and spiritual disciplines fundamental to a number of Asian religions such as Hinduism and Buddhism. For example, classical yoga, as described in the *Yoga Sutra,* an ancient text of yogic principles attributed to Patanjali, is composed of eight components, or limbs: moral principles, observances, posture, breath control, withdrawal of the senses, concentration, meditation, and pure contemplation (7). Here, *posture* refers to yogic exercises, or *asanas,* that originally were used to prepare for practicing breath control and meditation. In other words, yoga exercise was used as a means to an end, and the end was meditation and spiritual freedom. The physical arm of yoga, Hatha yoga, when coupled with a contemplative component is perhaps the most practiced form of mindful exercise in the West today.

Tai chi has a nearly 4,000 yr heritage and is derived from qigong (also called *chi kung),* which describes the entire tradition of spiritual, martial, and health exercises developed in China. Qigong is the primary Chinese methodology for activating the *medicine within,* or the natural self-healing resource. This ancient practice combines two ideas: Qi is the vital energy of the body, and gong is the skill of working with the qi (also called *chi).* Tai chi, the martial art derivative of qigong, is perhaps best described as a moving meditation. Most contemporary mind–body exercise programs (see later section on contemporary mindful exercise programs) are derived from early yoga and qigong.

Who, Where, and Why

Since the early 1990s there has been an explosive growth of mindful exercise programming in health clubs, fitness centers, and cardiovascular disease prevention and management programs (see Where Mindful Exercise Programs Are Taught). These programs often complement or substitute for conventional exercise programs. Fitness professionals need to have some understanding, if not a limited personal experience, with one or more of these movement forms, as Hatha yoga and Pilates were among the most frequently offered programs in fitness centers in 2005 (4). Nearly anyone can perform mindful exercise, as the exercises can be readily adapted to nearly any body type, functional capacity, or health status. This adaptation also depends on the skill and experience of the instructor. Common benefits to these programs are shown above.

Where Mindful Exercise Programs Are Taught

- Community fitness and wellness centers
- Athletic training programs
- Yoga studios and ashrams
- Personally individualized instruction and therapy on location (e.g., home, fitness center, or office)
- Professional fitness and sports medicine meetings
- Clinical rehabilitation programs (e.g., cardiac, pulmonary, musculoskeletal)
- Pain management programs
- Senior and retirement centers

Common Benefits of Mindful Exercise

- Reduced anxiety and mental tension
- Improved muscular fitness (muscular strength)
- Improved muscular flexibility
- Improved balance control
- Enhanced self-efficacy and mood
- Tendency to concomitantly improve other lifestyle behaviors (e.g., stress control and dietary behavior)

In recent years, mindful exercise programs have attracted three principal populations of individuals: young and middle-aged adults wishing to improve muscular fitness, flexibility, and stamina; older adults looking for physical activity programs that can be functionally tailored to their aging body and lifestyle; and individuals with stable chronic disease who are seeking a safe and individualized approach to exercise training and rehabilitation. Recent work by DiBenedetto and colleagues (3) underscores the potential utility of Iyengar yoga in improving ambulation in elderly populations. They trained 23 healthy elders with an 8 wk program of gentle Iyengar yoga and demonstrated improved hip extension, increased stride length, and decreased anterior pelvic tilt in the subjects. The common reason these groups cite for seeking mindful exercise, however, is to bring inner tranquility to the mind. Virtually all of the mindful exercise modalities discussed in this chapter can be readily adapted for cardiac, pulmonary, or musculoskeletal rehabilitation in either individualized therapy or therapy in small groups. Several forms of Hatha yoga may be difficult to modify for those with chronic disease; for example, Bikram yoga (because of the elevated ambient temperature) and a number of Hatha yoga poses, such as full inverted poses. Although nearly

Mindful Exercise and Rehabilitation

- Pulmonary rehabilitation: Yogic breathing therapy, yoga styles with particular emphasis on breath work such as Viniyoga, Integral yoga, Ashtanga, and Iyengar yoga
- Balance control (especially in elderly patients): tai chi, qigong, tai chi chih
- Cardiac rehabilitation (with emphasis on aerobic exercise): Neuromuscular Integrative Action (NIA)
- Musculoskeletal rehabilitation (e.g., sport rehab): Feldenkrais method, Alexander technique, therapeutic Iyengar yoga, individualized Pilates exercise
- Arthritis and carpal tunnel syndrome: Individualized therapeutic yoga
- Stress reduction: Virtually all forms of skillfully taught mindful exercise, particularly with yogic breathing, restorative yoga, qigong exercise, tai chi, and Ananda yoga
- Overall muscular fitness and flexibility: Iyengar yoga, Ashtanga yoga, Pilates

These forms of rehabilitation do not exclude other mindful exercise modalities.

any mindful exercise can serve in a therapeutic or rehabilitative role, several forms that may be more appropriate for particular disabilities or chronic medical conditions are shown in Mindful Exercise and Rehabilitation.

Essential Components of Mindful Exercise

The criteria for what constitutes mindful exercise are currently being debated by practitioners and researchers, and a unified set of definitive consensus standards awaits more controlled and adequately powered research trials. For now, mindful exercise should include the following criteria:

- Meditative or contemplative qualities. Mindful exercise includes a self-reflective, present-moment, and nonjudgmental sensory awareness which is process centered rather than strictly goal oriented.
- Proprioceptive awareness. Mindful exercise includes the perception of movement and spatial orientation arising from low-to-moderate muscular activity.
- Breath centering. In mindful exercise cognitive centering activity is focused on the breath and breath sounds. This breath centering process includes a variety of breathing techniques as employed in yoga, Tai Chi, and Qigong exercise.
- Anatomic alignment (e.g., of head, spine, trunk, and pelvis) or proper physical form. Disciplining oneself to follow a particular movement pattern or spinal alignment holds true for many forms of mindful exercise, but particularly for Hatha yoga, Alexander technique, Pilates, and tai chi. Not all mindful exercise utilizes a set sequential choreography or disciplined anatomical alignment. Exceptions include NIA and expressive ethnic dance exercise (e.g., Native American and Alaskan spiritual dance).
- Energycentric. The awareness of movement and flow of one's intrinsic energy, vital life force, chi, prana, or other positive energy is common to many classical mindful exercise programs (e.g., yoga).

The next section describes in detail the most prominent and classical forms of mindful exercise.

Key Point

Most mindful exercise today is inspired by classical, centuries-old forms such as Tai Chi and yoga. Mindful exercise has specific features, including meditative, proprioceptive, and breath work processes, that distinguish it from conventional exercise programs. The fitness professional interested in mindful exercise should acquire some understanding of the traditions from which many of the contemporary forms evolved. The central quality of all mindful exercise is the mindfulness, or nonjudgmental awareness, and without this feature it is merely a physical workout.

Yoga

Many contemporary mindful exercise programs we see today originated from the Eastern disciplines of yoga and qigong. "The word *yoga* is derived from the Sanskrit root yuj meaning to bind, join, attach and yoke, to direct and concentrate one's attention on, to use and apply. It also means union or communion" (16). The union refers to an integration of mind, body, and spirit. Yoga historically refers to the physical and spiritual disciplines fundamental to Buddhist, Jainism, and Hindu religious practices throughout Asia. There are at least eight branches of yoga, but for many people in the West, *yoga* means Hatha yoga. We must differentiate *yoga* from participation in Hatha yoga classes such as those taught in yoga centers and fitness centers in the United States. Hatha yoga may or may not include spiritual, moral, and related yogic lifestyle behaviors. Hatha yoga is the physical aspect of this discipline and includes a vast repertoire of physical postures, or *asanas,* that are performed while seated,

Factors Determining the Response to Hatha Yoga

Level of mental focus or kinesthesis
Position of the asana (e.g., head down or head up)
Duration of each asana
Pose sequence
Duration of entire pose sequence or yoga session
Breathing technique
Skill level of the student (i.e., years of yoga experience)
Anthropometric characteristics of the student (e.g., BMI, body structure, musculoskeletal health)

Popular Hatha Yoga Styles

- **Iyengar yoga.** Iyengar yoga was originally developed by B.K.S. Iyengar, who systematized over 200 classical asanas (poses), from very simple to very difficult. Iyengar yoga emphasizes precise anatomical alignment, which over the years has refined the therapeutic aspects of yoga. Iyengar also emphasizes breathing (pranayama).
- **Restorative yoga.** This style of Hatha yoga derives from the Iyengar yoga tradition and is perhaps most appropriate for those who are just embarking on a yoga program because it uses props (blankets, pillows, lumbar and neck rolls, bolsters) and elementary but progressive poses.
- **Ashtanga yoga.** This vigorous, more athletic style of yoga synchronizes a progressive series of postures with a specific breathing method (ujjayi pranayama). The asanas in Ashtanga yoga are sequenced in groups of poses which range from moderate to very difficult. The sequence pace and pose difficulty often characterize Ashtanga as power yoga.
- **Anusara yoga.** Founded by John Friend of Shenandoah, Texas, this form of Hatha yoga closely resembles Iyengar and stresses three focus points: attitude, alignment, and action. Participants are taught to be cognizant of their key power center, or focal point (the point at which most of the body weight or musculoskeletal force is placed during an asana).
- **Viniyoga.** This is a softer and more individualized method of Hatha yoga. It carefully integrates the flow of breath with movement of the spine. It is also known for therapeutic application of the classical asanas.
- **Kripalu yoga.** This is a three-level style of Hatha yoga customized to the needs of Western students. The Kripalu method blends the physical postures of Hatha yoga with the contemplative meditation of Raja yoga.
- **Integral yoga.** This is another gentle yoga form that gently stretches, strengthens, and calms the body and mind. It includes comfortable postures, deep relaxation, and breathing practices. It significantly emphasizes diet and is employed across the United States in Dr. Dean Ornish's heart disease reversal programs.
- **Bikram yoga.** Bikram yoga is a vigorous 90 min series of 26 poses designed to warm and stretch muscles, ligaments, and tendons in a particular sequence. Bikram classes are taught in a heated room, usually between 90 and 105 °F.
- **Kundalini yoga.** Also called the yoga of awareness, each class usually entails spine and flexibility warm-up, specific asana sequences commensurate with one's "coiled up energy," and relaxation. Each asana symbolizes life habits and emotion and a specific associated breath.
- **Sivananda yoga.** This is a style of classical yoga with traditional poses, breathing exercises, and relaxation. This style teaches 12 postures that constitute the sun salutation and can be readily adapted to beginners or those who have low functional capacities.
- **Ananda yoga.** This is a relatively gentle, nonathletic style of Hatha yoga. A unique feature of this system is that participants use silent affirmations while performing the asanas.

kneeling, standing, or lying prone or supine on the floor. Traditionally, Hatha yoga poses are used to ready the mind for meditation. Some of the more popular asanas in the West are named in Sanskrit, but their Western names include corpse pose, cobra, triangle, bridge, warrior, downward or upward facing dog, and the sun salutation (a sequence of 12 poses). The variables that determine the energy expenditure and psychophysiological responses to Hatha yoga are shown on page 347. The participant accrues optimal benefits from a Hatha yoga training program when the teacher specifically emphasizes each of these variables in a graduated and safe manner.

The styles of Hatha yoga better known in the West are shown on page 347. The principal challenge of nearly all styles is to become proficient at handling increasingly greater resistance (i.e., complexity and difficulty) in the various postures and breathing patterns while maintaining a homeostasis of mind and body—or the simultaneous quieting of thoughts and relaxing of body tension. The stamina and discipline required to attain the proper mental state and near-perfect stance and alignment can take many years to master. It is this mental and physical discipline that draws many to Hatha yoga practice, as this process can establish a template for other healthy lifestyle changes (e.g., regular meditation, healthier diet). Finally, it is paramount that yogic breathing, of which there are many techniques, be executed in synchrony with each pose during the asana. It may be difficult for fitness professionals to rationalize any breath holding, as they are essentially taught not to do this during the eccentric or concentric phases of muscular exercise for good reason. That said, the breath is held for brief periods of time with some forms of asana work (i.e., breath suspensions and retentions). Restorative yoga may be the safest and most productive starting point for those just learning yogic breathing and poses.

Key Point

Hatha yoga combines yogic breathing with yoga exercise in a very logical way. Whenever a yoga movement expands your chest or abdomen, you inhale. Conversely, when a movement compresses your chest or abdomen, you exhale.

Yogic Breathing (Pranayama)

In the yogic and qigong traditions, breathing functions as an intermediary between mind and body. Breath centering stands as an independent method of reducing mental tension and promoting relaxation in the short term and psychological well-being in the long term. There are many yogic breathing techniques, but the simplest is often the most beneficial. Simply focusing on the breath and breath sounds is often sufficient to calm the mind. Herbert Benson's classic book and technique *The Relaxation Response* is an excellent example of this integration of breath awareness and meditation (17).

Breathing is done through the nose during both inhalation and exhalation. Each breath is intentionally slow and deep with an even distribution, or smoothness, of effort. Sovik (14) recently published a helpful review on yogic breathing technique. He describes optimal yogic breathing as diaphragmatic, nasal, deep, smooth, even, quiet, and free of pauses.

In addition to reduced stress and mental tension, cardiovascular benefits result from yogic breathing. For example, Prakash (10) demonstrated that 10 subjects who had frequent premature ventricular contractions (PVCs) experienced a 50% reduction of PVCs after controlled deep yogic breathing at 6 breaths · min^{-1}. One of the mechanisms responsible for the mental quiescence experienced with yogic breathing is its stimulation of the parasympathetic nervous system. When fully stimulated by adequate yogic inspiration and expiration, mechanical receptors in pulmonary tissue (e.g., alveoli) activate parasympathetic nerves, which transiently reduces mental tension and increases relaxation response (9) (see figure 23.2). Acute reductions in blood pressure also have resulted from yogic breathing training (8).

Caution with beginner yogic breathers: Yogic breathing in itself is a very powerful exercise. Many people experience dizziness or lose consciousness while practicing beginning or advanced breathing techniques. It is strongly recommended that such techniques be initially taught and monitored by an experienced yogic breathing instructor. As with all cognitive approaches employed to facilitate relaxation, those utilizing yogic breathing therapy for this purpose should be aware of the contraindications of utilizing such therapy.

Yoga Teacher Standards

When choosing a yoga teacher, fitness instructors may wish to seek those with significant teaching experience. The Yoga Alliance's Experienced Registered Yoga Teachers (E-RYT) registry is one such resource of experienced teachers (www.yogaalliance.org/teacher_search.cfm). E-RYTs have significant teaching experience of at least 2 yr and 1,000 hr for an E-RYT 200 and at least 4 yr and 2,000 hr for an E-RYT 500. The 200 and 500 designations relate to the number of approved training contact hours the registered yoga teacher has completed. The 200 and 500 training hours include training from the following curriculum categories:

- Technique and practice (asanas, pranayamas, meditation)

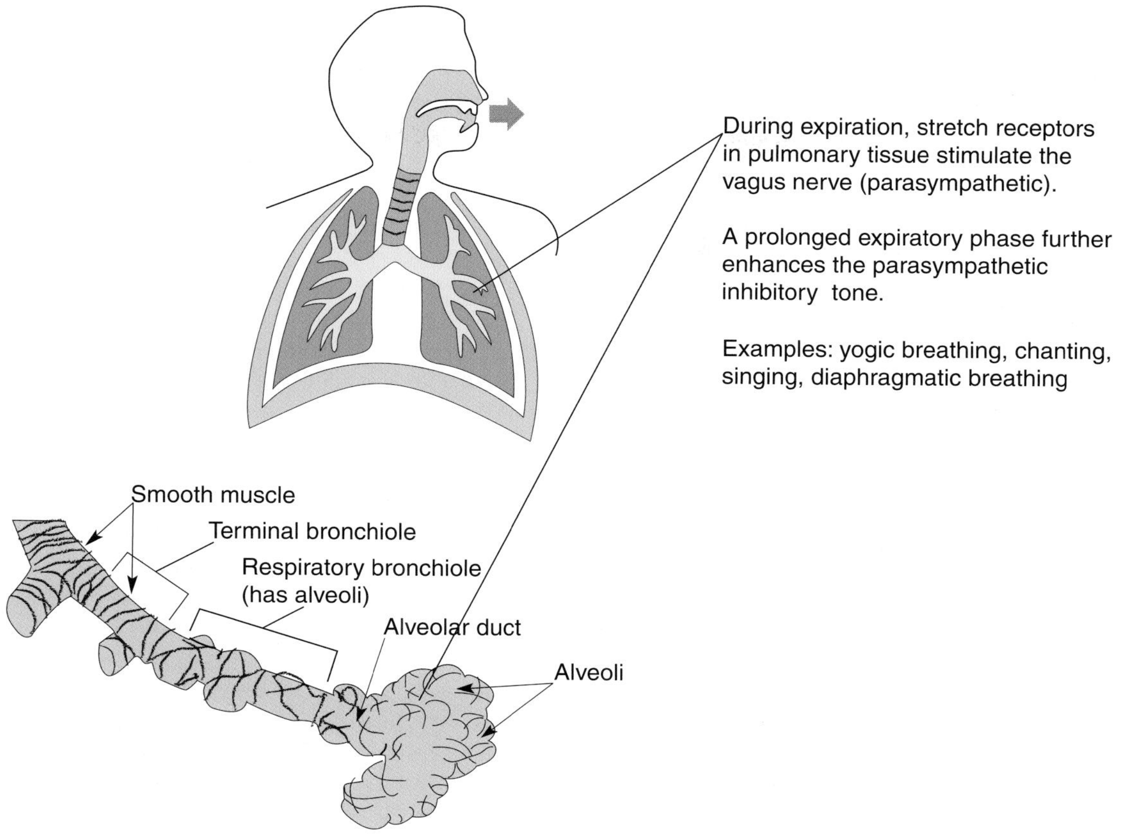
During expiration, stretch receptors in pulmonary tissue stimulate the vagus nerve (parasympathetic).
A prolonged expiratory phase further enhances the parasympathetic inhibitory tone.
Examples: yogic breathing, chanting, singing, diaphragmatic breathing
Smooth muscle
Terminal bronchiole
Respiratory bronchiole (has alveoli)
Alveolar duct
Alveoli

Figure 23.2 Yogic breathing and the parasympathetic nervous system.

- Teaching methodology (demonstration, observation, instruction)
- Anatomy and physiology (human anatomy and physiology, energy anatomy)
- Yoga philosophy (yoga history, lifestyle, ethics)
- Practicum (practice teaching, feedback, assisting students)

Key Point

It is important for the fitness professional to understand the origin and practice of yoga, which involves spiritual, meditation, and moral disciplines, versus Hatha yoga, which incorporates physical poses (asanas). The two terms *yoga* and *Hatha yoga* are not mutually exclusive. There are many styles of Hatha yoga ranging from the softer restorative yoga to the vigorous Ashtanga style. For participants to receive optimum benefit from Hatha yoga they must integrate appropriate asanas, yogic breathing, and meditative processes. Hatha yoga can improve muscular strength and flexibility and become a path for improved living habits, including stress reduction.

Qigong Exercise and Tai Chi

Possibly the simplest and the most practiced mindful exercise is qigong exercise. *Qigong* (pronounced "chee gung") refers to Chinese mental and physical exercises that cultivate the *qi (chi).* Qigong originates from Daoism and is often associated with healing, longevity, and enlightenment. *Qigong* is a combination of two Chinese characters. The second, the *gong,* refers to work or merit. The *qi,* however, is more complex. *Qi* is understood to be ever changing and ever flowing, a force at work in nature and society as well as in the human body. There are two types of qigong: internal and external. Internal qigong is practiced by individuals to promote self-healing. External qigong is a form of psychic therapy that involves the transfer of qi from a qigong master to another person. Tai chi is one form of qigong. The difference between qigong and tai chi is somewhat subtle but is discussed in the next section.

Qigong Exercise

Qigong exercise involves controlled breathing, soft flowing movements, and calm and careful focus. While these exercises are ancient, traceable to texts found in

Han period tombs from 2,000 yr ago, the term itself is relatively recent, not seen before the Ming period (1368-1644). Furthermore, before 1900, knowledge and dissemination of such exercises extended to the relative few who received training through traditional lineage holders. Only in the 1980s was qigong popularized to become the widespread exercise it is today.

Qigong exercise, also known as *Chinese health exercise,* dates back more than 3,000 yr. Qigong movements require very low energy expenditure, usually between 2 and 4 METs, and include standing, seated, and supine positions. (METs are multiples of resting energy expenditure; for example, 4 METs requires 4 times as much energy expenditure as resting.) For this reason qigong exercise is nearly perfectly suited to older people and people who have disabilities. The many qigong exercise styles are all based on balance, relaxation, breathing, and good posture. Some are named after animals whose movements they imitate (e.g., dragon, swan, crane, snake, wild goose, and animal frolics styles). Qigong culture holds that inhaling brings positive qi into your body and usually accompanies an opening movement (i.e., arms opening away from the body) while exhaling releases the negative qi and accompanies a closing movement (i.e., arms back to the body). Taiji qigong is ideal as a preparation for high-intensity conditioning exercise or as a cool-down. Taiji qigong consists of only 18 movements taken from the tai chi and qigong forms. It is recommended that this series be practiced once or twice a day for 15 to 20 min.

Research-Supported Medical Benefits of Qigong

- Reduced asthma-related symptoms (bronchospasm)
- Increased cerebral blood flow
- Reduced pain in patients with chronic pain
- Reduced mental tension and state anxiety
- Reduced blood pressure
- Increased bone density
- Improved cognitive performance
- Improved immunocompetence
- Reduced blood coagulation
- Reduced blood lipid levels (cholesterol and triglycerides)
- Improved sexual function
- Reduced risk of stroke

From K. Sancier and D. Holman, 2004, "Multifaceted health benefits of Qigong," *Journal of Alternative and Complementary Medicine* 10: 163-166.

Numerous published studies, mostly with small subject numbers, demonstrate many health benefits of qigong exercise.

Tai Chi

Tai chi (shorthand for tai chi chuan or taijiquan) is one form of the more ancient qigong (Chinese health exercise). Tai chi chuan is a complex martial arts choreography of over 100 flowing graceful movements which can be practiced for health, meditation, and self-defense. Tai chi is a form of qigong but not all qigong exercise is tai chi. Some qigong exercises are done while sitting or lying, and all tai chi exercises involve moving and standing. Some of the numerous styles of tai chi chuan are listed on page 351. Each form emphasizes a particular aspect, such as breathing, generating power, or relaxation. Some styles have a short form which may be more adaptable to people who have disabilities. In tai chi, students are taught to allow the practice to evolve into a free-flowing exercise such that the movements and breathing become one unified energy (qi) flow. Tai chi chih, developed by American Justin Stone, is a simpler form of tai chi chuan and consists of a series of 20 movements and one ending pose. Qigong exercise, described earlier, involves an even simpler set of movements than its martial arts relative tai chi involves.

Tai chi and qigong have a rich research-based tradition backed by several thousand published papers in international medical and sport science journals although most of these are not controlled, statistically powered trials (Qigong Database Version 7.3; www.qigonginstitute.org/html/database.php). One recently published paper that may be particularly helpful to fitness professionals systematically reviewed 47 studies of the physical and psychological effects of tai chi on various chronic medical conditions (15). This review indicated that tai chi was safe for a variety of chronic conditions and promoted balance

Key Point

The ancient qigong and tai chi practice has inspired many contemporary mindful exercise programs. The calming and introspective qualities of qigong and tai chi rank nearly highest among those of the mindful exercise modalities seen in the West today. Qigong exercise and tai chi are best suited for those who are older, those with low functional capacity, and those who wish to improve balance and coordination. Patient populations ideally suited for qigong and tai chi are cardiac rehabilitation patients, especially those in early phases following myocardial infarction or cardiovascular intervention procedures, hypertensive patients, and patients with stress-related disorders.

Forms of Tai Chi

- **Original Chen form.** The original Chen style (old form) is thought to be the template from which the more recent Wu, Yang, and Sung forms descended. Chen form is generally characterized by lower stances, constant twisting, varying speeds, and soft and more intense movements with power expression.
- **Yang style.** Yang style is the most widely practiced form of tai chi in the West today. The original Yang long form consists of 108 movements; however, the yang 24 short form is a popular modification practiced today.
- **Chang style.** Chang style is a relatively new style of tai chi developed by Chang Tung-Sheng in the 1930s. Chang style consists of more than 100 movements and is based on modifications to the Yang long form.
- **Wu style.** Wu style is an easier form of tai chi with smaller steps. Its movements, which involve less twisting, impose less stress on the legs and knees. The condensed Wu style includes 36 postures.
- **Sun style.** Sun style combines elements of the Wu and Yang styles. Sun style is characterized by very energetic steps.
- **Mulan Quan style.** This is a modern form based in traditional tai chi movement and wushu (Chinese martial arts). However, it adds aspects of Chinese folk dance and gymnastics for a very expressive movement process.

control, flexibility, and cardiovascular fitness, especially in older patients.

Contemporary Mindful Exercise Programs

Since the early 1980s numerous derivatives of mindful exercise have evolved from qigong, tai chi, and yoga. Some of these contemporary forms are neuromuscular integrative action (NIA), Gyrotonics, Chi Ball, walking meditation , E-Motion, Brain Gym, Yogarobics, Yogilates, aqua tai chi, yo chi, ChiRunning, ChiWalking, Flow Motion, mind–body circuit exercise, and many ethnic dance routines. The Asian martial arts (e.g., aikido, karate, taekwondo, kempo, and judo) also share many of the characteristics of early classical forms such as tai chi. Pilates, the Alexander technique, the Feldenkrais method, and various modern Hatha yoga styles have likewise matured as respected mindful exercise and rehabilitative methods as their techniques have been largely standardized over the last three decades.

Pilates

According to the Pilates Method Alliance (PMA), 9 million Americans practice Pilates and there are approximately 13,000 Pilates instructors in the United States, although many of these are not certified by the PMA or one of the several other Pilates organizations. In 2005, the PMA launched its certification exam for Pilates instructors. As of 2006 there is no one nationally recognized Pilates Instructor certification.

The Pilates method was developed by J.H. Pilates in the early 20th century. Pilates is an extremely orderly system of slow, controlled, distinct movements that demand a profound internal cognitive focus. This method is essentially divided into two modalities: floor or mat work and the work on the resistance equipment that Pilates developed (e.g., the Universal Reformer). Mat work is taught in either a group or a private setting, whereas work on the equipment is generally learned one on one or in small groups. Pilates is essentially a movement reeducation in which the student learns to overcome faulty compensatory movement patterns. These inefficient movement patterns are broken down into components by using a Reformer machine, which employs a series of levers and springs and changes the body's orientation to gravity. Pilates exercises facilitate more efficient movement by allowing the student to be in a position that minimizes undesirable muscle activity that can cause early fatigue and injury. Pilates equipment adapts to many human anatomic variations and can be adjusted such that similar movement sequencing can be applied to a variety of body types and limb and torso lengths. Pilates is advantageous for those who desire low-impact exercise to improve posture, flexibility, and functionality. Technique varies among Pilates training programs, most of which assert advantages over conventional strength and muscle reeducation training.

The main features of the Pilates method are mental concentration, fluid muscular contraction, breathing, alignment, and relaxation. The ultimate goal is to decompress the joints (especially the spine) and uniformly develop the body. Perhaps the most acclaimed benefit of Pilates training is improved core strength. This term connotes lumbar stabilization and motor control and has been promoted as a preventive and performance-enhancing regimen. In essence, core strengthening describes the muscular control required around the lumbar spine to maintain functional stability. Unfortunately, scientific reports of improvements in objective measures of core strength through Pilates training have been meager.

It is perplexing that considering its present popularity research studies evaluating Pilates remain scarce. A Medline search for research published from 1990 to 2005 identified only 18 papers of which nearly all were descriptive and observational studies. Segal, Hein, and Basforth (13) published one of the first studies quantifying improvements in flexibility (fingertip-to-floor distance) with Pilates; however, they reported no changes in body composition after 6 mo of Pilates mat exercise. Olson and coworkers at Auburn University performed a series of small uncontrolled studies on musculoskeletal and cardiovascular responses to Pilates mat exercises. These studies included EMG (electromyogram) evaluations validating the significant involvement of abdominal muscle groups in Pilates mat exercise. In the only studies on the energy requirements of Pilates, Olson evaluated eight women and two men (mean age 34 yr) to determine the energy cost of a Pilates mat workout across three different levels: a beginner workout (B), an intermediate workout (I), and an advanced workout (A). Normalized to a body weight of 75 kg, the caloric expenditure ($kcal \cdot min^{-1}$) was 8.0 for A, 6.5 for I, and 4.6 for B. This study showed that A and I were moderate-intensity activities. The B workout met the cutoff for classification as a low-to-moderate intensity activity (i.e., 3.5 METs was the cutoff) (information from paper presented by M. Olson at 2005 ACSM Health and Fitness Summit, Las Vegas, Nevada). The growing number of research studies on Pilates in the coming years should help separate claims from actual validated outcomes. The interested reader should please refer to Anderson and Specter's detailed scientific introduction to Pilates-based exercise and sport injury rehabilitation (1).

Neuromuscular Integrative Action (NIA)

Neuromuscular integrative action (NIA) was created by Debbie and Carlos Rosas in 1983. NIA is a composite of Eastern and Western mind–body exercise and has grown in popularity in many health clubs and fitness centers throughout the United States. NIA combines dance movements and moderately intense martial arts moves infused with subtle mindful techniques designed to heighten body awareness and what NIA professionals call *sensory IQ*. NIA is generally performed in bare feet and, through music and movement, each NIA session is "uniquely crafted to both calm and invigorate" (18).

NIA classes blend concepts from a diversity of cultures including tai chi, yoga, martial arts, Feldenkrais, and ethnic and modern dance. The NIA technique is based on a process termed *the body's way* and incorporates 9 movement energies, 13 principles, and 52 basic moves. Unlike other mindful exercise programs, NIA also includes a moderate aerobic component to address cardiorespiratory endurance. The aerobic segment fosters creativity and spontaneity rather than requires strict adherence to standard movement patterns. Participants are taught to move with self-expression and to couple movement tempo with their emotion.

Alexander Technique

The Alexander technique, as established by Frederick Matthias Alexander in the late 19th century, teaches the transformation of neuromuscular habits by helping an individual focus on sensory experiences. It is a simple and practical method for improving ease and freedom of movement, balance, support, and coordination. It corrects unconscious habits of posture and movement, which may be precursors to injuries. This method is useful for individuals with disc trouble, sciatica, low-back pain, whiplash injury, shoulder and arm pain, neck pain, or arthritis and athletes who wish to move with more ease and greater coordination. Cacciatore (2) recently published a detailed case study on low-back pain articulating a specific Alexander protocol that decreased pain and improved functionality. The Alexander technique is taught one on one or in small groups by a certified Alexander teacher.

Typical First Session in Alexander Technique

During the first lesson your teacher will observe your posture and movement patterns, for example, as you move out of a chair to the standing position. The teacher will also supplement the visual information by using her hands, gently placing them on your neck, shoulders, back, and so on. The teacher uses her hands in order to get more refined information about your patterns of breathing and moving. The teacher will ask you to perform some simple movements—perhaps walking, standing up, or sitting down in a chair—while she keeps her hands in easy contact with your body. At the same time the teacher's hands gather information, they will also convey information to you, gently guiding your body to encourage a release of restrictive muscular tension. In early stages of Alexander training, pupils are usually urged to come for lessons fairly frequently, perhaps 2 or 3 times a week (11).

Fitness instructors are encouraged to become familiar with referring to an Alexander teacher when advising individuals on improving faulty biomechanical habits or exercise performance, especially competitive performance, through more efficient postures and movement patterns. There are several thousand Alexander teachers worldwide. Most are members of one or more professional societies and most of these societies publish both a written and an online list of teachers. The Web site www.alexandertechnique.com/teacher/ publishes a teacher list by country and state.

Feldenkrais Method

The Feldenkrais method was developed by the Russian Moshe Feldenkrais (1904–1984) and consists of two interrelated, somatically based educational methods. The first, awareness through movement (ATM), is a verbally directed technique designed for group work. The second, functional integration (FI), is a nonverbal manual contact technique designed for people desiring more individualized attention. ATM incorporates active movements, imagery, and other forms of directed attention. These are gentle, nonstrenuous exercises that reeducate the nervous system and emphasize learning how to learn from the individual's own kinesthetic feedback.

Feldenkrais applications include pain management, sport performance improvement, performing arts improvement, stress relief, and confidence building. Activities that require significant coordination are prime examples of where the Feldenkrais method can be helpful (e.g., competitive running, golf, skiing, kayaking, rowing, horseback riding, and Hatha yoga). Sessions are taught individually or in small groups with the practitioner gently touching or moving the student to facilitate awareness and vitality. Like the Alexander technique, Feldenkrais teachings emphasize thinking rather than doing. A typical session might begin with the teacher observing movements associated with a specific sport or activity. The Feldenkrais teacher would systematically place his hands on the student to see which muscles were working, which ones weren't working, and which ones were not disengaging. From this the teacher can evaluate movement patterns and habits interfering with other movements. The ATM or FI method (a sequence of gentle reeducation movements) is then introduced and supervised. The Feldenkrais Educational Foundation of North America (Portland, Oregon) publishes a list of Feldenkrais teachers and is an excellent resource of professional publications on the Feldenkrais method.

Key Point

Contemporary styles of mindful exercise have markedly grown in popularity (number of forms and classes offered) over the last decade. Benefits of these programs depend on the energy expenditure, physical work, breathing technique, and meditative processes involved. Pilates in particular has grown in popularity to become a significant means to improve posture and core strength. The results of several small published trials on Pilates are promising, but more controlled research is clearly needed to support its utility in fitness and rehabilitation. The fitness professional should become knowledgeable of the Alexander and Feldenkrais instructions, as these relatively simple techniques address important deficiencies in skeletal mechanics, breathing, and anatomical alignment.

Mindful Exercise Outcomes

Monitoring responses to mindful exercise training is not as straightforward as monitoring outcomes in conventional exercise training. For example, during and after a 10 wk aerobics class you could show a measurable trend and objectively demonstrate reduced body fat and resting heart rate and improved exercise capacity. Assessing the benefits of a 10 wk Hatha yoga or tai chi program may require, in addition to measures of muscular fitness, more cognitive or affective outcome measures, considering that much of the training response is psychological. A number of indicators, including cognitive measures, helpful in evaluating the outcomes of mindful exercise classes are listed on page 354.

Mindful exercise induces relaxation from within by relaxing the muscles, slowing breathing, and, most importantly, calming the mind. Published scientific evidence shows that hypertension, insulin resistance, anxiety disorders, pain, cardiovascular disease risk factors, and depression all favorably respond to regular participation in mindful exercise, particularly tai chi, qigong exercise, and Hatha yoga (see page 355). Many of the extolled benefits of mindful exercise still lack objective research support. Quality published research on mindful exercise outcomes is progressing slowly, as most research published so far uses small subject numbers, is statistically underpowered, or suffers from inadequate controls. For example, Kirkwood and others (5) recently reviewed the existing research for hatha yoga and anxiety and found only eight studies that were reasonably well designed. Together these studies showed an encouraging trend for Hatha yoga to reduce anxiety, although it was not possible to say that yoga was clearly effective in treating anxiety. Another research issue is adequately measuring the muscular strength gained. For example, if Hatha yoga or Pilates was the primary intervention, is it valid to measure strength gains with a 1RM on a weight machine? There are no yoga, Pilates, or tai chi ergometers that specifically

Indicators for Mindful Exercise Outcomes

- Quality of life measures (e.g., SF-8, SF-12 quality of life scale instruments; SF = short form)
- Measures of mobility and physical function
- Flexibility and muscular strength measures that closely replicate the training program
- Resting blood pressure
- Forced expiratory volume in 1 sec (i.e., FEV_1)

  A measure for mindful activities focusing on breath work (e.g., yogic breathing, Hatha yoga)
- Balance control measures (e.g., standing balance test, backward tandem walk, Tinetti Balance Scale)

  A measure for mindful activities requiring neuromuscular balance (e.g., tai chi, qigong exercise)
- Mood alteration measures (e.g., state anxiety measures, Profile of Mood States)
- Pain or symptom measures
- Spirituality measures (e.g., Spiritual Well-Being Index, INSPIRIT)

replicate the exercise interventions associated with these modalities. Still, it is reasonable to state that the core benefits of mindful exercise programs are increased balance, muscular strength, and flexibility as well as immediate relaxation and mental quiescence.

Much has been written about the mechanisms responsible for the affective responses and mood alterations observed with meditation and mindful exercise. This issue is somewhat complicated by the fact that muscular exercise is conjoined with meditative activity such that our bodies have combined neuroendocrine and cognitive mechanisms. The following are some putative mechanisms that play a role in mindful exercise programs that have significant physical, breath work, and cognitive components (6):

- Psychological changes—expectancy (Rosenthal effect) and special attention (Hawthorne effect)
- Cortical and hemispheric lateralization changes in the brain
- Deactivation of the hypothalamic pituitary adrenal axis resulting in reduced catecholamine production (see figure 23.4)
- Central endorphinergic changes, or acute endorphin changes in the brain that act on neurotransmission
- Respiration-induced affective changes (e.g., pulmonary parasympathetic stimulation) (see figure 23.2)

Energy Cost of Hatha Yoga

When recommending mindful exercise modalities to inexperienced clients it may be helpful to start with forms requiring lower energy expenditure, such as qigong or restorative yoga. Figure 23.3 shows three levels of energy expenditure requirements by MET level and associated mindful exercise modalities. This figure is not based on actual comparative energy expenditure studies but is an approximation based on overall movement dynamics and case studies. Individual fitness, style proficiency and familiarity, and body mass all play roles in the energy expenditure requirements of each exercise form.

Level I ≤ 3 METs
Most restorative yoga asanas, some viniyoga, yogic breathing, Tai Chi Chih, most Qigong exercises, beginner Pilates mat exercise

Level II 3-5 METs
Some viniyoga asana sequences, many Iyengar and Bikram yoga asana sequences, Tai Chi Chuan, intermediate Pilates mat exercise

Level III ≥ 6 METs
Ashtanga asana sequences, some Iyengar and Bikram yoga asana sequences, advanced Tai Chi Chuan, NIA, advanced Pilates mat exercise

Figure 23.3 Approximate energy costs of mindful exercise modalities.

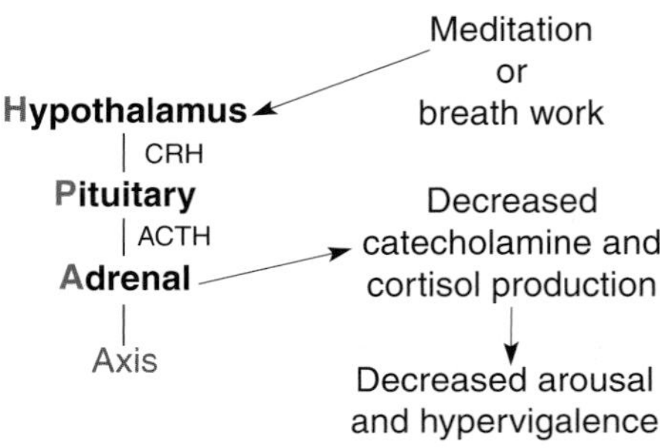

Figure 23.4 Hypothalamic, pituitary, and adrenal mechanisms involved in meditation and mindful exercise. CRH = corticotropin releasing hormone; ACTH = adrenal corticotropic hormone.

Research-Supported Benefits of Hatha Yoga and Tai Chi Exercise

Cardiorespiratory Benefits

- Lower resting systolic blood pressure
- Increased pulmonary function (e.g., FEV_1)
- Lower resting respirations
- Improved respiratory function in patients with asthma
- Increased parasympathetic tone
- Decreased resting blood lactate and resting oxygen consumption
- Enhanced arterial endothelial function
- Improved risk factor profile for cardiovascular disease (e.g., reduced blood lipids)
- Reduced cardiac ventricular arrhythmias

Musculoskeletal and Neuromuscular Benefits

- Increased muscular strength and flexibility
- Increased balance control
- Improved posture
- Decreased fracture risk and falls in older individuals
- Reduced low-back pain

Psychophysiological Benefits

- Increased cognitive performance
- Improved relaxation and psychological well-being
- Decreased stress hormones (e.g., norepinephrine, cortisol)
- Decreased state anxiety and depression scores
- Enhanced quality of life and decreased stress symptoms in breast and prostate cancer patients
- Reduced frequency of panic episodes
- Decreased symptoms associated with pain, angina, asthma, or chronic fatigue

Other Benefits

- Increased physical functioning in older persons
- Improved glucose tolerance
- Decreased HbA1c (glycated hemoglobin) and C-peptide levels in patients with type 2 diabetes
- Increased baroreflex sensitivity
- Decreased obsessive–compulsive disorder symptoms
- Decreased osteoarthritis symptoms
- Decreased carpal tunnel symptoms
- Adjunctive therapy for cancer and cardiovascular disease

From R. La Forge, 2003, Mind-body exercise for personal trainers. In *American Council on Exercise personal trainer manual*, 3rd ed. (San Diego, CA: American Council on Exercise).

Key Point

The benefits of mindful exercise can be measured by objective changes in quality of life, life stress, and stress-related symptoms. Depending on the type of mindful exercise, changes in muscular strength and flexibility may be difficult to quantify because many mindful exercise routines are largely nonstandardized and lack of objective musculoskeletal fitness assessment tools that quantify strength changes, e.g., evaluating strength gains with Hatha yoga poses. There is a clear need to develop and validate measures of muscular fitness outcomes for mindful exercise, particularly Pilates exercise. The mechanisms responsible for the affective changes observed with mindful exercise are complex and overlap with similar responses and mechanisms observed with aerobic exercise. One attribute of mindful exercise (e.g., qigong, tai chi, or restorative yoga) is that positive affective changes can occur at much lower energy expenditures with less risk of injury or cardiovascular complications.

- Musculoskeletal neural endocrine mechanisms, in which ascending neural pathways carry sensory information from the muscles and joints to a variety of thalamic and cortical structures of the brain that affect mood and cognition
- Thermic neuroendocrine affective changes induced by mindful exercise programs taught in high temperatures, as experienced with Bikram yoga

Mindful Exercise Training Resources

There are many training and certification programs for prospective tai chi, qigong, Pilates, NIA, and yoga teachers. Unlike some certification programs (e.g., of the American College of Sports Medicine and American Council on Exercise), most of the mindful instructor certification programs do not follow a standardized set of practice guidelines that cover a core curriculum such as exercise, preexercise assessment, program implementation, and exercise safety. This is not to imply that well-planned and professionally conducted Hatha yoga and tai chi teacher training programs do not exist. In the case of the classical forms (Hatha yoga and tai chi), standardizing practice guidelines will be difficult because some of these traditions steadfastly adhere to ethnic heritages and ancient teachings or sutras in an effort to maintain a purity and respect for the tradition. For yoga, one promising new professional body establishing teacher standards is the Yoga Alliance. This organization maintains a national registry of yoga teachers and schools that meet its recommended educational standards, and it strongly encourages the inclusion of core competencies. Select continuing education and training resources for mindful exercise include the following:

- Alexander Technique International. www.ati-net.com/contact.php. 888-668-8996.
- ChiRunning and ChiWalking instructor training. www.chirunning.com. 866-327-7867.
- Directory of qigong teachers and therapists (Qigong Institute, Menlo Park, California). www.qigonginstitute.org/listing/directory.php.
- Feldenkrais Educational Foundation of North America. www.feldenkrais.com. 503-221-6612.
- International Association of Yoga Therapists. www.iayt.org.
- Justin Stone's Tai Chi Chih. www.taichichih.org
- Kripalu Center for Yoga and Health. www.kripalu.org. 866-200-5203.
- National Qigong Association (United States). 888-815-1893.
- Pilates Method Alliance. www.pilatesmethodalliance.org/whatis.html.
- Qigong Institute. www.qigonginstitute.org. 415-323-1221.
- YogaFit International. www.yogafit.com. 888-786-3111.
- Yoga for the West Teacher Training Course by Mara Carrico. 760-942-4244.
- Yoga Alliance. 877-964-2255.

Case Studies

You can check your answers by referring to page 475 in appendix A.

1. A 38-yr-old apparently healthy woman who has been a personal training client of yours for 1 yr asks your opinion on starting a Hatha yoga program. She has improved her fitness level and lost weight but she still has metabolic syndrome (BMI 36, triglycerides 165 mg/dL, and borderline hypertension). What is your advice for her regarding a yoga program?
2. You are referred a competitive college-aged 10,000 m runner who wants to improve his running form, particularly during the sprint phase of a race (i.e., the last 200 m). Aside from specific resistance and running training, what mindful form of activity could you advise that may help his sprint technique?

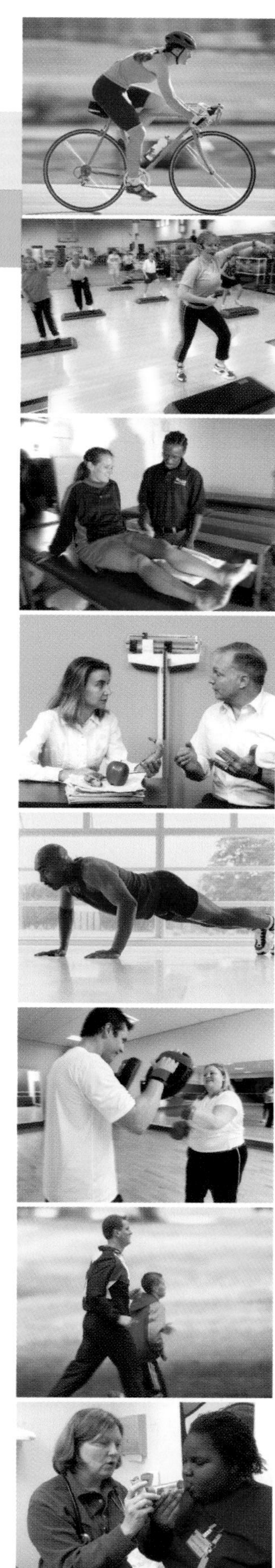

24 CHAPTER

Exercise Related to ECG and Medications

David R. Bassett Jr.

Objectives

The reader will be able to do the following:

1. Describe the basic anatomy of the heart.
2. Describe the basic electrophysiology of the heart.
3. Define the electrocardiogram (ECG) and identify the standard settings for paper speed and amplitude.
4. Identify the basic electrocardiographic complexes and calculate HR from ECG rhythm strips.
5. Describe the types of atrioventricular conduction defects and their probable effect on a subject's exercise response.
6. Identify the normal and abnormal cardiac rhythms and predict the probable effect of the abnormal rhythms on exercise performance.
7. Describe electrocardiographic signs and biochemical markers of a heart attack.
8. List the common categories of prescription medications used to treat cardiovascular diseases, some examples of each category, and the probable effect of these medications on exercise performance.

This chapter provides background information on the heart, electrocardiogram (ECG) analysis, and cardiovascular medications and how these factors affect exercise testing and prescription in the basically healthy population. This chapter is not intended to be a complete guide to ECG interpretation and cardiovascular medications; there are several excellent texts on these topics (4, 7, 9, 10).

Structure of the Heart

The heart is a muscular organ composed of four chambers: the right atrium, the right ventricle, the left atrium, and the left ventricle (see figure 24.1). The flow of blood through the heart is directed by pressure differences and valves between the chambers. Venous blood from the body enters the right atrium via the inferior and superior vena cava. From the right atrium, blood passes through the **tricuspid valve** into the right ventricle. The right ventricle pumps blood through the **pulmonary valve** into the pulmonary arteries leading to the lungs. In the lungs, blood gives up carbon dioxide and picks up oxygen. The oxygen-rich blood is returned to the heart via the pulmonary veins emptying into the left atrium. From the left atrium, blood passes through the **mitral valve** into the left ventricle. The left ventricle pumps oxygenated blood past the **aortic valve,** into the aorta and coronary arteries and to the rest of the body. The left ventricle, which generates more pressure than the right ventricle generates, is thicker.

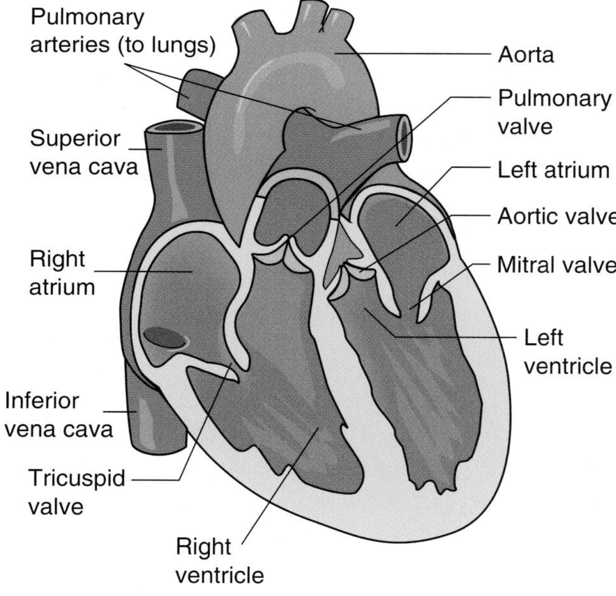

Figure 24.1 The chambers and valves of the heart.

Reprinted, by permission, from J.E. Donnelly, 1990, *Living anatomy,* 2nd ed. (Champaign, IL: Human Kinetics), 199.

Coronary Arteries

The heart muscle, or **myocardium,** does not receive a significant amount of oxygen directly from blood in the atria or ventricles. Oxygenated blood is supplied to the myocardium via the **coronary arteries,** which lie on the surface of the heart. There are two coronary artery systems (the right and left coronary arteries), which branch off the aorta at the coronary sinus. The left main coronary artery follows a course between the left atria and the pulmonary artery and branches off into the left anterior descending and left circumflex arteries (figure 24.2). The left anterior descending artery follows a path along the anterior surface of the heart and lies over the interventricular septum, which separates the right and left ventricles. The left circumflex artery follows the groove between the left atrium and left ventricle on the anterior and lateral surface of the heart. The right coronary artery follows the groove that separates the atria and ventricles around the posterior surface of the heart and forms the posterior descending artery. Numerous smaller arteries split off each of the major arteries, becoming smaller and smaller and finally forming the capillaries in the muscle cells of the heart, where gas exchange occurs. A major obstruction in any of these coronary arteries reduces blood flow to the myocardium **(myocardial ischemia)** and decreases the ability of the heart to pump blood. If the coronary arteries become blocked and the heart muscle does not receive oxygen, then a portion of the heart muscle might die, which is known as a **myocardial infarction (MI),** or heart attack.

Coronary Veins

Venous drainage of the right ventricle occurs via the anterior cardiac vein, which normally has two or three major branches and eventually empties into the right atrium. The venous drainage of the left ventricle occurs primarily through the anterior interventricular vein, which roughly follows the same path as the left anterior descending artery, eventually forming the coronary sinus and emptying into the right atrium.

Oxygen Use by the Heart

The myocardium is well adapted to use oxygen to generate adenosine triphosphate (ATP). Approximately 40% of the volume of a myocardial muscle cell is composed of mitochondria, the cellular organelle responsible for producing ATP with oxygen. The oxygen consumption of the heart in a resting person is about 8 to 10 ml · min^{-1} per 100 g of myocardium; in comparison, the total resting oxygen consumption for the body is about 0.35 ml · min^{-1} per 100 g of body mass (5). Myocardial oxygen consumption can increase six- to sevenfold during heavy

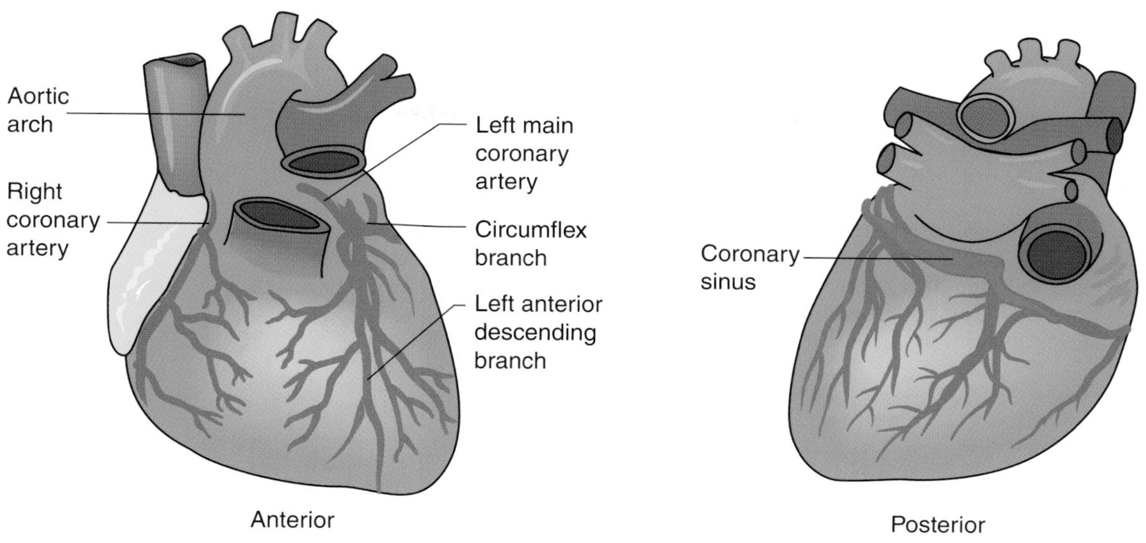

Figure 24.2 Coronary blood vessels.
Reprinted, by permission, from J.E. Donnelly, 1990, *Living anatomy*, 2nd ed. (Champaign, IL: Human Kinetics), 202.

exercise in adults, whereas in young people the total body oxygen consumption can easily increase 12 to 15 times. Heart muscle has a limited capacity to produce energy via anaerobic pathways and depends on the delivery of oxygen to the mitochondria to produce ATP. At rest, the whole body extracts only about 25% of the oxygen present in each 100 ml of arterial blood, and the body can meet an increased need for oxygen by simply extracting more from the blood. In contrast, the heart extracts about 75% of the oxygen available in the arterial blood. Consequently, an increase in the oxygen needs of the heart must be met by delivering more blood via the coronary arteries. An adequate oxygen supply to the heart is needed not only to allow the heart to pump blood but also to maintain normal electrical activity, which is covered in the next section.

Electrophysiology of the Heart

At rest, the insides of the myocardial cells are negatively charged and the exteriors of the cells are positively charged. When the cells are depolarized (stimulated), the insides of the cells become positively charged and the exteriors become negatively charged. If a recording electrode is placed on the chest so that the wave of depolarization spreads toward the electrode, the electrocardiogram (ECG) records a positive (upward) deflection. If the wave of depolarization spreads away from the recording electrode, a negative (downward) deflection occurs. When the myocardial muscle cell is completely polarized or depolarized, the ECG does not record any electrical potential but shows a flat baseline, known as the *isoelectric line*. After depolarization, the myocardial cell undergoes repolarization to return to its resting electrical state. The steps leading from rest (complete polarization) to complete stimulation (complete depolarization) back to rest (repolarization) are shown in figure 24.3.

Key Point

The heart is a muscular organ composed of four chambers: the right atrium, the right ventricle, the left atrium, and the left ventricle. The coronary arteries supply the heart muscle (myocardium) with blood, and the heart meets increasing oxygen demands by increasing blood flow.

Conduction System of the Heart

The **sinoatrial (SA) node** is the normal pacemaker of the heart and is located in the right atrium near the superior vena cava (figure 24.4). Depolarization spreads from the SA node across the atria and results in the P wave (see Basic Electrocardiographic Complexes on page 362). There are three tracts within the atria that conduct depolarization to the **atrioventricular (AV) node.** Impulses travel from the SA node through the atrial muscle and conduction tracts and enter the AV node, where conduction slows to allow the atrial contraction to empty blood into the ventricles before the start of ventricular contraction. The **bundle of His** is the conduction pathway

1 Completely polarized

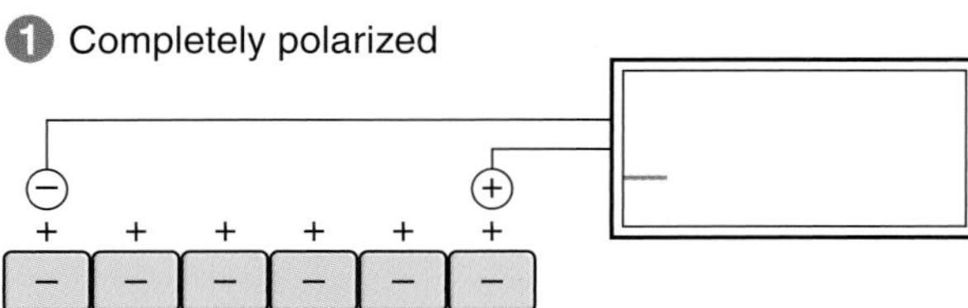

The myocardial cells shown on the left are at rest and are completely polarized. Because both of the recording electrodes are surrounded by positive charges, there is no voltage difference between them and the electrocardiogram shown on the right records the isoelectric line (0 mV).

2 Partially depolarized

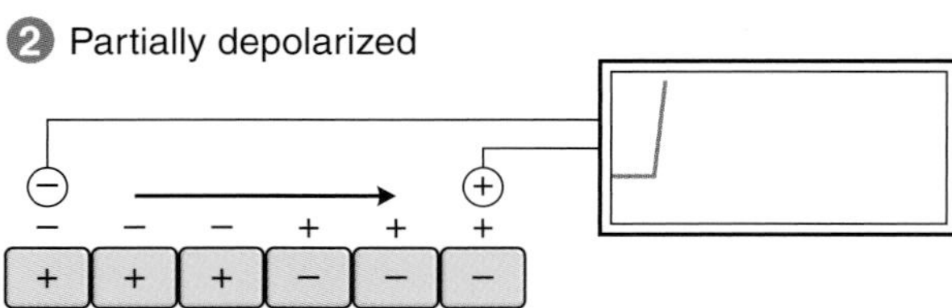

The process of depolarization (positive charges inside the cell and negative charges outside) is spreading from left to right. Because the electrode on the right is surrounded by positive charges, the ECG records a positive deflection. The amplitude of the deflection is proportional to the mass of the myocardium undergoing depolarization.

3 Completely depolarized

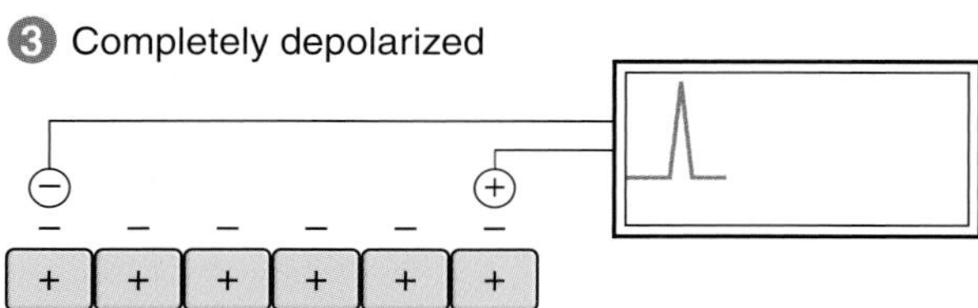

Depolarization is now complete, and both electrodes are surrounded by negative charges. Because there is no voltage difference between electrodes, the ECG is now recording 0 mV, or the isoelectric potential.

4 Partially repolarized

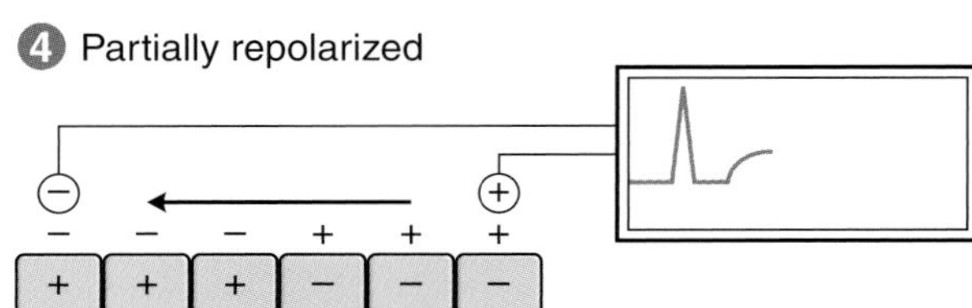

Repolarization has started from the right and is moving to the left. The ECG shows a positive (upward) deflection, because the right-hand electrode is surrounded by positive charges. Note that repolarization occurs in the opposite direction from depolarization in the human heart, and this is the reason the depolarization and repolarization complexes are both normally positive. If repolarization had started on the left and moved to the right, the ECG deflection would have been negative.

5 Completely repolarized

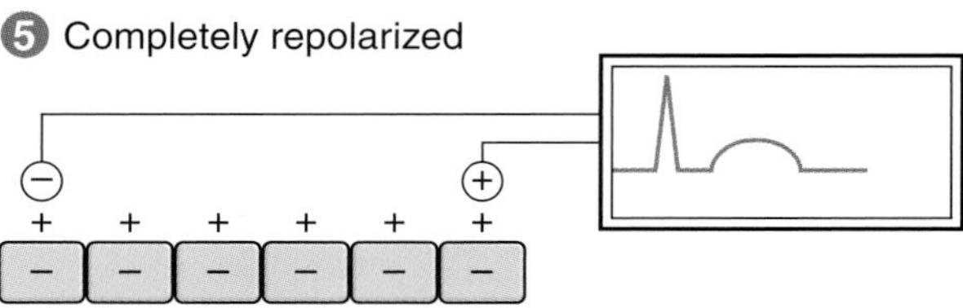

The muscle cells are now completely repolarized, or in the resting state, and the ECG records the isoelectric line. The myocardial cells are now ready to be depolarized again.

Figure 24.3 Steps in an electrocardiographic cycle.

that connects the AV node with **bundle branches** in the ventricles. The right bundle branch splits off the bundle of His and forms ever-smaller branches that serve the right ventricle. The left bundle splits into two major branches that serve the thicker left ventricle. **Purkinje fibers** are the terminal branches of the bundle branches and form the link between the specialized conductive tissue and the muscle fibers. Small electrical junctions between adjacent cardiac muscle cells, known as **intercalated disks,** allow the electrical impulses to pass from cell to cell. The intercalated discs allow for simultaneous contraction of the ventricular muscle fibers, which is needed for effective pumping of the heart.

Key Point

The electrical impulse originates in the SA node, located in the right atrium. From there the electrical impulse spreads to the AV node, the bundle of His, the left and right bundle branches, and the Purkinje fibers. Waves of depolarization then spread from cell to cell throughout the ventricular muscle. Any restriction in blood flow to the myocardium could upset the electrical activity of the heart or damage the myocardium itself.

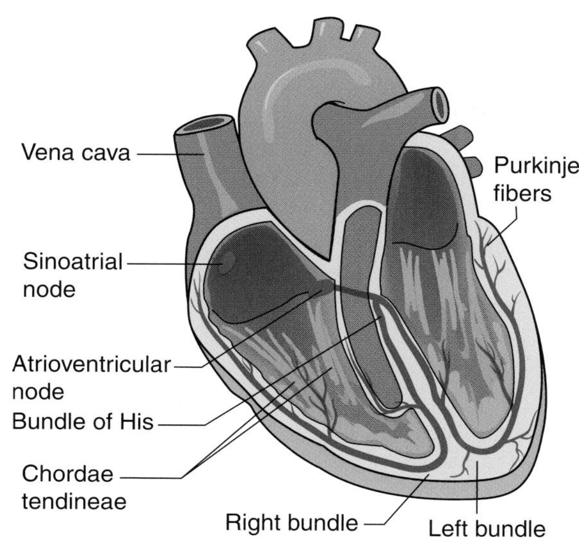

Figure 24.4 Electrical conduction system of the heart. These are the normal pathways used to ensure the rhythmic contraction and relaxation of the chambers of the heart.

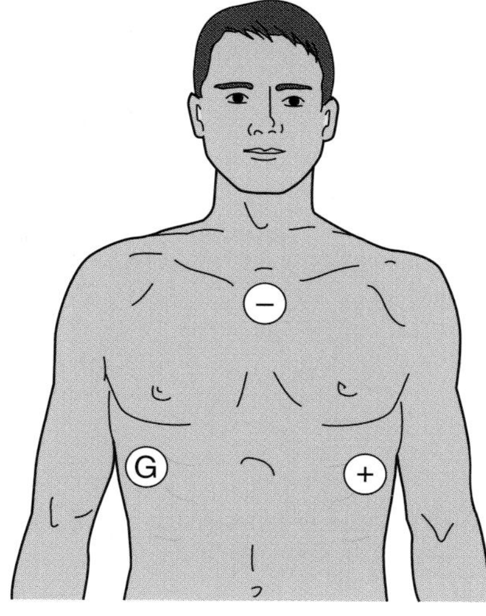

Figure 24.5 Lead placement for CM5: (–) negative electrode, (+) electrode, and (G) ground.
Adapted from M. Ellestad, 1994, *Stress testing: Principles and practice* (Philadelphia, PA: Davis).

Interpreting the ECG

This section on analyzing the electrocardiogram (ECG) may appear to go beyond what a fitness professional needs to know about the topic. The physician is the person to judge whether an ECG response is normal; however, the fitness professional must be aware of the basic ECG interpretation to communicate with the physician, program director, and clinical exercise specialist.

Systematically evaluating the ECG allows the examiner to determine the HR, rhythm, and conduction pathways and to search for signs of ischemia or infarction. Physicians normally evaluate a 12-lead ECG, but for our purposes a single ECG lead is adequate. A commonly used single ECG lead for exercise testing is the CM5 (see figure 24.5), which looks similar to lead V5 on a 12-lead ECG.

Defining the ECG

The **electrocardiogram (ECG)** is a graphic recording of the heart's electrical activity. As waves of depolarization travel through the heart, electrical currents spread to the tissues surrounding the heart and then travel throughout the body. If recording electrodes are placed on the skin, small voltage differences between various regions of the body can be detected. Thus, the electrocardiograph is a sensitive voltmeter that records the electrical activity of the heart.

Time and Voltage

ECG paper is standardly marked to allow measurement of time intervals and voltages. Time is measured on the horizontal axis, and the paper normally moves at 25 mm · sec^{-1}. Most ECG machines can run at 50 or 25 mm · sec^{-1}, so one must know the paper speed when measuring the duration of ECG complexes (see Basic Electrocardiographic Complexes on page 366). ECG paper is marked with a repeating grid (see figure 24.6). Major grid lines are 5 mm apart, and at a paper speed of 25 mm · sec^{-1}, 5 mm correspond to 0.20 sec. Minor lines are 1 mm apart, and at a paper speed of 25 mm · sec^{-1}, 1 mm equals 0.04 sec.

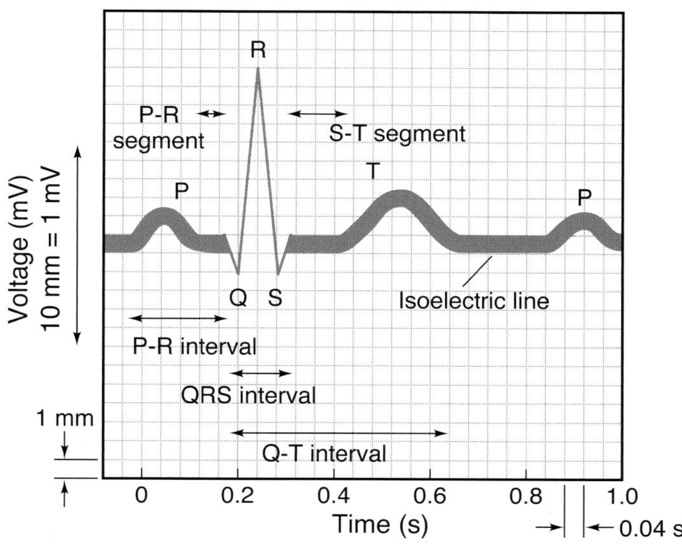

Figure 24.6 ECG complex with time and voltage scales.
Adapted, from M.J. Goldman, 1982, *Principles of clinical electrocardiography*, 11th ed. (Los Altos, CA: Appleton & Lange), with permission of the McGraw-Hill Companies.

Key Point

The pattern of electrical activity across the heart is called the *electrocardiogram (ECG).* The ECG is recorded with an electrocardiograph, and it provides information about the rhythm of the heart. The ECG paper speed is normally 25 mm · sec^{-1}, and at this speed each 1 mm mark represents 0.04 sec. The standard calibration factor is normally 0.1 mV per millimeter of deflection.

Voltage is measured on the vertical axis, and the standard calibration factor is normally 0.1 mV per millimeter of deflection. Most ECG machines can be adjusted to reduce this factor by 50% or to double it. You must know the voltage calibration before evaluating an ECG. All ECG measurements in this chapter refer to a paper speed of 25 mm · sec^{-1} and a voltage calibration of 0.1 mV · mm^{-1}.

Basic Electrocardiographic Complexes

The **P wave** is the graphic representation of atrial depolarization. The normal P wave lasts less than 0.12 sec and has an amplitude of 0.25 mV or less. The T_a wave is the result of atrial repolarization. It is not normally seen, because it occurs during ventricular depolarization and the larger electrical forces generated by the ventricles hide the T_a wave. The **Q wave** is the first downward deflection after the P wave; the Q wave signals the start of ventricular depolarization. The **R wave** is a positive deflection following the Q wave; it results from ventricular depolarization. If there is more than one R wave in a single complex, the second occurrence is called *R'*. The **S wave** is a negative deflection preceded by Q or R waves, and it is also the result of ventricular depolarization. The **T wave** follows these waves, which are collectively called the **QRS complex,** and it results from ventricular repolarization.

Electrocardiograph Intervals

The **R-R interval** is the time between successive R waves. When the heart rhythm is regular, the duration of an R-R interval can be used to determine the heart rate (beats · min^{-1}). If the heart rhythm is irregular, the R-R interval varies and you must determine HR from the number of R waves in a 6 sec time interval (see figure 24.7).

The P-P interval is the time between two successive atrial depolarizations. The **P-R interval** is measured from the start of the P wave to the beginning of the QRS complex. The interval is called *P-R* even if the first deflection after the P wave is a Q wave. Thus, the P-R interval includes the time periods corresponding to atrial depolarization and the delay in the electrical impulse at the AV node. The upper limit for the normal P-R interval is 0.20 sec, or 5 small blocks on the grid of the ECG paper.

The width of the QRS complex depends on the time for depolarization of the ventricles. A normal QRS complex lasts less than 0.10 sec, or 2.5 small blocks on the ECG paper. The **Q-T interval** is measured from the start of the QRS complex to the end of the T wave and corresponds to the duration of ventricular systole.

Segments and Junctions

The **P-R segment** is measured from the end of the P wave to the beginning of the QRS complex. This segment forms the isoelectric line, or baseline, from which S-T segment deviations are measured. The RS-T segment, or **J point,** is the point at which the S wave ends and the S-T segment begins. The **S-T segment** is formed by the isoelectric line between the QRS complex and the T wave. During an exercise test this segment is examined closely for depression or elevation, which may indicate the development of myocardial ischemia or perhaps MI. S-T segment deviation usually is measured 60 or 80 ms after the J point.

Key Point

The P wave signifies atrial depolarization, the QRS complex signifies ventricular depolarization, and the T wave signifies ventricular repolarization. If the rhythm is regular, HR can be determined by dividing 1,500 by the number of millimeters between successive R waves. HR also can be determined by starting with an R wave that falls on a thick black line and counting off the next six black lines as 300, 150, 100, 75, 60, and 50 and determining at which corresponding number the next R wave occurs. If the rhythm is irregular, HR can be determined by counting the number of R-R intervals in a 6 sec ECG strip and multiplying by 10.

Heart Rhythms

The ECG provides vital information about heart rhythms. Abnormalities in the electrical activity of the heart can be diagnosed from the ECG.

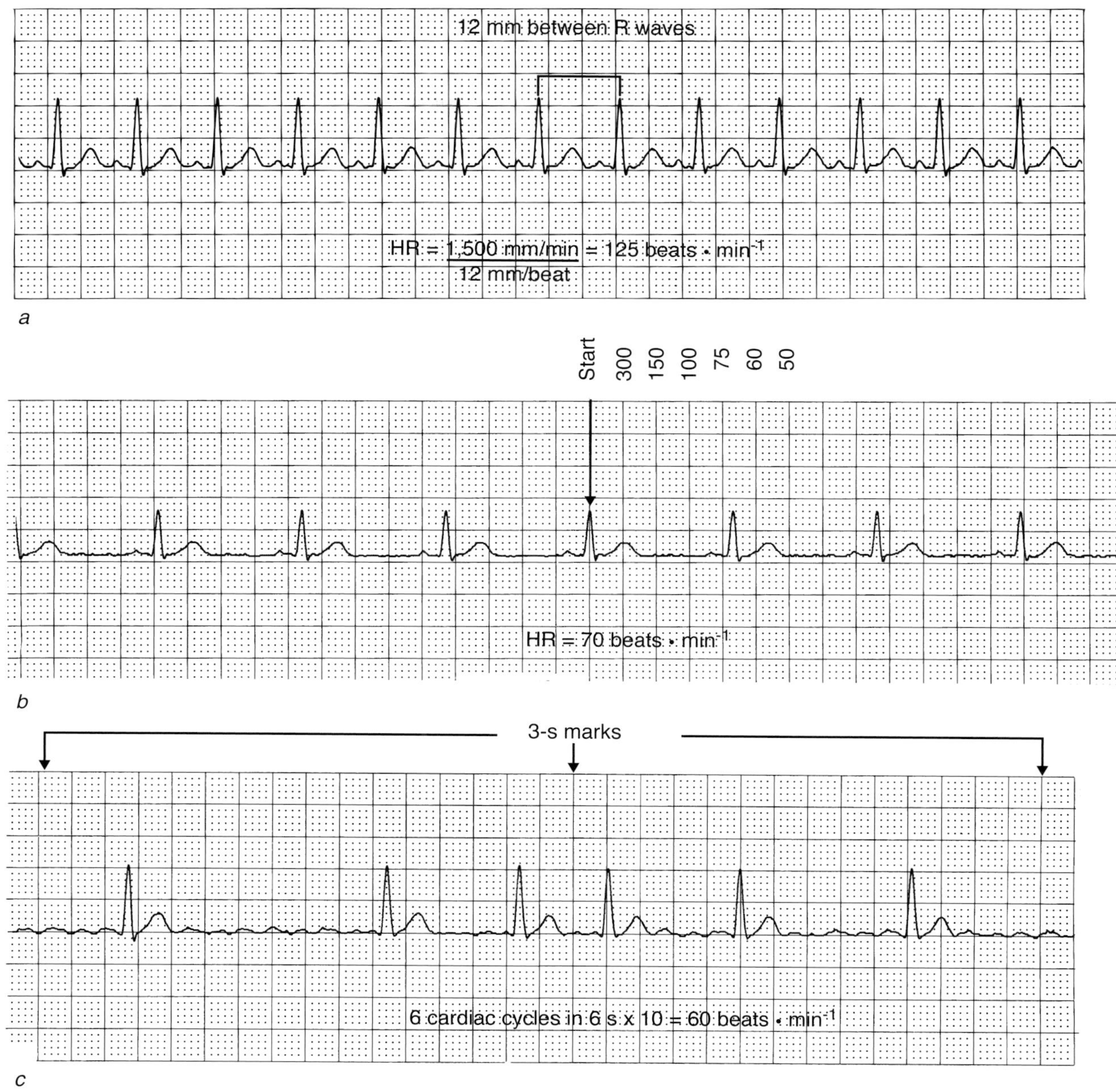

Figure 24.7 Three methods of determining heart rate from the electrocardiogram. *(a)* An approximate HR (beats · min^{-1}) can be determined by dividing 1,500 (60 sec at 25 mm · sec^{-1}) by the number of millimeters between adjacent R waves. *(b)* A second method is to begin with an R wave that falls on a thick black line. As you move to the right, count off the next six black lines as 300, 150, 100, 75, 60, and 50 (memorize these numbers). If the next R wave falls on one of these lines, the corresponding number indicates the HR. If the next R wave falls in between two thick black lines, you can estimate the HR by interpolation. *(c)* A third method is commonly used when the HR is irregular. With this method, you count the number of complete R-R intervals in a 6 sec ECG strip and multiply by 10.

Sinus Rhythm

Sinus rhythm is the normal rhythm of the heart (see figure 24.8). The HR is 60 to 100 beats · min^{-1} and the pacemaker is the sinus node.

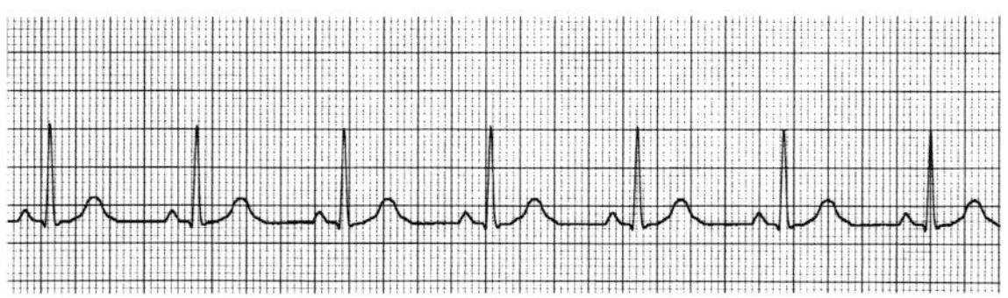

Figure 24.8 Normal sinus rhythm. In this example, the heart rate is 71 beats · min^{-1}.

Sinus Bradycardia

The heart rate in **sinus bradycardia** is less than 60 beats · min^{-1} (see figure 24.9). This is a normal rhythm, and it is often seen in conditioned subjects and patients taking beta-blockers.

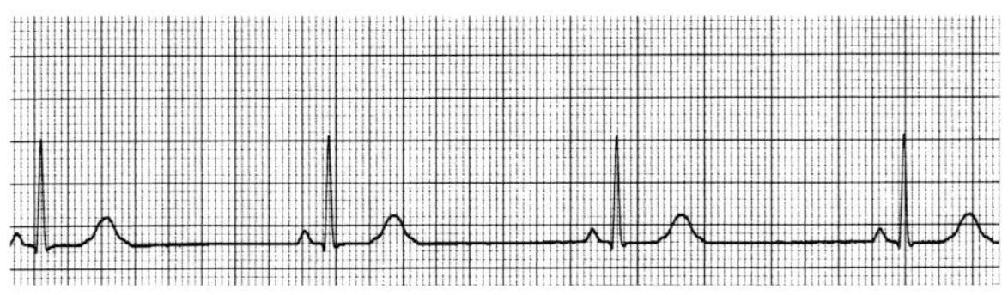

Figure 24.9 Sinus bradycardia. In this example, the heart rate is 35 beats · min^{-1}.

Sinus Tachycardia

Sinus tachycardia (HR >100 beats · min^{-1}) is normally seen during moderate and heavy exercise (see figure 24.10). Thus, exercise-induced sinus tachycardia is perfectly normal. Resting sinus tachycardia may be seen in deconditioned people or in patients who are apprehensive before exercise testing. In these heart rhythms, the SA node still functions as the pacemaker.

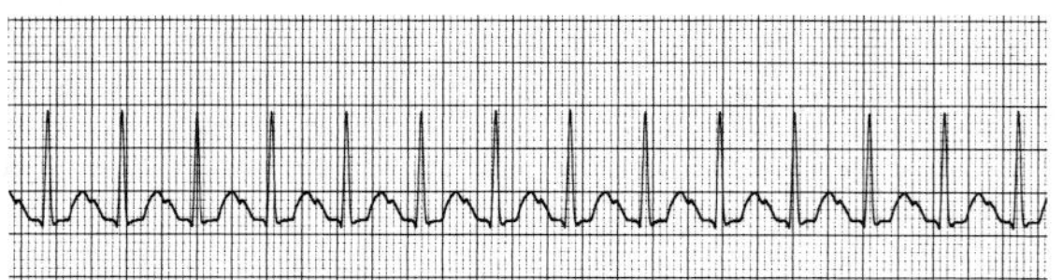

Figure 24.10 Sinus tachycardia. In this example, the heart rate is 143 beats · min^{-1}.

Key Point

If the SA node is pacing the heart and the HR is between 60 and 100 beats · min^{-1}, the heart is in normal sinus rhythm. Bradycardia is defined as an HR less than 60 beats · min^{-1}. Tachycardia is an HR greater than 100 beats · min^{-1} (normally seen during moderate and heavy exercise).

Atrioventricular Conduction Disturbances

Atrioventricular conduction disturbances refer to a blockage of the electrical impulse at the AV node. The blockage may be either partial or complete.

First-Degree AV Block

When the P-R interval exceeds 0.20 sec and all P waves result in ventricular depolarization, a **first-degree AV block** exists (see figure 24.11). Causes of a first-degree AV block include medications such as digitalis and quinidine, infections, and vagal stimulation.

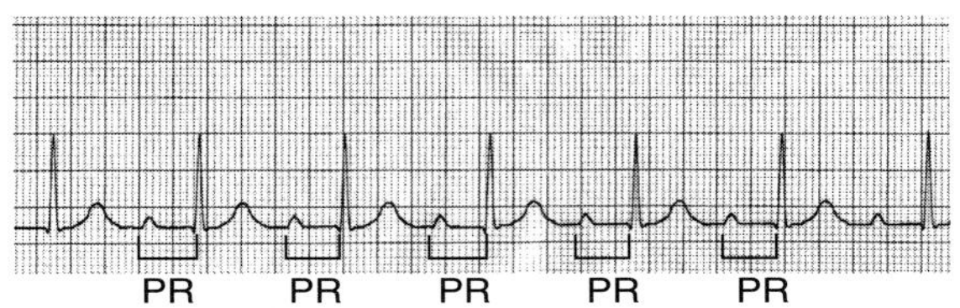

Figure 24.11 First-degree atrioventricular block. PR marks the prolonged P-R interval (0.28 sec in this example).

Second-Degree AV Block

The distinguishing feature of **second-degree AV block** is that some but not all P waves result in ventricular depolarization. There are two types of second-degree AV blocks: Mobitz type I and Mobitz type II. **Mobitz type I AV block,** or Wenckebach AV block, is characterized by a P-R interval that progressively lengthens until an atrial depolarization fails to initiate a ventricular depolarization and the QRS complex is skipped (see figure 24.12). This conduction disturbance is seen most commonly after an MI. The site of the block is within the AV node and is probably the result of reversible ischemia.

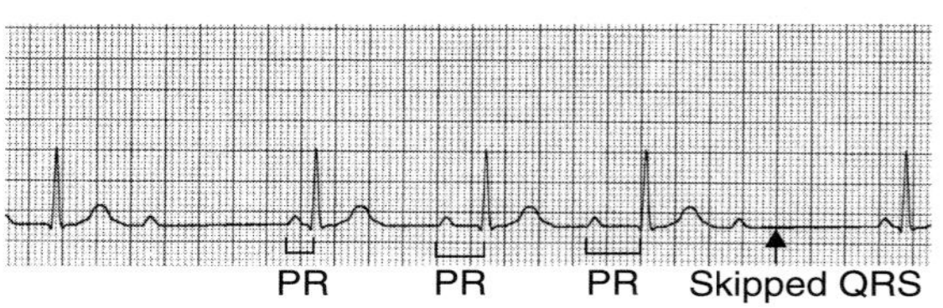

Figure 24.12 Mobitz type I (Wenckebach) AV block. The P-R interval (PR) gradually lengthens until finally a QRS complex is skipped.

Mobitz type II AV block is the more serious of the second-degree AV blocks, and it is characterized by atrial depolarization occasionally not resulting in ventricular depolarization, even though P-R intervals remain constant (i.e., do not lengthen; see figure 24.13). The site of the block is beyond the bundle of His, and it is usually the result of irreversible ischemia of the interventricular conduction system.

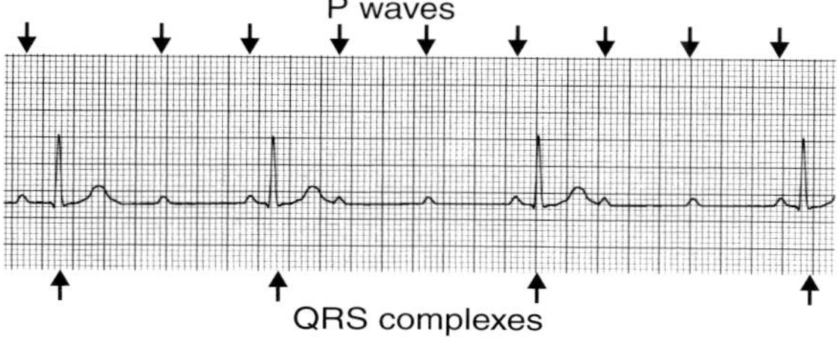

Figure 24.13 Mobitz type II AV block. Occasionally, and without lengthening of the P-R interval, QRS complexes are skipped.

Third-Degree AV Block

Third-degree AV block is present when the ventricles contract independently of the atria (see figure 24.14). The P-R interval varies and follows no regular pattern. The ventricular pacemaker may be the AV node, the bundle of His, Purkinje fibers, or the ventricular muscle, and it will almost always result in a slow ventricular rate of fewer than 50 beats · min^{-1}.

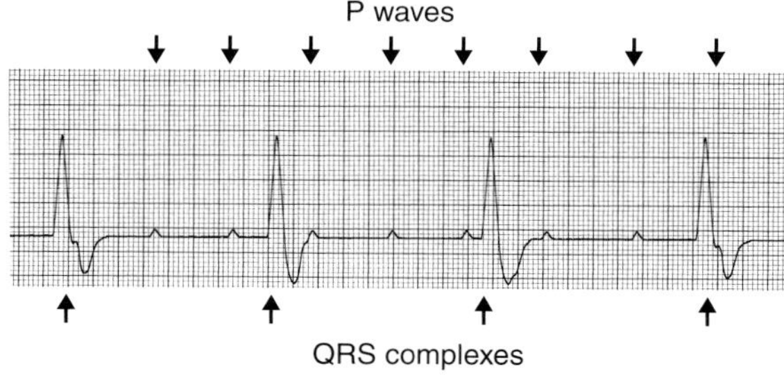

Figure 24.14 Third-degree AV block. There is no relationship between the atrial rate (e.g., 94 beats · min^{-1}) and the ventricular rate (e.g., 36 beats · min^{-1}), indicating complete blockage of the AV node.

Arrhythmias

An arrhythmia is an irregular heartbeat. Arrhythmias often arise when the myocardium becomes hyperexcitable because of a lack of blood flow or the use of stimulants.

Sinus Arrhythmia

Sinus arrhythmia is a sinus rhythm in which the R-R interval varies by more than 10% from beat to beat. In sinus arrythmia, a P wave precedes each QRS complex, but the QRS complexes are unevenly spaced. Sinus arrhythmia is seen often in highly trained subjects and occasionally in patients taking beta-adrenergic blocking medications. The rhythm may be associated with respiration because HR increases with inspiration and decreases with expiration.

Premature Atrial Contraction

In **premature atrial contractions,** the rhythm is irregular and the R-R interval is short between a normal sinus beat and the premature beat (see figure 24.15). The premature beat originates somewhere other than the sinus node and is known as an **ectopic focus** (an irritable spot on the myocardium that depolarizes on its own). An ectopic focus often is caused by stimulants (e.g., caffeine), antihistamines, diet pills, cold medications (e.g., ephedrine), and nicotine. Premature atrial contractions may be seen before exercise testing in apprehensive subjects.

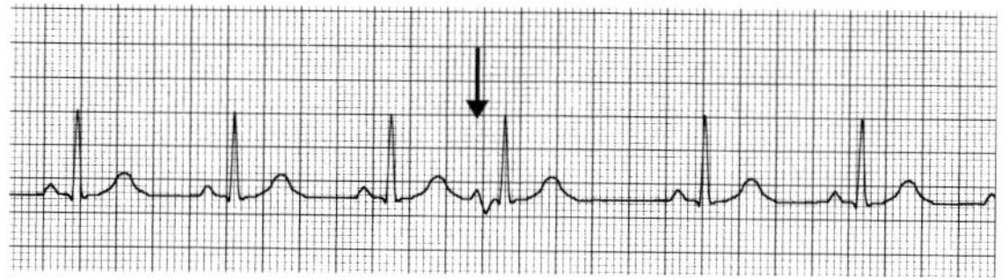

Figure 24.15 Premature atrial contraction. The arrow indicates a premature, diphasic P wave coming from an ectopic focus in the atria.

Atrial Flutter

During **atrial flutter,** the atrial rate is from 200 to 350 beats · min^{-1}, whereas the ventricular response is 60 to 160 beats · min^{-1}. The atrial rhythm is usually irregular, whereas the ventricular rhythm is either regular or irregular. The pacemaker site during atrial flutter is not the SA node but an ectopic focus, and so normal P waves are not present. F waves, resembling a sawtooth pattern, may be seen (see figure 24.16). The causes of atrial flutter include increased sympathetic drive, hypoxia, and congestive heart failure.

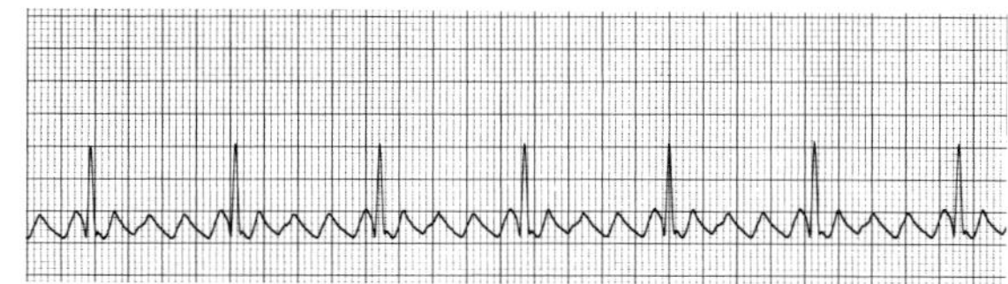

Figure 24.16 Atrial flutter. In atrial flutter, the atrial rate is 200 to 350 beats · min^{-1} (300 beats · min^{-1} in this example), but the ventricular rate is much slower.

Atrial Fibrillation

During **atrial fibrillation,** the atrial rate is 400 to 700 beats · min^{-1}, while the ventricular rate is usually 60 to 160 beats · min^{-1} and irregular. Multiple pacemaker sites are present in the atria, and P waves cannot be discerned (see figure 24.17). The significance of atrial fibrillation in exercise testing and training lies in its effect on ventricular function. During atrial fibrillation, the atria and ventricles are not coordinated, and the ability of the left ventricle to maintain an adequate cardiac output may be impaired. The causes of atrial fibrillation are essentially the same as those for atrial flutter.

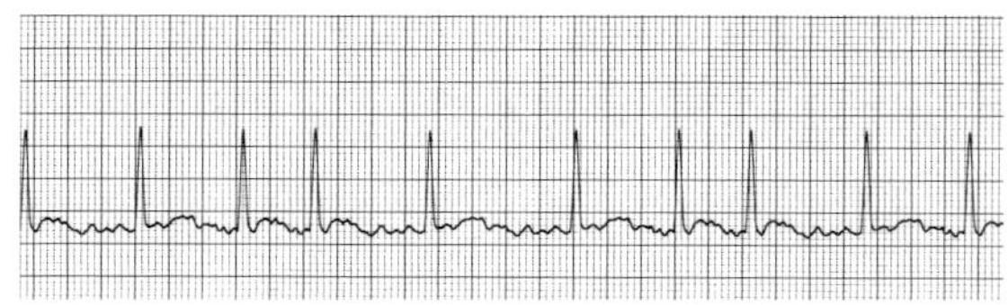

Figure 24.17 Atrial fibrillation. A jagged baseline and irregularly spaced QRS complexes are seen.

Premature Junctional Contraction

A **premature junctional contraction (PJC)** results when an ectopic pacemaker in the AV junctional area depolarizes the ventricles. Inverted P waves frequently accompany PJCs as the atrial depolarization proceeds in an abnormal direction (see figure 24.18). This characteristic of PJCs may distinguish them from premature atrial contractions, which frequently have diphasic P waves. If these two conditions cannot be distinguished, the more general term *premature supraventricular contraction* may be used to indicate an ectopic focus above the ventricles.

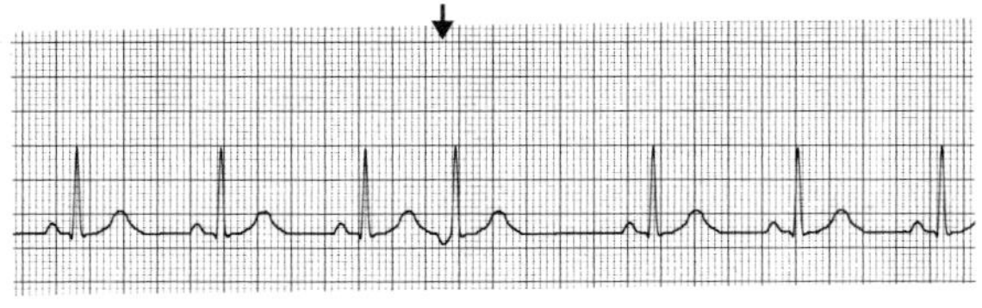

Figure 24.18 Premature junctional contraction. The arrow indicates a premature, inverted P wave coming from the AV node.

If the nodal tissue remains in the refractory phase after a PJC, then normally conducted waves of depolarization initiated from the sinus node will not pass into the ventricles and a compensatory pause will develop. PJCs usually result in a QRS complex of normal duration, or they may slightly prolong the QRS complex. PJCs may be caused by catecholamine-type medications, increased parasympathetic tone on the AV node, or damage to the AV node. PJCs are of little consequence, unless they occur very frequently (more than 4 to 6 PJCs · min^{-1}) or compromise ventricular function (9).

Although supraventricular arrhythmias may concern fitness professionals and patients, Ellestad (10) found that exercise-induced supraventricular arrhythmias do not seem to compromise the long-term prognosis of patients with CAD. The significance of the supraventricular arrhythmias lies in the uncoupling of the atria and ventricles and in the resulting effect on the ability of the ventricles to maintain an adequate cardiac output. Recurrent atrial fibrillation may have little effect on the exercise response of a person with good left ventricular function, but it may cause significant symptoms in a person with poor ventricular function.

Premature Ventricular Contractions

Premature ventricular contractions (PVCs) result from an ectopic focus in the His-Purkinje system, which initiates a ventricular contraction. PVCs have a QRS complex that is wide (>0.12 sec) and irregularly shaped (see figure 24.19). PVCs often result in the ventricles being in the refractory phase of depolarization when the normal sinus depolarization wave reaches the ventricle, and a compensatory pause develops. PVCs are among the most common arrhythmias seen with exercise testing and training in patients with CAD. If PVCs have the same shape, they originate from the same site (ectopic focus) and are called *unifocal.* Multiple-shape PVCs that originate from multiple sites in the ventricles are called *multifocal* and are much more serious than unifocal PVCs. The rhythm of normal contractions alternating with PVCs is called *bigeminy;* if every third contraction is a PVC, the rhythm is called *trigeminy.* Three or more consecutive PVCs are known as **ventricular tachycardia.** If a single PVC falls on the descending portion of the T wave, the ventricles may be thrown into fibrillation. Premature ventricular contractions adversely affect the prognosis of patients with CAD; generally, the more complex the PVC, the more serious the problem. Ellestad (10) showed that the combination of S-T segment depression and PVCs increases the incidence of future cardiac events.

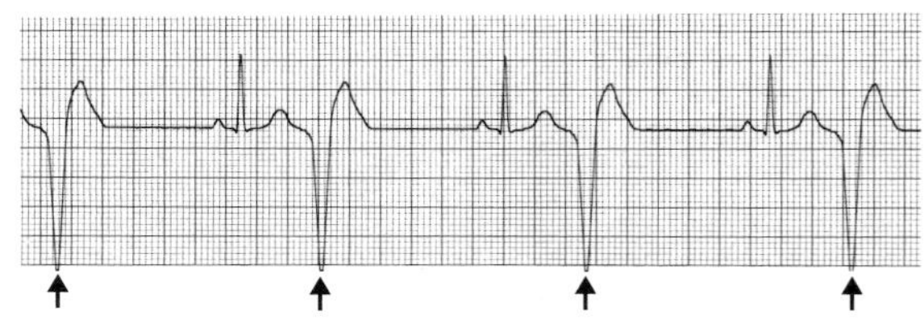

Figure 24.19 Premature ventricular contractions. The arrows indicate premature ventricular contractions coming from a single ectopic focus in the ventricles (unifocal PVCs).

If a PVC occurs during pulse counting, patients may report that the heart "skipped a beat" and may undercount their HR. They should be instructed to not increase the exercise intensity in an attempt to keep the HR in the target zone as a result of skipped beats. They should immediately reduce the exercise intensity and should report the appearance or increase of skipped beats to the fitness professional and physician.

Ventricular Tachycardia

Ventricular tachycardia is present whenever three or more consecutive PVCs occur (see figure 24.20). This situation is an extremely dangerous arrhythmia that may lead to ventricular fibrillation. The heart rate is usually 100 to 220 beats · min^{-1}, and the heart may be unable to maintain adequate cardiac output during ventricular tachycardia. Ventricular tachycardia may be caused by the same factors that initiate PVCs; it requires immediate medical attention.

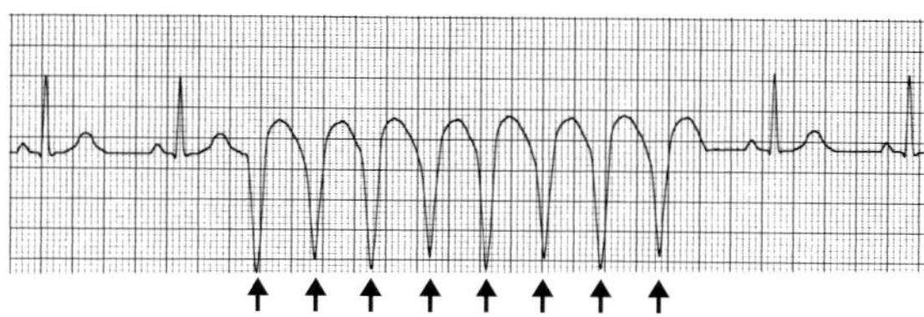

Figure 24.20 Ventricular tachycardia. A succession of three or more PVCs in a row is seen.

Ventricular Fibrillation

Ventricular fibrillation is a life-threatening rhythm, and it requires immediate cardiopulmonary resuscitation until a defibrillator can be used to restore a coordinated ventricular contraction; otherwise, death will result. A fibrillating heart contracts in an unorganized, quivering manner, and the heart is unable to maintain significant cardiac output. P waves and QRS complexes are not discernible; instead the electrical pattern is a fibrillatory wave (see figure 24.21).

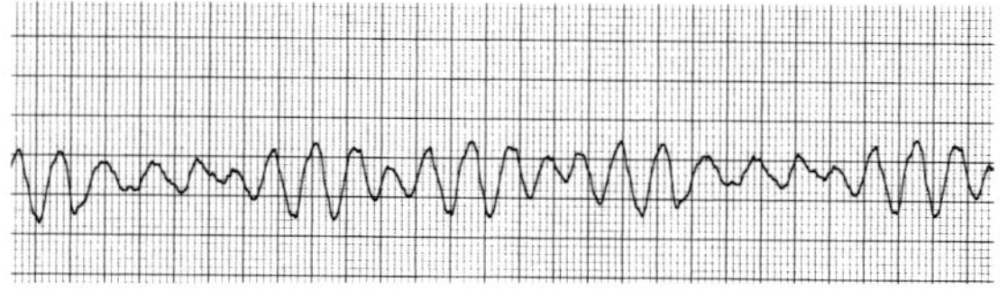

Figure 24.21 Ventricular fibrillation. When there are no discernible P waves or QRS complexes, the heart contracts in a disorganized, quivering manner.

> **Key Point**
>
> The ECG can be used to detect disturbances in the electrical conducting system of the heart, such as first-, second-, or third-degree AV block. The ECG can also indicate arrhythmias (abnormal heart rhythms), including sinus arrhythmia, premature beats, tachycardia, flutter, and fibrillation. Abnormal rhythms may limit exercise performance by decreasing cardiac output. In the case of severe arrhythmias, the fitness professional should terminate the exercise session and obtain immediate medical assistance.

Automated External Defibrillators

Defibrillators are devices used to treat ventricular fibrillation. They send a momentary electrical shock to the heart, often causing the heart to return to its normal rhythm. Recent technology has permitted the development of portable, battery-powered devices called automated external defibrillators (AEDs). The operator applies two surface electrodes to the person's chest. These electrodes are connected to the AED, which has computer software that is capable of determining the person's heart rhythm. If ventricular fibrillation is detected, the AED gives a command to stand clear and then signals the operator to deliver a shock by pushing a button. Police, fitness professionals, flight attendants, and even laypersons are receiving AED training by organizations such as the AHA and the American Red Cross. Research studies have shown that using AEDs hastens response time and greatly improves chances of survival (3).

Myocardial Ischemia

Myocardial ischemia is a lack of oxygen in the myocardium attributable to inadequate blood flow. Obstruction of the coronary arteries is the most common cause of myocardial ischemia. A coronary artery is significantly obstructed if more than 50% of its diameter is occluded. A 50% reduction in diameter equals a loss of 75% of the arterial **lumen** (12). An obstructed coronary artery may supply an adequate blood flow at rest, but it will probably be unable to provide enough blood and oxygen during increased demand such as during exercise. Ischemia often, but not always, results in angina pectoris.

Angina pectoris is defined as pain or discomfort caused by temporary, reversible ischemia of the myocardium that does not result in death or infarction of heart muscle. The pain often is located in the center of the chest, but pain may occur in the neck, jaw, or shoulders or may radiate into the arms and hands. Angina pectoris tends to be reproducible; patients often report anginal symptoms at roughly the same level of exertion. During exercise, a patient experiencing anginal discomfort may deny pain, but on further questioning, the individual will admit to the sensation of burning, tightness, pressure, or heaviness in the chest or arms. Patients frequently confuse angina pectoris with musculoskeletal pain and with the discomfort resulting from the sternal incision of coronary artery bypass surgery. Anginal pain generally does not alter with movements of the trunk or arms, whereas such movement may decrease or increase musculoskeletal pain. Discomfort is probably not angina if the pain changes in quality or intensity when you press on the affected area (12).

Myocardial ischemia may cause **S-T segment depression** on the ECG during an exercise test. S-T segment depression usually occurs at a relatively constant double product. The double product equals HR · SBP, and it is a good estimate of the amount of work the heart is doing. Three types of S-T segment depression are recognized: upsloping, horizontal, and downsloping (figure 24.22). Ellestad (10) and coworkers have shown that the prognostic implications of upsloping and horizontal S-T segment depression are roughly similar. Downsloping S-T segment depression, however, affects survival more adversely.

S-T segment elevation also may occur during exercise testing. S-T segment elevation during an exercise test usually indicates an **aneurysm,** or a weakened area of noncontracting myocardium or scar tissue.

Myocardial Infarction

If the myocardium is deprived of oxygen for a sufficient length of time, a portion of the myocardium dies; this partial death is known as a *myocardial infarction (MI).* Pain is the hallmark symptom of an MI. It is often very similar to anginal pain, only more severe, and may be described as a heavy feeling, a squeezing in the chest, or a burning sensation. Other symptoms that may accompany an MI are nausea, sweating, and shortness of breath.

S-T segment elevation is often the first ECG sign of an acute MI. Later, pronounced Q waves and T wave inversion may appear in certain leads. Over time, the S-T segment changes subside and the T wave returns to normal (see figure 24.23) (18). Other clinical signs of an acute MI include elevations in cardiac muscle enzymes (serum lactate dehydrogenase and creatine phosphokinase), which leak into the blood after the myocardium is damaged (12).

The Framingham Heart Study demonstrated that up to 25% of MIs may be silent infarctions, meaning that the infarction does not cause sufficient symptoms for the person to seek medical attention (13). These silent infarctions may be recognized later during routine ECG examinations by the presence of significant Q waves in certain leads.

Patients with CAD should be instructed how to differentiate anginal attacks from possible MIs. If an anginal attack occurs, the patient should stop the activity, if any, that precipitated the discomfort and should take a nitroglycerin (NTG) tablet under the tongue. If the anginal discomfort persists after 5 min, the patient takes a second sublingual NTG tablet. This procedure is repeated, if needed, one more time. If the pain persists 5 min after the third NTG tablet, the patient should seek immediate medical attention (4).

Key Point

Inadequate blood flow to the myocardium often, but not always, results in symptoms of chest pain (angina pectoris). S-T segment depression or elevation on the ECG can indicate inadequate blood flow (ischemia). Significant Q waves on the ECG can indicate that a portion of the heart muscle has died (MI).

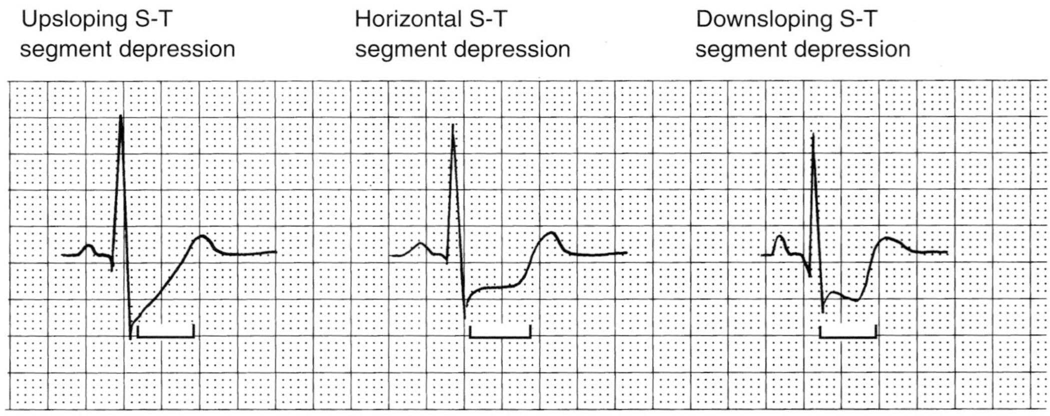

Figure 24.22 S-T segment depression.

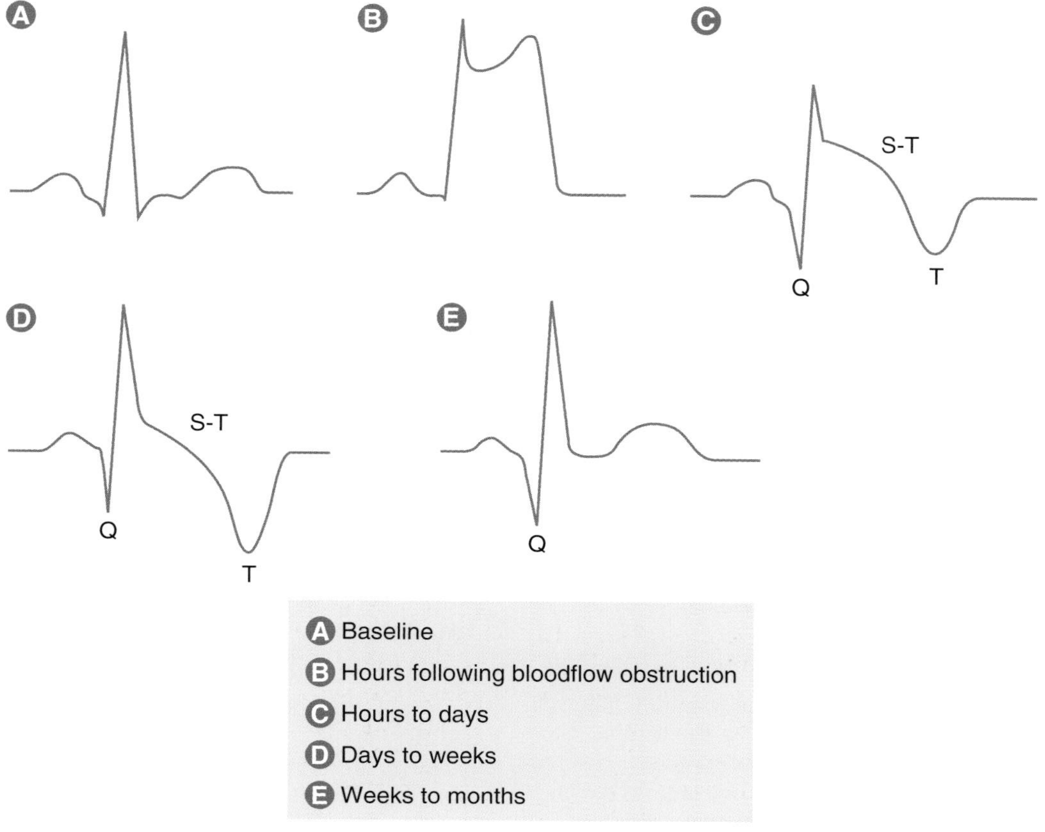

Figure 24.23 Evolution of ECG changes after obstruction of a coronary artery.
Reprinted, by permission, from E. Stein, 1992, *Rapid analysis of electrocardiograms*, 2nd ed. (Philadelphia, PA: Lea & Febiger), 150.

Cardiovascular Medications

A variety of medications are used to treat people with heart disease. Some control blood pressure, whereas others control heart rate or rhythm; still others affect the force of contraction of the ventricles. Other drugs the fitness professional will likely encounter include medications to control blood glucose concentrations, medications for patients with hyperlipidemia to control abnormal blood lipid levels, and bronchodilators for individuals with asthma. Fitness professionals do not prescribe medications or deal on a day-to-day basis with patients taking these medications, but they do encounter participants taking some of these medications. This section summarizes the major classes of drugs, describes how they affect the exercise HR response, and indicates possible side effects.

β-Adrenergic Blockers

β-adrenergic blocking medications (β-blockers) are prescribed commonly for patients with CAD or with hypertension and occasionally for patients with migraine headaches. They compete with epinephrine and norepinephrine for the limited number of **β-adrenergic receptors.** β-blockers are generally used to reduce the HR and the vigor of myocardial contraction, thus lowering the oxygen requirement of the heart. Because these medications influence submaximal and maximal HR, β-blockers have a profound effect on exercise prescription. Subjects should be tested while on β-blockers if they will be training while taking these medications. All β-blockers lower HR at rest and particularly during exercise, as seen in figure 24.24.

Two types of β-adrenergic receptors are recognized: β_1 and β_2. β_1 receptors are found mainly in the heart, and β_2 receptors are located primarily in the smooth muscle in the lungs, arterioles, intestine, uterus, and bladder. Some β-blockers selectively block the β_1 receptors in the heart. The β_1-selective (cardioselective) blockers include Sectral, Tenormin, Brevibloc, and Lopressor. Other β-blockers are less selective and act on both the β_1 and β_2 receptors. These nonselective β-blockers include Inderal, Corgard, Visken, and Blocadren. An undesirable side effect of the nonselective β-blockers is contraction of the smooth muscle surrounding the airways in the lungs

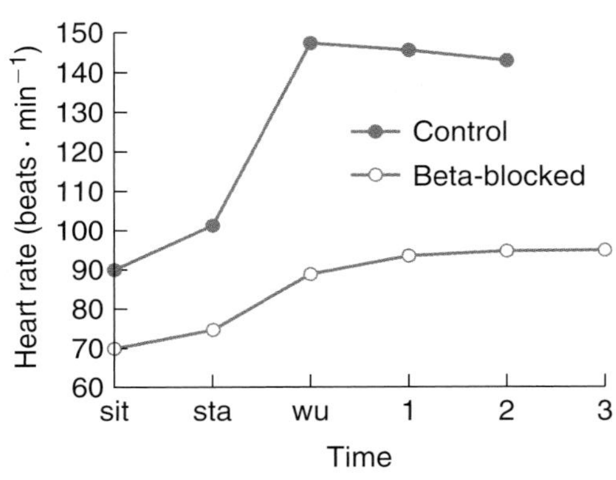

Figure 24.24 The heart rate before and after β-blockade (2 days of 40 mg of Inderal per day) in a very apprehensive patient undergoing treadmill testing; sit = sitting; sta = standing; wu = warming up at 1.0 mi · hr^{-1} (1.6 km · hr^{-1}), 0% grade. Min 1 and 2 are 2.0 mi · hr^{-1} (3.2 km · hr^{-1}), 0% grade. Minute 3 is 2.0 mi · hr^{-1} (3.2 km · hr^{-1}) and 3.5% grade.

and reduction of the airway lumens, which increases the work of breathing. This side effect can result in labored breathing, shortness of breath, and other asthma-like symptoms.

Indications for using β-blockers include hypertension, angina pectoris, and supraventricular arrhythmias. In addition, as previously mentioned, some β-blockers are used to treat migraine headaches. Nonselective β-blocking medications are not recommended for patients with asthma, bronchitis, or similar lung problems. β-blocking medications may also blunt some of the symptoms of hypoglycemia in people with insulin-dependent diabetes, an undesirable side effect (4).

Using Inderal and presumably other β-blocking medications does not invalidate the THR (target heart rate) method of prescribing exercise intensity. Hossack, Bruce, and Clark (11) showed that the regression equations relating %HRmax to %$\dot{V}O_2$max are similar in β-adrenergic blocked and nonblocked patients with CAD. Thus, the THR method of exercise prescription is assumed valid if the measured HRmax is determined while the patient is on β-blocking medications.

Because β-blockers lower HRmax, their use invalidates estimating THR by taking 70% to 85% of age-adjusted, predicted HRmax (predicted HRmax = 220 – age). For example, a 40-yr-old individual has a predicted HRmax of about 180, with an estimated 70% to 85% THR of 126 to 153 beats · min^{-1}. If this individual takes a β-blocker, HRmax could easily drop to 150 beats · min^{-1}. If the estimated THR of 126 to 153 beats · min^{-1} is used for training, this individual may be training at HRmax. HRmax must be measured to calculate an appropriate THR for anyone taking β-blockers, and this measurement should be repeated after any change in β-blocking medicines.

There has been some question as to whether β-blocking medicines reduce or block the effectiveness of endurance training. In general, work capacity and endurance training are impaired more after nonselective β-blockade than after β_1-blockade (19). Ades and coworkers (1) examined the effects of endurance training in 30 adults with hypertension taking a placebo, metoprolol (a β_1-selective blocker), or propranolol (a nonselective β-blocker). $\dot{V}O_2$max increased 24% in the placebo group and 8% in the metoprolol group but did not increase in the propranolol group. Pavia and coworkers (17) found that chronic use of a β_1-selective blocker (metoprolol) in postmyocardial patients did not interfere with the typical effects of endurance training. They observed similar increases in $\dot{V}O_2$peak in patients taking metoprolol and in those who were not on β-blockers.

Nitrates

The **nitrates** exist in several forms including patches, ointments, long-acting tablets, and sublingual tablets, and they are used to prevent or stop attacks of angina pectoris. Nitrates are produced from amyl nitrate (a volatile agent), which is rendered nonexplosive by adding an inert chemical such as lactose. Nitrate preparations relax venous smooth muscle, which reduces venous return and the quantity of blood the heart has to pump. Arterial smooth muscle is also relaxed, although to a lesser degree than venous smooth muscle, thus lowering the peripheral vascular resistance against which the heart has to pump. Both of the actions help reduce the work and oxygen requirement of the heart. Many patients use NTG (nitroglycerine) on a 24 hr basis with ointment or patches. Patients may take longer-acting tablet forms of NTG (Isordil, Sorbitrate, Dilatrate) before beginning activities that are likely to provoke anginal attacks, whereas sublingual tablets (Nitrostat) are used to treat acute anginal episodes. Headaches, dizziness, and hypotension are the main side effects of NTG (4). β-adrenergic blocking medications may potentiate the hypotensive actions of NTG.

Calcium Channel Blockers (Calcium Antagonists)

The **calcium channel blockers** currently include verapamil (Isoptin), nifedipine (Procardia), and diltiazem (Cardizem). These drugs interfere with the slow calcium currents that occur during depolarization in cardiac and vascular smooth muscle. Verapamil is used primarily to treat atrial and ventricular arrhythmias, whereas nifedipine and diltiazem are used to treat exertional angina and variant angina pectoris, or angina pectoris attacks that occur at rest (4).

The effects of calcium channel blockers on exercise prescription and training have been studied. Chang and Hossack (6) showed that the regression equations relating %HRmax and %$\dot{V}O_2$max are the same in patients taking diltiazem and in nonmedicated patients. Isoptin and Procardia are assumed not to alter the relationship between %HRmax and %$\dot{V}O_2$max. Calcium antagonists are not thought to adversely affect endurance training in healthy subjects or in patients with CAD (15). MacGowan and coworkers (16) showed that verapamil does not diminish training responses in healthy, young subjects.

Antiarrhythmic Medications

Common **antiarrhythmics** include Pronestyl, Norpace, Cardioquin, Quinaglute, Tambocor, Sectral, Cordarone, Tonocard, and the digitalis preparations. The β-blocking medications also are used to treat some types of arrhythmias. With the exception of the β-blockers, these medications have little influence on the HR response to exercise; in fact, the reduction in arrhythmias may improve work capacity.

Digitalis Preparations

The **digitalis** medications are used to increase the vigor of myocardial contractions (contractility) and treat atrial flutter and fibrillation (4). In individuals with poor ventricular function, the increased contractility resulting from digitalis preparations may increase work capacity. Digitalis medications are marketed under several trade names including Lanoxin, Lanoxicaps, Purodigin, and Crystodigin. Cardiac side effects of the digitalis group include premature ventricular contractions, Wenckebach AV block, and atrial tachycardia. Digitalis drugs can cause false-positive tests for coronary heart disease due to S-T segment depression during exercise testing (9). The side effects of the digitalis drugs can be potentiated by quinidine sulfate.

Antihypertensives

Antihypertensives can be broken down into five groups according to the mechanism of action. Drugs in the first group, *diuretics,* work by increasing the excretion of electrolytes and water. These drugs include Lasix, Diamox, Diuril, Esidrix, Enduron, HydroDIURIL, and many others. This group is often used as the first treatment for hypertension. Side effects include hypokalemia, or low blood levels of potassium. Hypokalemia can induce arrhythmias and is a potentially serious problem. Diuretic-induced hypokalemia often can be prevented by consuming more citrus fruits, which are high in potassium. If dietary sources of potassium prove to be ineffective, a prescription potassium supplement (K-Tab, Kay Ceil, or Slo-K) can be used (4). Alternatively, a potassium-sparing diuretic (Midamor, Aldactone, Dyrenium) can be prescribed.

The second group of antihypertensive medications comprises the *antiadrenergic agents.* These include drugs that act at the level of the central nervous system, such as clonidine (Catapres) and methyldopa (Aldomet), and they reduce sympathetic outflow from the brain. This group also includes drugs that act principally on α-adrenergic receptors to lower peripheral vascular resistance, such as prazosin (Minipress). In addition, this group includes those drugs that block β-adrenergic receptors (see previous section) to decrease cardiac output, renin release, and sympathetic outflow from the brain.

In an important side effect, the diuretics and β-blockers elevate triglyceride and cholesterol levels and impair glucose and insulin metabolism. Thus, although they effectively lower BP and reduce the incidence of stroke and of severe kidney disease, they have a less-than-predicted effect on preventing heart attacks.

Vasodilators make up the third group of antihypertensive medications. These medications decrease BP by relaxing vascular smooth muscle. Some of the brand names in this category are Apresoline, Vasodilan, and Loniten. Their side effects include hypotension, dizziness, and tachycardia. The active chemical in Loniten is also marketed under the name Rogaine as a topical solution for stimulating hair growth in male-pattern baldness. Rogaine has little or no antihypertensive effect.

Antihypertensive medications in the fourth group work through the renin-angiotensin system. These drugs lower BP by inhibiting angiotensin-converting enzyme (ACE), which converts angiotensin I to angiotensin II. They are called *ACE inhibitors* for that reason. Some of the brand names in this category are Vasotec, Zestril, and Capoten. The ACE inhibitors are expensive and may produce a dry cough in 5% to 10% of patients. They decrease left ventricular hypertrophy, reduce proteinuria in diabetic patients, and maintain blood lipid levels.

The fifth group of antihypertensive medications includes the *calcium antagonists* (calcium channel blockers; see previous section on page 370). As with the ACE inhibitors, drugs in this class do not adversely affect lipid, glucose, and insulin metabolism.

Lipid-Lowering Medications

The lipid-lowering medications (Questran and Colestid; Pravachol, Zocor, and Lescol; Lopid and Atromid-S; and nicotinic acid) lower cholesterol and triglycerides in individuals who are unable to adequately control lipids through diet and exercise. These lipid-lowering medications are unlikely to have any substantial effects on exercise testing or training. Patients taking these medications need to be closely monitored by their physician because of potential toxic effects on the liver. Some lipid-lowering agents (Lopid, Atromid-S) can potentiate anticoagulants and make participants in exercise programs more susceptible to bruising.

Anticoagulants

The **anticoagulants** delay blood clotting. Oral anticoagulants include Dicumarol and Coumadin. These medications are unlikely to directly affect exercise testing or training, but they do increase the risk of bruising. Aspirin and some other medications (e.g., nonsteroidal anti-inflammatory drugs such as Motrin, Advil, and Nuprin) can potentiate anticoagulants and increase the risk of bruising with minimal trauma.

Nicotine Gums and Patches

Nicotine gums and patches are used as smoking substitutes for people who are trying to stop smoking. With **nicotine gum,** the nicotine is absorbed through the oral mucosa, providing sufficient plasma nicotine concentrations to curb the craving to smoke. Nicotine gums are marketed under the names Bantron and Nicorette. With transdermal nicotine patches, the nicotine is absorbed through the skin. Nicotine may affect the exercise response, particularly if a person chews nicotine gum but also continues to smoke. Nicotine may increase heart rate and blood pressure as well as the incidence of cardiac arrhythmias (2).

Bronchodilators

The **bronchodilators** relax smooth muscle surrounding airways in the lungs and relieve the symptoms of asthma, bronchitis, and related lung disorders. These medications can be taken orally or from an inhaler. The inhalers are generally used for acute asthma episodes, whereas long-term bronchodilation is usually obtained with oral preparations. Most of these drugs stimulate the β_2 receptors that relax bronchial smooth muscle and increase the airway lumen. Because of their β-adrenergic stimulating effect, they can increase HR and BP, although most of their effect focuses on the smooth muscle found in airways. Some of the inhaler brand names include Brethaire Inhaler, Ventolin, Alupent, Maxair, and others. The oral bronchodilators include Theobid, Aminophyllin, Theo-Dur, and many others (4).

Oral Antiglycemic Agents

A substantial number of obese participants in fitness programs have hyperglycemia, or elevated levels of blood glucose. In this condition the pancreas is able to produce insulin, but it is unable to produce sufficient quantities to maintain normal blood glucose control. This condition is called non-insulin-dependent diabetes mellitus; often this condition can be controlled with **oral antiglycemic agents.** The oral antiglycemic medications stimulate the pancreas to secrete more insulin, which facilitates tissue uptake of glucose. The stimulating action of the oral antiglycemic medications requires a functioning pancreas. Brand names include DiaBeta, Diabinese, Glucotrol, Micronase, Orinase, and Tolinase. These drugs are in the sulfonylurea class (4). Recently, a new type of oral antiglycemic drug has become available (Glucophage, in the metformin class). Metformin reduces insulin resistance, thereby lowering blood sugar. A serious side effect of these drugs is hypoglycemia, or low blood sugar. Hypoglycemia is potentially dangerous, and the fitness professional should be cognizant of any changes in alertness and orientation in patients taking any medication that can lower plasma glucose concentrations.

Insulin-dependent diabetes mellitus is a more serious disorder of carbohydrate metabolism and is characterized by an absence of insulin and requires frequent insulin injections. Insulin cannot be taken orally because it is a protein and would be inactivated by the digestive process. When working with an insulin-dependent diabetic who is taking insulin, the fitness professional should be aware of the possibility of hypoglycemia. Signs of hypoglycemia include bizarre behavior and slurred speech. When individuals with insulin-dependent diabetes mellitus are exercising, it is a good idea to have a source of sugar readily available in the event of a hypoglycemic episode. See chapter 20 for additional details on diabetes.

Depressants

Tranquilizers reduce anxiety. Minor tranquilizers may lower HR and BP by controlling anxiety, but otherwise the exercise response is not affected. With major tranquilizers, HR may increase while BP either drops or remains

Key Point

Medications are prescribed for a variety of reasons: high BP, abnormal heart rhythms, elevated blood lipids, asthma, and other medical concerns. Appendix D summarizes the common categories of prescription medicines for cardiovascular and related diseases, lists some of the members of each category, and describes their effects on exercise performance.

unchanged (2). **Alcohol** is a depressant that can affect the exercise test by impairing motor coordination, balance, and reaction times. Chronic alcohol consumption tends to elevate resting and exercise BP. The acute effects of alcohol ingestion on the exercise response have been examined. During brief maximal exercise, small to moderate doses of alcohol do not affect oxygen uptake, stroke volume, ejection fraction, cardiac output, arteriovenous oxygen difference, and peak lactate concentration (20). However, higher doses (blood alcohol content = 0.20 mg · dl^{-1}) may impair myocardial function, as shown by a 6% decrease in ejection fraction (14). Alcohol intake can provoke arrhythmias at rest and during exercise.

Case Studies

You can check your answers by referring to pages 475 and 476 in appendix A.

1. The following ECG tracing (see case study figure 24.1) was obtained on a 38-yr-old female before she took a GXT on the treadmill.
    a. Determine the HR (beats per minute) and the durations of the P-R interval, QRS complex, and Q-T interval (in seconds).
    b. What condition does she have?
    c. What factors might cause this condition?

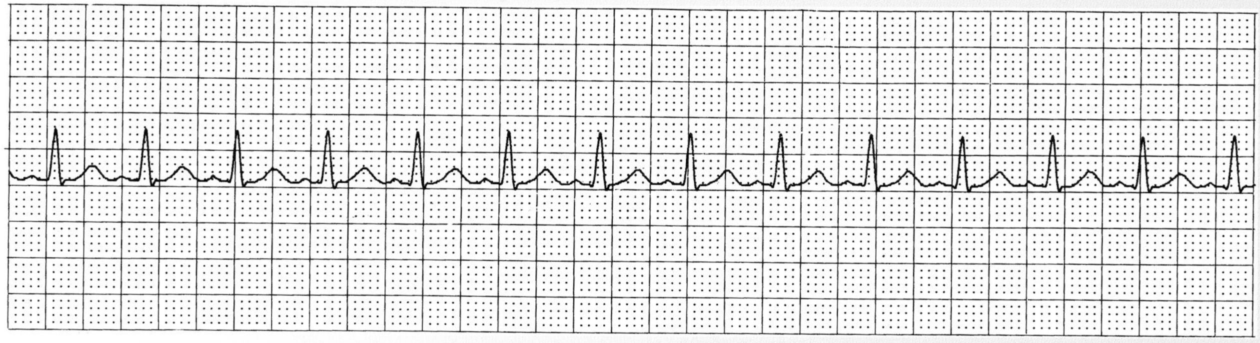

Case study figure 24.1.

2. A 21-yr-old male college student, taking a cold medication containing ephedrine, showed the following ECG tracing at rest (see case study figure 24.2).
    a. What type of arrhythmia does he have?
    b. What is the ventricular rate?

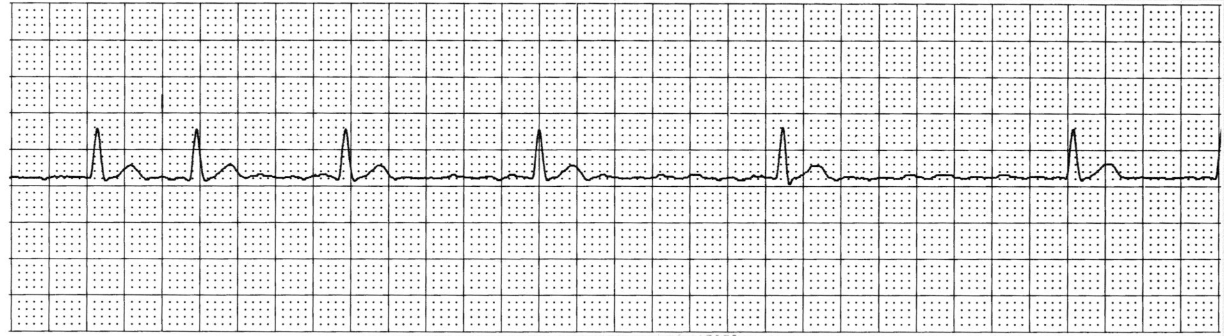

Case study figure 24.2.

3. A 57-yr-old participant in your exercise program showed the following ECG tracing (see case study figure 24.3) while she was exercising at 3.5 mi · hr^{-1} on a 6% grade on the treadmill.
    a. What ECG abnormality is shown here?
    b. What action should be taken?

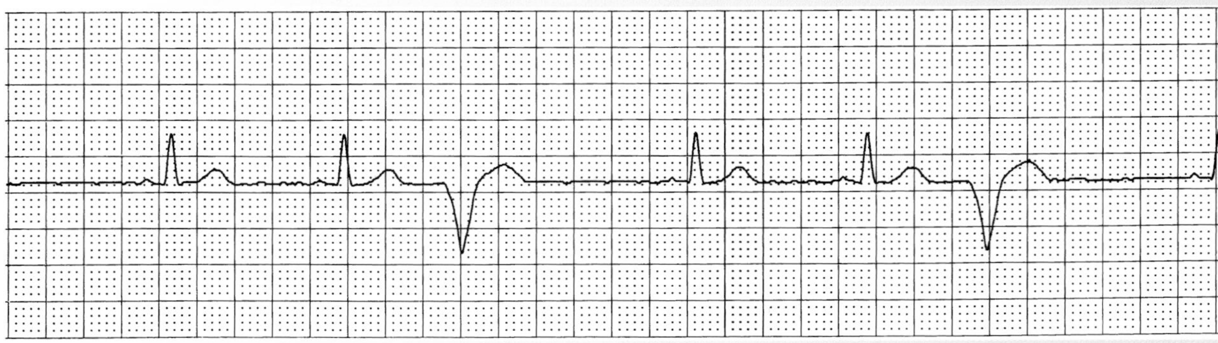

Case study figure 24.3.

4. A 55-yr-old, apparently healthy male is referred to your facility for an exercise program and brings with him the results of his most recent exercise test. You notice that the participant was taking Coumadin and Inderal when he took his exercise test. Since the test, his physician has stopped the Inderal. What effect, if any, would this change in medication have on the exercise prescription? (See appendix D.)
5. A participant in your exercise program has been taking a β-blocking medication for several years without experiencing any significant side effects. He was recently given a prescription for Isordil and now reports that he often becomes dizzy upon standing suddenly. Could this be related to his medication? If so, why? (See appendix D.)

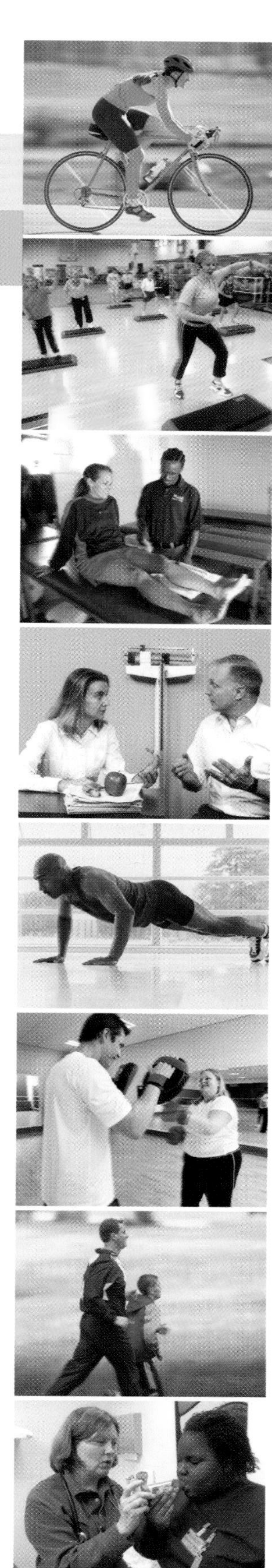

25 CHAPTER

Injury Prevention and Treatment

Sue Carver

Objectives

The reader will be able to do the following:

1. Describe ways to minimize injury risk and prevent the transmission of blood-borne pathogens.
2. Describe the signs and symptoms of soft-tissue injuries (sprains, strains, contusions, and heel bruises), how to initially treat injuries, and when to use heat in long-term treatment.
3. Identify signs, symptoms, and proper treatment for bone injuries, wounds, and common skin irritations.
4. Describe the causes of heat-related disorders, how to prevent heat illness, and how to treat a heat-related emergency; provide guidelines for fluid replacement before and after exercise.
5. Explain the causes of cold-related disorders and how to prevent frost nip, superficial and deep frostbite, and hypothermia; explain how to treat a cold-related emergency.
6. Distinguish between the signs and symptoms of diabetic coma and those of insulin shock and describe the proper treatment for each.
7. Identify common cardiovascular and pulmonary complications resulting from exercise participation.

(continued)

8. Identify the signs, symptoms, and management of common orthopedic problems; classify injuries as mild, moderate, and severe; and recommend appropriate modification of exercise programs when injury occurs.
9. Describe procedures to check vital signs.
10. Describe artificial respiration and cardiopulmonary techniques for adults.

The fitness professional must be prepared to safely handle an emergency medical situation. This chapter discusses injury prevention, injury recognition, and common treatment approaches as well as planning for and handling a medical emergency.

Preventing Injuries

Certain inherent risks are associated with participating in physical activity. The fitness professional should be aware of those risks and control factors that increase the risk of injury. Advanced planning, training in injury recognition and emergency care, adequate equipment and facilities, and counseling in activity selection all help reduce the possibility of injury. The following is a brief discussion of factors contributing to injury and steps that can be taken to reduce injury risk (3-9, 11-12, 14-16, 19, 21-22, 24, 28, 32).

Controlling Injury Risk

Injury risk in competitive athletic events is controlled by game rules. In exercise programs where games are used for aerobic activity, injury risk may be reduced by controlling the tempo of the activity or by modifying existing rules to enhance participant safety (e.g., limiting body contact, using a softer ball).

The fitness professional should encourage participants to seek professional advice regarding the selection and fitting of proper exercise equipment. The equipment most commonly used, and most widely abused, is footwear. Inadequately protecting the foot is a major contributor to a variety of leg and low-back problems. Improperly maintained exercise equipment and facilities also contribute to higher overall injury risk.

In this age of concern over blood-borne pathogens such as the **human immunodeficiency virus (HIV)** and **hepatitis B virus (HBV)**, precautions should be taken to protect both the participant and the fitness professional. Open cuts should be covered, and clothing that is saturated with blood should be changed. Necessary supplies should be available to care safely for an open wound, including protective gloves, biohazard containers, antiseptic solution, dressings, disinfectant, and a sharps container if applicable. Participants should be instructed to report all wounds immediately. The fitness professional should know **universal precaution** guidelines for managing acute blood exposure as well as appropriate cleaning and disposal policies for contaminated areas.

Contributing Factors to Injury

Activity implies movement, and with increased movement comes a corresponding increase in the risk of injury. In fitness programs, the incidence of injury increases when the frequency of the exercise sessions increases and when the intensity of the exercise is maintained at the high end of the target heart rate (THR) zone (figure 25.1). The risk of injury is also heightened by faster movements, as found in competitive activities; by quick changes in direction, as found in fitness games; and by increased focus on smaller muscle groups. Environmental conditions such as extreme heat or cold can also increase the risk associated with physical activity. Lack of proper adaptation to the environment, as well as lack of education in prevention, recognition, and treatment of problems associated with these extreme environments, can lead to devastating results.

Age, sex, and body structure influence the risk of injury. In general, the very young and the very old are at the greatest risk, and older individuals usually require longer recovery times. Because of differences in body structure and strength, females are often more susceptible to injury in coed activities and games requiring quick

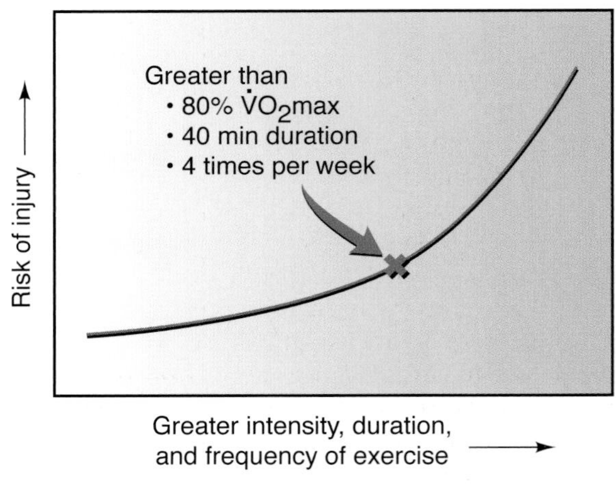

Figure 25.1 Risk of injury increases with too much activity.

changes of direction or body contact. For either males or females, a lack or an imbalance of muscle strength, a lack of joint flexibility, and poor CRF increase the chance of injury. Obese individuals may not only have low CRF but also have excess weight that additionally stresses weight-bearing joints. Participants with specific medical problems such as asthma, diabetes, or known allergic reactions may need special attention to avoid potentially serious complications.

Reducing Injury Risk

Screening participants before they begin any physical activity program can help reduce injury risk. The screening should highlight the major areas that increase health risk, assist the participant in recognizing problems, and alert the fitness professional to potential problems that could occur in an exercise session (e.g., asthma attack, diabetic shock). Proper planning for emergency situations lowers overall risk. Individuals who cannot be properly supervised or given adequate care for their physical problems should be referred to a program or facility that can provide the needed services. Policies to handle such referrals and all major emergency situations should be written and communicated to all fitness professionals in a fitness center.

A major factor in reducing the risk associated with physical activity is the design and implementation of an individual's exercise program. The program can focus on problems encountered in the preliminary tests, which might include the following:

- Flexibility measures
- Assessment of body composition
- Evaluation of muscular strength, power, and endurance
- Posture assessment
- Cardiovascular fitness evaluation

The way the fitness professional conducts the exercise program has a major bearing on the risk of injury to the participant. To highlight this point, figure 25.2 contrasts the "train, don't strain" fitness goal with the "train hard, train smart" performance goal. Educating participants about the proper intensity of the exercise session (i.e., to stay in the THR zone) and how to recognize the signs and symptoms of overuse helps reduce injury risk. The fitness professional should emphasize that the entire program and each individual session are graduated so the participant will avoid doing too much too soon. This precaution is especially true for people who have not been involved in a regular exercise program and who tend to overestimate their abilities. Overexertion can lead to chronic overuse injuries, extreme muscle soreness, and undue fatigue.

In educating participants about the signs and symptoms of overuse, the fitness professional should distinguish between simple muscle soreness and injury. Muscle soreness tends to peak 24 to 48 hr following exercise and dissipates with use and time. The signs and symptoms of injury include the following:

- Exquisite point tenderness
- Pain that persists even when the body part is at rest
- Joint pain
- Pain that does not go away after warming up

Key Point

The fitness professional should be aware of inherent risks associated with activity and minimize risk by planning in advance, using proper equipment and facilities, educating participants regarding injury recognition and care, evaluating participants to determine fitness needs or special health problems that may need monitoring, and giving clear guidelines for graduating activity. The fitness professional should follow universal precaution guidelines and use appropriate gloves, biohazard containers, sharps containers, and disinfectant to reduce the spread of blood-borne pathogens.

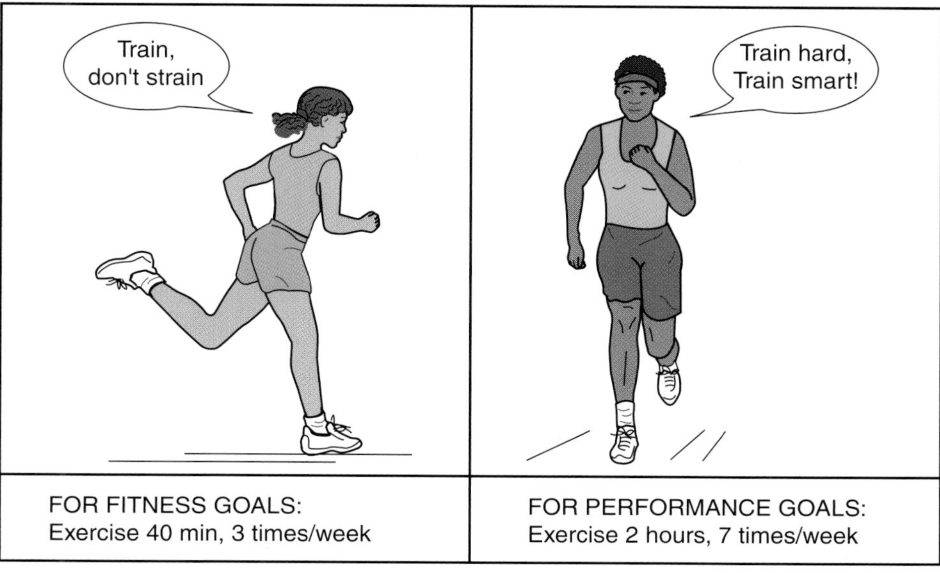
Train, don't strain
Train hard, Train smart!
FOR FITNESS GOALS: Exercise 40 min, 3 times/week
FOR PERFORMANCE GOALS: Exercise 2 hours, 7 times/week

Figure 25.2 Fitness training versus performance training.

- Swelling or discoloration
- Increased pain with weight-bearing activities or with active movement
- Changes in normal bodily functions

Injury Treatment

Treating an injury depends on the type and severity of the injury. This section describes approaches to take with injuries that are common to fitness programs and sports (2, 3, 5-8, 10-13, 16-22, 25-27).

Treating Soft-Tissue Injuries

Sprains (overstretching or tearing of **ligamentous** tissue) and strains (overstretching or tearing of muscle or **tendon**) are common injuries associated with adult fitness programs. Most significant injuries to joint structures or to soft tissue require protection, rest, and the immediate application of ice, compression, and elevation (known by the acronym *PRICE).* Figure 25.3 reinforces the **PRICE** concept. Usually, a wet wrap is applied first to give compression. Start distal to the injury and wrap toward the heart. Compression should be firm but not tight. When a joint structure is involved, apply a wet compression wrap and surround the entire area with ice. Secure with another elastic wrap. If the injury involves a contusion (bruise) or strain to a muscle belly, put the muscle on mild stretch before applying a wet compression bandage and ice. If possible, elevate the injured part above heart level to minimize the effect of gravity and reduce bleeding into tissues. With any injury, shock is a possibility, and the fitness professional should be prepared to handle this situation.

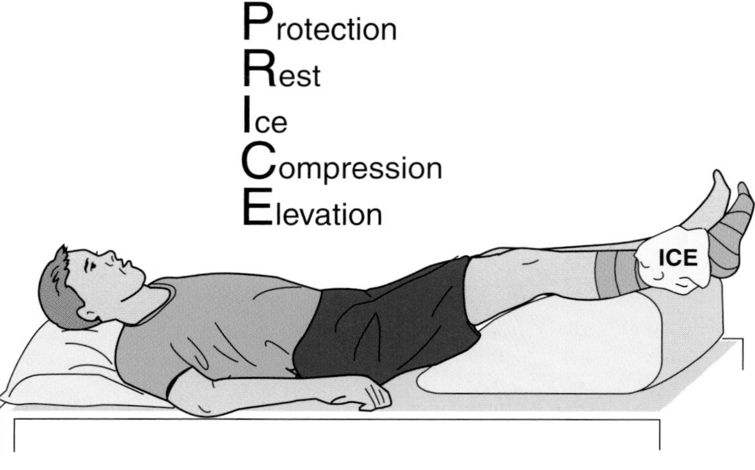

Figure 25.3 The PRICE method for treating sprains and strains.

In most cases, the participant should be instructed to continue applying ice anywhere from 24 to 72 hr, depending on the severity of the injury. Ice causes vasoconstriction of the blood vessels, thus helping to control bleeding into tissues. Ice also reduces the sensation of pain. Standard treatment times with ice are 15 to 20 min, with reapplication hourly or when pain is experienced. If the possibility of bleeding into the tissues still exists and ice is not being used, the compression bandage should be in place to minimize swelling. Using ice or compression at bedtime is not necessary unless pain interferes with sleep. If this occurs, applying ice frequently (every 1-2 hr) may help control the pain. Physician referral is recommended in cases of moderate or severe injury.

An injured participant may want to apply heat sooner than is warranted. Heat usually is applied in the later stages of an acute injury, when the risk of bleeding into tissues is minimal. In contrast, heat is a common treatment for chronic inflammatory conditions as well as generalized muscle soreness. Heat causes a vasodilation of the blood vessels and reduces muscle spasm. Standard treatment time for a moist heat pack is 15 to 20 min. When in doubt about which mode of treatment to use, ice is the safer choice. Table 25.1 outlines common soft-tissue injuries, signs and symptoms, and immediate care.

Key Point

When soft tissues are injured, proper assessment and initial treatment can reduce the possibility of further trauma and can aid in the healing process (see table 25.1 for details). Protection, rest, ice, compression, and elevation (PRICE) are the important steps for immediate care of most musculoskeletal and joint injuries. Heat is often used in chronic inflammatory conditions or with general muscle soreness and should be applied only in the later stages of an acute injury when the risk of bleeding into tissues is minimal.

Treating Fractures

Fractures, or injury to bone, should be suspected if there is exquisite point tenderness over a bone, visual or palpable deformity, or referred pain to an area of bone upon percussion or vibrational stress. X rays should be taken if a fracture is suspected. If deformity is present, do not push the bone back into place. Splint and refer to a physician. Table 25.2 gives additional procedures to follow when treating a fracture.

• Table 25.1 Soft-Tissue Injuries and Their Treatment •

Injury	Signs and symptoms	Immediate care
Sprain—stretching or tearing of ligamentous tissue **Strain**—overstretching or tearing of a muscle or tendon **Contusion**—impact force that results in bleeding into the underlying tissues; a bruise	1st degree—mild injury resulting in overstretching or minor tearing of tissue; range of motion limited, minimal point tenderness, no swelling 2nd degree—moderate injury resulting in partial tearing of tissue; limited function, point tenderness and probable muscle spasm, painful ROM, swelling or discoloration (probable if immediate first-aid care is not given) 3rd degree—severe tearing or rupture of tissue; exquisite point tenderness, immediate loss of function, swelling and muscle spasm likely to be present with discoloration appearing later, possible palpable deformity	Protection, rest, ice, compression, and elevation. Usual treatment time: 15 to 20 min ice bag 5 to 7 min ice cup or ice slush How often: Moderate and severe—every hour, or when pain is experienced Less severe—as symptoms necessitate Continue with ice treatments at least 24 to 72 hr, depending on the severity of the injury. Refer to a physician if function is impaired. Mild to moderate strains—gradual stretching to the point of discomfort is recommended.
Heel bruise (stone bruise)—sudden abnormal force to heel area that results in trauma to underlying tissues		Protection, rest, ice, compression, and elevation. Pad for comfort when weight bearing is resumed.

Information from 1-2, 11-16, 18, 21, 23, 25, 26, 35.

• Table 25.2 Fractures and Their Treatment •

Injury	Signs and symptoms	Immediate care
Fracture—disruption of bone with or without loss of continuity or external exposure, ranging from periosteal irritation to complete separation of bony parts **Simple**—bone fracture without external exposure **Compound**—bone fracture with external exposure	Acute: Direct trauma to bone resulting in disruption of continuity and immediate disability; deformity or bony deviation, swelling, pain, palpable tenderness, referred pain crepitus, false joint, discoloration (usually becomes apparent later)	Acute: Control bleeding—elevation, pressure points, direct pressure. Treat for shock. If an open fracture, control bleeding and apply a sterile dressing, prevent further disruption and infection; do not move bones back into place. Control swelling with pressure and ice, if wound is closed. Splint above and below the joint and apply traction if necessary. Protect body part from further injury. Refer to physician.
	Chronic: Low grade inflammatory process causing proliferation of fibroblasts and generalized connective tissue scaring, pain progressively worsens until present all the time, direct point tenderness	Chronic: Rest. Heat. Refer to physician.

Information from 1, 2, 7, 12, 13, 23, 25-26.

Treating Wounds and Other Skin Disorders

Wounds are also common injuries associated with activity programs. The major concern with an open wound is bleeding. Once bleeding is controlled, further care can be given. This may consist of protecting the wound from infection, covering the wound with a bandage, treating the participant for shock, or referring the participant immediately to a physician for suturing. In minor cases, a thorough cleansing and application of a sterile dressing may be all that is needed. The fitness professional should use safety measures to prevent risk from exposure to blood. Internal bleeding is a very serious condition. The fitness professional should treat for shock and obtain medical assistance immediately.

Shearing and pressure forces are attributable to poorly fitting shoes and socks, poorly conditioned or sensitive skin, and incorrect foot biomechanics that lead to friction and compression injuries of the foot. Hand calluses and other skin irritations can develop from friction during activities that require frequent gripping (e.g., of a tennis racket or a bat) or rubbing of body parts against each other or another object (as is frequently the case in gymnastics or wrestling, for example).

Table 25.3 outlines guidelines for immediate care of wounds. Table 25.4 discusses care of common skin irritations. The fitness professional should use universal precautions in treating an open wound. Protective gloves should be worn when handling potentially infectious materials. Proper disposal of infectious materials and decontamination of infected areas should be a routine policy.

Table 25.3 Wounds and Their Treatment

Injury	Signs and symptoms	Immediate care
Incision—cutting of skin resulting in an open wound with cleanly cut edges and exposure of underlying tissues	Smooth edges that may bleed freely Signs of infection (see Laceration)	Clean wound with soap and water, moving away from injury site. Minor cuts can be closed with a butterfly bandage or steri-strip. Apply a sterile dressing. Refer to a physician if wound needs suturing (e.g., facial cuts and large or deep wounds) or signs of infection are present.
Laceration—tearing of skin resulting in an open wound with jagged edges and exposure of underlying tissues	Jagged edges that may bleed freely Signs of infection: redness; swelling; increase in skin temperature; tender, swollen, and painful lymph glands; mild fever; and headache	Soak in antiseptic solution such as hydrogen peroxide to loosen foreign material. Clean with antiseptic soap and water using sterile technique and moving away from the injury site. Apply a sterile dressing. Instruct individual to seek medical attention if signs of infection are recognized. Usually refer to a physician; a tetanus shot or sutures may be needed. If injury is extensive, control bleeding, cover with thick sterile bandages, and treat for shock. Refer to a physician.
Puncture—direct penetration of tissues by a pointed object	Small opening that may bleed freely Signs of infection (see Laceration)	If object is embedded deeply: Protect body part and refer to physician for removal and care. Treat for shock. Clean around wound, moving away from injury site. Allow wound to bleed freely to minimize risk of infection. Apply a sterile dressing. Puncture wounds are usually referred to a physician. A tetanus shot may be needed. Instruct individual to seek medical attention if signs of infection are present.

Injury	Signs and symptoms	Immediate care
Abrasion—scraping of tissues resulting in removal of the outermost layers of skin and the exposure of numerous capillaries	Superficial, reddish, irregular surface Oozing or weeping from underlying capillaries May contain dirt, debris, or bacteria embedded in tissue	Debride and flush with antiseptic solution such as hydrogen peroxide; then cleanse with soap and water. Apply a petroleum-based antiseptic agent to keep wound moist. This allows healing to take place from the deeper layers. Cover with non-adherent gauze. Instruct person to seek medical help if signs of infection are recognized.
Excessive bleeding—internal or external bleeding that results in massive loss of circulating blood volumes; often results in shock and can lead to death	External hemorrhage 1. Arterial Color: bright red Flow: spurts, bleeding usually profuse 2. Venous Color: dark red Flow: steady, oozing	Elevate affected part above heart. Put direct pressure over the wound, using a sterile compress if possible. Apply a pressure dressing. Use pressure points. Treat for shock. Refer to a physician.
Internal bleeding—bleeding within the deep structures of the body (chest, abdominal, or pelvic cavity) and bleeding of any of the organs contained within these cavities	Internal hemorrhage—bleeding into chest, abdominal, or pelvic cavity and bleeding of any of the organs contained within these cavities Generally, no external signs, except when an individual coughs up blood or finds blood in the urine or feces or experiences the following: Restlessness Thirst Faintness Anxiety Cold, clammy skin Dizziness Pulse—rapid, weak, and irregular Blood pressure—significant fall	Treat for shock. Refer to hospital immediately. Don't give water or food.
Shock caused by bleeding	Restlessness Anxiety Pulse—weak, rapid Skin temperature—cold, clammy, profuse sweating Skin color—pale, later cyanotic Respiration—shallow, labored Eyes—dull Pupils—dilated Thirsty Nausea and possible vomiting Blood pressure—marked fall	Maintain an open airway. Control bleeding. Elevate lower extremities approximately 12 in. (31 cm) (exceptions: heart problems, head injury, or breathing difficulty—place in comfortable position, usually semireclining, unless spinal injury is suspected, in which case do not move). Splint any fractures. Maintain normal body temperature. Avoid further trauma. Monitor vital signs and record at regular intervals—every 5 min or so. Do not feed or give any liquids.

Information from 1-2, 7-9, 11-17, 19, 23-25, 32, 34.

• Table 25.4 Skin Irritations and Their Treatment •

Skin irritation	Signs and symptoms	Immediate care
Blister—a collection of serum just below the superficial layer of skin	Defined area of fluid accumulation under skin Feels hot Painful to touch	Prevent by engaging in heavy activity slowly and toughening skin by use of astringents (tannic acid or salt water). Stop activity if friction area develops, apply ice, and cover irritation with a friction-proofing material or donut pad. Prevent contamination of torn blister; clean with soap and water. Refer to physician if signs of infection are present.
Callus—markedly thickened area of skin, usually over an area of pressure	Visible and excessive callus formation: May be painful May have cracks or fissures May become infected May develop blisters	Prevent excessive callus formation by using an emery callus file. Take measures to reduce friction by wearing properly fitted shoes and socks, using powder or lubricant, and correcting abnormal biomechanical foot faults with orthotics. Protect susceptible areas by using special protective devices such as gloves, tape, or pad. Prevent infection by keeping callus trimmed down and using a lubricant to prevent cracks and tears in callus.
Corns **Hard corn**—thickening of skin located on toes **Soft corn**—circular area of thickened white macerated skin between toes and proximal head of phalanges	Local pain Inflammation and thickening of soft tissue Generally seen on top of toes and associated with hammer toe deformity Pain and inflammation	Prevent by wearing properly fitted shoes or fitting with orthotics if cause is due to abnormal foot biomechanics. Prevent with properly fitted shoes, and control moisture accumulation by keeping skin dry between toes. Separate toes with cotton or lamb's wool.
Ingrown toenail—leading side edge of toenail grows into soft tissue	Severe inflammation, pain, and infection	Apply hot antiseptic soaks for 20 min, 2 to 3 times a day, at 110 to 120 °F (43.4-48.9 °C). When toenail is pliable, insert wisp of cotton under leading edge of toenail and lift from soft tissue beneath. Refer to physician or podiatrist if signs of infection are present.
Intertrigo—chafing due to excessive rubbing of body parts in combination with perspiration	Pain, inflammation, burning, itching, moistness, cracking, lesion	Cleanse frequently. Use medicated drying powder.
Plantar wart—viral infection on foot, leading to a localized overgrowth of skin; can be confused with callus	Distinct edge with central core Sometimes appears to be growing inward; small black dot in center surrounded by clearer callus area Excessive thickening of skin	Use donut to take pressure off of wart. Keep callus area around wart filed down (do not file down wart). See physician or podiatrist for cure or removal.

Information from 11-15, 16-17, 23, 25, 30, 32, 34.

Key Point

The steps for dealing with simple and compound fractures, wounds (and excessive bleeding), and other skin disorders are listed in tables 25.2, 25.3, and 25.4.

Environmental Concerns

The environment can play an important role in the development of serious problems related to maintaining normal body temperature during exercise. This section examines the factors related to an increased risk of heat- and cold-related injuries.

Heat-Related Problems

Heat illness can strike anyone. Poor physical condition, although a contributing factor, is not the primary cause. Even the most highly conditioned athlete can experience a heat-related disorder. The exercise and the environment can place large heat loads on an individual. Excessive heat loads overstimulate sweat because **evaporation** of sweat is the major mechanism for cooling the body. As a result, large amounts of water may be lost during physical activity, causing an increase in the core body temperature **(hyperthermia).** If too much water is lost, circulatory collapse and death can occur. The following information outlines methods of recognizing dehydration (excessive loss of body fluids) and preventing heat illness.

A water loss up to 3% of body weight is considered safe. A 3% to 5% loss is considered borderline, and more than a 5% loss is considered serious. Water loss can be monitored by weighing participants before and after activity. Individuals who are outside the 3% range from one workout to the next may have an increased risk of heat injury and should be monitored carefully if allowed to participate.

The practical experience of military and athletic teams working in the heat and humidity has led to guidelines for preventing heat injury. Applying these guidelines to adult fitness programs will enhance participants' enjoyment and safety. Participants should do the following to prevent heat injury:

- Acclimatize to heat and humidity by gradually increasing training intensity and duration over 7 to 10 days.
- Hydrate before activity and frequently during activity.
- Decrease the intensity of exercise if the temperature or humidity is high; use THR as a guide.
- Monitor weight loss by weighing before and after workouts. Consume fluids if more than 3% of body weight is lost during activity. Minimize participation until weight is within the 3% range.
- Consume a diet high in carbohydrate; carbohydrate has a high water content and helps to maintain fluid balance.
- Wear appropriate clothing for hot or humid weather conditions. Expose as much skin surface as possible.

Further precautions include wearing light-colored clothing because lighter colors do not retain as much heat as darker colors. Cotton materials absorb sweat and allow evaporation to occur. Certain synthetic clothing and materials with paint screens do not absorb sweat and should be avoided.

Participants should be educated to recognize symptoms of overexertion: nausea or vomiting, extreme breathlessness, dizziness, unusual fatigue, muscle cramping, and headache. Symptoms related to heat illness include hair standing on end on the chest or upper arms, body chills, headache or throbbing pressure, nausea or vomiting, labored breathing, dry lips or extreme cotton mouth, faintness (heat syncope) or muscle cramping (heat cramps), and cessation of sweating. Heat rash can also be a symptom and is attributable to inflamed sweat glands. It usually occurs in children who have sweated profusely. If these symptoms are present, the risk for developing heat exhaustion or heatstroke rises dramatically, and participants should stop activity and get into the shade. In addition, participants should be instructed to ask for help if they are disoriented or if the symptoms are severe. The fitness professional should provide fluids and encourage all individuals to drink.

Individuals who experience heatstroke may sustain permanent damage to their thermoregulatory system. People who do not have efficient cooling mechanisms may be highly susceptible to heat injury. People who take medications such as antihistamines or diuretics, use high quantities of salt in their diet or consume salt tablets, or drink alcohol in large quantities (particularly before activity) will have a higher risk of heat injury. Furthermore, people who participate in physical activity while experiencing fever could elevate their body temperature to dangerous levels. Table 25.5 outlines the various stages of heat illness, the signs and symptoms associated with each, and guidelines for immediate care.

Be aware of environmental factors such as relative humidity and temperature. The relative humidity can be calculated by measuring dry-bulb and wet-bulb atmospheric temperatures (see chapter 10) using a sling psychrometer. As mentioned earlier, evaporation of sweat is a primary means to lose heat during exercise.

• Table 25.5 Heat-Related Problems and Their Treatment •

Heat illness	Signs and symptoms	Immediate care
Heat cramps—spasmodic muscular contractions caused by exertion in extreme heat	Muscle cramping (calf is very common location) Multiple cramping (very serious)	Isolated cramps: Apply pressure to the cramp and release, stretch muscle slowly and gently, apply gentle massage, and ice. Hydrate by drinking lots of water. Multiple cramps: Danger of heatstroke; treat as heat exhaustion.
Heat exhaustion—collapse with or without loss of consciousness, suffered in conditions of heat and high humidity, largely resulting from the loss of fluid and salt by sweating	Profuse sweating Cold, clammy skin Normal or slightly elevated temperature Pale Dizzy Weak, rapid pulse Shallow breathing Nausea Headache Loss of consciousness Thirst	Move individual out of the sun to a well-ventilated area. Place in shock position, with feet elevated 12 to 18 in. (31-46 cm); prevent heat loss or gain. Gently massage the extremities. Apply gentle ROM movement to the extremities. Force consumption of fluids. Reassure the individual. Monitor body temperature and other vital signs. Refer to a physician.
Heatstroke—final stage of heat exhaustion in which the thermoregulatory system shuts down to conserve depleted fluid levels	Generally no perspiration Dry skin Very hot Temperature as high as 106 °F (41.1 °C) Skin color bright red or flushed (dark-pigmented individuals will have ashen skin) Rapid, strong pulse Labored breathing Change in behavior Unresponsive	Treat as an extreme medical emergency. Transport to hospital quickly. Remove as much clothing as possible without exposing the individual. Cool quickly, starting at the head and continuing down the body; use any means possible (fan, hose down, pack in ice). Wrap in cold, wet sheets for transport. Treat for shock; if breathing is labored, place in a semi-reclining position.
Heat syncope—fainting or excessive loss of strength because of excessive heat	Headache Nausea	Normal intake of fluids.

Information from 1-2, 11-15, 30-35.

This fluid loss must be replaced to minimize health risk and maximize safe and enjoyable participation in an exercise program. For most individuals who participate in CRF programs, thirst is an adequate indicator of when to hydrate. Generally, replacing fluids as they are used is the best way to meet the demands of the body. When extreme sweating or dry atmospheric conditions are present, however, the thirst mechanism may not keep up with the need for fluid intake.

Normal daily fluid intake for the sedentary individual is between 60 and 80 oz (1.8-2.4 L). The actual fluid requirement depends on too many factors to establish a single recommendation for maintaining hydration. However, drinking 8 to 10 oz (240-300 ml) of fluid before heavy exercise, in addition to drinking frequently during activity, helps prevent heat illness.

Salt and other minerals may be lost during prolonged exercise, particularly during hot and humid weather. Even so, using **salt tablets** is not recommended unless accompanied by a large intake of water. Water with a 0.1% to 0.2% salt solution may be given to individuals with high water loss. Consuming more salt at mealtimes and a high intake of water throughout the day, however, generally meets the body's need for sodium and fluid replacement.

Most **electrolyte** drinks are diluted solutions of glucose, salt, and other minerals, with added artificial flavoring. Some brands also contain as much as 200 to 300 kcal in 1 qt (946 ml) of solution. Other than sodium, the minerals provided by an electrolyte solution do not provide much benefit. When sweating is profuse, large amounts of electrolyte solution may serve the same function as a diluted salt solution. In cases of mild to moderate sweating, the normal intake of salt in food adequately replaces sodium. The main advantage of using a flavored solution is that the individual might drink more than if ingesting plain water or a salt solution. However, considering the prices of commercially prepared electrolyte solutions, plain water or homemade solutions, such as the one presented next, are much more economical.

Homemade Electrolyte Solution

1 qt (946 ml) water

1/3 tsp. (5 ml) salt

0.5 to 1.5 tbsp. (7-22 ml) sugar for flavoring

Fluids at a temperature of 5 to 15 °C (41-59 °F) are absorbed faster than fluids at other temperatures.

Key Point

Inefficient body cooling mechanisms, certain medications, high intake of salt or alcohol, and exercising with a fever or in high heat and humidity may cause heat-related disorders. Heat illness is potentially deadly, and the fitness professional must be aware of ways to prevent it and must be able to recognize the signs of heat illness and act on them (see table 25.5). Proper hydration, evaluated through a weight chart, is a good first step in prevention. Provide water before, during, and after activity to prevent dehydration.

Cold-Related Problems

Exercising in cold, windy weather can cause problems if certain precautions are not taken. Considerable heat loss can occur through convective heat loss from the skin and evaporation of skin moisture. Hypothermia occurs when body heat is lost at a faster rate than it is produced and core body temperature drops below 35 °C (95 °F). Peripheral blood vessels in cold areas constrict, which conserves body heat but increases the risk of frostbite. Exercising in cold, rainy weather can compound the problem by increasing the rate of evaporation. Windchill is another factor that must be taken into account. A high windchill factor can result in severe loss of body heat even when the air temperature is above freezing. Additionally, body temperature drops even more quickly in cold water than in air of the same temperature. Cold-related problems are preventable if participants follow these precautions:

- Avoid exercising outdoors in extreme cold and wind.
- Layer clothing and remove layers as needed to avoid sweating.
- Warm up before exercise and avoid bouts of inactivity.
- Stay dry.
- Cover the face, nose, ears, fingers, and head (a great deal of heat is lost when the head is exposed).
- Avoid swimming or exercising in cold water, particularly when the surrounding air temperature is low.

Table 25.6 describes how to recognize and treat cold-related problems.

Key Point

Exercising in cold, rainy weather or when the windchill factor is high, as well as exercising in cold water, may lead to cold-related disorders. Precautionary measures such as avoiding exposure to extreme cold, wearing removable layers, warming up before activity, remaining constantly active, and understanding the effect of windchill on air temperature can help prevent cold-related problems. See table 25.6 for specific advice on how to treat cold-related problems.

Medical Concerns

Some individuals have controlled medical conditions that might be aggravated by exercise. In addition, it is important to recognize major cardiovascular and respiratory problems. This section summarizes common medical concerns.

Diabetic Reactions

The fitness professional should be familiar with the signs and symptoms of diabetic coma and insulin shock (see table 25.7). When an emergency arises and a person with diabetes is conscious, she is usually able to name the problem. If the individual cannot tell you the problem, then ask when food was last eaten and whether insulin was taken that day. If the person has eaten but has not taken insulin, then he is probably going into a

Table 25.6 Cold-Related Problems and Their Treatment

Cold-related problems	Signs and symptoms	Immediate care
Deep frostbite—freezing of deep tissue, including muscle and bone	Hard, cold, numb, pale, or white area Permanent damage to tissue may be sustained	Protect body part. Remove jewelry from injured part. Remove from further cold exposure. Handle gently. Refer to a physician. Rapid re-warming is necessary.
Frost nip—freezing of tips of extremities such as ears, nose, or fingers, involving only the surface of the skin	Skin firm and cold Burning, itching, local redness Skin may peel or blister in a day or two	Re-warm by applying firm pressure over the affected area, blowing warm air over the area, submerging in warm water 100 to 105 °F (37.8-40.6 °C), and holding frost-nip area against body.
Superficial frostbite—freezing of layers of skin and subcutaneous tissue	Pale, waxy, and cold skin Purple coloring Following re-warming there may be swelling and superficial blisters Stinging, burning, and aching may be present for several days or weeks	Remove from cold. Re-warm area.
Hypothermia—core body temperature drops below 95 °F (35.0 °C)	Shivering Impairment of neuromuscular function Decreased ability to make decisions Muscle rigidity Hypotension Shock Death	Treat as a medical emergency. Remove from cold. Treat for shock. Immediately transport to hospital.

Information from 1-2, 11-15, 30-34.

Table 25.7 Diabetic Reactions and Their Treatment

Diabetic reaction	Signs and symptoms	Immediate care
Diabetic coma/ hyperglycemia—loss of consciousness caused by too little insulin	Headache Confused Disoriented Stuporous Nauseated coma Skin color—flushed Lips—cherry red Body temperature—decreased; skin—dry Breath odor—sweet, fruity Vomiting Abdominal pain Air hunger Rapid, weak, thready pulse Normal or slightly low BP Unconsciousness	Call for medical assistance. Little can be done unless insulin is at hand. If medical assistance is not quickly available, 1. treat as shock; 2. administer fluids in large amounts by mouth, if individual is conscious; 3. maintain an open airway; 4. turn the head to the side to prevent aspirating vomitus if individual is nauseated; and 5. do not give sugar, carbohydrates, or fats in any form. Recovery—gradual improvement over 6 to 12 hr. Fluid and insulin therapy should be directed by a physician.

Diabetic reaction	Signs and symptoms	Immediate care
Insulin shock/ hypoglycemia—anxiety, excitement, perspiration, delirium, or coma caused by too much insulin or not enough carbohydrates to balance insulin intake	Skin color—pale (dark-pigmented individuals will appear ashen) Skin temperature—moist and clammy; cold sweat Pulse—normal or rapid and bounding Blood pressure—normal or slightly elevated Breathing—normal or shallow and slow Weakness on one side of the body No odor of acetone on breath Intense hunger Possible double vision Unusual behavior—confused, aggressive, lethargic Fainting, seizure, coma, or unconsciousness	Administer sugar as quickly as possible (e.g., administer orange juice, candy). If individual is unconscious, place sugar granules under the tongue. If individual is unconscious or recovery is slow, call for medical assistance. Recovery—generally quick; 1 or 2 min. Refer to a physician if still unconscious or recovery is slow.

Information from 1-2, 11-15, 21, 23.

diabetic coma, a condition in which there is too little insulin to fully metabolize the carbohydrate consumed (hyperglycemia). If the individual has taken insulin but has not eaten, then she probably is experiencing insulin shock, a condition in which there is too much insulin or not enough carbohydrate to balance the insulin intake (hypoglycemia).

If the individual lapses into unconsciousness, check for a medical-alert identification tag to try to identify the problem. If you don't know whether the individual is suffering from diabetic coma or insulin shock, give sugar. Brain damage or death can occur quickly if insulin shock is left untreated; it is a far more critical state than diabetic coma. If the problem is insulin shock, the individual should respond quickly, within 1 to 2 min; at that point transport the person to a hospital as quickly as possible. If the individual is in a diabetic coma, there is little chance of seriously worsening the condition by giving sugar. Several hours of fluid and insulin therapy will be needed, under a physician's direction. Table 25.7 outlines the diabetic reactions, their signs and symptoms, and the immediate care of each.

Cardiovascular and Pulmonary Complications

Cardiovascular complications can occur with injury because of decreased circulating blood volumes, as may occur with bleeding, hyperthermia or hypothermia, shock, or heart attack. The fitness professional should be able to recognize and deal with potential complications such as **tachycardia** (excessively rapid heartbeat), **bradycardia** (abnormally slow heartbeat), hypertension (high blood pressure), and **hypotension** (low blood pressure).

Key Point

Diabetic coma results from hyperglycemia, and insulin shock is attributable to hypoglycemia.

Pulmonary complications may be observed more readily. **Apnea,** or temporary cessation of breathing, can be caused by an obstructed airway, allergic reaction, drowning, or intrathoracic injury. Dyspnea, or labored breathing, can be caused by hyperventilation, asthma, and chest or lung injury. **Tachypnea,** excessively rapid breathing, may be a sign of overexertion, shock, or hyperventilation. The fitness professional should feel comfortable assessing circulation and respiration and have the knowledge and skills to perform appropriate emergency procedures.

Most common respiratory disorders include hyperventilation, asthma, and airway obstruction. Hyperventilation can occur with heavy exhalation or rapid breathing, resulting in breathing out too much carbon dioxide (CO_2) and thereby reducing CO_2 levels in the blood. Low CO_2 levels may cause dizziness, faintness, chest pains, and tingling in the feet and hands. Reassuring the person in a calm manner, encouraging a slower breathing rate, and helping the person breathe into a paper bag or into hands cupped over the nose and mouth will help restore CO_2 levels.

Asthma is a condition in which the smooth muscles of the bronchial tubes go into spasm; edema and inflammation of the mucous lining are triggered by exercise, changes in barometric pressure or temperature, virus, emotional upset, and noxious odors. The affected individual may appear anxious, pale, and sweaty; may cough or wheeze; and may seem short of breath. Hyperventilation may occur, resulting in dizziness, and, because of mucous secretions, the individual may frequently try to clear the throat.

The fitness professional should be prepared to handle an asthma attack. Generally, people with asthma know how to care for themselves and carry medication. Individuals with exercise-induced asthma are often prescribed medication to take before activity. Encourage people with asthma to drink water, and promote relaxation and breathing exercises. Remove any known irritants from the environment if possible. If bronchial spasm is excessive, seek medical attention.

Airway obstruction can occur when a foreign object or the tongue blocks the airway. If breathing is labored but the person is coughing forcefully, stay with the person and encourage continued coughing. If, however, the person is unsuccessful in expelling the object or the airway becomes totally blocked, have someone call for an ambulance and begin abdominal thrusts (**Heimlich maneuver**). In an unconscious person, visually checking the airway passage or performing a finger sweep or Heimlich maneuver may dislodge a known obstruction. Generally, moving the lower jaw forward or tilting the head and lifting the chin will open an airway blocked by the tongue. **Rescue breathing** should be performed if the person has stopped breathing and repositioning the head does not change the status.

Respiratory shock, a condition in which the lungs are unable to supply enough oxygen to the circulating blood, can result in a medical emergency. Signs and symptoms include paleness of skin or cyanosis; weak, rapid pulse; rapid, shallow breathing; decreased BP; changes in personality including disinterest, irritability, restlessness, and excitement; extreme thirst; and in severe cases, urinary retention and fecal incontinence.

Treatment includes maintaining body heat and elevating feet and legs 12 to 18 in. (31-46 cm). If head or neck injury is suspected, protect the involved area and raise the head and shoulders by placing a pillow or rolled up blanket underneath the individual. Keep the participant warm, reassure them and seek medical attention. Employ cardiopulmonary resuscitation (CPR) techniques (see pages 393 and 395).

Key Point

Common cardiovascular complications from exercise include excessively rapid or abnormally slow heartbeat and high or low BP. Pulmonary complications include temporary cessation of breathing, labored breathing, and airway obstruction.

Common Orthopedic Problems

Many injuries that are commonly referred to an orthopedic physician for diagnosis and treatment result from overuse or irritation of a chronic musculoskeletal problem. In most instances, the injuries do not immediately incapacitate the participant. It may be weeks or months after the onset of pain before the participant seeks medical consultation. By this time, the inflammation is severe and generally prevents normal function of the part involved. In many cases, a severe injury can be avoided if proper care is initiated early. Table 25.8 outlines common orthopedic problems, their causes, their signs and symptoms, and general treatment guidelines.

Shin Splints

Shin splint is a catchall expression used to describe a variety of conditions of the lower leg. The term shin splints is often used to define any pain located between the knee and the ankle (usually anterior medial and lateral). Diagnosis of shin splints should be limited to conditions involving inflammation of the musculotendinous unit caused by overexertion of muscles during weight-bearing activity. A more specific diagnosis is preferred over the general term *shin splint.* In any event, the physician must rule out the following conditions: stress fracture, metabolic or vascular disorder, **compartment syndrome,** and muscular strain. The physical complaints often accompanying shin splint pain include the following:

- A dull ache in the lower leg after workouts
- Decreased performance and work output because of pain
- Soft-tissue pain
- Mild swelling along the area of inflammation
- Slight temperature elevation at the site of inflammation
- Pain when moving the foot up and down

People with shin splints usually have no history of trauma. The symptoms start gradually and progress if activity is not reduced. The following is the usual symptomatic treatment:

- Rest in the acute stage; reduce weight-bearing activity.
- In mild cases brought on by overuse, decrease or modify activity for a few days (e.g., choose swimming or bicycle workouts instead of running).
- Apply heat or ice before activity; use ice after activity. Heat treatments may consist of applying moist heat packs for 15 to 20 min or using a whirlpool. The temperature of the whirlpool water should

be approximately 100 to 106 °F (37.8-41.1 °C). Treatment time is usually 15 to 20 min. Ice treatment may consist of applying an ice bag for 15 to 20 min or applying ice massage or ice slush for 5 to 7 min.

Treatment should begin at the first sign of pain. If pain is extreme, the participant should see a doctor. Determining and treating the cause, in addition to symptomatic treatment, are necessary to prevent recurrence. Table 25.9 cites the major causes for shin splints as well as the signs and symptoms and steps that can be taken to prevent the onset or recurrence of lower-leg pain.

Exercise Modification

Most orthopedic injuries can be classified as mild, moderate, or severe. When in doubt, conservative treatment is recommended. Any injury that results in acute pain or affects performance and any injury in which the individual hears or feels a pop at the time of injury should be referred to a physician. If conservative measures fail to improve the condition within a reasonable time (2-4 wk), physician consultation is again recommended.

Other conditions may call for modifying the exercise program. The participant may be obese or arthritic or may have a history of musculoskeletal problems. Exercise in a pool is often employed with such individuals since warm water is therapeutic, supports the body weight, and generally allows for a greater range of movement. In any case, the activity should suit the condition. Anyone who requires exercise modification should be monitored closely. Table 25.10 summarizes the general guidelines for classifying injuries and offers suggestions for modifying activity.

Table 25.8 Common Orthopedic Problems and Their Treatment

Injury	Common causes	Signs and symptoms	Treatment
Inflammatory reactions **Bursitis—** inflammation of bursa (sac between a muscle and bone that is filled with fluid, facilitates motion, pads and helps to prevent abnormal function) **Capsulitis—**inflammation of the joint capsule **Epicondylitis—** inflammation of muscles or tendons attached to the epicondyles of the humerus **Myositis—**inflammation of voluntary muscle **Plantar fasciitis—** inflammation of connective tissue that spans the bottom of the foot **Tendinitis—**inflammation of a tendon (a band of tough, inelastic, fibrous tissue that connects muscle to bone) **Tenosynovitis—** inflammation of a tendinous sheath **Synovitis—**inflammation of the synovial membrane (a highly vascularized tissue that lines articular surfaces)	Overuse Improper joint mechanics Improper technique Pathology Trauma Infection	Redness Swelling Pain Increased skin temperature over the area of inflammation Tenderness Involuntary muscle guarding	Ice and rest in the acute stages. If chronic, generally use heat before exercise or activity, followed by ice after activity. Massage. Perform muscle stretching exercises. Correct the cause of problem. If correction of the cause and symptomatic treatment do not relieve symptoms, refer to a physician; anti-inflammatory medication is usually prescribed. If disease process or infection is suspected, refer to a physician immediately.

(continued)

• Table 25.8 Common Orthopedic Problems and Their Treatment *(continued)* •

Injury	Common causes	Signs and symptoms	Treatment
Tennis elbow—inflammation of the musculotendinous unit of the elbow extensors where they attach on the outer aspect of the elbow (lateral epicondylitis)	Faulty backhand mechanics—faults may include leading with the elbow, using an improper grip, dropping the racket head, or using a topspin backhand with a whipping motion Improper grip size— usually too small Racket strung too tightly Improper hitting— hitting off center, particularly if using wet, heavy balls Overuse of forearm supinators, wrist extensors, and finger extensors	Pain directly over the outer aspect of the elbow in region of the common extensor origin Swelling Increased skin temperature over the area of inflammation Pain on extension of the middle finger against resistance with the elbow extended Pain upon racket gripping and extension of the wrist	Ice and rest in the acute stages. If chronic, generally use heat before exercise or activity, followed by ice after activity. Apply deep friction massage at the elbow. Perform strengthening and stretching exercises for the wrist extensors. Correct the cause of problem: 1. Use proper techniques. 2. Use proper grip size (when racket is gripped, there should be room for one finger to fit in the gap between the thumb and fingers). 3. Use racket that is strung at the proper tension (usually between 50 and 55 lb, or between 22.7 and 25.0 kg. 4. Avoid stiff rackets that vibrate easily. Keep elbow warm, particularly in cold weather. Use a counter force brace, a circular band that is placed just below the elbow (to reduce the stress at the origin of the extensors). If correction of cause and symptomatic treatment do not relieve symptoms, refer to a physician; anti-inflammatory medication is usually prescribed.

Injury	Common causes	Signs and symptoms	Treatment
Mechanical low-back pain— low-back pain that results from poor body mechanics, inflexibility of certain muscle groups, or muscular weakness	Tight low-back musculature Tight hamstrings Poor posture or postural habits Weak trunk musculature, particularly abdominal muscles Differences in leg length because of a structural or functional problem Structural abnormality Obesity	Generalized low-back pain, usually aggravated by activity that accentuates the curve in the low back (e.g., hill running) Muscle spasm Palpable tenderness that is limited to musculature and not located directly over the spine Possible difference in pelvic height or other signs that indicate a possible leg-length discrepancy Muscle tightness, particularly of the hamstrings, hip flexors, and low back	Refer any individual with acute onset of low-back pain or any signs of nerve impingement to a physician for evaluation and X ray. Rule out structural abnormalities such as spondylolisthesis, ruptured disc, fracture, neoplasm, or possible segmental instability before instituting a general exercise program. Further diagnostic procedures may be warranted. Symptomatic treatment consists of ice application and referral to physician in acute cases. Chronic cases are generally treated with moist heat to reduce muscle spasm and ice after activity. Correct the causes of low-back pain: 1. Stretch tight muscles. 2. Strengthen weak muscles. 3. Thoroughly warm up before activity and cool down following activity. 4. Correct leg-length differences. 5. Emphasize correct postural positions. 6. If possible, correct or compensate for structural abnormalities (e.g., orthotics for a biomechanical problem).

Information from 11, 14-16, 26.

• Table 25.9 Shin Splint Syndrome •

Injury	Common causes	Signs and symptoms	Treatment
Shin splints— inflammatory reaction of the musculotendinous unit, caused by overexertion of muscles during weight-bearing activity (following conditions must be ruled out: stress fracture, metabolic or vascular disorder, compartment syndrome, muscular strain)	Prominent callus in metatarsal region Fallen metatarsal arch Weak longitudinal arch Muscular imbalance Poor leg, ankle, and foot flexibility Improper running surface Improper running shoes Overuse Biomechanical problems or structural abnormalities Improper running or skills technique Training in poor weather	Lower longitudinal arch on one side in comparison to the opposite side Tenderness in arch area Abnormal wear patterns of shoes	Keep callus filed down. Wear a metatarsal arch pad. Conduct strengthening exercises for toe flexors. Wear longitudinal arch tape for support. Wear arch supports. Conduct strengthening exercises for the dorsiflexors and inverters. Exercise to increase ROM. Avoid hard surfaces. Avoid changing from one surface to another. Select a shoe that absorbs shock well; be sure that the shoe is properly fitted. Be flexible about changing the training program if there are signs that a great deal of physical stress is occurring. Encourage year-round conditioning. Always warm up properly. Refer to podiatrist or other professional specializing in foot care; orthotics may be indicated. Design a special training program to allow for individual differences (e.g., increase intensity of workouts and reduce duration). Correct technique. Perform specific stretching or strengthening exercises as well as technique work. Use common sense when training in cold or foul weather. Dress properly to maintain warmth. Warm up and cool down properly.
Stress fracture— bone defect that occurs because of overstress to weight-bearing bones, which accelerates the rate of remodeling; inability of bone to meet the demands of the stress results in loss of continuity in the bone and periosteal irritation Tibial stress fractures—more common in individuals with high arches in feet Fibula stress fractures—more common in pronators	Overuse or abrupt change in training program Change in running surface Change in running gait	Referred pain to the fracture site when a percussion test is used (e.g., hitting the heel may cause pain at the site of a tibial stress fracture) Pain usually localized to one spot and exquisitely tender to palpation Pain generally present all of the time but increases with weight-bearing activity; no lessening of pain after warm-up	Refer to physician. X rays should be obtained. Usually no crack is detected in the bone. A cloudy area becomes visible when the callus begins to form. Often this does not show up until 2 to 6 wk after onset of pain. Early detection can usually be made through a bone scan or thermogram. If a stress fracture is suspected but not diagnosed, treat as a stress fracture. Running and other high-stress, weight-bearing activities should not be allowed until the fracture has healed and the bone is no longer tender to palpation. Tibial stress fractures usually take 8 to 10 wk to heal; fibula stress fractures take approximately 6 wk. When acute symptoms have subsided, bicycling and swimming activities can usually be initiated to maintain cardiovascular levels. This should be cleared with the supervising physician. If a specific cause is attributed to the development of a stress fracture, steps should be taken to correct the cause.

Information from 3, 7-8, 11-17, 20-26, 29, 31.

Cardiopulmonary Resuscitation (CPR) and Emergency Procedures

All fitness professionals should be well versed in **cardiopulmonary resuscitation** (CPR) techniques. (Courses are generally available through the local American Heart Association [AHA] or the American Red Cross [ARC].) In an emergency situation there is little time to think, and most reactions occur automatically. Having a plan of action and routinely practicing the plan help to ensure that proper **emergency procedures** are followed in these situations (1-15).

Basic Emergency Plan

First, *be prepared.* Carry a cell phone, or make sure a phone is available for use during the exercise class, and know where the phone is located. If a phone is not available, have an alternative emergency plan in mind. The fitness professional should identify the **emergency medical system (EMS)** and services (e.g., ambulance, hospital, doctor) that are to be used and keep a phone list in a convenient location. Decide who is to phone for medical help in an emergency situation, and make sure that person knows how to direct help to the location of the injured individual. All necessary medical information (e.g., release forms, medical history forms) should be readily available, and all emergency equipment and supplies (e.g., stretcher, emergency kit and supplies, automated external defibrillator, splints, ice, inhaler, money for phone call, blanket, spine board) should be easily accessible. The equipment should be checked periodically to ensure that it is in proper working order, and the supplies should be up to date. And, of course, know where the fire alarms and fire exits are located.

Remain calm to reassure the injured person and help prevent the onset of shock. Clear thinking allows for sound judgment and proper execution of rehearsed plans. In most instances, speed is not necessary. Cases of extreme breathing difficulty, stopped breathing or circulation, choking, severe bleeding, shock, head or neck injury, heat illness, and internal injury are exceptions and require urgent action. Otherwise, careful evaluation and a deliberate plan of action are desirable. The fitness professional should have a system for evaluating and dealing with life-threatening situations. All procedures should be conducted calmly and professionally.

Determine the history of the injury from direct observation of what happened, the injured person's account of what happened, or a witness's account of the injury. If the injured person is unconscious or semiconscious

Table 25.10 Injury Classification Criteria and Exercise Modifications

Criteria	Modifications
Mild injury Performance is not affected. Pain is experienced only after athletic activity. Generally, no tenderness is felt on palpation. No or minimal swelling is present. No discoloration is apparent.	Reduce activity level, modify activity to take stress off of the injured part, treat symptomatically, and gradually return to full activity.
Moderate injury Performance is mildly affected or not affected at all. Pain is experienced before and after athletic activity. Mild tenderness is felt on palpation. Mild swelling may be present. Some discoloration may be present.	Rest the injured part, modify activity to take stress off of the injured part, treat symptomatically, and gradually return to full activity.
Severe injury Pain is experienced before, during, and after activity. Performance is definitely affected because of pain. Movement is limited because of pain. Moderate to severe point tenderness is felt on palpation. Swelling is most likely present. Discoloration may be present.	Rest completely and see a physician.

From D.D. Arnheim, 1987, *Essentials of athletic training* (St. Louis: Times Mirror/Mosby).

and no cause is determined, check for a medical-alert identification tag.

Check vital signs—heart rate (HR), breathing, blood pressure (BP), and bleeding—to determine the seriousness of the situation. This evaluation will identify a course of action.

Checking Vital Signs

The following paragraphs describe vital signs and how to monitor each. Important vital signs to check include the pulse, color, body temperature, mobility, and BP of the injured person.

Check HR. Use light finger pressure over an artery to monitor pulse rate. The most common sites for checking HR are the carotid, brachial, radial, and femoral pulses. If there is no pulse and the individual is unconscious, begin CPR. The average heart rate for an adult is between 60 and 100 beats · min^{-1}.

Assess color. For light-pigmented individuals, if skin, fingernail beds, lips, sclera of eyes, and mucous membranes are red or flushed, heatstroke, high blood pressure, carbon monoxide poisoning, fever, and sunburn are possible. If the person is pale or ashen, changes in skin color could be attributable to shock, fright, insufficient circulation, heat exhaustion, insulin shock, or a heart attack. If the person is bluish, the poor oxygenation of the blood could be the result of airway obstruction, respiratory insufficiency, heart failure, or some poisonings. For dark-pigmented individuals, assess nail beds, the inside of the lips, the mouth, and the tongue. Pink is the normal color for these; a bluish cast suggests shock. A grayish cast suggests shock from **hemorrhage.** A red flush at the tips of the ears suggests fever.

Take body temperature. Normal body temperature is 98.6 °F (37.0 °C). Record temperature with a thermometer placed under the tongue (for 3 min); in the axilla, or armpit (10 min); or in the rectum (1 min). Cool, clammy, damp skin suggests shock or heat exhaustion; cool, dry skin indicates exposure to cold air; and hot, dry skin suggests fever or heatstroke.

Check mobility. Inability to move (paralysis) suggests injury or illness of the spinal cord or brain.

Take blood pressure (BP). BP usually is taken at the brachial artery with a BP cuff and sphygmomanometer. The following results will help determine the problem:

- Normal BP—in men, systolic blood pressure SBP, the pressure during the contraction phase of the heart, is equal to 100 plus the age of the individual up to 140 to 150 mmHg; diastolic blood pressure (DBP), the pressure during the relaxation phase of the heart, is equal to 65 to 90 mmHg. In women, both readings are generally 8 to 10 mmHg lower.
- Severe hemorrhage, heart attack—marked decrease (20-30 mmHg) in BP.
- Damage or rupture of vessels in the arterial circuit—BP is abnormally high (>150 SBP/>90 DBP).
- Brain damage—increase in SBP with a stable or falling DBP.
- Heart ailment—decrease in SBP with an increase in DBP.

Questions to Determine Action

Ask the following questions to help determine a course of action for treating injured participants.

Is the individual conscious? If not, a head, neck, or back injury is possible. If you are unsure as to why the individual is unconscious, check for a medical-alert identification tag. Assess airway, breathing, and circulation. Do not use ammonia capsules to arouse the person; he may jerk the head backward in response, causing additional injury. If breathing has stopped and the individual is in a prone position, log-roll as carefully as possible, keeping the head, neck, and spine in the same relative position, to begin CPR.

If the individual is unconscious but breathing, protect against further injury. Do not move the person unless their life is in danger. Wait for medical assistance to arrive. Systematically evaluate the entire body and perform necessary first-aid procedures.

Is the individual breathing? If not, establish an airway and administer artificial respiration. Summon medical help. The following information will aid in determining why the person has stopped breathing.

- Normal respiration—20 breaths · min^{-1}
- Respiration in well-trained individuals—6 to 8 breaths · min^{-1}
- Shock—rapid, shallow respiration
- Airway obstruction, heart disease, pulmonary disease—deep, gasping, labored breathing
- Lung damage—frothy sputum with blood at the nose and mouth, accompanied by coughing
- Diabetic acidosis—alcoholic or sweet, fruity odor to breath
- Cessation of breathing—abdomen and chest movement and airflow at nose and mouth have ceased

Is the individual bleeding profusely? If so, control bleeding by elevating the body part; applying direct pressure over the wound or at **pressure points;** and, as a last resort, putting on a tourniquet. A tourniquet should only be used in life-threatening situations in which risking a limb is a reasonable action to save a life. Treat for shock.

Key Point

When an exercise participant is injured, check for consciousness, breathing, and bleeding as well as head, neck, or back injuries. Take a pulse, temperature, and BP reading according to the guidelines in the previous section.

Is there evidence of a head injury? Head injury is indicated by a history of a blow to the head or a fall on the head, deformity of the skull, loss of consciousness, clear or straw-colored fluid coming from the nose or ears, unequal pupil size, dizziness, loss of memory, and nausea. Prevent any unnecessary movement. If it is necessary to move the person, use a stretcher and keep the individual's head elevated. If the individual is unconscious, assume there is also a neck injury. Summon medical help immediately. The following information will help determine the reason for head injury:

- Drug abuse or nervous system disorder—constricted pupils
- Unconscious, cardiac arrest—dilated pupils
- Head injury—pupils are unequal size
- Disease, poisoning, drug overdose, injury—pupils do not react to light
- Death—pupils widely dilated and unresponsive to light

Is there evidence of a neck or back injury? The history of the injury may provide a clue. Other indications of a possible neck or back injury include pain directly over the spine, burning or tingling in the extremities, and loss of muscle function or strength in the extremities. When in doubt, assume there is a neck or back injury. The following information will aid in determining the injury:

- Probable injury of spinal cord—numbness or tingling in the extremities
- Occlusion of a main artery—severe pain in the extremity, with loss of cutaneous sensation
- Hysteria, violent shock, excessive drug or alcohol use—no pain

Rescue Breathing, CPR, and Using the Automated External Defibrillator

Cardiac arrest is the single leading cause of death in the United States, leading to more than 350,000 deaths each year. An abnormal, chaotic heart rhythm known as *ventricular fibrillation* (see chapter 24) keeps the heart from filling with blood. When started early enough, CPR can keep oxygen flowing to the brain, but it cannot correct or restore a normal heartbeat. Shocking the heart with an electrical impulse often restores the sinus rhythm. The sooner the shock is delivered, the greater the chance of survival. The automated external defibrillator (AED) allows rescuers with limited experience and training to defibrillate a heart. The AED has significantly increased the survival rate of individuals experiencing myocardial infarction (MI). In another situation, the participant may stop breathing and not be undergoing cardiac arrest. In this case, rescue breathing (RB) helps restore breathing, but pulse should also be checked to ensure that the heart is pumping blood throughout the body. A pulse may be faint or undetectable and the rescuer may believe that an individual requires both CPR and the AED or just one or the other. If no pulse is found, CPR should be started until the AED is available. The AED allows the rescuer to prepare to shock but has a safety device to ensure that a shock is not delivered unless needed. The fitness professional should be trained and prepared to use any of the previously mentioned techniques, CPR, RB and the AED, to restore breathing and blood flow in a potentially fatal situation involving a participant. The following discussion outlines the steps the American Heart Association teaches for RB, CPR, and using the AED. The fitness professional should review current recommended techniques (4).

If a participant appears to have stopped breathing, RB should be initiated. If the fitness professional finds that breathing has stopped and there is no pulse, the AED (if readily available) should be used or CPR should be started immediately. Although the steps for RB and CPR techniques are for adults only, the fitness professional should review current recommended techniques for all age categories (adults, children, and infants). The following is a list of steps to use in rescuing an unconscious person:

1. Check the scene for safety and to help determine probable cause for collapse.
2. Check the person for injuries and responsiveness as well as for any additional clues about the cause of collapse.
3. Determine responsiveness by gently shaking or tapping the individual and asking if he is OK.
4. If you are alone and the person is unresponsive, immediately call for help, get any needed supplies and the AED if close by, and determine whether the person should be moved before you begin the rescue attempt. If there are other people around, instruct one bystander to call for help and another

to get needed supplies and the AED, and cautiously move the individual if safety dictates moving. Then begin the rescue attempt, following basic precautions for preventing disease transmission.

5. Look, listen, and feel for breathing. If the person is not breathing, and if necessary, move the individual to a face-up position while supporting the head and neck. Reposition the neck by using a head tilt and chin lift or jaw thrust and reassess. If the person is still not breathing, pinch the nose shut, cover the mouth with yours, and give two slow breaths. Then assess circulation by sliding the index and middle finger of one hand into the groove at the side of his neck closest toward you. Take no more than 10 sec to check the carotid pulse.
6. If there is a pulse but the person is still not breathing, initiate RB at a rate of one breath every 5-6 sec. Recheck for signs of circulation and breathing every 2 min.
7. If there is no breathing but circulation is still present, continue RB.
8. If there is no breathing or pulse, begin using the AED and CPR; if the AED is not readily available, begin CPR and continue until the AED arrives.
9. If CPR is initiated, place two fingers above the xiphoid process at the lower end of the sternal notch, place the heel of one hand above the two fingers in the middle of the sternum, and place the second hand on top. Interlace fingers and lift off of the chest wall. With your shoulders positioned over your hands, compress the chest 1.5 to 2 in. (3.8-5.1 cm). Give 30 compressions and two rescue breaths at a rate of 100 compressions $\cdot$ min^{-1} for an adult. Continue for five cycles or 2 min and recheck for signs of circulation. If there is no circulation, continue CPR, checking circulation every few minutes. If the AED is ready to use, recheck the pulse, and if you find no pulse, follow the steps as outlined next.
10. Turn on the AED. Do not use the AED near alcohol or any other flammable material, in a moving vehicle, on a person lying on a conductive surface or in water.
    - Use caution when using an AED on an individual weighing less than 55 lb (24.9 kg) or less than 8 yrs old. Try 5 cycles or 2 min of CPR before using the AED.
    - Use children's pads and a child's shock dosage if available. If using adult pads, the pads should not touch
    - Do not use cellular phones within 6 ft (1.8 m) of the AED.
    - To use the defibrillator, perform the following steps:
      1. Wipe the person's chest dry.
      2. Remove any metal on or around the person, including a bra with underwire and clothing with metal hooks.
      3. Remove any patches on chest, such as a transdermal medication patch, with a gloved hand.
      4. Attach the pads as instructed, one to the upper right of the chest and the other on the individual's lower left side.
      5. Plug the electrode into the AED. Follow the instructions as the computerized voice runs you through the various steps in using the AED.
      6. Be ready to analyze the person's heart rhythm.
      7. Make sure no one is touching the individual; advise people to stand clear; push the analyze button.
      8. The AED will analyze the rhythm and will instruct to shock or to begin CPR.
      9. If a shock is advised, anyone near the scene should be instructed to stand back; deliver the shock by pushing the shock button.
      10. The AED will then analyze the rhythm again.
      11. If the AED advises that no shock is needed, check the pulse again; if there is no pulse, begin CPR until the AED reanalyzes.

If a second rescuer is available and the initial rescuer gets tired, the second rescuer can prepare the AED (if available) for use or can take over CPR at the end of a cycle of 30 compressions. Two person CPR is conducted in a cycle of 15 compressions and 2 breaths at a rate of 100 compressions $\cdot$ min^{-1}.

Emergencies are difficult to predict. Therefore, all individuals of qualifying age should go through basic life saving training techniques through a reputable organization such as the American Heart Association or the American Red Cross and maintain current certification. Because recommendations may change based on current research, it is important to learn correct techniques to avoid unnecessary injuries to the victim and to have optimal outcomes.

Key Point

Fitness professionals should update their training regularly to keep informed about the latest technology for dealing with these emergency situations.

Case Studies

You can check your answers by referring to page 476 in appendix A.

1. You are instructing an aerobics class when a participant collapses. On approaching the individual, you note that breathing is shallow and slow and that the skin color is pale, moist, and clammy. The individual is conscious but not alert, reports double vision and an intense hunger, and is wearing a medical-alert tag.
    a. What illness do you suspect?
    b. What questions do you ask?
    c. What action should you take?
2. You are leading an aerobics class and a participant collapses. You observe that the participant's skin is dry and red, breathing is labored, and pulse is rapid and strong. No trauma was experienced.
    a. What heat-related illness should be suspected?
    b. What is the immediate care?
    c. What emergency planning should be in effect?

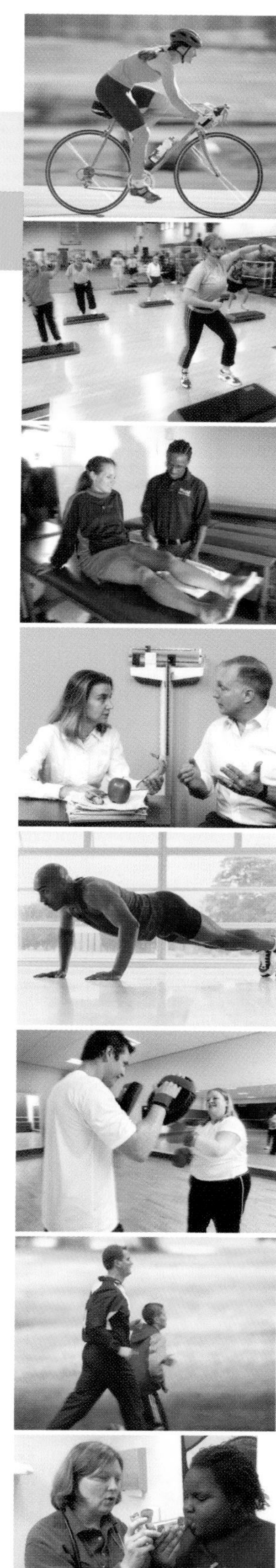

CHAPTER 26

Program Administration and Management

Michael Shipe

Objectives

The reader will be able to do the following:

1. Describe the necessity and application of long-term planning for fitness facilities.
2. Describe the personnel and working environment recommended for a fitness program.
3. Identify the five aspects of a comprehensive fitness program.
4. Address potential legal issues for fitness programs.
5. Explain capital and operating budgets.
6. Describe the recommended equipment for a fitness program.
7. Describe the importance of proper documentation for all fitness programs.

The fitness industry has grown prodigiously during the last 20 yr. Today, fitness facilities operate in a highly competitive marketplace, in either direct or indirect competition with locally or regionally based facilities, national franchises, and hospital-based exercise facilities. The keys to success for today's exercise facilities include exemplary customer service, a certified and well-trained staff, programming for a variety of populations, and a vast array of exercise equipment provided in a safe and meticulous facility. Altogether, these services must be offered at a monthly fee commensurate with those of competing fitness facilities. An outline of how the fitness facility will excel in each of these components should be provided in a strategic operational plan, which should state contemporary (1 yr) and long-term (3-5 yr) objectives. Facility staff members should understand how their job responsibilities assist the overall goals for the facility. Based on the fitness facility's target population, varying standards of screening, supervision, and equipment availability are necessary. This chapter outlines successful program administration for facilities with predominantly healthy populations.

Strategic Operational Planning

If you have a large source of raw materials and instructions to build a house, the next logical step is to design a blueprint to guide the construction process. In kind, proper planning is essential to any successful business. The following sections address the various areas that, when managed properly, can lead to successful daily and long-term fitness facility operations. These recommendations consider successful program administration as well as facility guidelines championed by the AHA and ACSM (2, 3, 4).

In most fitness facilities, the program director is an experienced fitness professional who manages a staff of 8 to 20 employees. The director's typical job responsibilities entail the following:

- Developing and implementing a sound capital and operational budget
- Hiring, supervising, training, and evaluating personnel
- Delineating the protocols for preparticipation screening, equipment orientation, and exercise prescription for new members, including special populations
- Determining where, when, and what programs and classes will be offered for specific populations
- Ensuring a safe and clean exercise environment
- Encouraging continual communication among staff members as well as between staff members and exercise participants
- Maintaining quality control

All organizations maintain a mission statement that clearly defines their purpose and operational objectives. Proper management comes from following a systematic approach designed to increase the effectiveness and efficiency of operations in order to accomplish the goals of the facility more readily (7). A program director should devise contemporary and long-term plans for successfully meeting the facility's mission statement.

Long-Term Planning

Long-term plans should address goals (e.g., greater revenue generation), resources required to accomplish these goals (e.g., capital expenditures and personnel), and explicit plans to attain these objectives (e.g., exercise programs focusing on the facility's target population, retention programs). Essentially, the program director needs to draw a map that directs the employees and programs of the facility from where they presently are to where they should be in the next 3 to 5 yr.

An example of a fitness facility developing long-term planning may involve how they can increase their annual revenues during the next 3 yr. To obtain this goal, they identify the best target population—the senior population. Next, the facility designs specific programs to attract this population, such as a warm water based group exercise program, PACE (people with arthritis can exercise) classes, and monthly education classes addressing common challenges for this population. The financial cost of each program should be determined as well. These programs can be implemented incrementally and should be evaluated annually to determine their financial viability and their ability to attract new participants as well as their contribution to customer satisfaction.

Directors should plan in conjunction with the administration of the facility and consider input from pertinent employees and participants. Program administrators must understand what their supervisors want to achieve while simultaneously understanding what their participants desire for customer service. Knowing the requirements of the administrators and customers determines what the facility will offer regarding facility layout, exercise program, equipment, personnel, and supplies. Depending on how capital intensive a given plan is, it may not be implemented for months or even years, while others can be offered immediately.

Short-Term Planning

Short-term plans form a subset of the facility's long-term plans. Adhering to a short-term planning structure ensures that contemporary plans are consistent with the mission statement for the facility. For instance, if facility utilization is a long-term, ongoing objective, what programs can be developed and implemented in the next month to achieve this goal? A program designed to reward participants who utilize the facility 12 or more times in the next 30 days would be feasible and would help improve facility utilization. Each participant who meets the program's attendance criteria could be entered in a drawing to win a gift certificate to a local business. Rather than always seeking the administration's input for short-term planning, program directors should work closely with their staff and participants to determine what they can do to improve customer satisfaction immediately. Short-term planning is akin to the protocol addressed for long-term planning (e.g., specific goals, resources, and programs should be determined), but the plans must be practical in the consideration that resources are smaller and planning time is significantly shorter.

Key Point

Short- and long-term strategic operational planning provides the framework for how the facility will achieve its mission. The program director should compile recommendations from administration, employees, and participants to design the current programs that will help attain the long-term goals.

Quality and Program Assessment

Exercise facilities continually change the programs they offer in order to improve their customer service and retention rates. The program administrator must decide which programs should be continued, revised, or eliminated. Program decisions can be facilitated by performing annual program quality assessments. Ideally, each program will make a profit while fulfilling the facility's mission statement. Formal evaluation criteria should be developed to determine each program's specific contribution to the facility. Examples of health and fitness facility program quality evaluations may entail direct (e.g., revenue, lower health care costs, less absenteeism from work) and indirect (e.g., client satisfaction, safety, contribution of program to customer service) monetary contribution criteria (3). Many indirect benefits of an exercise program are not readily quantifiable, and they must be estimated. Thus, administrators should focus on direct monetary program contributions when they are attempting to financially justify a given program. Altogether, the program administrator must judge the value of a specific program's benefits using the best information available including financial records, employee input, and customer feedback. Each program's evaluation outcomes should be considered in the context of whether or not it satisfies the facility's mission statement. By doing so, the facility will provide programs which increase its client population, improve customer service and help ensure the safety and efficacy of its services (3).

Key Point

Evaluating a fitness program is a continual process to ensure that the program significantly contributes to the facility's mission statement.

Managing and Evaluating Personnel

Given that program directors often spend considerable time addressing administrative responsibilities, it is imperative that they hire staff who not only are qualified professionally but demonstrate exemplary interpersonal skills. Successful managers dedicate a significant amount of time to recruiting, hiring, supporting, and evaluating their personnel. By doing so, they work toward the mission of the facility while fostering the professional growth of their employees.

Finding Qualified Staff

After determining what programs to offer, program directors must decide how to staff each program. A typical fitness facility requires the following personnel:

Full-Time

- Wellness director
- Fitness director
- Fitness specialist
- Membership or marketing manager
- Secretary

Part-Time

- Medical advisor (typically available only in clinic based programs)
- Dietitian (typically available only in clinic based programs)
- Health educator
- Receptionist for front desk
- Equipment technician
- Cleaning staff

Contract

- Instructors for leading group exercise
- Fitness professionals

Specific qualifications required of all personnel should be established, including education, professional experience, certifications (if necessary), and interpersonal skills. The minimum requirements for a certain position can be derived from an appropriate certification (e.g., ACSM, NSCA) for that position (see Sample Job Description). Establishing uniform qualifications for each type of position helps to ensure that all personnel are adequately qualified, to enhance the professionalism of the facility, and to assure the participants that they are receiving accurate exercise prescription and supervision (7).

Each position should have a detailed job description, addressing the major categories listed in the sample job description, that covers the responsibilities for the

Sample Job Description

Job title: Fitness Coordinator

Reports to: Wellness Director

Qualifications

- BS in exercise science, exercise physiology, or related field; MS preferred
- ACSM health fitness instructor or exercise specialist certification
- CPR and first-aid certification
- Three to five years experience in evaluating health status, administering fitness assessment, and developing and implementing exercise prescriptions for generally healthy and special populations
- Ability to communicate effectively verbally and in writing with fellow employees and participants

Client Assessment and Orientation Responsibilities

1. Administers physical fitness tests for generally healthy and special populations.
2. Develops and implements appropriate exercise prescriptions based on participant's fitness test results and personal goals.
3. Supervises the daily operations of the fitness floor including managing personnel, offering programs for healthy and special populations, maintaining equipment, and ensuring proper supervision of the exercise area.
4. Plans and conducts exercise and health education programs for various populations.
5. Devises and implements quality assessment protocols for each fitness program.

Client Rights and Organizational Ethics

1. Identifies and respects the participant's rights and their role in meeting the participant's needs.
2. Provides informed consent.
3. Maintains confidentiality of personal health information.
4. Complies with standards of ethical practice in relation to the ethics of the organization.

Leadership

1. Supports the organization administration.
2. Supports the mission of the facility.
3. Develops and adheres to a capital and operational budget.

Improving Performance

1. Attends annual safety training.
2. Evaluates competency of staff in following emergency procedures and in readily identifying contraindications to exercise testing.
3. Conducts monthly staff meetings to inform staff of overall performance and solicits input to improve customer satisfaction.
4. Maintains effective and appropriate communication with staff and participants.

position. This document should classify the employee's regular responsibilities into several categories such as organizational ethics, participant assessment, exercise prescription, and leadership skills. Categories that include the most important or commonly performed daily responsibilities should account for the majority of the participant's evaluation score. Although facilities should have standard job descriptions, the descriptions may be modified based on the needs of the facility and skill of the employee.

The fitness industry is driven by customer service. Although prospective employees may have the professional experience and academic knowledge requisite for the position, their ability to work effectively with participants is equally important. The simple adage, "Customers don't care how much you know until they know how much you care," captures this notion. Thus, the program administrator should thoroughly assess the prospective employee's interpersonal skills during the interview, perhaps by simulating difficult customer interactions (e.g., role-playing) and assessing the employee's responses, inquiring how the employee has successfully addressed challenging customer situations in the past, and allowing other staff members to address these categories as well. Overall, these interactions will provide greater insight into the prospective employee's interpersonal skills and can serve as the decisive factor of whether to hire someone.

Evaluating Personnel

As previously noted, a job description details each employee's specific professional responsibilities. This information should be shared with employees when they begin their employment. Employees should understand that their job description will serve as the basis for their annual evaluation and possible merit raise.

Formal evaluations are likely to be performed biannually or only once a year, yet prudent supervisors provide pertinent employee performance feedback regularly. Feedback opportunities present themselves when employees contend with customer service issues. For instance, a supervisor observes an employee who handles a participant's complaint about a poor equipment orientation by promptly scheduling another one and explaining they will make certain the participant is satisfied with their command of the equipment when it is completed. The supervisor should quickly provide some positive verbal or written remark for addressing the situation professionally and improving the customer's satisfaction with the facility. When employees handle customer service issues poorly, the supervisor should address the issue in a private setting. Depending on the extent and importance of the customer issue, the employee's actions may only warrant a short discussion of how to better address a similar customer service situation in the future or require a formal written reprimand. The supervisor should document positive and negative customer service instances in the employee's personnel file, which may be utilized in their next formal evaluation.

As a supervisor, the program administrator must rate the employees on their pertinent job responsibilities. The administrator may do so by assigning concise, quantifiable measures to each of the responsibilities (organized by category) in the employee's job description. For instance, each responsibility may be rated on a scale of 1 to 5 (1 representing unsatisfactory performance, 5 indicating exemplary performance). Given that each category is weighted by importance, adding the results for each category together will produce the employee's overall job performance. A uniform protocol for job performance evaluation quantifies an employee's professional performance and shows the employee which areas and responsibilities need improvement.

Cultivating a Good Working Environment

Fitness facilities with employees who are properly trained, supervised, and evaluated tend to provide a warm and welcoming environment for their members. In addition, each fitness facility should provide equipment that is properly functioning, safe, clean, and readily repaired when it malfunctions. Achieving these objectives cultivates a successful work environment and is accomplished in part by maintaining effective communication among the program administrator, staff, and participants. Effective communication with all three parties requires multiple channels. Channels of communication may consist of annual performance evaluations, feedback from members (via surveys) regarding fitness testing and equipment orientation satisfaction, or allowing employees to make suggestions to improve the facility's operations.

Providing consistent and accurate information is imperative so that employees understand their specific job requirements, how well they are meeting these requirements, and what they should do to address any professional shortcomings. The program administrator can meet these objectives by regularly supervising the employees as they work or during one-on-one meetings to discuss their professional progress or common challenges in customer service. In addition, monthly staff meetings enhance overall communication. During these meetings, the department's contribution (e.g., financial, service) to the facility's objectives should be discussed. Further, employees should be encouraged to provide input on improving future programming. Not only will they provide valuable insight, they will appreciate the opportunity to share their ideas with administrative staff.

Aside from employee input, the program administrator should also seek the opinions of the participants on program offerings and day-to-day customer service, possibly by administering a structured survey to members who have used the facility for a standard length of time (e.g., 3 mo), calling randomly selected members each week to inquire about their satisfaction with the facility, or simply maintaining a participant suggestion box. Suggestions should be addressed with the participant either in person or via a telephone call. The program administrator may also politely ask participants while they are exercising if there is anything the facility can do to improve their exercise experience. Establishing rapport with participants provides them with a greater sense of customer service that transcends simply providing a safe, clean exercise facility with an array of equipment.

Key Point

Full-time and part-time personnel with the requisite professional and interpersonal qualifications are necessary for a successful fitness facility. Each employee should have a specific job description that serves as a tool for evaluating professional performance.

Developing a Successful Program

The ACSM guidelines for facilities list five aspects of interaction between the fitness program and the participants: screening, testing, exercise prescription, delivery of the fitness program, and counseling (2).

Participant Screening

Facilities that offer exercise equipment should provide cardiovascular screening to prospective members before they undergo fitness testing or begin a fitness program (4). Chapter 3 addresses the criteria for admitting participants to various exercise programs. These guidelines from the AHA and ACSM reduce the chance that people with contraindications to exercise testing and participation are allowed in fitness programs designed for apparently healthy individuals (2, 3). The program administrator should develop a standardized screening process to ensure that employees use uniform guidelines to assess the health of prospective participants. Further, the administrator should regularly test employees to ensure they can readily recognize signs and symptoms of health problems that require special attention.

After health status has been determined but before fitness tests are administered, participants must be furnished with **informed consent.** Before administering fitness tests, it is imperative to obtain adequate informed consent in order to satisfy both ethical and legal considerations (2). This document should include enough information to ensure that the participant understands the objectives, attendant risks, and protocols of the fitness tests to be performed (see form 26.1). In addition, participants should understand that they may stop any test at any time if they desire to do so. The facility's administration and legal counsel should be consulted regarding the design and proper administration of the informed consent (9).

Participants should understand the content of the consent form. In order to ensure this understanding, the fitness professional should read the informed consent out loud and then allow the participant to reread it. Next, the fitness professional should inquire if the participant has any questions about what he is consenting to before they both sign the form. The fitness professional should record any pertinent questions from the participant and document the accompanying answers on the form. If the participant is a minor, a legal guardian or parent must sign the consent form. A copy of the informed consent should be provided to the participant (8).

Properly designed and administered informed consent notifies the participant about the format of the fitness tests and the voluntary risk she assumes. A signed informed consent does not absolve the fitness professional and the facility from legal action in the case of a fatal event during exercise testing. However, it does greatly minimize the chances of allegations regarding negligence and malpractice (6).

Testing

After participants' health status has been ascertained and they have made an informed consent, they may undergo fitness testing. Fitness testing helps determine if participants can begin their exercise program immediately, if they require physician consent before exercising regularly, or if they should not be permitted to join the facility (see chapter 3). Fitness tests provide a baseline quantification of aerobic fitness, body composition, muscular strength and endurance, and flexibility. These initial results should be compared to subsequent fitness tests in order to gauge improvements in each category. The test results positively reinforce regular physical activity as well as form the basis for modifying the exercise prescription. Fitness test procedures are included in chapters 3, 5, 6, 8, and 9.

Exercise Prescription, Orientation, and Counseling

The participant's health status, personal goals, and fitness test results should be considered when designing the exercise prescription. Chapters 10, 11, 12, and 13 address exercise prescription for aerobic fitness, weight

FORM 26.1 Sample Informed Consent for Fitness Test Participation

Testing objectives: In order to more safely participate in an exercise program, I hereby consent, voluntarily, to a series of exercise tests. Each test will assist in the determination of my overall physical fitness and will assess the following: cardiovascular fitness, body composition, muscular strength and endurance, and flexibility. I shall perform a graded exercise test (GXT) by walking on a treadmill or riding a cycle ergometer. The GXT will begin at a low level and gradually increase in difficulty until my target heart rate is achieved. The test may be stopped at any time because of feelings of significant fatigue or for any other personal reason. Body composition will be determined using skinfold tests. Muscular strength and endurance will be assessed with proper resistance training equipment. A sit-and-reach test will ascertain the flexibility of the hip joint.

Risk and discomforts: I understand that the risks of the GXT or other test procedures may include abnormal heart rhythms, abnormal blood pressure response, fainting, and very rarely a heart attack. Every professional effort will be made to minimize these risks through proper administration of a completed health status questionnaire (HSQ) as well as assessment of relevant health questions and supervision during the tests.

Responsibilities of the participant: I acknowledge that I have completed the HSQ and answered any attendant health questions accurately. During the GXT or other tests, I will report any heart-related symptom (i.e., pain, pressure, tightness, or heaviness in the chest, neck, jaw, back, or arms) immediately. I have reported all medications (including nonprescription medications) taken on a regular basis, including today, to the appropriate staff member.

Benefits to be expected: I desire to pursue a GXT and additional fitness tests so that I may obtain better advice regarding my present level of cardiovascular fitness and overall physical fitness. This information will be used to prescribe an appropriate individualized exercise program. I understand that this test does not entirely eliminate risk in the proposed exercise program.

Inquiries: I understand that I can withdraw my consent or discontinue participation in any aspect of the fitness testing at any time without penalty or prejudice toward me. I have read the above statements and have had all of my questions answered to my satisfaction.

Use of medical records: I have been informed that the information obtained from the fitness tests is privileged and confidential as described in the Health Insurance Portability and Accountability Act of 1996. It will not be disclosed to anyone other than my physician or individuals responsible for designing and supervising my exercise program, without my express written permission.

______________________________________ ______________________

Signature of participant Date

______________________________________ ______________________

Signature of witness Date

From Edward T. Howley and B. Don Franks, 2007, *Fitness Professional's Handbook*, 5th ed. (Champaign, IL: Human Kinetics).

management, muscular strength and endurance, and flexibility and low-back function for generally healthy adults. In addition, chapters 15 through 21 suggest exercise prescriptions for special populations.

After writing the personalized exercise prescription, the participant should be given a simple-to-follow workout card. The card should contain pertinent equipment information including the order in which exercises or machines should be used, seat heights, and the recommended weight to be used. Next, the fitness professional should orient the participant to the equipment that will be used during the exercise program. The fitness professional should demonstrate how to use the equipment properly, including how to modify seat heights, ROM, and the amount of weight to be used. Since few participants will be able to recall all of the equipment instructions they received, a brief follow-up orientation may be scheduled to ensure the participant is comfortable operating the equipment. In addition, the orientation provides an opportunity for the fitness professional to develop personal rapport with the participant. The personal information obtained during this interaction can be used to initiate future discussions. Engendering a professional relationship with the participant increases the likelihood that they will reveal any difficulties experienced with the exercise program (e.g., if it is exceptionally challenging or progressing too slowly). Thus, the fitness professional can readily modify the exercise program to address the participant's concerns and ensure greater customer satisfaction. Establishing solid fitness professional-customer relationships also is conducive to selling additional facility services such as personal training or sessions with a massage therapist.

Participants should be given reasonable goals for the expected outcomes of their exercise program, periodic reassessment of their physical progress, and educational information that enhances their understanding of the health benefits of regular physical activity. Educational information should be tailored to the individual's health history. For example, people with type 2 diabetes can be given a handout (1-2 pages) detailing the benefits of exercise in managing blood sugar levels and providing useful eating tips for weight management. Seminars, bulletin boards, newsletters, Web sites, and e-mail can all be used to share knowledge on the benefits of regular physical activity in preventing and managing common health problems. Overall, the health information should be accurate, concise, and readily understandable for a population that is likely to have little, if any, physiology or nutrition background.

Key Point

A successful fitness program employs appropriate protocols for screening, informed consent, fitness testing, exercise prescription, and subsequent program modification. These protocols coupled with educational counseling should provide an exemplary exercise program tailored to each participant's personal goals and health history.

Safety and Legal Concerns

An overriding objective for each fitness facility should be to provide a safe exercise environment. This objective is initially addressed with the proper screening of exercise participants and is sustained by employing trained and experienced staff members who provide appropriate informed consent, exercise prescriptions, equipment orientations, and supervision (9). Providing a safe exercise environment helps legally protect the fitness facility.

Liability

The legal system has established that "members of health clubs are owed a duty of reasonable care to protect them from injury on the premises and this duty includes a general responsibility to ensure that their members know how to properly use gym equipment" (10). Reasonable care for club participants includes appropriate fitness screening, informed consent, equipment orientation, and exercise supervision. Fitness professionals should also maintain current CPR certification and adhere to the facility's standards for emergency procedures. Providing reasonable care helps readily identify health problems (e.g., contraindications) that preclude exercise testing or participation and minimizes the likelihood of adverse events during exercise, which reduces legal **liability** (6).

All fitness professionals should know how to prevent and manage common injuries and emergencies, including CPR and hypoglycemia incidents, that arise in fitness facilities. Chapter 25 provides detailed protocols for injury prevention and treatment.

The program administrator should be aware of common liability problems. Legal experts consider exercise facilities to be liable when they fail to do any of the following (adapted from references 11 and 15):

- Monitor or stop a GXT using professional judgment.
- Evaluate participants' functional abilities or impairments that require special attention.
- Recommend safe ranges of exercise intensity.
- Instruct participants on safe exercise activities.

- Supervise exercise participation and advise individuals how to restrict or modify exercise not performed under supervision.
- Assign participants to levels of monitoring, supervision, and emergency medical support commensurate with health status.
- Refrain from giving advice construed to represent diagnosis of a medical condition.
- Refer participants for physician consent or to other medical professionals given appropriate signs and symptoms.
- Maintain proper and confidential records in accordance with the 1996 Health Insurance Portability and Accountability Act (HIPAA).

Undoubtedly, minor and major health incidents will occur. A survey of over 200 exercise facilities indicated that in the last year, 25% of them experienced *at least* one medical emergency requiring an ambulance (12). The program administrator should make certain that each fitness professional has the requisite certification (CPR and BLS [basic life support]) and training to deal with major health incidents. In addition, fitness professionals (especially those who work on contract) should be encouraged to carry liability insurance. Most organizations have an insurance policy that includes liability coverage for their employees. Fitness professionals can consult national organizations (e.g., ACSM and NSCA) that have established arrangements with insurance carriers for the provision of individual liability insurance.

Fitness facilities should regularly inspect exercise equipment for proper function and maintenance. Each inspection and equipment maintenance or repair should be documented and kept on file for reference.

All fitness facilities should establish protocols designed to provide a safe exercise environment for participants. Employees who fail to provide reasonable care can be guilty of **negligence.** If injury or death occurs as a result of negligence, the fitness professional and facility are legally liable. Facilities whose professional operations meet the standard of care and adhere to accepted emergency procedures for their participants on a daily basis are significantly less likely to be negligent (10).

Emergency Procedures

The AHA and ACSM state that "all health facilities must have written emergency policies and procedures that are reviewed and practiced regularly" (6). Consulting local emergency services will help establish the proper procedures. All staff members should be trained periodically (e.g., quarterly) to ensure they understand and properly adhere to the facility's established emergency protocols (5). This training may involve simulating common health incidents and grading the response of the staff members. The sample emergency procedures on page 408 can be modified appropriately to meet the requirements of individual exercise facilities. A prudent emergency procedure for cardiac arrests follows the AHA chain of survival, which includes four steps: early access to care and calling 911, early cardiopulmonary resuscitation (CPR), early defibrillation, and early advanced care (5). Procedures for common emergencies along with telephone numbers for emergency assistance should be clearly posted or in a visibly accessible area near a telephone (2).

An exercise facility that serves generally healthy participants needs the following minimum emergency equipment: a telephone, signs indicating the possible hazards of using the exercise equipment, a stethoscope, and a sphygmomanometer (6). Increasingly, exercise facilities serve participants with type 2 diabetes. Thus, having a glucose meter and blood sugar test strips available is necessary for checking the blood sugar of participants experiencing hypoglycemic symptoms.

The AHA and ACSM recommend that larger fitness facilities (2,500 members or more), facilities with programs for seniors, and facilities whose emergency response time to a cardiac arrest is greater than 5 min are equipped with an AED (6). In some states (e.g., Illinois, New York, Rhode Island, and Louisiana), AEDs are mandatory in all exercise facilities (1). These devices have been proven to make a critical difference in the chances of surviving cardiac arrest. Survival rates as high as 90% have been reported where defibrillation is achieved within the first minute after cardiac arrest (5). AEDs are designed to detect arrhythmias and will only shock rhythms that respond favorably to defibrillation (e.g., ventricular tachycardia and fibrillation), ensuring their safe use.

Key Point

Fitness facilities should maintain a comprehensive safety program that includes properly trained personnel, participant screenings, informed consent, appropriate exercise supervision, and adherence to standard emergency procedures. Altogether, these activities help the fitness facility attain the legal standard of care for their participants.

Budgeting

A sound **budget** is essential to successful strategic planning. Program administrators should maintain a short-term

Sample Emergency Response Protocol

Cardiac Emergency

1. The first person on the scene will assess the seriousness of the cardiac event. Do not move the participant, unless to move the participant into a lying position.
2. If warranted, begin proper CPR procedures by calling 911 to report the location and nature of the emergency. If the exercise program is in a medical facility, contact and inform the operator that a cardiac event has taken place so that the designated code team is summoned.
3. Check for breathing and pulse; if absent, begin CPR immediately.
4. If an automatic external defibrillator (AED) is available, administer the AED and CPR according to established American Red Cross or American Heart Association external defibrillation algorithms.
5. Additional staff members should assist with CPR, monitor and record vital signs, and prevent bystanders from interfering with the participant's treatment.
6. Continue CPR until medical personnel arrive, and then follow their instructions.
7. Immediately fill out an incident report and send it to the proper department for review.

Additional Serious Emergencies

Following is the procedure for treating these injuries:

Breathing problems
Neck or back injuries
Unconsciousness
Limb injury with obvious deformity
Head injury
Severe chest pain
Bleeding from ear, nose, or mouth

1. Do not move the participant, unless to move the participant into a lying position, with feet elevated (unless you suspect a back injury).
2. Contact 911 as in cardiac emergencies.
3. Treat for shock.
4. Control bleeding.
5. Do not manage the injury beyond the basic standards of first aid or the standards set by governing or certifying organizations, unless properly licensed, registered, or certified and acting under the written referral of a licensed physician.
6. Continue first aid until medical personnel arrive, and then follow their instructions.
7. Immediately fill out an incident report and send it to the proper department for review.

Other Accidents and Minor Injuries

The following procedure is for treating injuries without gross swelling, deformity, or noticeable discoloration:

1. Do not allow a sick or injured person to sit, stand, or walk until you are certain that the condition warrants it.
2. If the individual complains of "feeling bad," instruct individual to cease the workout and to sit where you can readily ascertain and monitor vital signs.
3. If the individual has questionable symptoms or unusual vital signs (e.g., low blood pressure or very faint heart rate), monitor them until they stabilize.
4. If warranted, use the most readily available first-aid kit for treatment.
5. Immediately fill out an incident report and send it to the proper department for review.

Adapted from U.S. Public Health Service, 2001, "Guidelines for public access defibrillation programs in federal facilities," *Federal Register* 66(100): 28495-28511.

(annual) and long-term (3-5 yr) budget so that they can assess the financial standing of their facility. Ideally, a budget allows for exemplary customer service, equitable reimbursement for employees, and contemporary exercise equipment in the context of practical facility capital expenditures. The facility's budget should be feasible in regard to containing conservative revenue goals and realistic expense figures. Most budgets are predicated on the previous year's revenue and expense results with slight modifications to account for equipment upgrades, changes in programming, facility maintenance, and so on. Based on the facility's financial performance, years of operation, and future growth considerations, annual budgets will differ significantly in their scope and financial magnitude. Form 26.2 outlines a suggested budget.

A well-designed budget not only indicates if specific financial goals are being attained but also answers the following questions: How many memberships need to be sold to meet financial objectives? Is the profit goal realistic? Is enough money available to enhance existing program offerings? Is it feasible to give staff members the pay increases they have requested? The answers to these questions should guide the program administrator's immediate and long-term plans for the facility. Further, a budget can translate the policy of a facility into financial terms. A budget may be divided into two segments: capital and operational (13).

Capital Budget

A capital budget for a fitness facility typically allocates money for treadmills, elliptical trainers, bikes, resistance machines, computers, office furniture, and essentially any equipment that costs more than $500 and has a useful life of at least 1 yr. The serial number, repairs, expected useful life, and depreciation for each piece of equipment should be inventoried and recorded annually. The program administrator should arrange to verify this information during an annual inspection of all exercise equipment. Performing these activities gives a contemporary assessment of the facility's equipment and provides a good estimate for future capital needs. For instance, if a facility has 20 treadmills (with an expected useful life of 5 yr) and 4 of them have been owned for 4 yr, then the program administrator should designate money for 4 new treadmills in the next annual capital budget (13).

Operational Budget

The operational budget constitutes the expenses of providing day-to-day services for participants, including labor and program costs and maintenance and utility expenses. Given that many of these expenses change regularly, the program administrator should regularly update this budget. Development of the operational budget may be divided into four distinct phases: research, goal and objective determination, administration review, and implementation (13). Review form 26.3 for additional information concerning each phase.

The research phase includes analyzing the objective and the financial viability of each program. Every fitness facility should offer a regular program for weight loss, while other programs, such as dance classes, may be offered only 4 wk once a quarter. Goal and objective development entails the realistic financial and customer service requirements you want to develop during the next fiscal year. As stability balls have become increasingly popular, would a group class using this equipment be profitable and benefit the facility's participants? The program administrator should implement strategies that helped new programs succeed in the past as well as employee and participant feedback (via direct questions, surveys, or suggestions) to assist with this component of the operational budget. Next, a well-organized draft should be developed. The accuracy of the draft depends on how well the first two phases of the budget were conducted. The draft budget should clearly delineate the differences between the current year and the upcoming one (see form 26.3). Again, this information should be shared with staff members since they have contributed to the budget's development and are aware of and agree upon the financial goals for the facility (12, 14).

The completed operational budget should be presented to upper management at least 1 mo before the end of the fiscal year. Undoubtedly, the administration will make several adjustments to the original budget. After the changes have been incorporated, the final operational budget should be implemented at the beginning of the fiscal year. During monthly staff meetings, the program administrator can use a monthly operational budget to demonstrate where the facility is succeeding financially and to receive employee feedback on how to address programs not succeeding as projected.

Budgeting for Personnel and Facilities

The largest portion of the operational budget concerns personnel salary and benefits. In larger facilities, the human resources department will establish salary ranges for each position. In contrast, a smaller operation may survey the salaries offered by similar businesses in the region to establish a reference point for determining salaries of various positions. The facility should offer a competitive base salary and pertinent benefits. An attractive benefit could be the opportunity to pursue reimbursable continuing education (certifications and university courses). Fitness facilities attempting to minimize operational costs by offering substandard salaries and benefits will quickly experience a high staff turnover rate, which undermines customer service and ultimately revenues.

FORM 26.2 Sample Determination of an Operational Budget

1. What are the purposes for each program? ______________________________

2. Describe the current program, including successful and unsuccessful components.

3. What are your current expenditures?
   A. Personnel salaries (full-time, part-time, contract) __________
   B. Marketing and advertising __________
   C. Facilities
      (1) Loan repayment __________
      (2) Insurance __________
      (3) Maintenance and repairs __________
      (4) Utilities __________
      (5) Taxes __________
   D. Supplies __________
   E. Other (e.g., travel expenses, continuing education) __________
4. What are your current revenue sources?
   A. Membership dues, including initiation fees __________
   B. Insurance (third-party reimbursement) __________
   C. Gifts __________
   D. Special programs (e.g., massage, pro shop) __________
   E. Other __________
5. What are upcoming changes?
   A. What changes should be made in your department over the next 5 yr, including changes in personnel, equipment, new programs, old programs, and renovation or repair of the facility? __________
   B. Regarding each of these changes, indicate the change in cost and potential profit.
   C. Provide logical incremental steps by which the changes can be incorporated.
6. What are future revenue considerations?
   A. What are the potential sources of increased revenue? __________
   B. What will be required to achieve this increased revenue, including additional costs?
   C. What will be the net contribution margin for each potential revenue source?
7. What is a reasonable revenue projection for each year over the next 3 to 5 yr?
8. What aspects of the program can be supported with this income? __________
9. If revenue exceeds expectations, where will the additional revenue be allotted?
10. If revenue does not meet expectations, what aspects of the programs can be reduced or eliminated?

FORM 26.3 Sample Monthly Operational Budget Report

Item	Month		Year to date	
	Budgeted	Actual	Budgeted	Actual
Revenues				
Membership dues	______	______	______	______
Fitness tests	______	______	______	______
Group programs	______	______	______	______
Special programs	______	______	______	______
Other	______	______	______	______
Total	______	______	______	______
Expenses				
Salaries	______	______	______	______
Administrative	______	______	______	______
Full-time	______	______	______	______
Part-time	______	______	______	______
Contract	______	______	______	______
Materials	______	______	______	______
Fitness testing	______	______	______	______
Clerical	______	______	______	______
Cleaning	______	______	______	______
Other	______	______	______	______
Overhead	______	______	______	______
Telephone	______	______	______	______
Maintenance	______	______	______	______
Utilities	______	______	______	______
Rent	______	______	______	______
Contracts	______	______	______	______
Other	______	______	______	______
Total	______	______	______	______
Balance	______	______	______	______
Versus last year	______	______	______	______

From Edward T. Howley and B. Don Franks, 2007, *Fitness Professional's Handbook*, 5th ed. (Champaign, IL: Human Kinetics).

Key Point

Proper financial management is an integral part of the short-term (annual) and long-term (3-5 yr) strategic planning process. The budget should be divided into capital and operational components. Capital budget considerations include significant monetary expenditures such as exercise equipment. In contrast, the operational budget concentrates on daily operational expenses such as labor, program, and maintenance costs.

FORM 26.4 Sample Incident Report

Personal Information

Name: ______________________________ Date: ________________

Address: ____________________________ Phone: ________________

Age: ______________ Male ( ) Female ( ) Client ( ) Visitor ( )

Type of Occurrence

With injury ( ) Without injury ( ) Property damage ( ) Missing article ( ) Complaint ( )

Breach of confidentiality ( ) Forward to human resources if confidentiality breached ( )

Other (specify): ____

Occurrence Documentation

Location of occurrence: ____

Describe exactly what happened in detail, including the nature of the injury or health problem and how the incident occurred. If property or equipment damage occurred, describe damage and quote approximate value of the loss.

____

____

List, in order, the things the first responder or other staff members did in response to the incident.

____

____

Witnesses

If employee(s), state name and department

Name:______________________________________

Address: ____________________________________ Phone: ________________

Name:______________________________________

Address: ____________________________________ Phone: ________________

Treatment

Did the individual refuse examination or treatment? Yes ( ) No ( ) N/A ( )

Was the individual seen by a physician? Yes ( ) No ( ) N/A ( )

If yes, was an X ray, MRI, or PET scan performed? Yes ( ) No ( )

If yes, describe findings: ____

____

____________________________________ ________________

Signature and title of employee preparing the report Date of report

____________________________________ ________________

Signature of department head/administration supervisor Date of report

A copy of this form should be kept on file and the original sent to quality management within 24 hours.

Each employee should undergo an annual evaluation that quantifies professional performance in order to determine salary adjustment.

Equipment and Record Keeping

Most fitness facilities offer a variety of aerobic and resistance training equipment from various manufacturers. The program administrator should develop a rapport with each equipment vendor. Vendors can provide information on contemporary product offerings, consultation for common equipment problems, and discounts on certified pre-owned exercise equipment or other capital expenditures.

Equipment for Exercise and Fitness Testing

Although participants value a wide selection of exercise equipment, proper maintenance and cleanliness are equally important. A maintenance log should be maintained that details when a piece of equipment malfunctioned, the specific problem, what was required to repair the machine, and when the machine was returned to service. Inoperable machines should always be unplugged (if necessary) and visibly labeled with a sign stating that it is out of order. This sign may also indicate the expected date of repair. If possible, the inoperable equipment should be removed from the exercise area. The facility should maintain a list of local technicians to contact when a machine malfunctions. These individuals should be contacted promptly to ensure the machine is readily repaired. This practice will reduce member complaints regarding the amount of time it takes to repair equipment. The program administrator should also develop a daily cleaning schedule for all equipment to ensure it is presentable as well as to maximize its longevity.

Additional equipment is necessary to conduct appropriate fitness tests. The extent and quality of this equipment vary with the exercise facility's program options. Table 26.1 recommends the minimum and advanced equipment for testing and exercise.

Record Keeping

Fitness facilities that conduct proper participant screenings, informed consent, and fitness tests collect a wealth of personal health information. Personal health information is protected under the HIPPA of 1996 and therefore must remain confidential. This information should be systematically organized and kept in a secure area that only designated employees can access. Increasingly, fitness test results are stored digitally and thus require safeguards to ensure they remain private. The program administrator should also keep records of all staff meetings, job evaluations, and training (including the demonstration of competence in emergency procedures).

An incident form (form 26.4) should be used to document all accidents and injuries. The original completed forms should be kept in a secure area and copies forwarded to the appropriate administrator or department.

Table 26.1 Exercise Equipment for Fitness Testing

Area	Minimum	Advanced
Testing equipment		
Health status	HSQ	Computer-based health assessment
Cardiorespiratory	Walking or running track Bench RPE scale Blood pressure	Cycle ergometer Treadmill Oxygen analysis ECG Lipid analysis Glucose meter
Body composition	Scale Tape measure Skinfold calipers Bioelectrical impedance analyzer	Underwater tank
Abdominal strength and endurance	Mat	
Midtrunk flexibility	Sit-and-reach box	
Upper-body strength and endurance	Bench and free weights	Stack weight machines

(continued)

Table 26.1 Exercise Equipment for Fitness Testing *(continued)*

Area	Minimum	Advanced
Exercise equipment		
Cardiorespiratory	Walking or running track Treadmill with flat grade only	Treadmill with incline option Upright and recumbent cycle ergometer Elliptical and cross trainers Rowers NuStep Arm ergometers
Resistance training	Bench Free weights	Stack weight machines Free weights Pneumatic resistance Isokinetic machines Freemotion machines

RPE = rating of perceived exertion; ECG = electrocardiogram.

This information is essential if subsequent questions are raised about an accident. Regardless of the extent of the injury, the injured participant should be contacted within 48 hr to determine the recovery status. Any relevant information acquired during the follow-up contact should be documented as well. Further, any instances involving breach of confidentiality should be sent to human resources immediately.

Key Point

Exercise and testing equipment should be properly inventoried, maintained, and replaced on a regular basis. In addition, the program administrator should ensure the confidentiality of all personal health information and incident reports.

Case Studies

You can check your answers by referring to page 476 in appendix A.

1. The wellness director informs you that, as the supervisor, you are responsible for evaluating three full-time fitness professionals and two part-time fitness instructors. What steps would you take to carry out the evaluation?
2. The board of directors asks you to evaluate the objectives for the fitness facility, including the extent to which they are being achieved. What resources would you use in providing the answer?

PART VI

Scientific Foundations

Part VI provides the basic scientific foundation for understanding the structure and function of the human body. In chapter 27, we review the bones, joints, and muscles of the body and their biomechanical functions during common physical activities. In chapter 28, we cover the basic concepts of energy, muscle function, and the physiological response to acute and chronic physical activity. Differences due to gender, type of exercise, and temperature are described.

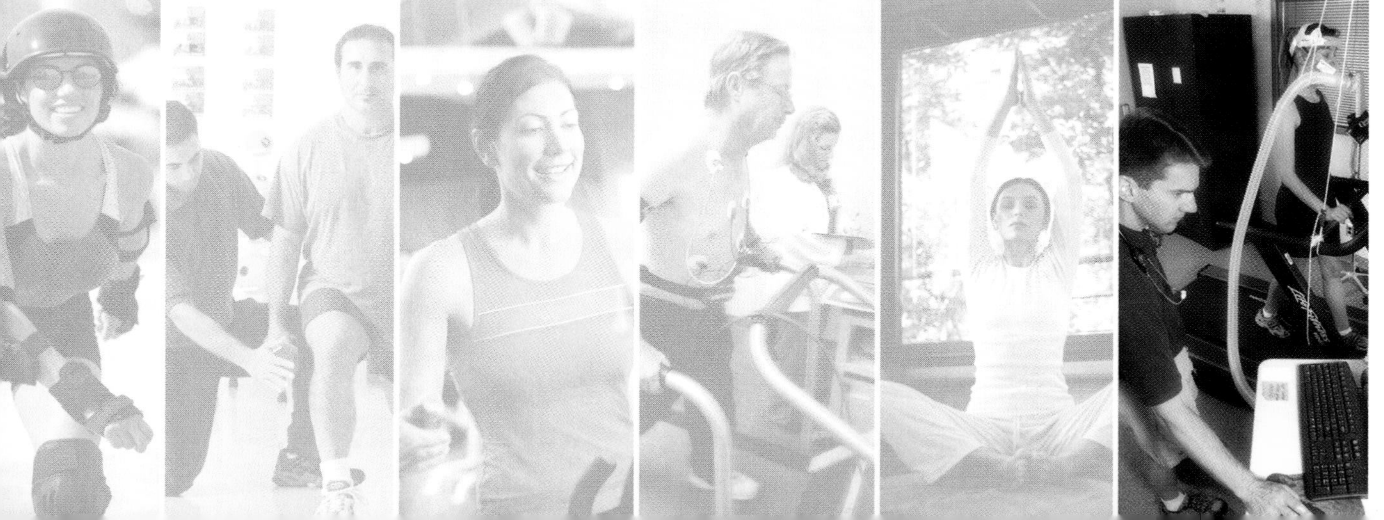

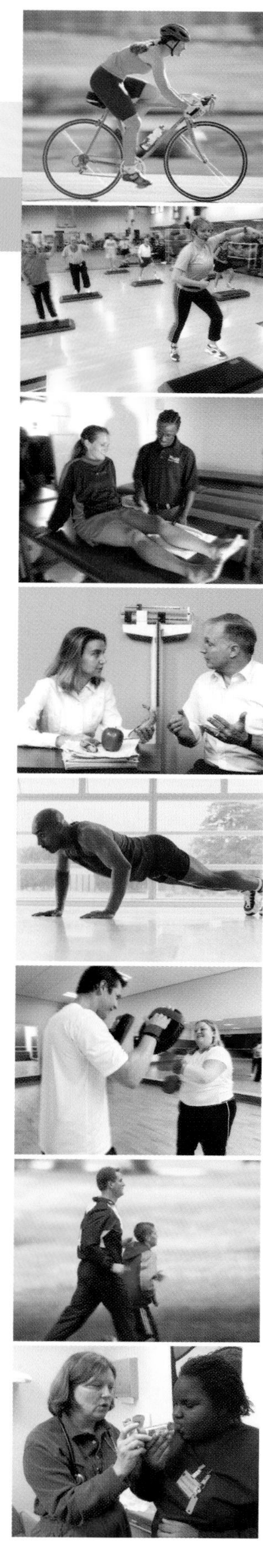

27 CHAPTER

Functional Anatomy and Biomechanics

Jean Lewis

Objectives

The reader will be able to do the following:

1. Describe the structure of long bones.
2. Identify the major bones of the skeletal system and classify them by shape.
3. Describe ossification of long bones.
4. Distinguish between synarthrodial, amphiarthrodial, and diarthrodial joints, both structurally and functionally, and identify the structures of a diarthrodial joint.
5. List the factors that determine the range and direction of motion at the joints.
6. Name and demonstrate the movements possible at each joint.
7. Describe forces that can cause joint movement and that can resist movement caused by another force.
8. Describe the gross structure of a muscle.
9. Explain how muscle tension increases.
10. Describe the phases of a ballistic movement, including the muscle action.

(continued)

Objectives (continued)

11. Explain the differences among concentric, eccentric, and isometric muscle actions.
12. Describe the roles of muscles.
13. List the major muscles in each muscle group, and identify the major actions and joints involved in the following muscles: trapezius, serratus anterior, deltoid, pectoralis major, latissimus dorsi, biceps brachii, brachialis, triceps brachii, flexor and extensor carpi radialis and ulnaris, rectus abdominis, external oblique, erector spinae, gluteus maximus, gluteus medius, iliopsoas, rectus femoris, vasti muscles, hamstring muscles, tibialis anterior, soleus, and gastrocnemius.
14. Cite specific errors occurring during exercise involving the vertebral column, lumbosacral joints, and knee joint.
15. Analyze locomotion, throwing, cycling, jumping, and swimming for movement and muscle involvement.
16. Describe good lifting techniques.
17. Describe the three factors that determine stability; identify the interrelationships among line of gravity, base of support, balance, and stability; and describe the practical applications of these interrelationships during physical activity.
18. Describe torque and its relationship to muscle actions.
19. Describe how an exerciser can change positions of body segments to alter the resistive torque.
20. Explain how the mechanical principles of rotational inertia and angular momentum apply to movement.
21. Discuss the common errors seen in locomotion, throwing, and striking.

The fitness professional must have knowledge of the bones, joints, and muscles; must understand muscle forces and other forces; and must be able to apply biomechanical principles to human movement. With this knowledge and understanding, the instructor is better equipped to direct safe physical activity for participants seeking the health-related effects of exercise. This knowledge also helps the instructor earn the respect of clients, who will view the instructor as a professional in the field rather than a technician who may know what to do but not why. This chapter is merely a summary; for greater detail on anatomy and biomechanics, see the references (1-9).

Skeletal Anatomy

Most of the 200 distinct bones in the human skeleton help produce movement. Their high mineral component gives them rigidity; their protein component makes them resistant to tension. The two types of bone tissue are (a) compact tissue, which is the dense, hard, outer layer of bone, and (b) spongy, or cancellous, tissue, which has a lattice-like structure to provide greater structural strength along the lines of stress while reducing the weight of the bone. Bones are divided into four classifications according to their shape: long, short, flat, and irregular.

Long Bones

The long bones, found in the limbs and digits, serve primarily as levers for movement. Each long bone consists of the **diaphysis,** or shaft, which is made up of thick, compact bone surrounding the hollow medullary cavity; the **epiphyses,** or expanded ends, composed of spongy bone with a thin, outer layer of compact bone; the **articular cartilage,** a thin layer of hyaline cartilage covering the articulating surfaces (the surfaces of a bone that meet or come into contact with another bone to form a joint) that provides a frictionless surface and helps absorb shock; and the **periosteum,** a fibrous membrane covering the entire bone (except where the articular cartilage is present) to serve as an attachment site for many muscles (see figure 27.1).

Short, Flat, and Irregular Bones

In addition to long bones, the skeleton is made up of short bones, flat bones, and irregularly shaped bones (see figure 27.2).

The tarsals (in the ankle) and carpals (in the wrist) are the short bones. Their composition (spongy bone with a thin outside layer of compact bone) provides greater strength, but their cubic shape decreases their movement potential.

Key Point

The structures of a long bone include the diaphysis, or shaft; the epiphyses, or expanded ends; the periosteum, which covers the bone except at the articulating surfaces; and the articular cartilage, which covers the articulating surfaces to provide a frictionless surface and help absorb shock.

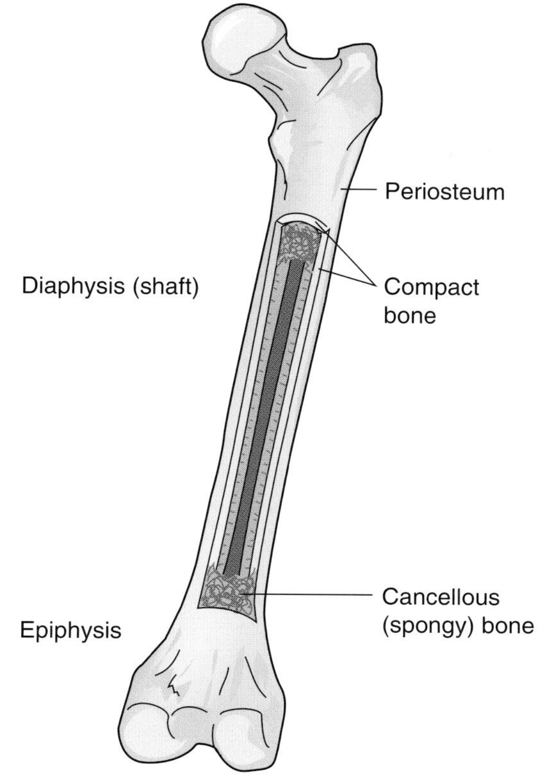

Figure 27.1 The femur, an example of a long bone.

The flat bones, such as the ribs, ilia, and scapulae, serve primarily as broad sites for muscle attachments and, in the case of the ribs and ilia, to enclose cavities and protect internal organs. These bones are also spongy and covered with a thin layer of compact bone.

The ischium, pubis, and vertebrae are irregularly shaped bones that protect internal parts and support the body in addition to being sites for muscle attachments.

Ossification of Bones

The skeleton begins as a cartilaginous structure, which is replaced gradually by bone in a process known as **ossification.** This process begins at the diaphysis of long bones (in centers of ossification) and spreads toward the epiphyses. The **epiphyseal plates** between the diaphyses and epiphyses are the growth areas where the cartilage is replaced by bone; bone growth in length and width continues until the epiphyseal plates are completely ossified. During growth, additional cartilage is laid down to be replaced eventually by bone. When no further cartilage is produced, and the cartilage present is replaced by bone, growth ceases. Other secondary centers of ossification develop in the epiphyses and in some bony protuberances, such as the tibial tuberosity and the articular condyles of the humerus. Short bones have one center of ossification. Dates of closure vary. Although bone fusion at some centers of ossification may occur by puberty or earlier, most of the long bones do not completely ossify until the late teens. Premature closing, which results in a shorter bone length, can be caused by trauma, abnormal stresses, malnutrition, and drugs.

Key Point

Ossification is the replacement of cartilage with bone. Generally, bone growth is completed by the late teens.

Structure and Function of the Joints

Joints, which are the places where bones meet, or articulate, are often classified according to the amount of movement that can take place at those sites. Joints are synarthrodial, amphiarthrodial, or diarthrodial. The **synarthrodial joints** are the immovable joints. The bones merge into each other and are bound together by fibrous tissue that is continuous with the periosteum. The sutures, or the lines of junction, of the cranial (skull) bones are prime examples of this type of joint. The **amphiarthrodial,** or cartilaginous, **joints** allow only slight movement in all directions. Usually a fibrocartilage disk separates the bones, and movement can occur only by deformation of the disk. Examples of these joints are the tibiofibular and sacroiliac joints and the joints between the bodies of the vertebrae in the spine. **Ligaments,** which are tough, fibrous bands of connective tissue, connect the bones to each other, not only in this type of joint but in all joints.

Diarthrodial, or synovial, **joints** (see figure 27.3) are freely movable joints that allow greater movement direction and range; most of the joint movements during physical activity occur at diarthrodial joints. The diarthrodial joints are the most common type and include most joints of the extremities. Strong and fairly inelastic ligaments, along with connective and muscle tissue crossing the joint, maintain the stability of the joint. Diarthrodial joints have distinct physical characteristics that differentiate them from the other types of joints. The articulating surfaces of the bones are covered by articular cartilage, a type of hyaline cartilage that reduces friction and acts somewhat as a shock absorber. Each joint is enclosed by an **articular capsule,** a ligamentous structure that may be fairly thin or may be thick enough to be considered a separate ligament. The **synovial membrane** lines the inner surface of the capsule. It secretes synovial fluid into the **joint cavity,** the space enclosed by the articular capsule, to bathe (or lubricate) the joint to ease movement.

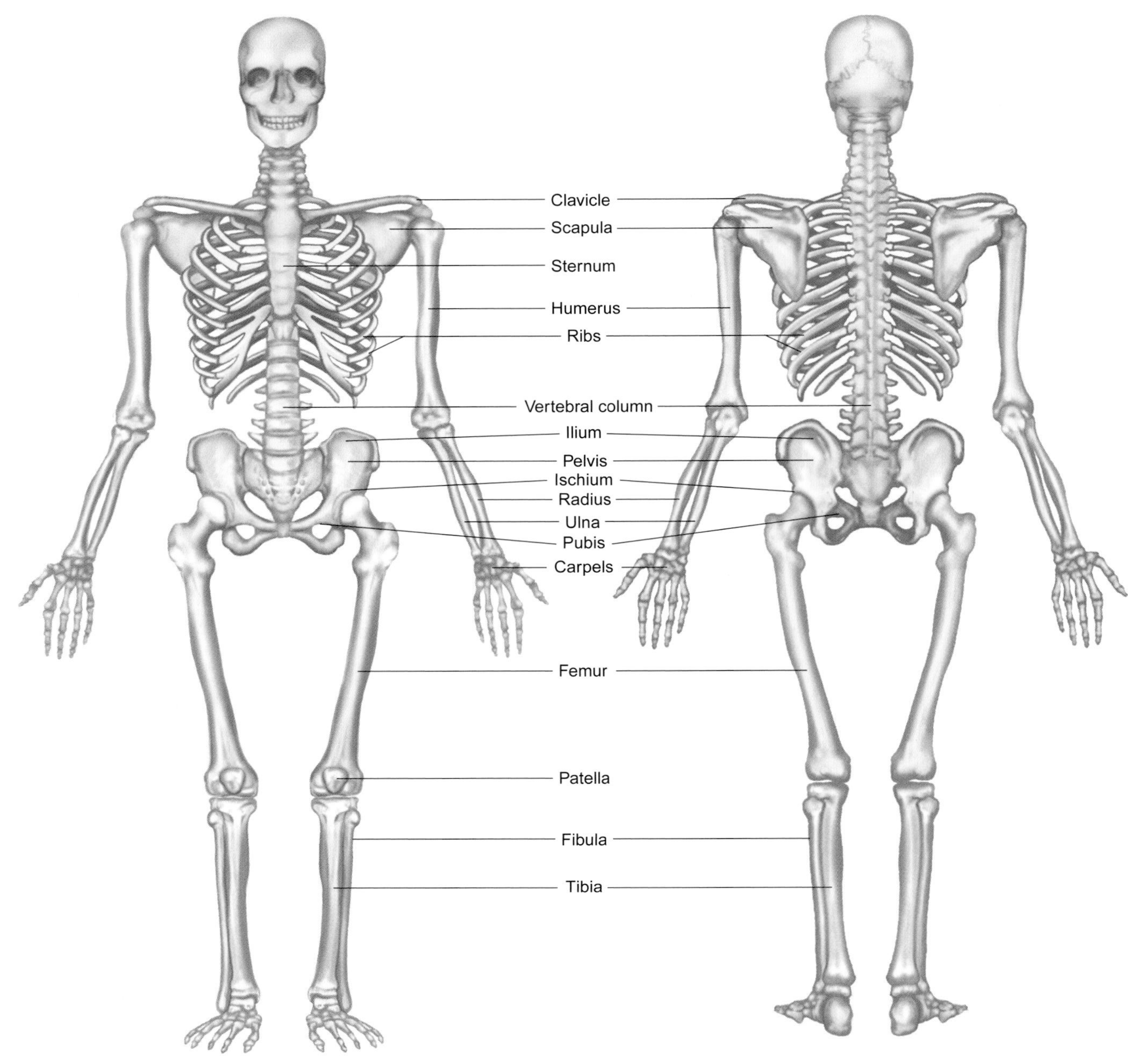

Figure 27.2 Front and back view of the human skeleton.

Normally, the joint cavity is small and therefore contains little synovial fluid, but an injury to the joint can increase the secretion of synovial fluid and cause swelling. Some diarthrodial joints, such as the sternoclavicular, distal radioulnar, and knee joints, also have a partial or complete fibrocartilage disk between the bones to aid shock absorption and, in the case of the knee, to give greater stability to the joint. The partial, semilunar-shaped disks between the femur and the tibia at the knee are called **menisci.**

To reduce frictional rubbing that occurs as the tendons change length during muscle action, tendons often are surrounded by tendinous sheaths—cylindrical, tunnellike sacs lined with synovial membrane. For example, the two proximal tendons of the biceps brachii muscle pass through these tunnels in the bicipital groove of the humerus. **Bursae,** or sacs of synovial fluid that lie between muscles, tendons, and bones, also reduce friction between the tissues and act as shock absorbers. Many bursae are found around the shoulder, elbow, hip, and knee. Bursitis, or the inflammation of a bursa, can result from repeated friction or mechanical irritation or from inflammatory or degenerative conditions of the tendons.

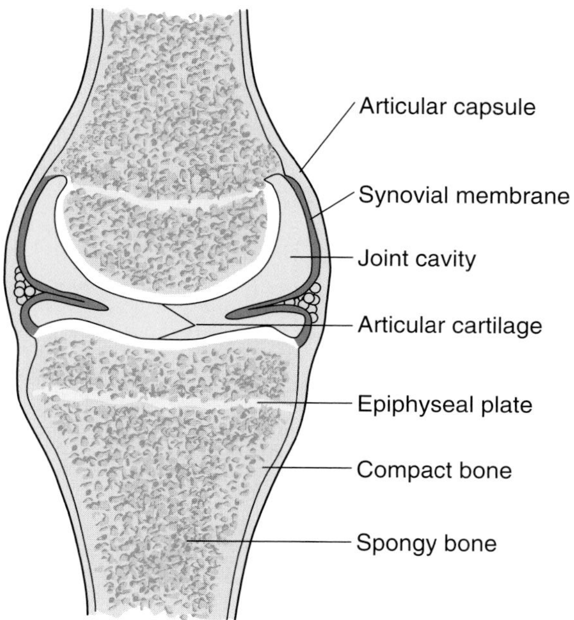

Figure 27.3 A diarthrodial, or synovial, joint.

Key Point

The three types of joints are synarthrodial, which do not allow movement; amphiarthrodial, which allow only slight movement; and diarthrodial, or synovial, which allow a wide range of movement and are characterized structurally by articular cartilage, articular capsule, synovial membrane, and synovial fluid within the joint cavity.

Factors Determining Direction and Range of Motion

Most of the movement at a joint is rotary: The bone moves around a fixed axis, the joint. The structures of the bones at and near their articulating ends largely determine both the direction and the range of movement. Ball-and-socket joints, which are found at the hip and shoulder, allow a wide range of movement in all directions, but a hinge joint, such as the elbow joint, restricts both direction and range of movement because bone impinges on bone. The length of the ligaments and to a lesser extent their **elasticity,** or ability to lengthen (stretch) passively and return to their normal length, also affect range of movement. For example, the iliofemoral ligament at the anterior hip joint is a strong but short ligament that prohibits much hip hyperextension. Elasticity can be changed by exercise; the amount of elasticity is determined by the amount and type of physical activity in which an individual engages.

Key Point

The potential range and direction of motion relate to the shape of the articulating ends of the bones, the length of ligaments, and the elasticity of connective tissue.

Specific Joint Movements

Specific terminology is used to describe the direction of movement at the different joints. The anatomical position (standing with arms at sides and turned so the palms of the hands face forward) serves as a point of reference. Although terminology may differ for specific joints, **flexion** in general refers to anterior or posterior movement from the anatomical position that brings two bones together, **extension** is the return from flexion, and **hyperextension** is the continuation of extension past the anatomical position. **Abduction** is the movement of a bone laterally from the anatomical position; **adduction** is the return back toward the anatomical position. **Rotation** occurs when the bone spins around its longitudinal axis so that its surface faces a different direction.

Shoulder Girdle This joint complex includes the articulations between the sternum and the clavicle and between the clavicle and the scapula. Rotary joint movement occurs at those articulations, but the movement terms *elevation, depression, abduction, adduction,* and *upward* and *downward rotation* describe the resulting movements of the scapulae (see figure 27.4). Abduction, adduction, and scapular elevation and depression all can occur without shoulder joint movement but may enhance it. Upward and downward rotation can occur only when the humerus is moved upward, outward, and downward. If the scapulae cannot rotate upward, the arms cannot lift sideways above the horizon (beyond 90°).

Shoulder Joint Because of its ball-and-socket structure, the shoulder joint can move in all directions—flexion, extension, hyperextension, abduction, adduction, lateral (outward, away from the midline) and medial (inward, toward the midline) rotation, and circumduction (the circular movement of the arm in a wide arc). Horizontal extension and horizontal flexion are movements of the arm parallel to the ground (see figure 27.5).

Scapular movements can enhance movements at the shoulder joint. As the arm flexes or horizontally flexes,

Adduction
a
Abduction
b
Upward rotation
Downward rotation
c

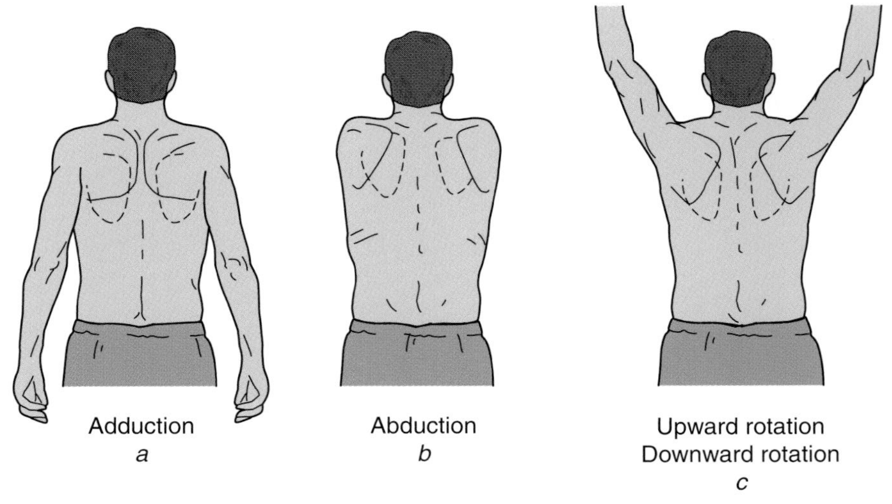

Figure 27.4 Movements of the scapulae.

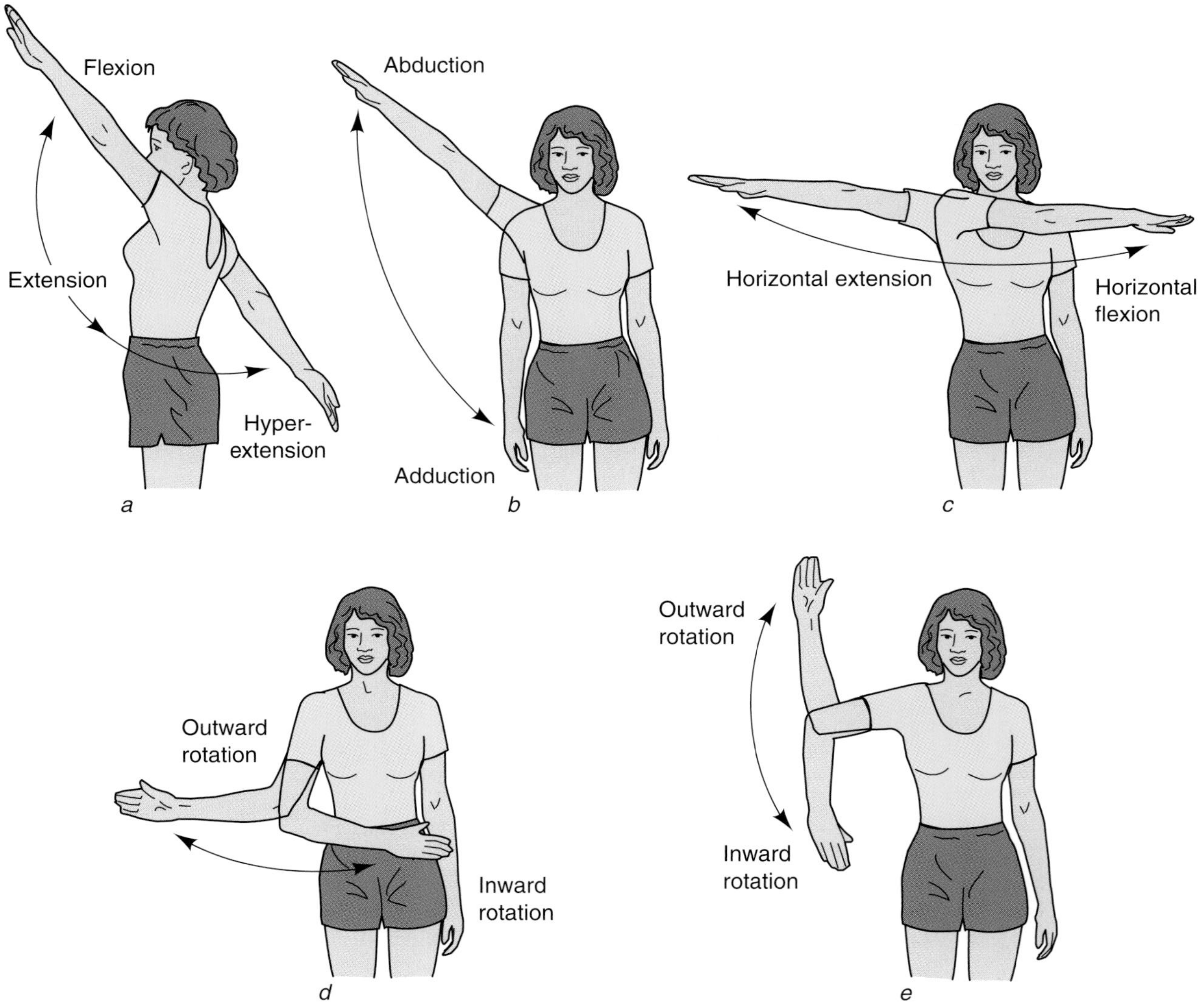

Flexion
Extension
Hyper-
extension
a
Abduction
Adduction
b
Horizontal extension
Horizontal
flexion
c
Outward
rotation
Inward
rotation
d
Outward
rotation
Inward
rotation
e

Figure 27.5 Movements of the shoulder joint.

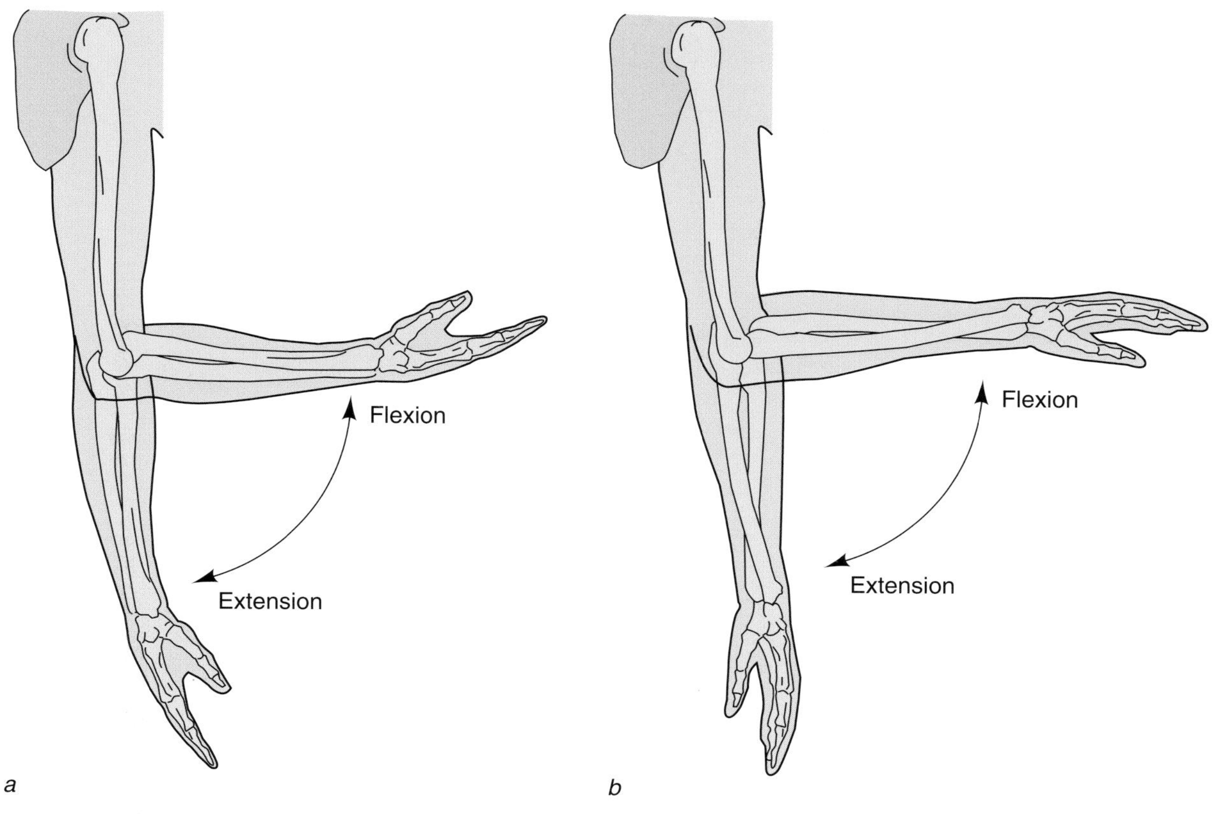

Figure 27.6 Movements of the elbow joint.

scapular abduction can move the hand out farther in front. Scapular adduction can allow the arm to move farther back during hyperextension and horizontal extension. Elevation of the scapula can allow the hand to reach higher. Medial rotation may be accompanied by scapular abduction; lateral rotation may be accompanied by scapular adduction.

Elbow Joint Sometimes referred to as the humeroulnar joint because of the bones involved in movement at the elbow joint, the elbow joint allows only flexion and extension because of its bony arrangement (see figure 27.6). The ability of some individuals to hyperextend the elbow joint is attributable to the shape of the articulating surfaces.

Radioulnar Joints Pronation and supination describe the movements of the radius around the ulna in the lower arm (see figure 27.7). Although the wrist is not involved in these movements, the position of the radioulnar joints can be identified by the direction the palm of the hand faces. When the arms hang down alongside the trunk, the palm faces forward in the supinated position and toward the back in the pronated position. In the supinated position, the radius and ulna are parallel to each other; in the pronated position, the radius lies across and on top

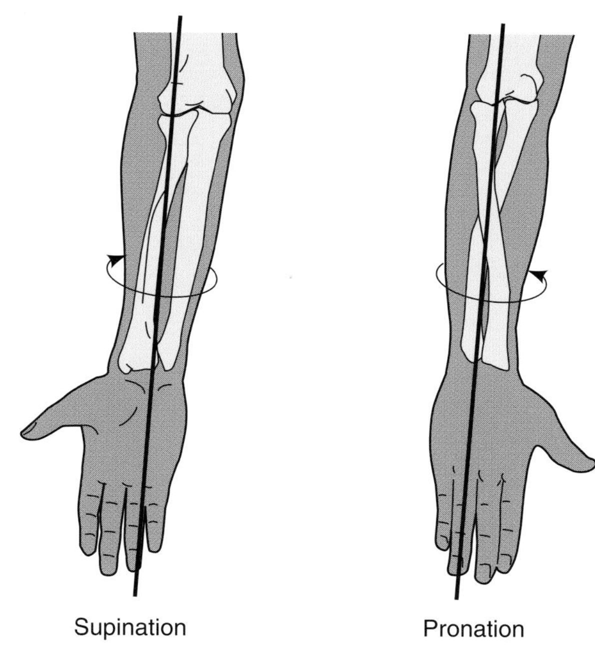

Figure 27.7 Movements of the radioulnar joints.

of the ulna. Pronation combined with shoulder joint medial rotation and supination combined with shoulder joint lateral rotation move the hand even farther around the midline.

Wrist Joint Movement at the wrist joint can occur in two planes of direction. Flexion, extension, and hyperextension occur in the one plane; abduction (radial flexion) and adduction (ulnar flexion) occur in the other (see figure 27.8).

Metacarpophalangeal and Interphalangeal Joints The second through the fifth metacarpophalangeal joints allow flexion and extension as well as abduction and adduction of the fingers. The metacarpophalangeal joint of the thumb allows only flexion and extension, but it is the only digit that also allows movement at the carpometacarpal joint (which gives the thumb its movement ability). All the interphalangeal joints of the fingers and toes only flex and extend.

Vertebral Column Movements of the trunk—flexion, extension, hyperextension, lateral flexion, and rotation—occur at all the joints of the vertebral column (see figure 27.9).

Lumbosacral Joint: Pelvis Movement The pelvis (see figure 27.10) tilts mainly at the joint formed by the fifth lumbar vertebra and the pelvis. The reference point for the direction of the tilt is the iliac crest. As the crest moves forward and down, the pelvis has a forward, or anterior, pelvic tilt; as the crest rotates toward the back, the pelvis has a backward, or posterior, tilt. The anterior pelvic tilt usually is accompanied by a hyperextension of the lumbar vertebrae, whereas a backward tilt usually results in a flattening out of the lumbar vertebrae.

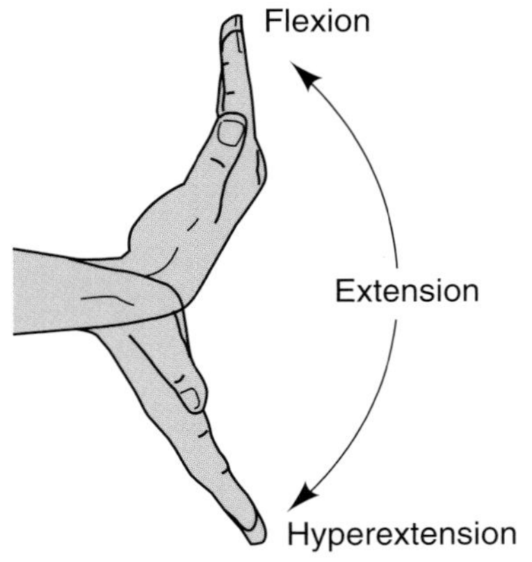

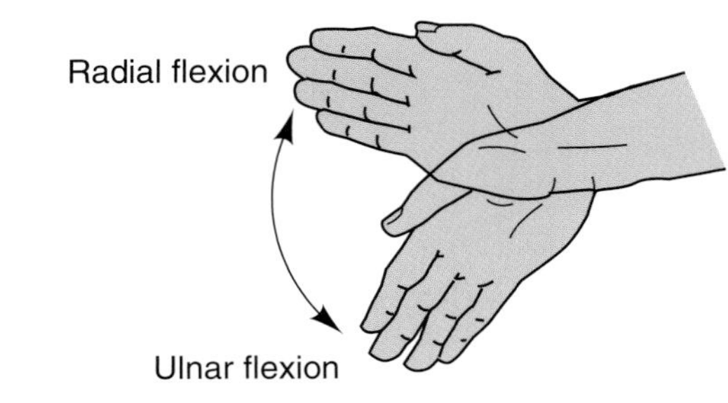

Figure 27.8 Movements of the wrist joint.

Hip Joint

The structure of the hip joint is similar to that of the shoulder joint, a ball-and-socket arrangement, and the hip and shoulder joints share the same possible movements (see figure 27.11). Because of the deepness of the socket and the tightness of the ligaments at the hip joint, range of motion (ROM) at this joint, especially

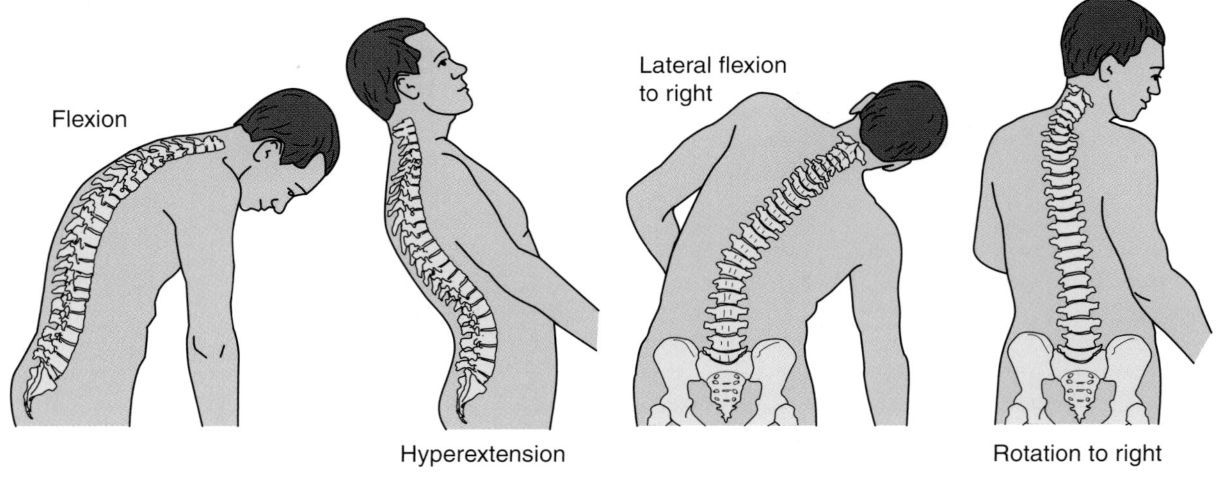

Figure 27.9 Movements of the vertebral column.

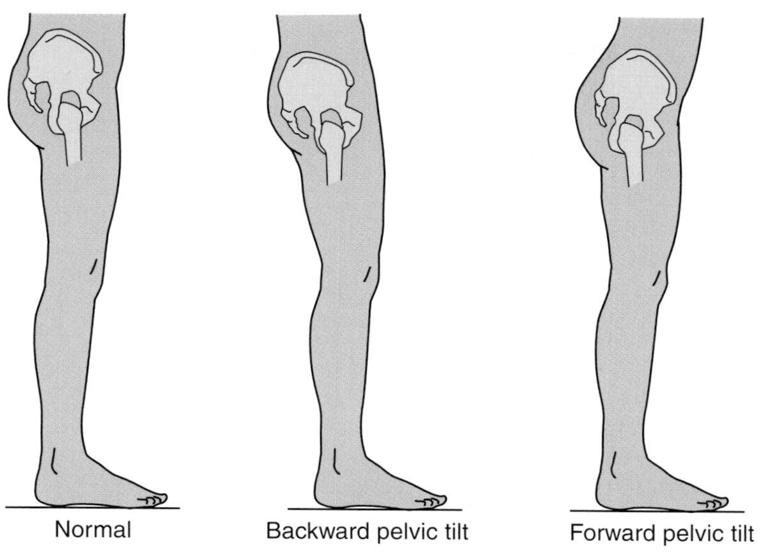

Figure 27.10 Movements of the lumbosacral joint.

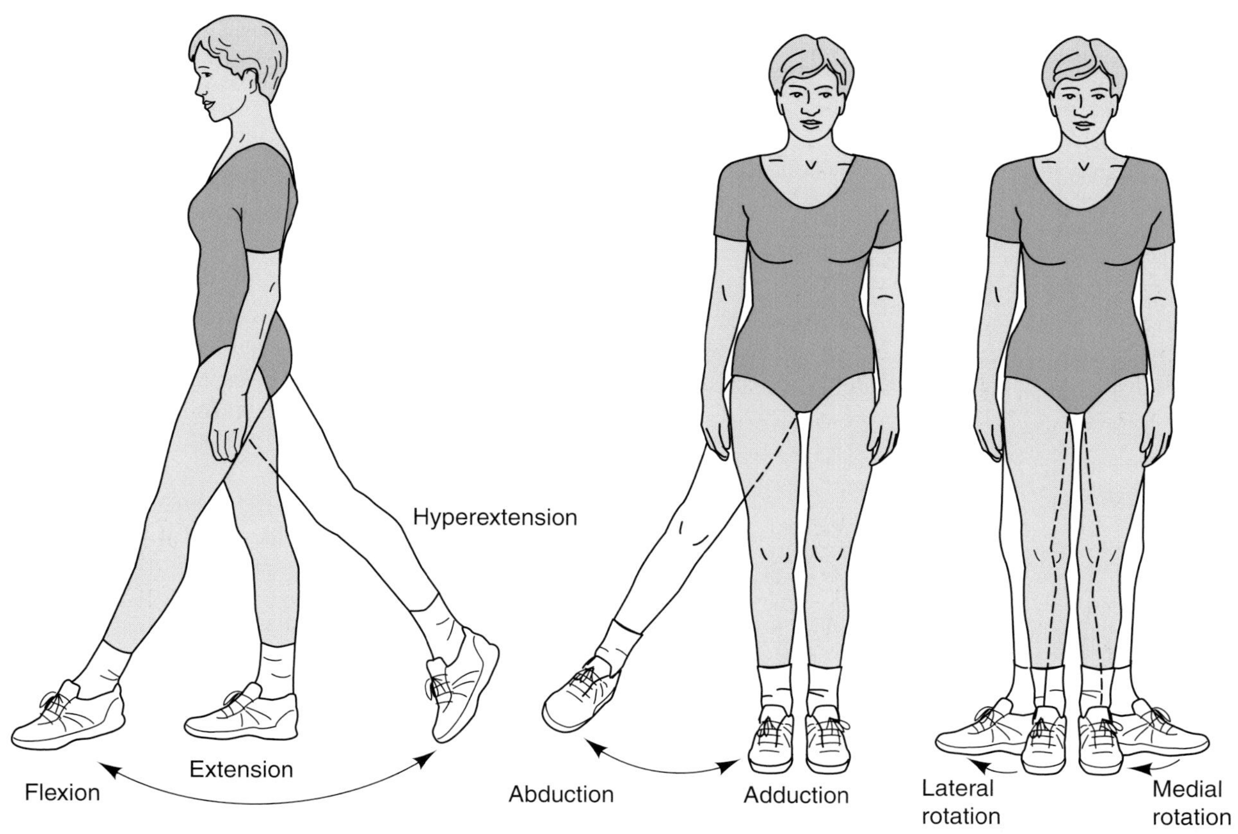

Figure 27.11 Movements of the hip joint.

for hyperextension, is less at the hip than at the shoulder joint. True hip abduction is also limited to about 45° by bony impingement. The leg can be abducted higher only by rotating the hip laterally.

Knee Joint Flexion and extension are the major movements at the knee. Although some hyperextension may be possible, it should be avoided (see figure 27.12). When the knee is in a flexed position, limited rotation, abduction, and adduction are possible.

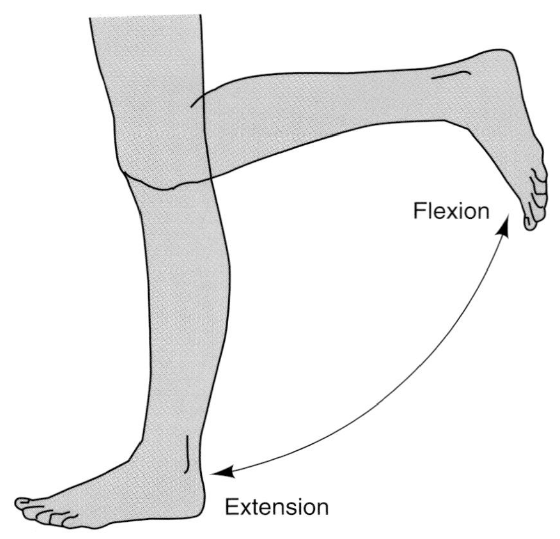

Figure 27.12 Movements of the knee joint.

Ankle Joint Also called the **talocrural joint,** the ankle joint is limited to movement in one plane only. Plantar flexion (pointing the toes downward) is still sometimes referred to as *extension;* dorsiflexion (flexing the toes back) is also referred to as *flexion* (see figure 27.13).

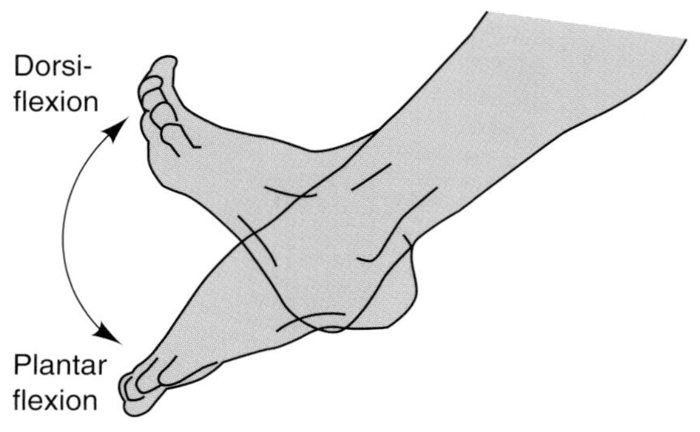

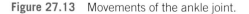

Figure 27.13 Movements of the ankle joint.

Intertarsal Joints The sideways movements of the foot occur between the different tarsal joints in the foot (see figure 27.14). Inversion can be considered a combination of pronation and adduction; eversion is a combination of supination and abduction.

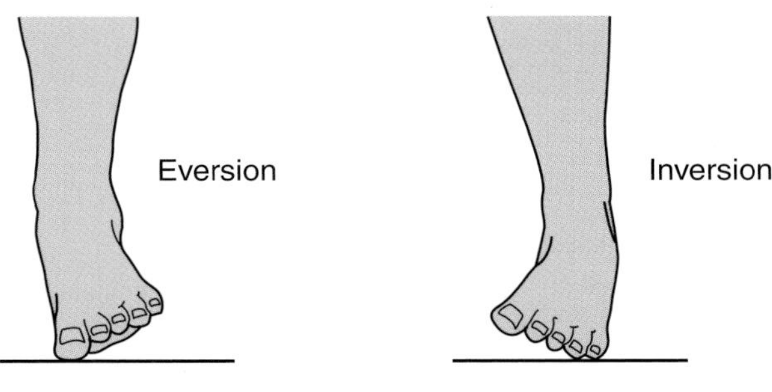

Figure 27.14 Movements of the intertarsal joints.

Forces That Cause Movement

Joint movement is caused primarily by either muscle shortening or gravitational pull, although other forces, such as another person pushing or pulling on a body part, may cause joint movement. Whether a muscle action causes the movement depends on the force of that action and the amount of resistance from the other forces.

Forces That Resist or Prevent Movement

The same forces that can cause movement also resist or prevent movement. Joint movement caused by gravity can be resisted or decelerated by eccentric muscle action (which lengthens the muscle; see the section on eccentric action later in the chapter). Gravity always resists movement occurring in the direction away from the earth. Other forces that can resist movement include internal tissue restriction by tight ligaments and tendons, exercise bands, hydraulic or air pressure devices on resistance training equipment, and the drag provided by air and water against bodies moving through them.

Key Point

Forces that can both cause and resist joint movements include muscle action and gravity.

Voluntary (Skeletal) Muscle

A skeletal muscle involved in joint movements consists of thousands of muscle fibers (e.g., the brachioradialis

Key Point

The possible movements at each joint are summarized in this table.

Joint	Movements
Shoulder girdle	Elevation, depression; abduction, adduction; upward rotation, downward rotation
Shoulder joint	Flexion, extension, hyperextension; abduction, adduction; medial rotation, lateral rotation; horizontal flexion, horizontal extension
Elbow joint	Flexion, extension
Radioulnar joint	Pronation, supination
Wrist joint	Flexion, extension, hyperextension; radial flexion, ulnar flexion
Metatarsophalangeal joints	Flexion, extension; abduction, adduction
Vertebral column	Flexion, extension, hyperextension; lateral flexion; rotation
Lumbosacral joint	Forward pelvic tilt, backward pelvic tilt
Hip joint	Flexion, extension, hyperextension; abduction, adduction; medial rotation, lateral rotation
Knee joint	Flexion, extension
Ankle joint	Plantar flexion, dorsiflexion
Intertarsal joint	Eversion, inversion

has approximately 130,000 fibers; the gastrocnemius has more than 1 million) and connective tissue. Each fiber is enclosed by the connective tissue endomysium. The **fasciculi,** or bundles of fibers grouped together, are surrounded by the **perimysium,** and the entire muscle is enclosed by the **epimysium.** The **tendon** is the passive part of the muscle made up of elastic connective tissues. Each muscle attaches to the bone itself; to the periosteum of the bone; or to deep, thick fascia by tendons and the perimysium and epimysium connective tissues. The sizes and shapes of the tendons vary and depend on their functions and the shape of the muscle itself. Some tendons (e.g., the hamstring muscle tendons found at the sides of the posterior knee and the Achilles tendon) are obvious and significant parts of the entire muscle, but other muscles such as the supraspinatus and infraspinatus (muscles that abduct and rotate the arm) seem to lie directly on the bone with no observable tendon. Many of the distal attachments (attachments farthest away from the body part being moved) that are usually found on bones that show the largest movements have more defined tendinous structures than the proximal attachments (attachments nearest to the body part being moved). Broad and flat tendons, such as the proximal tendinous sheath of the latissimus dorsi, are **aponeuroses.** Refer to figure 27.15 for anterior and posterior views of surface muscles. Other muscles lie underneath the surface muscles.

Muscle Action

Each muscle fiber is innervated, or receives stimuli, by a branch of a motor neuron. A **motor unit** consists of a single motor neuron and its branches and all the muscle

Key Point

The structures associated with muscle include fasciculi, perimysia, epimysia, tendons, and aponeuroses.

Key Point

The motor unit consists of a single motor neuron and its branches and all the muscle fibers innervated by that motor neuron. Muscular tension is increased by recruitment and summation.

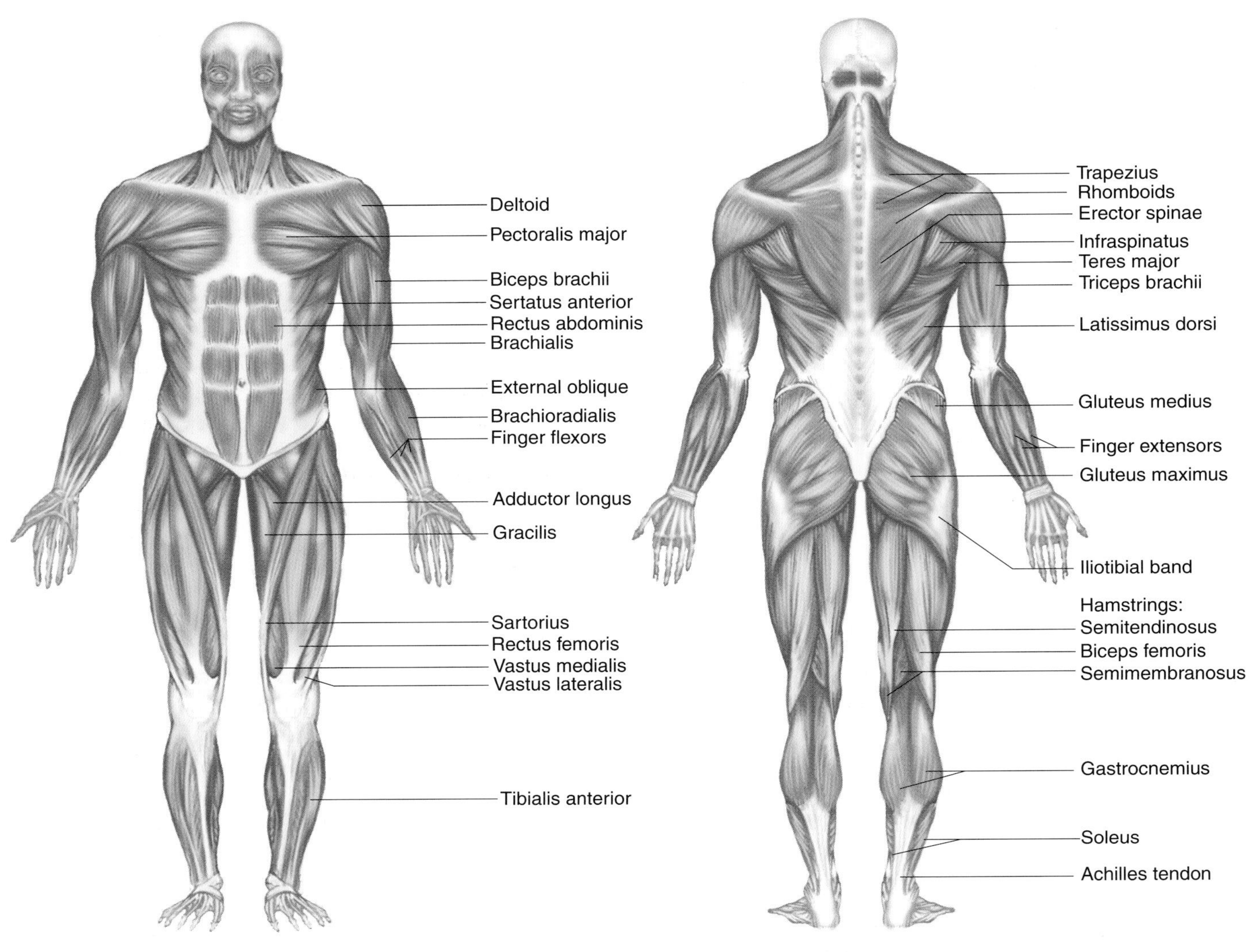

Figure 27.15 Front and back views of the surface muscles of the human body.

fibers innervated by that motor neuron. With a sufficiently strong stimulus, each muscle fiber within that motor unit responds maximally; muscular tension increases as a result of the stimulation of more motor units (**recruitment**) or an increased rate of stimulation (summation). A muscle whose primary purpose is a strength or power movement (like the gastrocnemius) rather than a delicate movement (like the finger muscles) has a large number of muscle fibers and also has many muscle fibers per motor unit. When a muscle develops tension, it tends to shorten toward the middle, pulling on all of its bony attachments. Whether the attached bones move as a result of that muscle action depends on the amount of the force of the action and the resistance to that movement from other forces. The three major muscle actions are concentric actions, eccentric actions, and isometric actions.

Concentric Action

Concentric action occurs when a muscle acts forcibly enough to actually shorten. This shortening pulls the bones of attachment closer to each other, causing movement at the joint. Figure 27.16 illustrates elbow flexion against gravity as a result of a concentric action: The muscles responsible for the flexion act with sufficient force to shorten, which pulls the lower arm toward the humerus. Although the pull is on all the bones of attachment, usually only the bone farthest from the trunk (e.g., a limb) moves during a concentric action. To stand up from a semisquat position, the body must extend at the hip joints and knee joints, but gravity resists that extension. The muscles must develop sufficient force to overcome the gravitational force; if sufficient force is developed, the muscle shortens in a concentric action, pulling on the bones to cause extension. Resistance training with free weights

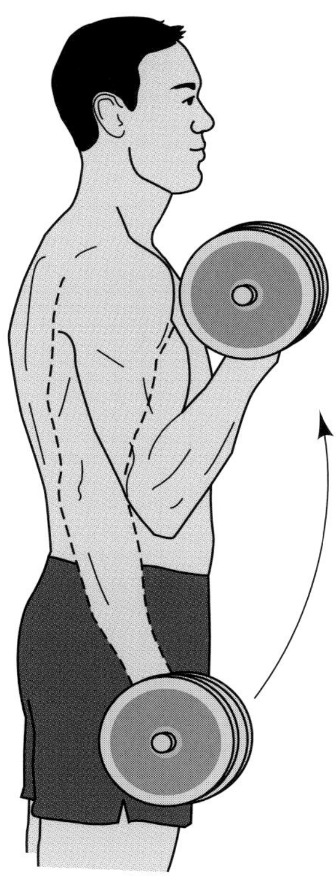

Figure 27.16 Concentric action by the elbow flexors.

uses gravitational pull as the resistance; the use of pulleys changes the direction of the gravitational pull, offering resistance to movement in other directions. Water resists movement of submerged body parts in all directions.

To exercise muscles by using gravity as the resisting force, the movements must be done in the direction opposite the pull of gravity (i.e., away from the earth). Arm abduction from a standing position occurs opposite the pull of gravity, so a concentric action is required by the muscles that will pull the humerus into the abducted position. Movements such as shoulder horizontal flexion and horizontal extension (see figure 27.5) executed from a standing position occur parallel to the ground and therefore are not resisted by gravity. Internal tissue friction is the only resistance, but concentric action by the muscles responsible for these movements is still necessary. During these movements, gravity is still trying to draw the arm toward the earth, but it is not interfering with the horizontal movement. To perform horizontal flexion and extension against the resistance of gravity, the performer must get into a position in which these movements are away from the pull of gravity. To horizontally extend the shoulder joints against gravity, the performer can lie prone on a bench or floor or stand with the trunk flexed at the hip. Horizontal flexion against gravity can be done from a supine position on the floor.

A concentric action is also necessary for a rapid movement, regardless of the direction of other forces. When an external force could cause the desired movement without any muscular action, but too slowly, concentric actions produce the desired speed. An example of this is seen in the arm movements during the second count of a jumping jack, when the arms adduct from their abducted position: Gravity would adduct the arms, but concentrically acting muscles speed up the adduction.

A muscle that is very effective in causing a certain joint movement is a prime mover, or **agonist.** Assistant movers are muscles that are not as effective for the same movement. For example, the peroneus longus and brevis are prime movers for eversion of the intertarsal joints, but they assist plantar flexion of the ankle joint only a little. During a concentric action, muscles that act opposite to the muscles causing the concentric action, the **antagonist** muscles, are basically passive and lengthen as the agonists shorten. For example, for the elbow to flex against gravity, the muscles responsible for elbow flexion act concentrically, while the antagonists, or the muscles responsible for elbow extension, relax and lengthen passively. In some fitness activities, such as aerobic dance, however, the antagonist muscles can offer more resistance to the concentrically acting muscles. This resistance occurs when all the muscles are activated (as in a bodybuilder's pose) during the movements.

Eccentric Action

An **eccentric action** occurs when a muscle generates tension that is not great enough to cause movement but instead brakes the speed of movement caused by another force (see figure 27.17). The muscle exerts force, but its length increases. Arm abduction requires a concentric action of muscles; gravity will adduct the arm back down to the side. To adduct the arm more slowly than gravity does, the same muscles that acted concentrically to abduct the arm now act eccentrically to control the speed of the lowering arm. Eccentric actions also may occur when a muscle's maximum effort is not great enough to overcome the opposing force; movement will be caused by that force despite the maximally activated muscle, which is still lengthening. An example of this may occur when a person with the elbow joint flexed to 90° is handed a heavy weight. The exerciser tries to flex the elbow joint or even maintain the 90° position but lacks the strength to do so. The elbow joint extends despite the efforts to flex it. Muscles antagonist to the eccentrically acting muscles passively shorten during the movement.

Ballistic Movements and Muscle Action

A **ballistic,** or fast, **movement** occurs when resistance is insignificant, as in throwing a ball, and requires a burst of concentric actions to initiate the movement.

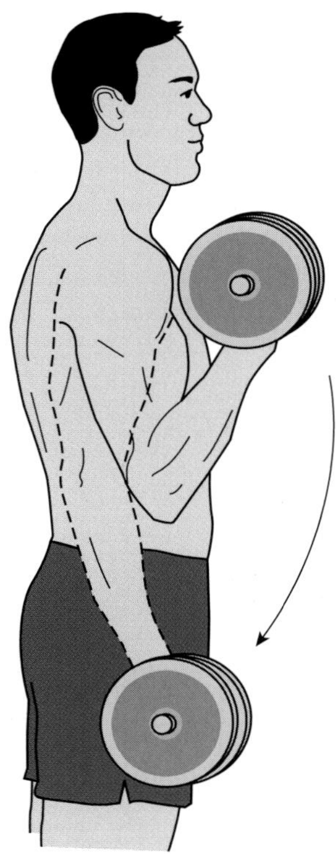

Figure 27.17 Eccentric action by the elbow flexors.

Once movement has begun, the muscles that caused the movement basically shut down; any further action slows the movement. Other muscles actively guide the movement in the appropriate direction. Eccentric actions of muscles that are antagonist to the muscles that initiated the movement decelerate and eventually stop the movement. For example, one of the most important movements in throwing is medial rotation of the shoulder joint. The muscles responsible for medial rotation act quickly and concentrically to begin the throwing motion. After the ball is released, the muscles responsible for lateral rotation act eccentrically to slow and eventually stop the movement; this is called the follow-through. The reverse is true for the windup, or preparation for the actual throw. All of this occurs in an exceedingly short time.

Key Point

A ballistic movement is a rapid movement that begins with the agonist muscles acting concentrically to initiate movement, followed by coasting, in which there is minimal muscle activity, and then by follow-through, with the antagonist muscles acting eccentrically to decelerate the movement.

Jumping jacks require repeated ballistic movements in which opposing muscles come into play. The arm movements require concentric action by the agonist muscles to initiate the rapid movement. Once the movement is initiated, these muscles basically shut down. To stop the abduction movement and initiate the arm movement in the opposite direction, muscles antagonistic to those that acted concentrically act eccentrically to decelerate the movement and then act concentrically to initiate the next arm movement (adduction).

Isometric Action

During an **isometric,** or static, **action,** the muscle exerts a force that counteracts an opposing force. The muscle length does not change, so no movement occurs, and the joint position is maintained. The contractile part of the muscle shortens, but the elastic connective tissue lengthens proportionately, so there is no overall change in the entire muscle length. Holding the arm in an abducted position or maintaining a semisquat position requires isometric action, producing just enough muscle force to counteract the pull of gravity and resulting in no movement. The effort involved in trying to move an immovable object (e.g., pushing against a wall) is another example of isometric actions; although the amount of muscular force can be maximal, the joint does not move (see figure 27.18).

A backward pelvic tilt desired during some exercises is maintained by isometric action of the abdominal muscles after they have acted concentrically to tilt the pelvis backward. During all resistance exercises that involve the arms or legs, the trunk muscles should act isometrically to stabilize the trunk and help prevent injury.

Roles of Muscles

As previously mentioned, muscles can act in several ways and have several functions. They can cause movement

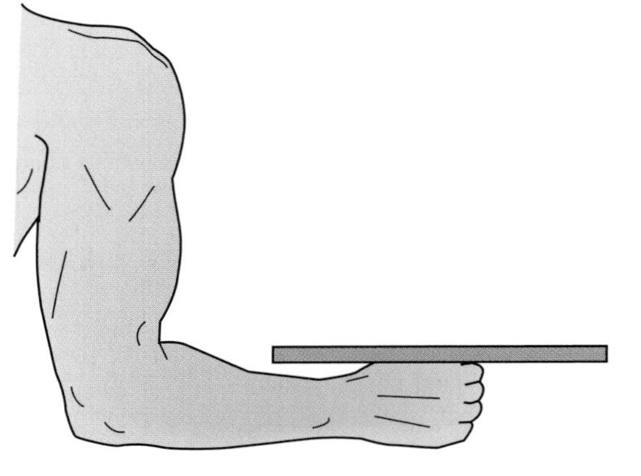

Figure 27.18 Isometric action by the elbow flexors.

Key Point

A concentric action, which shortens the muscle and therefore pulls the bones of attachment, is necessary to effect joint movement in a direction opposite another force, such as gravity, as well as rapid joint movement regardless of the direction of any other forces. An eccentric action, which lengthens the muscle, controls the velocity of movement caused by another force. An isometric action, which does not change the length of a muscle, prevents movement.

(concentric action), decelerate movement caused by another force (eccentric action), or prevent movement (isometric action). Muscles may also act isometrically to stabilize or prevent undesirable movement. For example, during a push-up exercise, gravity tends to cause the vertebral column and hip joint to hyperextend. Isometric action of the abdominal muscles prevents this sagging; activating the abdominal muscles stabilizes the trunk in its proper position.

Another function of the muscle is to counteract an undesirable action caused by the concentric action of another muscle. The concentric action of most muscles causes more than one movement at the same joint or causes movement at more than one joint. If only one of those movements is intended, another muscle must act to prevent the undesirable movement. For example, concentric action of the upper trapezius fibers both elevates and somewhat adducts the scapula. If only adduction is desired, the lower trapezius fibers, which cause depression and adduction, neutralize the undesirable elevation to avoid unnecessary discomfort. In this example, the different fibers of the trapezius neutralize the unwanted action and help the desired action. The biceps brachii muscle causes both elbow flexion and radioulnar supination; for only flexion to occur, the pronator teres counteracts the supination.

Key Point

The major roles of the muscles are to cause movement (concentric action) regardless of an opposing force, decelerate or control the speed of movement (eccentric action) caused by another force, and prevent movement (isometric action). Other muscle functions include counteracting an undesirable action caused by the concentric action of another muscle and guiding movements initiated or caused by another muscle.

Muscles also guide movements initiated or caused by other muscles. During activities against a great resistance, such as lifting free weights, muscles help maintain balance or proper direction of the movement. After muscle force has initiated a ballistic movement, other muscles can help guide the movement in the proper direction.

Muscle Groups

A **muscle group** includes all of the muscles that cause the same movement at the same joint. The group is named for the joint where the movement takes place and for the movement commonly caused by the concentric action of those muscles. The elbow flexors, for example, are a muscle group composed of the specific muscles responsible for flexion at the elbow joint when the muscles act concentrically. Table 27.1 lists the muscles that are prime (and assistant) movers of the muscle groups. A movement being observed at a joint does not necessarily involve the muscle group for the movement that is occurring. The muscle group responsible for the opposite action may be acting eccentrically to control the movement. For example, the elbow flexor muscle group flexes the elbow joint during the elbow curl exercise. To return to the starting position, the pull of gravity extends the joint to the original position, but the elbow flexor muscle group is still exerting force to eccentrically control the speed of that movement. To maintain the elbow in a flexed position requires an isometric action by those same elbow flexors.

Specific muscles that cause more than one action at a joint or cause movement at more than one joint belong to more than one muscle group. For example, the flexor carpi ulnaris muscle belongs in both the wrist flexor and wrist adductor muscle groups. The biceps brachii is part of the elbow flexor and radioulnar supinator muscle groups.

Key Point

A muscle group includes all the muscles that act concentrically to cause a specific movement at a specific joint.

Tips for Exercising Muscle Groups and Common Exercise Mistakes

Many of the errors in exercise and movement result from a lack of knowledge rather than a lack of muscular strength or coordination. By applying basic knowledge,

• Table 27.1 Prime Movers (and Assistant Movers) •

Joint	Prime movers (and assistant movers)
Shoulder girdle	Abductors—serratus anterior, pectoralis minor
	Adductors—middle fibers of trapezius, rhomboids (upper and lower fibers of trapezius)
	Upward rotators—upper and lower fibers of trapezius, serratus anterior
	Downward rotators—rhomboids, pectoralis minor
	Elevators—levator scapulae, upper fibers of trapezius rhomboids
	Depressors—lower fibers of trapezius, pectoralis minor
Shoulder joint	Flexors—anterior deltoid, clavicular portion of pectoralis major (short head of biceps brachii)
	Extensors—sternal portion of pectoralis major, latissimus dorsi, teres major (posterior deltoid, long head of triceps brachii, infraspinatus/teres minor)
	Hyperextensors—latissimus dorsi, teres major (posterior deltoid, infraspinatus, teres minor)
	Abductors—middle deltoid, supraspinatus (anterior deltoid, long head of biceps brachii)
	Adductors—latissimus dorsi, teres major, sternal portion of pectoralis major (short head of biceps brachii, long head of triceps brachii)
	Lateral rotators—infraspinatus*, teres minor* (posterior deltoid)
	Medial rotators—pectoralis major, subscapularis*, latissimus dorsi, teres major (anterior deltoid, supraspinatus*)
	Horizontal flexors—both portions of pectoralis major, anterior deltoid
	Horizontal extensors—latissimus dorsi, teres major, infraspinatus, teres minor, posterior deltoid
Elbow joint	Flexors—brachialis, biceps brachii, brachioradialis (pronator teres, flexor carpi ulnaris and radialis)
	Extensors—triceps brachii (anconeus, extensor carpi ulnaris and radialis)
Radioulnar joint	Pronators—pronator quadratus, pronator teres, brachioradialis
	Supinators—supinator, biceps brachii, brachioradialis
Wrist joint	Flexors—flexor carpi ulnaris, flexor carpi radialis (flexor digitorum superficialis and profundus)
	Extensors and hyperextensors—extensor carpi ulnaris, extensor carpi radialis longus and brevis (extensor digitorum)
	Abductors (radial flexors)—flexor carpi radialis, extensor carpi radialis longus and brevis (extensor pollicis)
	Adductors (ulnar flexors)—flexor carpi ulnaris, extensor carpi ulnaris
Lumbosacral joint	Forward pelvic tilters—iliopsoas (rectus femoris)
	Backward pelvic tilters—rectus abdominis, internal oblique (external oblique, gluteus maximus)
Spinal column (thoracic and lumbar areas)	Flexors—rectus abdominis, external oblique, internal oblique
	Extensors and hyperextensors—erector spinae group
	Rotators—internal oblique, external oblique, erector spinae, rotatores, multifidus
	Lateral flexors—internal oblique, external oblique, quadratus, lumborum, multifidus, rotatores (erector spinae group)
Hip joint	Flexors—iliopsoas, pectineus, rectus femoris (sartorius, tensor fascia latae, gracilis, adductor longus and brevis)
	Extensors and hyperextensors—gluteus maximus, biceps femoris, semitendinosus, semimembranosus
	Abductors—gluteus medius (tensor fascia latae, iliopsoas, sartorius)
	Lateral rotators—gluteus maximus, the six deep lateral rotator muscles (iliopsoas, sartorius)
	Medial rotators—gluteus minimus, gluteus medius (tensor fascia latae, pectineus)
Knee joint	Flexors—biceps femoris, semimembranosus, semitendinosus (sartorius, gracilis, gastrocnemius, plantaris)
	Extensors—rectus femoris, vastus medialis, vastus lateralis, vastus intermedius
Ankle joint	Plantar flexors—gastrocnemius, soleus (peroneus longus, peroneus brevis, tibialis posterior, flexor digitorum, flexor hallucis longus)
	Dorsiflexors—tibialis anterior, extensor digitorum longus, peroneus tertius (extensor hallucis longus)
Intertarsal joint	Inverters—tibialis anterior, tibialis posterior (extensor and flexor hallucis longus, flexor digitorum longus)
	Everters—extensor digitorum longus, peroneus brevis, peroneus longus, peroneus tertius

*Rotator cuff muscles.

an exerciser can perform better and more safely. This section offers specific tips for each major muscle group.

Shoulder Girdle and Shoulder Joint Complex

Movement can be enhanced and more muscles involved if shoulder girdle movements are deliberately incorporated with shoulder joint movements. These muscles can be optimally involved in the following exercises and movements:

- *Forward reaching.* Flexion can be accompanied by scapular abduction if the exerciser reaches the fingertips as far forward as possible.
- *Push-up.* At the completion of a push-up, the scapulae can be abducted to raise the chest a little bit more off the floor.
- *Overhead reaching.* Normally, some scapular elevation is involved when the arm is overhead. A conscious effort to reach as high as possible will involve the scapulae elevators more; conversely, a deliberate attempt to keep the shoulders down for a long-neck look requires concentric action by the scapulae depressors.
- *Sideward arm reaching.* During horizontal extension at the shoulder joint, the arm can be moved farther back with scapular adduction.

Elbow and Radioulnar Joints

Flexion against resistance requires concentric action of the flexor muscles at the elbow joint. The position of the radioulnar joints, whether the arm is supinated or pronated, does not affect the involvement of the elbow joint muscles. The degree to which these muscles are strengthened, however, is affected by supination and pronation—a good point to remember when instructing participants on how to perform curls. Normally, elbow flexion with the radioulnar joint in a pronated position (a reverse curl) is a weaker movement because the biceps brachii muscle cannot act as strongly as when the radioulnar joints are in a supinated position. (The distal tendon of the biceps brachii muscle is wrapped around the radius somewhat in the pronated position, which diminishes its pulling force.) The brachialis muscle, though, is not affected by the radioulnar joint position because it is attached to the ulna, which is the nonmoving bone in radioulnar joint movements. Further, the brachioradialis muscle can act with more force when the radioulnar joint is in a semipronated, semisupinated position. None of the elbow extensor muscles are affected by the position of the radioulnar joint, but the radioulnar joint position affects the amount of weight that may be pressed (moved) on the lat machine because of strength limitations of the wrist muscles. Triceps push-downs, in which elbow extension occurs with the radioulnar joints in the pronated position, require the wrist flexors to stabilize the wrist joint; triceps pull-downs (supinated position) utilize the wrist extensors, which are usually much weaker than the flexors. Exercisers who want to concentrate on building the elbow extensors should perform triceps push-downs.

Wrist Joint

During wrist flexion and extension curl exercises, the wrist muscles are affected by the position of the radioulnar joints. Gravity acts as a resistance for wrist flexion when the radioulnar joints are in the supinated position and as a resistance for extension when the radioulnar joints are in the pronated position. Remind exercise participants that the position of the radioulnar joints affects which wrist muscles are strengthened during these exercises.

Vertebral Column and Lumbosacral Joints

In general, neither neck hyperextension nor neck hyperflexion is desirable. The same pairs of muscles that act concentrically to cause flexion and extension can be strengthened or stretched, one side at a time, by cervical lateral flexion and rotation. Participants should tilt or turn the head from side to side rather than bend the neck forward or backward. Although hyperextension may not be contraindicated for the young, no benefits can be gained and it teaches bad habits.

Many exercises require appropriate positioning of the lumbosacral joint and lumbar vertebrae and actions by the abdominal muscles for either movement or stabilization. An abdominal curl-up or crunch exercise should begin with a backward pelvic tilt that is maintained throughout the curl-up and return movement. If the backward pelvic tilt cannot be maintained or the exerciser feels tightness or an ache in the lumbar area, the exercise should be stopped. If the problem is inadequate strength to maintain the backward tilt, the exercise should be modified to one that requires less abdominal muscle strength—one that the exerciser has sufficient abdominal strength to perform correctly.

A full curl-up, in which the exerciser comes up to a sitting position, requires hip flexion by the hip flexor muscles during the last stages of the exercise. Initially, the abdominal muscles concentrically tilt the pelvis backward and then flex the vertebral column. Once flexion is achieved, these muscles act isometrically to keep the pelvis tilted backward and the trunk in a flexed position. During a full curl-up, the exerciser can feel a sticking point that occurs when the trunk flexion is complete and the hip flexors begin to bring the trunk to an upright position. Doing partial curl-ups or crunches helps eliminate the role of the hip flexors and maintain focus solely on strengthening the abdominals.

The leg lift exercise is considered an abdominal exercise, but it is often not taught correctly. From a supine position on the floor, the legs are lifted and held up by concentric and then isometric action of the hip flexors. Some of the hip flexor muscles also pull the lumbosacral joint into a forward-tilted position. The abdominal muscles must prevent that forward tilt and maintain a flattened lumbar spine and posterior pelvic tilt. The backward pelvic tilt should precede the hip flexion, and, as in the case of the curl-up, if the proper tilt cannot be maintained, the exercise should not be done in that fashion.

The pelvis also tends to tilt forward during overhead arm movements from a standing position. This can be prevented by keeping the arms in front of the ears and by flexing the knees slightly.

When weights are lifted from a supine position, as in the bench press, there is a tendency to hyperextend the lumbar spine and tilt the pelvis forward. Although this tendency can allow the exerciser to lift a somewhat heavier weight, it does not increase the work of the arm and chest muscles, and it puts the low back into a compromising position. Bench presses are best done with the hips and knees in a flexed position and the feet on the bench or a bench extension. Upright presses are best done seated with the back supported.

Hip Joint

A common error during side-lying leg raises that exercise the hip abductors is the attempt to move the foot as high as possible. Because the ROM for true abduction is limited (about 45°), the exerciser often rotates the top leg laterally, which turns the foot out and allows it to go higher. However, this rotation changes the muscle involvement more to the hip flexors. To exercise the primary abductor muscles, the leg should not be rotated; the toes should face forward, not up. Turning the feet out comes from lateral rotation of the hip; there should be no attempt to rotate the knee or the ankle joints.

In backward leg movements for strengthening the gluteus muscles, hyperextension is limited primarily by the tightness of the hip ligaments. A leg can appear to be more hyperextended if it is accompanied by a forward pelvic tilt. The exerciser should be cautioned to keep the pelvis in its proper neutral position, even though some apparent hip hyperextension is lost.

A common exercise position is standing with feet shoulder-width apart. The exerciser should have the feet turned slightly outward (from hip lateral rotation). Too much rotation is potentially dangerous. During any squatting or standing movement, the knee should be directly over the foot (not in front of the foot) to prevent strain to the lateral and medial knee ligaments. Although during the squat the knee can be kept over the foot even in the toe-out position, some individuals tend to let the knees move toward the inside of the feet. It is easier to determine whether the knee position is correct when the feet are almost parallel with each other. During the squat, the exerciser should be able to see the big toe on each foot.

Knee Joint

Hyperflexion can strain and stretch knee ligaments and put pressure on the menisci; therefore, fully squatting below a 90° angle at the knee joint, especially when using additional weight, should not be attempted, nor should sitting on the lower legs. During any lunging movements or forward–back stride positions in which the front knee is flexed, the knee should be over or in back of the foot and not in front. Any knee position that puts a twisting pressure on the knee joint should also be avoided. The hurdler position, with one leg out to the back and side with a flexed knee, should be avoided; that leg should also be in front.

Ankle Joint

If the squat exercise is performed with the heels of the feet resting on a low block, the soleus muscles are exercised more than they would be if the feet were flat. This position with the heels up shortens the gastrocnemius muscles even more (they are already shortened by the flexed knee), limiting their ability to generate force. The soleus muscles, which do not cross the knees, aren't shortened to the extent that it affects force generation. The gastrocnemius muscles are weaker in this position, so more of the work is done by the soleus muscles. To increase the force production of the gastrocnemius muscles, the squat could be done with the balls of the feet on the block. A mountain climber especially would benefit from this modification because it mimics the knee and ankle joint positions in climbing.

Intertarsal Joints

Walking on the insides or outsides of the foot should never be done. Doing so not only stresses the knees but also causes ankle sprains. A better way of exercising the invertors and evertors is to walk back and forth, instead of up and down, across a ramp or hill.

Muscle Group Involvement in Selected Activities

Human movement is caused or controlled by muscle forces. The following sections briefly analyze the

Key Point

During exercises involving the vertebral column and lumbosacral joints, participants should remember the following:

- Maintain backward pelvic tilt during the abdominal crunch or curl-up.
- Tilt the pelvis backward before hip flexion in the curl-up and leg lift.
- Keep the pelvis tilted backward during overhead arm movements performed in a standing position.
- Keep the lumbar spine flat on bench during weightlifting in a supine position.

For exercise involving the knee, participants should remember the following:

- Keep the knee over the foot (not beyond) during lunging and squatting movements.
- Maintain foot and knee alignment.

involvement of muscle groups in some common physical activities.

Walking, Jogging, and Running

Jogging can be looked at as modified walking, and running can be viewed as a fast jog. The different phases and the muscle groups involved in walking, jogging, and running are similar, but more forceful muscle actions are needed to increase speed. The three basic phases of these movements are the push-off, recovery of the push-off leg, and landing.

The push-off is accomplished by the concentric action of the hip hyperextensors, the talocrural plantar flexors, and, to a lesser extent, the foot metatarsophalangeal flexors (see the back leg in figure 27.19). Because the knee of the back leg is almost extended at push-off, little work is done by the knee extensors to help propel the body forward. The gluteus maximus may assume a greater role in hip hyperextension as speed increases. Medial rotation takes place at the hip joint, but because the foot is fixed on the ground, this movement is seen at the pelvis.

At the beginning of the recovery phase, the hip flexors act concentrically to begin the forward leg swing. This is basically a ballistic movement, so the momentum initiated by the hip flexors continues the motion. The knee flexors bend the knee at the beginning of hip flexion, the extensors initiate the straightening of the knee, and the flexors then work eccentrically to control the knee extension at the end of the recovery phase. The talocrural joint is dorsiflexed to clear the foot from the ground and prepare for the landing (see the recovery leg in figure 27.19). Running speed is a product of stride length and stride frequency. To increase both factors in running, the hip flexes to a greater extent and with a much greater velocity (see figure 27.20, the recovery leg).

Just before landing, the hip extensors act eccentrically to decelerate the forward leg swing. On contact, the knee extensors act eccentrically to cushion the impact. The heel should touch the ground first during walking and jogging; as running speed increases, the ball of the foot or the entire foot may make contact. During the landing phase in walking and jogging, the talocrural dorsiflexors

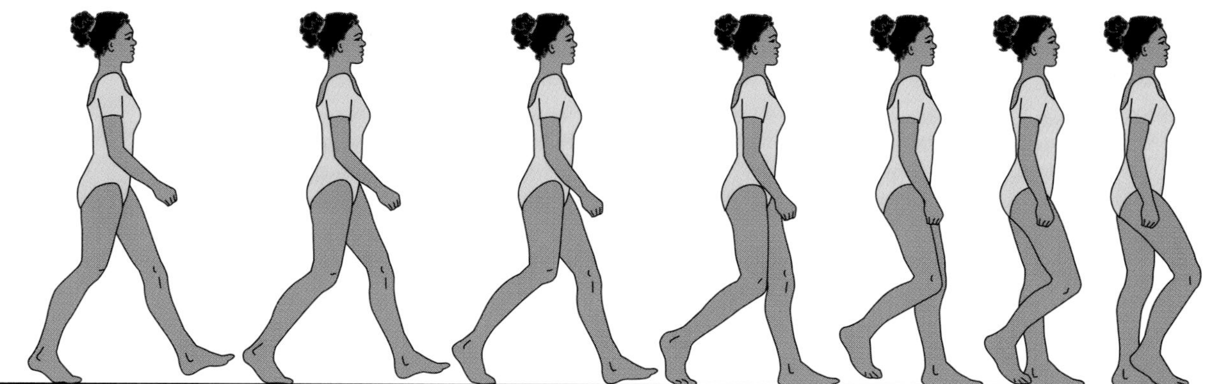

Figure 27.19 Walking movements.

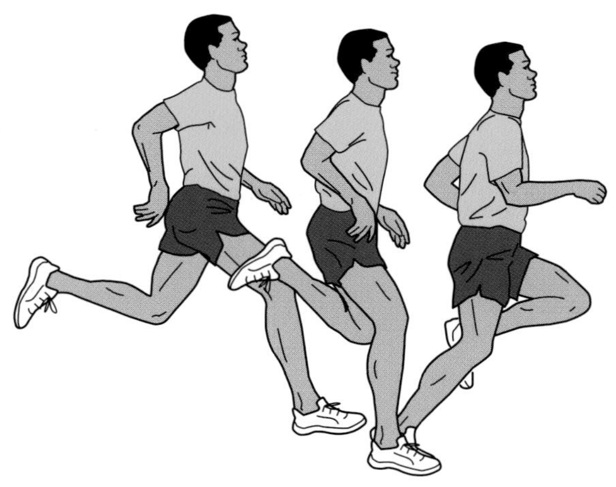

Figure 27.20 Running movements.

act eccentrically to control the speed of movement of the ball of the foot to the ground.

The arm swing requires shoulder flexion and extension to hyperextension. As speed increases, the swing becomes more vigorous, and there is more elbow flexion. For the greatest efficiency, the arms should move anteriorly and posteriorly. To increase the involvement of the upper limbs for exercise, a walker can exaggerate the flexion and hyperextension movements or can abduct and adduct or horizontally flex and extend the shoulder joint.

Walking or running up an incline elicits greater action from the gluteus maximus muscle at the hip and from the knee extensors. The talocrural dorsiflexors are more active immediately before landing in order to match the position of the talocrural joint to the angle of the incline. Because the talocrural joint is in a more dorsiflexed position, the plantar flexors begin acting during push-off from a more stretched position. For these reasons, hill climbing requires greater flexibility in the plantar flexors, especially the soleus muscle, and greater strength in the dorsiflexors. There is also more eccentric action by the knee extensors during landing in downhill than in uphill running. As a result, these muscle groups are more apt to become fatigued and to be sore afterward.

Jogging in place requires the talocrural plantar flexors to propel the body upward; they work more than any of the other lower-extremity muscle groups in this activity. The knee extensors are primarily involved in eccentric action to cushion the landing. During walking and jogging, the heel is the first part of the foot to make contact with the surface, but during jogging in place, the ball of the foot touches first. The plantar flexors therefore are also active during the landing, acting eccentrically to control the speed and amount of dorsiflexion. It is better to have sufficient dorsiflexion so the heel touches the ground briefly rather than to always stay up on the toes, which can strain the plantar flexors. Additional muscles can be involved in moving the leg immediately after push-off and before the foot lands again: hip flexion with flexed or extended knee, hip hyperextension with flexed or extended knee, hip abduction and adduction, hip lateral rotation along with hip and knee flexion that brings the foot to the front of the trunk, and medial rotation with knee flexion that brings the foot behind and to the side of the trunk.

Cycling

The main force in cycling comes from the hip and knee extensors during the downward push. With toe clips, riders can use the hip flexors and talocrural dorsiflexors to help return the pedal to the up position, but only if they make a conscious effort to do so.

Jumping

The hip and knee extensors, followed by the talocrural plantar flexors, forcibly propel the body upward. The lean of the trunk primarily determines the angle of takeoff. The trunk extends, and the arms flex from a hyperextended position just before the leg action. If the reach height of the arms is important, as in a jump ball in basketball or in a tennis smash, the scapulae elevate. During the landing, the hip and knee extensors and the talocrural plantar flexors act eccentrically.

Overarm Throwing

There are three phases in throwing: the windup, or preparation; the execution, or actual throw; and the follow-through, or recovery. Figure 27.21 illustrates the sequence of the actual throw.

In preparation for throwing, the weight shifts to the back foot, the back leg medially rotates (because the leg is fixed to the ground, rotation is seen at the pelvis), the trunk rotates and somewhat laterally flexes and hyperextends, the shoulder laterally rotates, and there is some horizontal extension of the throwing arm accompanied by adduction of the scapula, flexion of the elbow, and hyperextension of the wrist. The movements of the throwing arm are all ballistic. The lateral rotation at the shoulder is remarkably fast and powerful. Toward the end of the windup, the medial rotators begin to act eccentrically to decelerate the rotation in preparation for the actual throw.

The weight shift forward is the initial movement in the throw. This is accomplished by the hip abductors, hyperextensors, and lateral rotators; the talocrural plantar flexors; and the intertarsal everters of the back leg. The front hip rotates laterally. The trunk then flexes laterally in the direction opposite that of the windup and rotates, beginning at the lumbar area and continuing through the thoracic vertebrae, and then flexes. There is a forcible medial rotation of the shoulder, along with scapular abduction. Although there is some horizontal flexion, most of the force of the shoulder in an overhand throw comes from this medial rotation. The elbow extends, and the wrist moves toward flexion. Depending on the desired spin on the ball, the radioulnar pronators and the wrist abductors or adductors also may be involved.

Because the actions at the shoulder and elbow joints are vigorous ballistic movements, the shoulder lateral rotators and horizontal extensors act eccentrically to decelerate the movements; the elbow flexors act eccentrically to prevent elbow hyperextension.

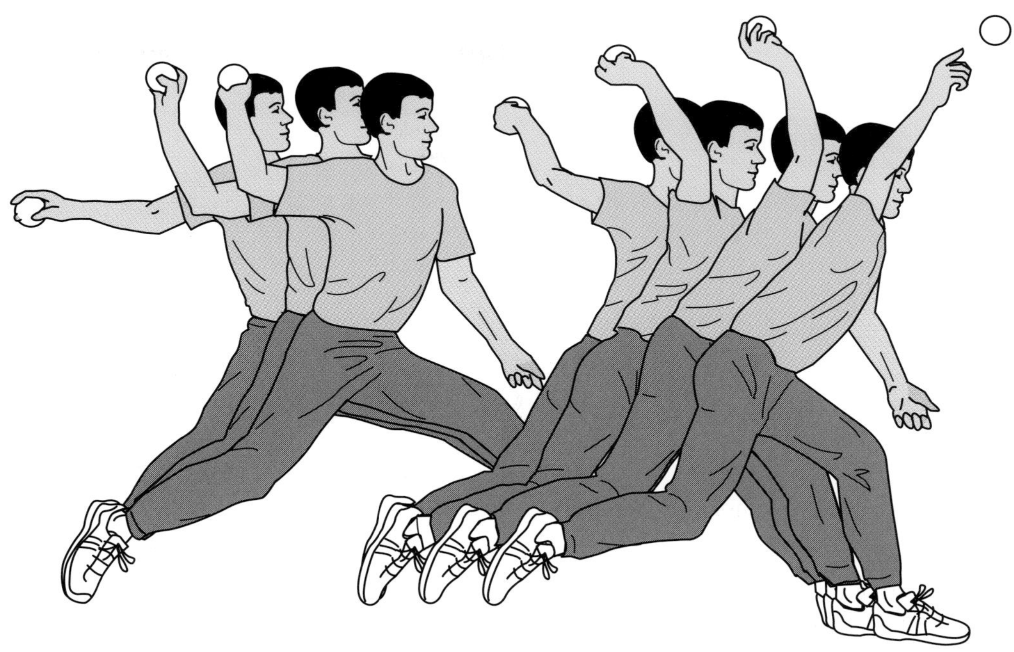

Figure 27.21 Overarm throwing movements.

Swimming and Exercise in Water

Swimming is a unique activity because water resists movement of submerged body parts in all directions and at all speeds. Exercises or movements performed in water demand concentric actions. Gravity is less of a factor in water, so less stress is put on the weight-bearing joints.

Lifting and Carrying Objects

The weight to be lifted from the ground should be located close to the lifter's spread feet; the lifter squats, keeping the trunk as erect as possible. The actual lifting should be accomplished by the legs rather than the spine or arms. Proper lifting is begun by moving the trunk to a position as perpendicular to the floor as possible and then tilting the pelvis backward and keeping the abdominal muscles activated; the knee extensors along with the hip extensors then act concentrically. The lift should be slow, not jerky (see figure 27.22). Insufficient leg strength can result in incorrect lifting. The weight should be carried close to the body, with the trunk assuming a position that allows the line of gravity to fall well within the area of the base. The trunk lateral flexors are more active when the weight is carried on one side, the extensors are more active when the weight is in front, and the abdominals are more active when the weight is carried across the top of the back, as in backpacking.

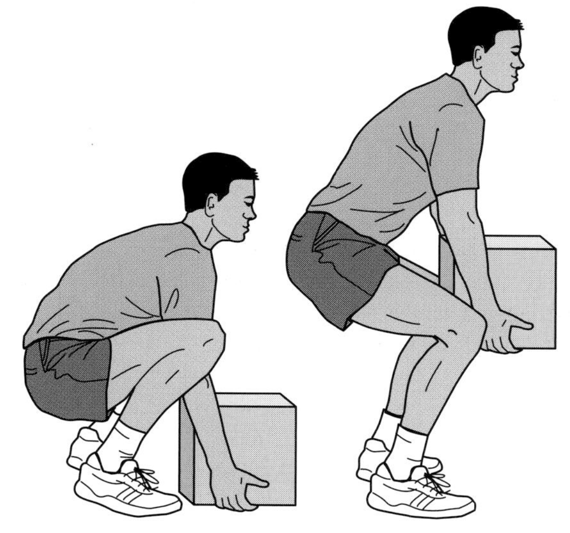

Figure 27.22 Lifting technique.

Key Point

The steps in proper lifting are to place the feet close to the object, move the vertebral column to an upright position perpendicular to the floor, tilt the pelvis backward, and slowly extend the hips and knees while activating the abdominals.

Key Point

The movements and muscles involved in locomotion, throwing, cycling, jumping, and swimming are summarized here.

Major muscle group	Movement task
Hip extensors	Locomotion—push-off; cycling; jumping; swimming—front crawl, back crawl, sidestroke
Hip flexors	Locomotion—recovery; swimming—front crawl, back crawl, sidestroke
Hip abductors	Swimming—breaststroke; throwing
Hip adductors	Swimming—breaststroke
Hip lateral and medial rotators	Throwing
Knee extensors	Locomotion—landing; cycling; jumping
Knee flexors	Locomotion—recovery
Talocrural plantar flexors	Locomotion—push-off, landing; jumping
Talocrural dorsiflexors	Locomotion—recovery
Shoulder joint flexors	Underhand throwing
Shoulder joint extensors	Swimming—front crawl
Shoulder joint medial and lateral rotators	Throwing
Anterior shoulder joint muscles	Swimming—back crawl; sidestroke lead arm; throwing
Posterior shoulder joint muscles	Swimming—sidestroke trail arm, breaststroke; throwing—windup
Shoulder girdle upward and downward rotators	Swimming—breaststroke, sidestroke lead arm, front crawl, back crawl
Shoulder girdle abductors	Swimming—back crawl; throwing
Shoulder girdle adductors	Swimming—front crawl, breaststroke Throwing—windup
Shoulder girdle elevators	Swimming—front crawl, back crawl, sidestroke lead arm, breaststroke
Elbow flexors	Throwing
Elbow extensors	Throwing
Trunk flexors	Throwing
Trunk rotators	Throwing

Basic Mechanical Concepts for Human Movement

Knowing the principles of mechanics is also necessary to understand human movement. Some of these basic but important concepts are described next.

Achieving Stability

In order to maintain balance, an individual's line of gravity must fall within the area of the base of support. Figure 27.23*a* illustrates the area of the base of support in a standing position with feet together; figure 27.23*b* illustrates a position with feet apart and forward and back.

Stability, or the ease with which balance can be maintained, is proportional to the distance from the line of gravity to the outer limits of the base that is farthest from a potentially upsetting force. Figure 27.24 compares more stable positions with less stable positions. A wide base of support usually, but not necessarily, ensures greater stability. With the feet apart, if one leans so that the line of gravity falls directly over one foot and a pushing force is applied in the same direction of the lean, there is less stability than if the feet were together but with the line of gravity along the edge of the foot closer to the applied force.

Stability is also indirectly proportional to the height of the center of gravity, which is approximately at the level of the naval when a person is standing. The lower the center of gravity over the feet, the greater the force needed to upset the stability. Stability is also directly proportional to body weight. With all other factors

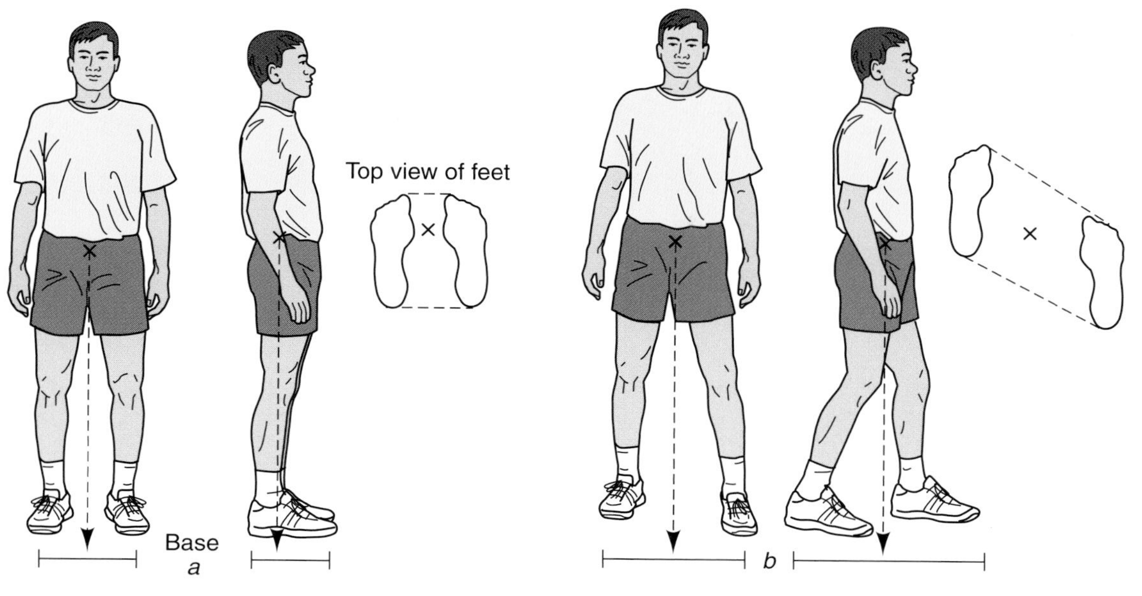

Figure 27.23 Bases of support.

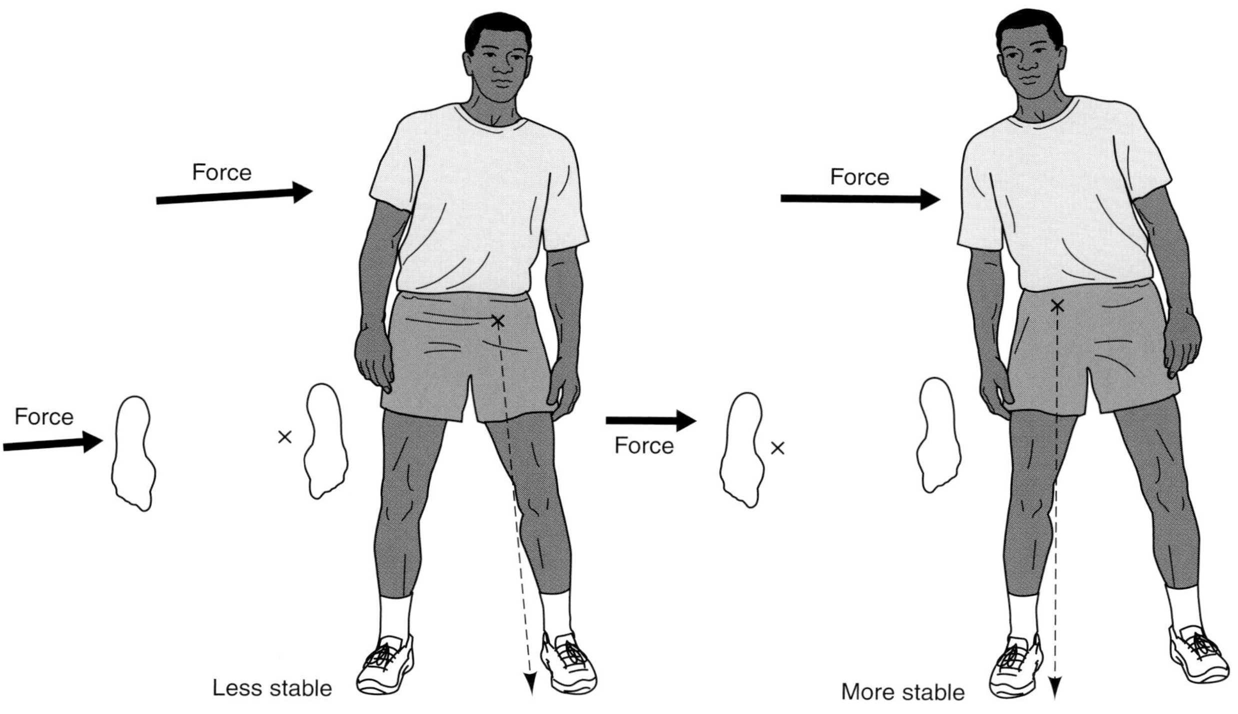

Figure 27.24 Relationship between the line of gravity and the outer limits of base of support.

being equal, a heavy person is more stable than a lighter one.

Stability may be increased by moving the feet apart to widen the base of support and by flexing the knees and hips to lower the center of gravity. During standing exercises that require balance, stability can also be aided by holding or pushing against a nearby object such as a wall or chair. Many exercises can be executed from a sitting position, which increases the base and lowers the center of gravity. To help maintain stability against a potentially upsetting force, the weight should be shifted toward that force. Just before locomotion begins, a position close

> **Key Point**
>
> Stability in humans is directly proportional to the distance of the line of gravity from the limits of the base, indirectly proportional to the height of the center of gravity above the base, and directly proportional to the weight of the body. For stability during standing, the knees should be flexed to lower the center of gravity, the feet should be apart in the direction of an oncoming force to increase the distance between the line of gravity and the outer limits of the upsetting force, and the weight of the body (line of gravity) should be shifted toward the force.

to instability is attained by shifting the line of gravity closer to the outer limits of the base (which is the area of the push-off foot in walking or the hands in a track start position) in the direction of the intended movement. During locomotion, as the line of gravity moves outside the limits of the base, a new base is established when the other foot lands and stability is maintained. If something prevents the foot from establishing a new base, stability is lost. A basketball guard, in taking a charge from a forward, will fall down quicker and easier if in an unstable position—standing fairly erect with feet closer together and weight on heels—at the collision.

Torque

A force is any push or pull that causes movement. The effect produced when a force causes rotation is called **torque (T).** It is the product of the magnitude of the force *(F)* and the **force arm (FA),** which is the perpendicular distance from the axis to the direction of the application of that force. Torque can be expressed as follows:

$$T = F \cdot FA$$

When two opposing forces act to produce rotation in opposite directions, one of the forces often is designated as the **resistance force (R);** its force arm is called the **resistance arm (RA).** When we consider the torque produced by muscle to cause movement against gravity or some other external force, *F* and *FA* are designated for the muscle and *R* and *RA* for the gravitational or other opposing force.

Applying Torque to Muscle Action

Muscle action can be considered the force; the *FA* is the perpendicular distance from the joint (axis) to the direction of the force from its point of application (where the muscle attaches to the bone being moved). Figure 27.25 illustrates the direction of pull of the biceps brachii on the radius; *FA* is the perpendicular distance from the elbow joint to this line of force. If the muscle insertion were closer to the joint, the same force would produce less torque because of the shorter force arm and more muscle force would be required to produce the same torque.

Joint position also affects torque. Figure 27.26 shows the direction of pull by the biceps brachii but with the elbow in a less flexed position. This shortens *FA,* so the same muscle force produces less torque at that joint angle.

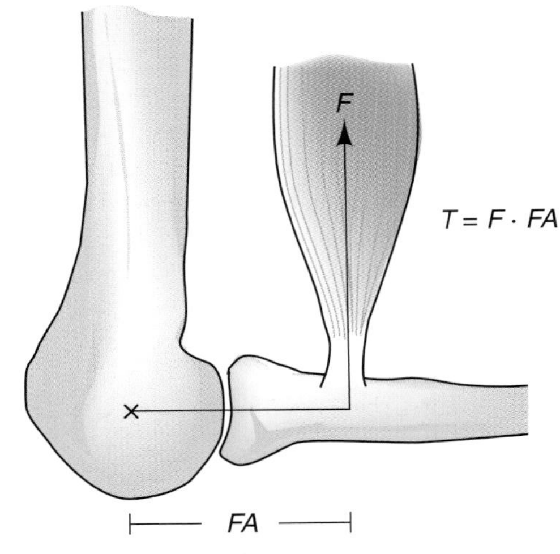

Figure 27.25 Force *(F)* and force arm *(FA)* of the biceps brachii.

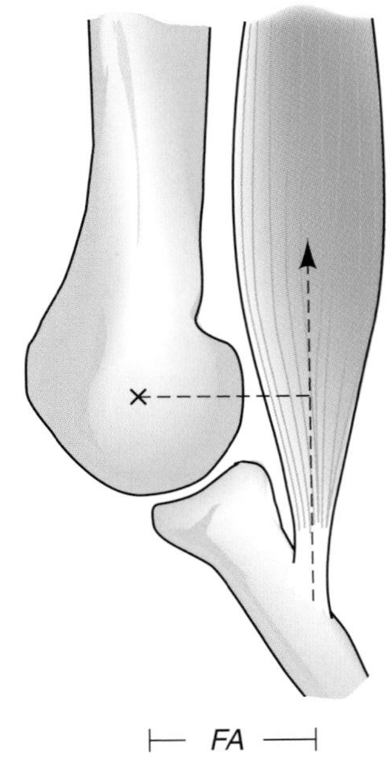

Figure 27.26 Effect of less flexion at the elbow joint on the force arm *(FA)* of the biceps brachii.

Torque Resulting From Other Forces

The force from gravitational pull is treated as a resistance force. The resistance *(R)* produced by gravity pulling on a body part is the weight of the object; the resistance arm *(RA)* is the perpendicular distance from the axis of rotation to the point of the object that represents its center of gravity. The torque is the product of *R* and *RA*. Figure 27.27 illustrates the torque produced by gravity acting on the arm. The torque that opposes limb movements can be increased by adding weight to increase both the magnitude of force and the length of the resistance arm or by moving the weight farther from the axis. The resistance arm of a force applied by someone pushing or pulling on a limb is the perpendicular distance from the axis to the point of application of the push or pull.

For muscle action to move a bone, the muscle force must produce a torque greater than the opposing or resistance torque; the muscle action is concentric. A greater resistance torque results in movement, and the muscle acts eccentrically. Technically, it can be argued that the muscle force during an eccentric action should be considered the resistance, and the external force causing the movement should be considered the force. When the muscular torque equals the resistance torque, no movement occurs; the muscle acts isometrically.

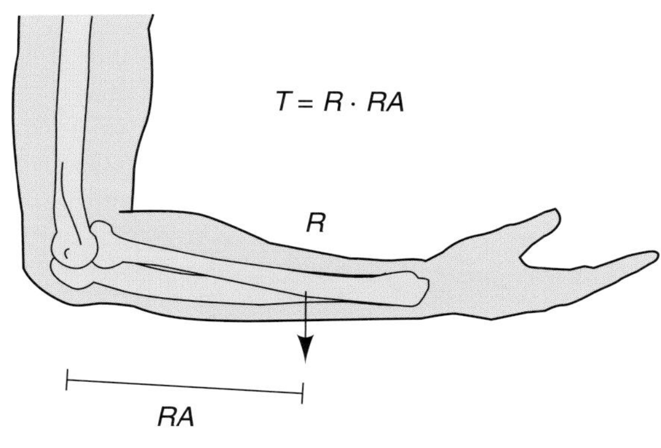

Figure 27.27 Resistance *(R)* and resistance arm *(RA)* of lower arm.

> **Key Point**
>
> Torque can be expressed as $T = F \cdot FA$ for the torque that produces the movement or as $T = R \cdot RA$ for the torque that opposes the movement. A concentric action produces a torque that is greater than the resistive torque. An eccentric action produces a torque that is less than the opposing torque. An isometric action produces a torque that equals the opposing torque.

Applying Torque to Exercising

Knowledge of torques can be used to modify exercises for different people. The amount of muscular action required by the exercise can be tailored to an individual's needs by altering the amount of resistance or the resistance arm or both in order to change the resistive torque. For example, resistive torque can be increased with external weights so that it requires stronger muscle actions. The resistance torque also can be changed by altering the position of the body parts. Figure 27.28 shows an exerciser reducing the required muscle force by not using the weight to decrease both the resistance and the resistance arm and by flexing the elbow to shorten the resistance arm.

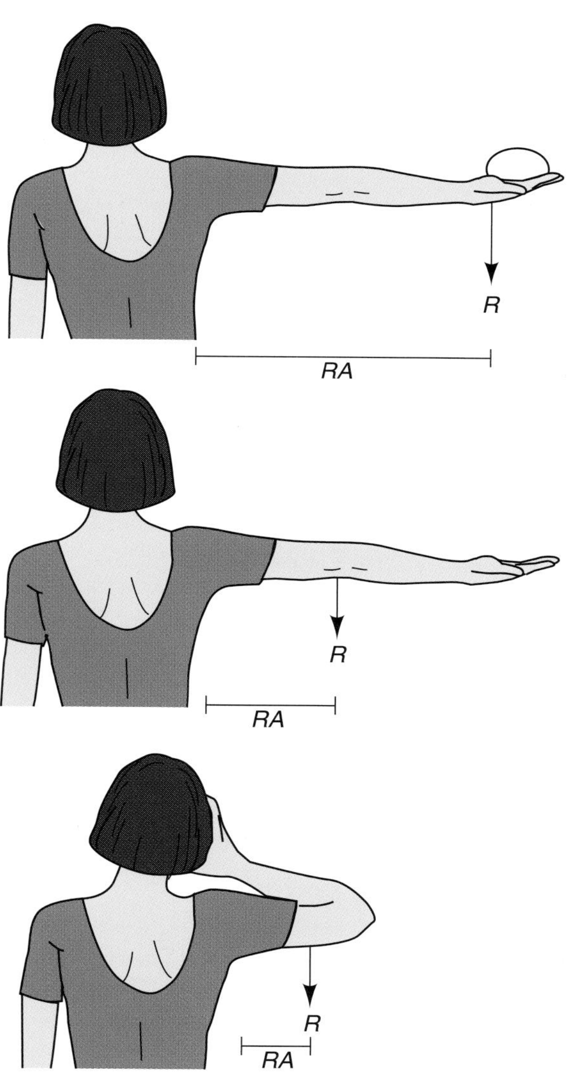

Figure 27.28 Modifying resistive torque.

> **Key Point**
>
> The torque that resists limb movements can be altered by modifying the amount of the resistive force and changing the position of the resistive force relative to the joint to change the resistance arm.

During a curl-up, the position of the arms determines the length of *RA* and therefore the amount of resistance torque against which the abdominal muscles have to work. The arms may be held at the sides of the body to bring the upper-body mass closer to the axis of rotation to reduce the required muscle force, or the arms can held overhead with hands on the scapulae or straight out to increase the resistive torque, therefore increasing the required muscle force. Lessening the resistance torque does not necessarily make the exercise easy for everyone. If an exerciser with less strength finds the resistive torque too great to overcome for a sufficient number of repetitions, he can change limb positions to reduce the torque against which he has to work; however, this individual is still working as hard, relative to his maximal ability, as a stronger individual who did not have to reduce the resistive torque.

Rotational Inertia

Rotational inertia (also referred to as the *moment of inertia),* or the reluctance of a body segment to rotate around an axis or a joint, depends on the body's mass and the distribution of that mass around the joint. A leg, for example, has more rotational inertia than an arm not only because it is heavier but also because its mass is concentrated a greater distance away from its axis. A softball bat held by its fat end has less rotational inertia than a bat grasped in the usual manner.

The rotational inertia of body segments before or during movement depends on the mass of the segments, which cannot be changed, and on the distribution of the mass around the joints, which can be manipulated. For example, an arm with the elbow, wrist, and fingers extended has a greater rotational inertia than an arm with the elbow, wrist, and fingers flexed; a leg with an extended knee and ankle has more inertia than a leg with the knee flexed and ankle dorsiflexed. The amount of muscular force necessary to cause rapid limb movement is proportional to the rotational inertia of the limb to be moved. During jogging, in which speed is not a factor, the knee of the recovery leg is flexed to reduce the leg's rotational inertia around the hip joint. Less muscular force is needed to swing the recovery leg forward, which reduces the possibility of local fatigue of the hip flexors. In sprinting, the quicker the recovery leg is brought forward, the faster the running speed. Powerful actions of the hip flexors, along with greater knee flexion, result in the recovery leg coming through sooner and thus in increased overall speed. Another example of rapid movement to which this principle can be applied is jumping jacks. Keeping the elbow flexed reduces the rotational inertia. This may reduce the amount of muscle force produced by the shoulder abductor and adductor muscle groups to maintain a certain cadence or, if maximum muscle force is still applied, result in faster movements.

Angular Momentum

Angular momentum, or the quantity of angular motion, is expressed as the product of the angular velocity and the rotational inertia, which is determined by both the mass of the moving body part and the distribution of the mass around the joints. A moving body part possesses angular momentum; the faster it moves and the greater its rotational inertia, the greater the angular momentum. The amount of force necessary to change angular momentum is proportional to the amount of the momentum.

Applying Angular Momentum to Exercising

The concept of angular momentum can be applied to ballistic limb movements during exercise. A fast-moving body segment is decelerated by eccentric muscle actions; a faster movement, a greater mass, or a greater desired deceleration requires greater muscle force to be applied to decelerate the body segment. Care must be taken when performing rapid ballistic limb movements, especially when using added weight. The movements may generate great momentum, and considerable muscle strength may be required to decelerate and eventually stop them.

Transfer of Angular Momentum

Transfer of angular momentum from one body segment to another can be achieved by stabilizing the initial

> **Key Point**
>
> Rotational inertia created during fast limb movements can be decreased by moving the mass of the limb closer to the axis or joints. The amount of angular momentum depends on the rotational inertia and angular velocity of a moving body segment. The amount of eccentric force necessary to decelerate the angular velocity of a body segment is proportional to the amount of the angular momentum of the body segment. Angular momentum can be transferred from one body segment to another by stabilizing the initial moving body part at a joint.

moving body part at a joint, which causes angular movement of another body part. For example, when an athlete performs a curl-up to exercise the trunk flexors, flinging the arms forward from an overhead position transfers their momentum to the trunk. This decreases the amount of muscular action needed by the trunk flexors and makes the exercise seem easier, but the abdominal flexors do not work as hard. In another example, a jump with a turn in the air can be better achieved if, just before takeoff, the arms are swung forcibly across the body in the intended direction of the spin.

Common Mechanical Errors in Locomotion, Throwing, and Striking

Success in physical activities depends in part on properly executing movement. Some of the more common errors that violate the laws of mechanics are discussed in the next sections.

Errors in Locomotion

Some beginning joggers have a tendency to run stiff legged, or with insufficient knee flexion of the recovery leg. This results in a greater rotational inertia of the leg; the hip flexors must exert greater force than they would exert if the knee were more flexed to bring the mass of the leg closer to the hip axis.

Another potential problem is direction of the arm and leg movements. All movements should be executed in the anterior and posterior directions. Swinging the hands across the trunk rotates the upper trunk; in reaction, the lower trunk rotates in the opposite direction. The recovery leg may also rotate medially at the hip; this swings the recovery foot to the outside. The touchdown foot should land in a forward–backward direction and not pointed to the outside. Sometimes runners are not aware of this tendency, and the fitness professional should instruct them to "toe in" somewhat when landing, which corrects the foot alignment.

Some joggers and runners propel themselves too high off the ground during the airborne phase; this shortens stride length. Although the length of time the body is airborne may be the same as when running with less lift, less horizontal distance is covered.

Overstriding, in which the line of gravity from the runner's center of gravity falls in front of the touchdown foot, can decrease running speed. No propulsion force against the ground for forward movement can take place until the line of gravity is over and ahead of the foot. Under-striding, in which the line of gravity falls well in back of the foot at touchdown, shortens the time during which the propulsion muscles can work.

Errors in Throwing and Striking

A ball is thrown for accuracy, speed, or distance, which depends in part on the speed of the ball when it leaves the hand. The speed of the ball in the hand just before release is the speed of the ball immediately after it leaves the hand. The more joints that are involved in the throwing motion, the greater the speed of the ball when it is released. Proper throwing and striking techniques are the same for females and males. Most throwing problems that result in low velocity, such as pushing the ball rather than throwing it, stem from a lack of trunk rotation or from poor timing of this rotation with the movements of the shoulder joint. The thrower should rotate the trunk and hips during the windup so that the pelvis is sideways to the intended direction of the throw and the shoulders are rotated even more to the back. As the hips and then the different sections of the spinal column rotate back to begin the throw, the arm lags behind. This sets up a whiplike action of the arm and allows adequate time for the important medial rotation. Without this trunk rotation, the resulting inadequate arm rotation produces a pushing motion during the throw. The vertebral column also has to rotate in a wavelike fashion, with the thoracic vertebrae being the last to rotate.

The same sequence of motion applies to striking events, such as tennis and badminton stroking and softball batting. A common fault in learning how to serve a tennis ball or smash a birdie is insufficient trunk rotation. It is easier to hit an object without trunk rotation, but less trunk rotation lessens the impact of the racket on the projectile. In batting, a common error is the lack of fluid timing among movements of the different body segments. The hip, trunk, and arm movements follow one another so the bat is moving with great velocity on contact with the ball. Beginners often stop one motion before beginning the next.

Key Point

Common mechanical errors in locomotion include running stiff legged, toeing out, swinging the arms across the trunk, overstriding, under-striding, and lifting too high off the ground. The most common mechanical errors in throwing and striking are insufficient trunk rotation and poor timing among the trunk, hip, and arm movements.

Case Studies

You can check your answers by referring to page 476 in appendix A.

1. You are supervising the resistance training area when you hear a lot of clanging noise coming from the vicinity of the seated leg press. You discover that the exerciser at that machine is not controlling the descent of the weights. You suggest that he slowly return the weights rather than letting them drop. He asks you why—he doesn't see any benefit in a controlled return other than reduced noise. What do you tell him?
2. Alice wants to know why she can move a heavier weight when she does wrist curls with her palms up than with her palms down and why she can do more pull-ups with her palms facing her than with her palms facing away. How would you answer her?
3. José complains that his lower back aches somewhat when he reaches overhead while standing in place during the cool-down portion of an aerobics class. What would you suggest he do during this movement to prevent the aching?

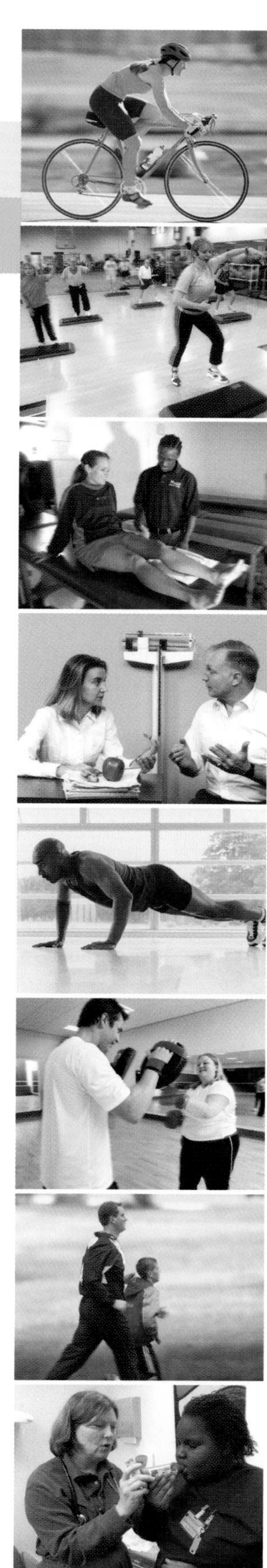

28 CHAPTER

Exercise Physiology

Objectives

The reader will be able to do the following:

1. Explain how muscle produces energy aerobically and anaerobically and evaluate the importance of aerobic and anaerobic energy production in fitness and sport.
2. Describe the structure of skeletal muscle and the sliding-filament theory of muscle contraction.
3. Describe the power, speed, endurance, and metabolism of the different types of muscle fibers.
4. Describe tension development in terms of twitch, summation, and tetanus, and describe the recruitment of muscle fiber types in exercise of increasing intensity.
5. Describe the various fuels for muscle work and how exercise intensity and duration affect the respiratory exchange ratio.
6. Describe how exercise tests, training, heredity, sex, age, altitude, carbon monoxide, and cardiovascular and pulmonary diseases influence $\dot{V}O_2$max.
7. Describe how the ventilatory threshold and the lactate threshold indicate fitness as well as predict performance in endurance events.
8. Explain how heart rate, stroke volume, cardiac output, and oxygen extraction change during a graded exercise test and during training, and link the variation in $\dot{V}O_2$max in the population to differences in maximal cardiac output and oxygen extraction.

(continued)

9. Summarize the effects of endurance training on muscular, metabolic, and cardiovascular responses to submaximal work and on $\dot{V}O_2max$, and describe how reducing or ceasing training affects $\dot{V}O_2max$ and the degree to which endurance training effects are specific to the muscles involved in the training.
10. Describe how men and women differ in their cardiovascular responses to graded exercise.
11. Contrast the importance of the different mechanisms for heat loss during heavy exercise and during submaximal exercise in a hot environment. Describe how training in a hot and humid environment affects heat tolerance.

Fitness professionals need to know basic exercise physiology to prescribe appropriate activities, deal with weight loss concerns, and explain to participants what happens when training in a hot and humid environment. This chapter can't possibly cover the extensive detail found in texts devoted to exercise physiology; instead, we summarize major topics and, where possible, apply the discussion to exercise testing and prescription. We refer the interested reader to the texts on exercise physiology listed in the references (2, 8, 22, 41, 46, 49, 52, 64).

Energy and Work

Energy is what makes the body go. Several kinds of energy exist in biological systems: electrical energy in nerves and muscles; chemical energy in the synthesis of molecules; mechanical energy in the contraction of muscle; and thermal energy, derived from all of these processes, that helps maintain body temperature. The ultimate source of the energy found in biological systems is the sun. The radiant energy from the sun is captured by plants and used to convert simple atoms and molecules into carbohydrate, fat, and protein. The sun's energy is trapped within the chemical bonds of these food molecules.

For the cells to use this energy, they must break down the foodstuffs in a manner that conserves most of the energy contained in the bonds of the carbohydrates, fats, and proteins. In addition, the final product of the breakdown must be a molecule the cell can use—adenosine triphosphate (ATP). Cells use ATP as the primary energy source for biological work, whether this work is electrical, mechanical, or chemical. In ATP, three phosphates are linked by high-energy bonds. When a bond between the phosphates is broken, energy is released and may be used by the cell. At this point the ATP has been reduced to a lower energy state, becoming adenosine diphosphate (ADP) and inorganic phosphate (P_i).

When a muscle performs work, ATP is constantly converted to ADP and P_i. The ATP must be replaced as fast as it is used if the muscle is to continue to generate force. The muscle cell has a great capacity to replace ATP under a variety of work circumstances, from a short dash to a marathon. Edington and Edgerton (18) devised a logical approach to studying the energy supplied for muscle contraction. They divided the energy sources (ATP sources) into immediate, short term, and long term.

Immediate Sources of Energy

The very limited amount of ATP stored in a muscle might meet the energy demands of a maximal effort lasting about 1 sec. **Creatine phosphate (CP),** another high-energy phosphate molecule stored in the muscle, is the most important immediate source of energy. CP can donate its phosphate molecule (and the energy therein) to ADP in order to make ATP, allowing the muscle to continue producing force.

$$CP + ADP \rightarrow ATP + C$$

This reaction takes place as fast as the muscle forms ADP. Unfortunately, the CP store in muscle lasts only 3 to 5 sec when the muscle is working maximally. This process does not require oxygen and is one of the **anaerobic energy** (without oxygen) mechanisms for producing ATP. CP is the primary source of ATP during a shot put, a vertical jump, or the first seconds of a sprint.

Short-Term Sources of Energy

As the muscle's store of CP decreases, the muscle fibers break down glucose (a simple sugar) to produce ATP at a very high rate. The glucose is obtained from blood or the muscle's glycogen store. The multienzyme pathway for glucose metabolism is called **glycolysis,** and it does not require oxygen to function (like the breakdown of CP, it too is an anaerobic process).

$$\text{Glucose} \rightarrow 2 \text{ pyruvic acid} + 2 \text{ ATP}$$

In glycolysis, glucose is broken down into two molecules of pyruvic acid; in the process, ADP is converted to ATP, allowing the muscle to maintain a high rate of work. But glycolysis can only continue for a limited time. When glycolysis operates at high speed, pyruvic acid is converted to lactic acid, and lactic acid (lactate) accumulates in the muscle and the blood. This accumulation of lactic acid in the muscle slows the rate of glycogen metabolism and actually may interfere with the mechanism involved in muscle contraction. Supplying ATP via glycolysis has its shortcomings, but it does allow a person to run at fast speeds for short distances. This short-term source of energy is of primary importance in events involving maximal work lasting about 2 min.

Long-Term Sources of Energy

The long-term source of energy involves the production of ATP from a variety of fuels, but this method requires the utilization of oxygen (it is **aerobic**). The primary fuels include muscle glycogen, blood glucose, plasma free fatty acids, and intramuscular fats. Glucose is broken down in glycolysis (as described previously), but in this case the pyruvic acid is taken into the **mitochondria** of the cell, where it is converted to a 2-carbon fragment (acetyl CoA) that enters the Krebs cycle. Fats are taken into the mitochondria, where they are also broken down into acetyl CoA, which again enters the Krebs cycle. The energy originally contained in the glucose and fats is extracted from the acetyl CoA and is used to generate ATP in the electron transport chain in a process called *oxidative phosphorylation,* which requires oxygen.

$$\text{Carbohydrate and fat} + O_2 \rightarrow \text{ATP}$$

ATP production via aerobic mechanisms is slower than production from the immediate and short-term sources of energy, and during submaximal work it may be 2 or 3 min before the ATP needs of the cell are met completely by this aerobic process. One reason for this lag is the time it takes for the heart to increase the delivery of oxygen-enriched blood to the muscles at the rate needed to meet the ATP demands of the muscle. The aerobic production of ATP is the primary means of supplying energy to the muscle in maximal work lasting more than 2 min and in all submaximal work.

Interaction of Exercise Intensity, Duration, and Energy Production

The proportion of energy coming from the anaerobic sources (immediate and short-term energy) is very much influenced by the intensity and duration of the activity. Figure 28.1 shows that during an all-out activity lasting less than 1 min (e.g., a 400 m dash), the muscles obtain most of their ATP from anaerobic sources. In a 2 min maximal effort, approximately 50% of the energy comes from anaerobic sources and 50% comes from aerobic sources; in a 10 min maximal effort, the anaerobic component drops to 15%. For a 30 min all-out effort, the anerobic component is about 5%, and is even smaller in a typical submaximal 30 min training session.

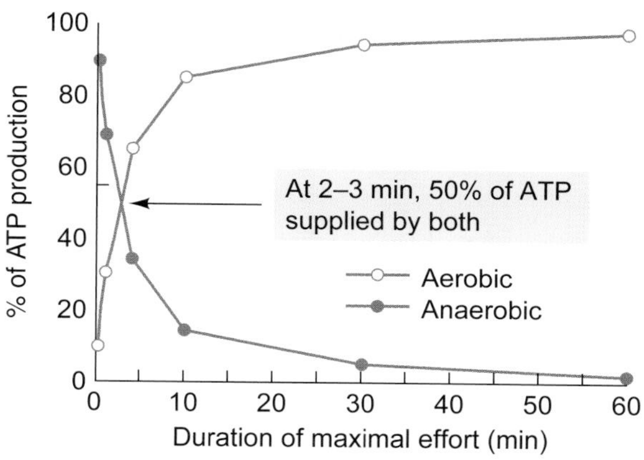

Figure 28.1 Percent of aerobic and anaerobic contributions to total energy supply during maximal work of various durations (49).

Key Point

ATP is supplied at a high rate by the anaerobic processes: CP breakdown and glycolysis. Anaerobic energy is important in short, explosive events (e.g., shot put) and in athletic competitions requiring maximal effort for less than 2 min. ATP is supplied during prolonged exercise by the aerobic metabolism of carbohydrate and fat in the mitochondria of the muscle. This is the primary means of supplying energy to the muscle in maximal work lasting more than 2 min and in all submaximal work.

Understanding Muscle Structure and Function

Exercise means movement, and movement requires muscle action. To discuss human physiology related to exercise and endurance training, we must start with skeletal muscle, the tissue that converts the chemical energy of ATP to mechanical work. How does a muscle do this?

Figure 28.2 shows the structure of skeletal muscle, from the intact muscle to the smallest functional unit within the muscle. A **muscle fiber** is a cylindrical cell that has repeating light and dark bands, giving it the name *striated muscle.* The striations are attributable to a more basic structural component called the **myofibril,** which runs the length of the muscle. Each myofibril is composed of a long series of **sarcomeres,** the fundamental units of muscle contraction. Figure 28.2 shows that the sarcomere contains the thick filament **myosin** and the thin filament **actin** and is bounded by connective tissue called the **Z line** (63).

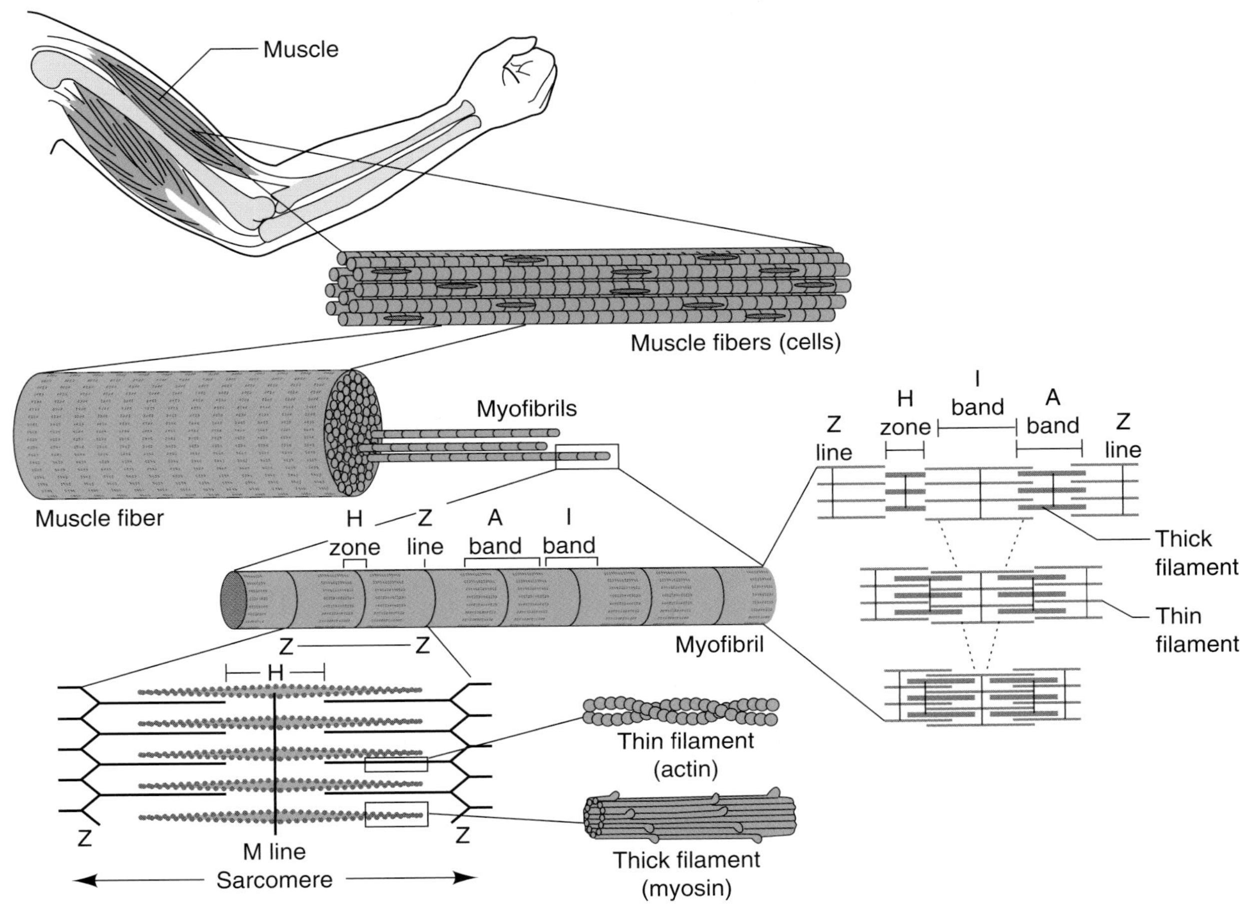

Figure 28.2 Levels of fibrillar organization within a skeletal muscle, and changes in filament alignment and banding pattern in a myofibril during shortening.
Reprinted from A.J. Vander, J.H. Sherman and D.S. Luciano, 1980, *Human physiology*, 3rd ed. (New York, NY: McGraw-Hill, Inc.), 212, 216, with permission of the McGraw-Hill Companies.

An enlargement of two sarcomeres in figure 28.2 shows the **A band, I band,** and **H zone** and the changes that take place when the sarcomere moves from the resting state to the contracted state. The I band is composed of actin and is bisected by the Z line, and the A band is composed of myosin and actin. According to the **sliding-filament theory** of muscle contraction, the thin actin filaments slide over the thick myosin filaments, pulling the Z lines toward the center of the sarcomere. In this way the entire muscle shortens, but the contractile proteins do not change size. So how does the muscle release the energy in ATP for shortening?

If ATP is the energy supply, then an ATPase (an enzyme) must exist in muscle to split ATP and release the potential energy contained within its bonds. The ATPase is found in an extension of the thick myosin filament, the **cross bridge,** which also can bind to actin. Figure 28.3 shows how ATP, the cross bridge, and actin interact to shorten the sarcomere (63).

Why aren't the cross bridges always moving and the muscle always in contraction? At rest, two proteins that are associated with actin block the interaction of myosin with actin: **troponin,** which has the capacity to bind calcium, and **tropomyosin.** Figure 28.4 shows that when a muscle is depolarized (excited) by a motor nerve, the action potential spreads over the surface of the muscle fiber and enters the fiber through special channels called **transverse tubules** (this process is step 1 in the figure). Once inside the muscle fiber, this wave of depolarization spreads over the **sarcoplasmic reticulum (SR),** a membrane that surrounds the myofibril, and the SR releases calcium (Ca^{2+}) into the sarcoplasm (step 2 in the figure). When the calcium binds with troponin, the tropomyosin aligns the cross-bridge binding site on the actin so that the myosin cross bridge can interact with it (step 3 in the figure). When the cross bridge binds to actin, energy is released, the cross bridge moves, and the sarcomere shortens (step 4 in the figure). This sequence repeats as

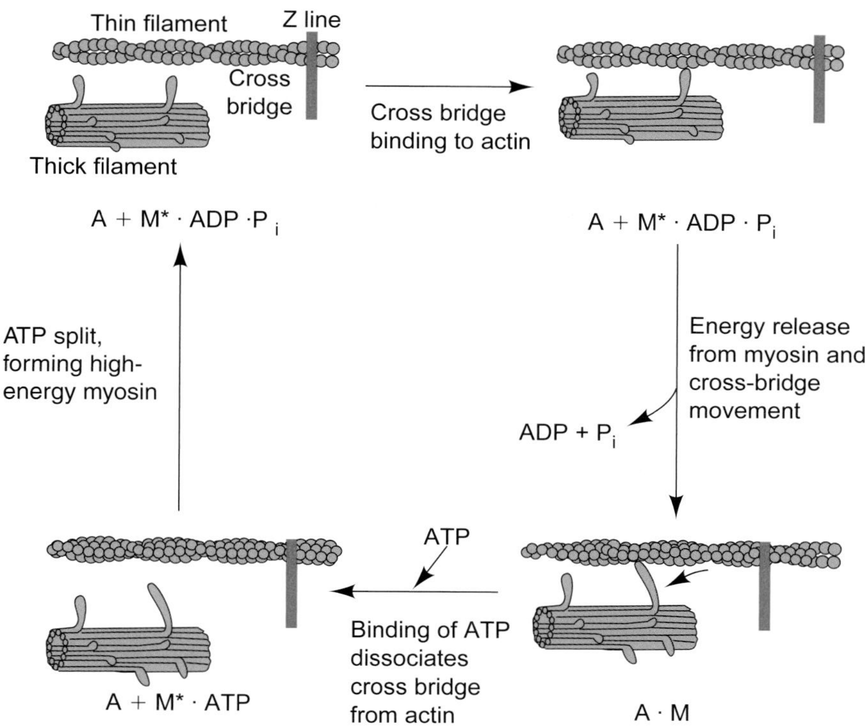

Figure 28.3 Chemical and mechanical changes during the four stages of a single cross-bridge cycle. Begin reading the figure at the lower left. A = actin; M* = energized form of myosin; ATP = adenosine triphosphate; ADP = adenosine diphosphate; P_i = inorganic phosphate.

Reprinted from A.J. Vander, J.H. Sherman and D.S. Luciano, 1985, *Human physiology*, 4th ed. (New York, NY: McGraw-Hill, Inc.), 263, with permission of the McGraw-Hill Companies.

long as calcium is present and the muscle can replace the ATP it uses. The muscle relaxes when the calcium is pumped back into the sarcoplasmic reticulum and troponin and tropomyosin can again block the interaction of actin and myosin (steps 5 and 6 in the figure) (63). The muscle needs ATP for moving the cross bridge, pumping the calcium back to the SR, and maintaining the resting membrane potential that allows the muscle to be depolarized.

Key Point

A muscle contracts when ATP is split to form a high-energy myosin-ATP cross bridge, the myosin-ATP cross bridge binds to actin and releases energy, the cross bridge moves and pulls actin toward the center of the sarcomere, and, finally, ATP binds to and releases the cross bridge from actin to start contracting again. Calcium release from the sarcoplasmic reticulum blocks inhibitory proteins (troponin and tropomyosin) and allows the cross bridge to bind to actin to begin moving. Relaxation occurs when calcium is pumped back into the sarcoplasmic reticulum and ATP binds to the cross bridge.

Muscle Fiber Types and Performance

Muscle fibers vary in their abilities to produce ATP by the different aerobic and anaerobic mechanisms described earlier in the chapter. Some muscle fibers contract quickly and have an innate capacity to produce great force, but they fatigue quickly. These muscle fibers produce most of their ATP by CP breakdown and glycolysis, and they are called **fast glycolytic,** or **type IIx,** fibers. Other muscle fibers contract slowly and produce little force, but they have great resistance to fatigue. These fibers produce most of their ATP aerobically in the mitochondria and are called **slow oxidative,** or **type I,** fibers. These fibers have many mitochondria and a relatively large number of capillaries helping to deliver oxygen to the mitochondria. Last, there is a fiber with both type I and type IIx characteristics. It is a fast-contracting muscle fiber that not only produces great force when stimulated but also resists fatigue because of its large number of mitochondria and capillaries. These fibers are called **fast oxidative glycolytic,** or **type IIa,** fibers.

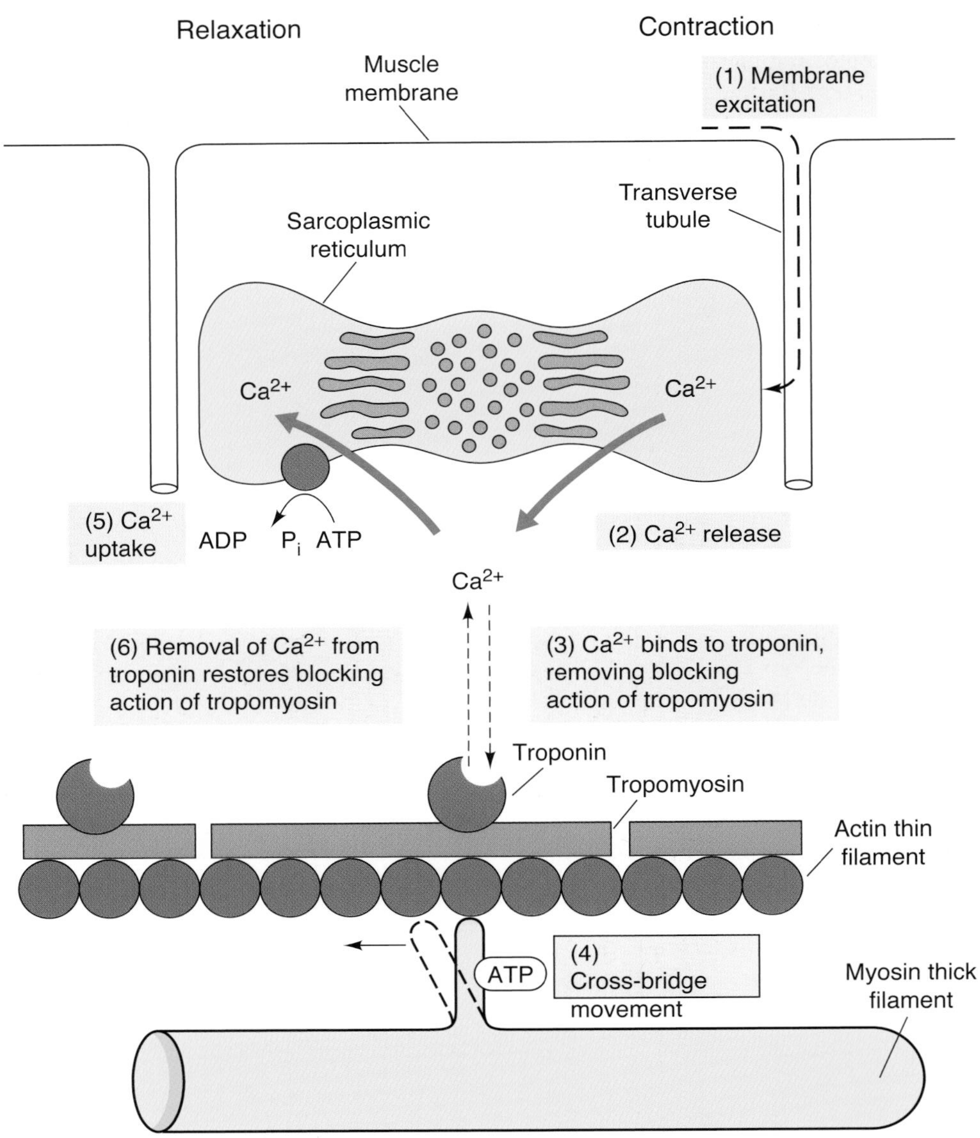

Figure 28.4 Role of calcium in muscle excitation–contraction coupling. ADP = adenosine diphosphate; P_i = inorganic phosphate; ATP = adenosine triphosphate; Ca^{2+} = calcium ions.

Reprinted from A.J. Vander, J.H. Sherman and D.S. Luciano, 1985, *Human physiology*, 4th ed. (New York, NY: McGraw-Hill, Inc.), 263, with permission of the McGraw-Hill Companies.

Muscle Fiber Types: Genetics, Sex, and Training

In the average male and female, about 52% of the muscle fibers are type I, with the fast-twitch fibers divided into approximately 33% type IIa and approximately 13% type IIx (57, 58). The distribution of fiber types in the overall population greatly varies, however. From studies comparing identical to fraternal twins, the distribution of fast and slow fibers seems to be genetically fixed. In addition, fast-twitch fibers cannot be converted to slow-twitch fibers, or vice versa, with endurance training (3). In contrast, the capacity of the muscle fiber to produce

Key Point

Muscle fibers differ in speed of contraction, force, and resistance to fatigue. Type I fibers are slow, generate low force, and resist fatigue. Type IIa fibers are fast, generate high force, and resist fatigue. Type IIx fibers are fast twitch, generate high force, and easily fatigue.

ATP aerobically (its oxidative capacity) seems to be easily altered by endurance training. In fact, in some elite endurance athletes, type IIx fibers can't be found; they have been converted to the oxidative version, type IIa (57). The increase in mitochondria and capillaries in endurance-trained muscles allows an individual to meet ATP demands aerobically, with less glycogen depletion and lactate formation (30).

Tension (Force) Development in the Muscle

The tension, or force, generated by a muscle depends on more than the fiber type. When a single threshold-level stimulus excites a muscle fiber, a single, low-tension twitch results—a brief contraction followed by relaxation. If the frequency of stimulation increases, the muscle fiber can't relax between stimuli, and the tension of one contraction adds to tension from the previous one. This addition process is called **summation.** A further increase in the frequency of stimulation results in the contractions fusing together into a smooth, sustained, high-tension contraction called **tetanus.** Muscle fibers typically develop tension through tetanic contractions. In addition to frequency of stimulation, the force of contraction depends on the degree to which the muscle fibers contract simultaneously (synchronous firing) and the number of muscle fibers recruited for the contraction. The latter factor, muscle fiber recruitment, is the most important.

Figure 28.5 shows the order in which the different muscle fiber types are recruited as the intensity of exercise increases. The order is from the most to the least oxidative, from the slowest to the fastest fiber (type I to type IIa to type IIx) (55). Consequently, at higher work rates when the type IIx fibers are recruited, there is a greater chance of producing lactic acid. Although chronic light exercise (less than 40% $\dot{V}O_2$max) recruits and causes a training effect in only the type I fibers, exercise beyond 70% $\dot{V}O_2$max involves all fiber types. This fact has important implications in the specificity of training and the potential for transferring training effects from one activity to another. Obviously, if you don't use a muscle fiber, it can't become trained.

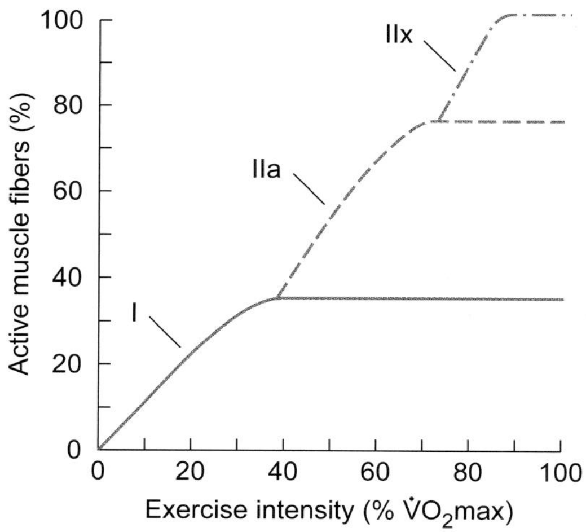

Figure 28.5 Recruitment of muscle fiber types in exercise of increasing intensity.

Reprinted, by permission, from D.G. Sale, 1987, "Influence of exercise and training on motor unit activation," *Exercise and Sport Sciences Reviews* 15: 99.

Key Point

Muscle tension depends on the frequency of the stimulation leading to a tetanus contraction, the synchronous firing of muscle fibers, and the recruitment of muscle fibers. The order of recruitment of muscle fibers is from the most to the least oxidative. Light to moderate exercise uses type I muscle fibers, whereas moderate to vigorous exercise requires type IIa fibers. Both favor the aerobic metabolism of carbohydrate and fat. Heavy exercise requires type IIx fibers that favor anaerobic glycolysis, which increases the likelihood of lactate production.

Metabolic, Cardiovascular, and Respiratory Responses to Exercise

A primary task of the fitness professional is to recommend physical activities that increase or maintain cardiorespiratory function. Activities that demand aerobic energy (ATP) production automatically cause the circulatory and respiratory systems to deliver oxygen to the muscle to meet the demand. The selected aerobic activities must be strenuous enough to challenge and thus improve the cardiorespiratory system. This crucial link between aerobic activities and cardiorespiratory function provides the basis for much of exercise programming. The following sections summarize selected metabolic, cardiovascular, and respiratory responses to submaximal work and to a maximal GXT. We begin by discussing how oxygen uptake is measured.

Measuring Oxygen Uptake

How does oxygen get to the mitochondria? Oxygen enters the lungs during inhalation; it then diffuses from the alveoli of the lungs into the blood. Oxygen is bound to hemoglobin in the red blood cells, and the heart delivers the oxygen-enriched blood to the muscles. Oxygen then diffuses into the muscle cells and reaches the mitochondria, where it is used (consumed) in the production of ATP. So how is oxygen consumption measured during exercise?

Oxygen consumption ($\dot{V}O_2$) is measured by subtracting the volume of oxygen exhaled from the volume of oxygen inhaled.

$$\dot{V}O_2 = \text{volume } O_2 \text{ inhaled} - \text{volume } O_2 \text{ exhaled}$$

In the classic approach to measuring $\dot{V}O_2$, the subject breathes through a two-way valve that allows the lungs to inhale room air (containing 20.93% O_2 and 0.03% CO_2) while directing exhaled air to a meteorological balloon, or Douglas bag (see figure 28.6). A volume meter measures the liters of air inhaled per minute, which is called the **pulmonary ventilation.** The exhaled air contained in the meteorological balloon is analyzed for its oxygen and carbon dioxide content, and the oxygen consumption (uptake) is calculated by multiplying the volume of air breathed by the percentage of oxygen extracted. Oxygen extraction is the percentage of oxygen extracted from the inhaled air, the difference between the 20.93% of O_2 in room air and the percentage of O_2 in the meteorological balloon.

The following is a simplified presentation of the steps used to calculate $\dot{V}O_2$; a more detailed presentation is found in appendix B.

$$\dot{V}O_2 = \text{pulmonary ventilation } (L \cdot min^{-1}) \cdot O_2 \text{ extraction.}$$

If ventilation = 60 $L \cdot min^{-1}$, and exhaled O_2 = 16.93%, then
$\dot{V}O_2 = 60\ L \cdot min^{-1}\ (20.93\%\ O_2 - 16.93\%\ O_2)$, and
$\dot{V}O_2 = 60\ L \cdot min^{-1}\ (4.00\%\ O_2) = 2.4\ L \cdot min^{-1}$.

CO_2 is produced in the mitochondria and diffuses out of the muscle into the venous blood, where it is carried back to the lungs. There it diffuses into the alveoli and, in this example, is exhaled into the meteorological balloon. CO_2 production ($\dot{V}CO_2$) can be calculated as described for the $\dot{V}O_2$:

If ventilation = 60 $L \cdot min^{-1}$, and exhaled CO_2 = 3.03%, then
$\dot{V}CO_2 = 60\ L \cdot min^{-1}\ (3.03\%\ CO_2 - 0.03\%\ CO_2)$, and
$\dot{V}CO_2 = 60\ L \cdot min^{-1}\ (3.00\%\ CO_2) = 1.8\ L \cdot min^{-1}$.

The ratio of CO_2 production ($\dot{V}CO_2$) to oxygen consumption ($\dot{V}O_2$) at the cell is called the **respiratory quotient (RQ).** Because $\dot{V}CO_2$ and $\dot{V}O_2$ are measured at the mouth rather than at the tissue, this ratio is called the **respiratory exchange ratio (R).** R tells us what type of fuel is being used during exercise (see the next section, Fuel Utilization During Exercise).

$$R = \dot{V}CO_2 \div \dot{V}O_2$$

Using the values already calculated,

$$R = 1.8\ L \cdot min^{-1} \div 2.4\ L \cdot min^{-1} = 0.75.$$

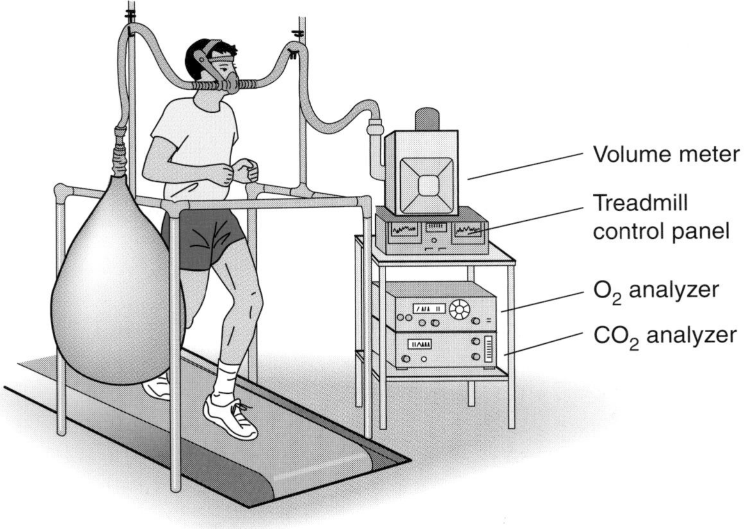

Figure 28.6 Conventional equipment for measuring oxygen uptake.

Fuel Utilization During Exercise

In general, protein contributes less than 5% to total energy production during exercise, and for the purpose of our discussion it will be ignored (49). Ignoring protein leaves carbohydrate (muscle glycogen and blood glucose, which is derived from liver glycogen) and fat (adipose tissue and intramuscular fat) as the primary fuels for exercise. The ability of R to provide good information about the metabolism of fat and carbohydrate during exercise stems from the following observations about the metabolism of fat and glucose.

When R = 1.0, 100% of the energy is derived from carbohydrate, 0% from fat; when R = 0.7, the reverse is true. When R = 0.85, approximately 50% of the energy comes from carbohydrate and 50% comes from fat (see Respiratory Quotients for Carbohydrate and Fat on page 453). For the R measurement to be correct, the subject must be in a steady state. If lactic acid is increasing in the blood, the plasma bicarbonate (HCO_3^-) buffer store reacts with the acid (H^+) and produces CO_2, which must be exhaled so that the exerciser is stimulated to hyperventilate:

$$H^+ + HCO_3^- \rightarrow H_2CO_3 \rightarrow H_2O + CO_2$$

This CO_2 does not come from the aerobic metabolism of carbohydrate and fat, and so when the CO_2 is exhaled, it results in an overestimation of the true value of R. During strenuous work, lactic acid is produced in great amounts, and R can exceed 1.0.

Effect of Exercise Intensity on Fuel Utilization

Figure 28.7 shows how R changes during progressive work up to $\dot{V}O_2$max. In the progressive test, R increases

Respiratory Quotients for Carbohydrate and Fat

For glucose ($C_6H_{12}O_6$),

$$C_6H_{12}O_6 + 6\,O_2 \rightarrow 6\,CO_2 + 6\,H_2O + \text{energy}$$

$$R = \frac{6\,CO_2}{6\,O_2} = 1.0.$$

For palmitate ($C_{16}H_{32}O_2$, a fatty acid),

$$C_{16}H_{32}O_2 + 23\,O_2 \rightarrow 16\,CO_2 + 16\,H_2O + \text{energy}$$

$$R = \frac{16\,CO_2}{23\,O_2} = 0.7.$$

at about 40% to 50% $\dot{V}O_2max$, indicating that type IIa fibers are being recruited and carbohydrate (CHO) is becoming a more important fuel source. Using carbohydrate provides an adaptive advantage—the muscle obtains about 6% more energy from each liter of O_2 when carbohydrate is used (5 kcal $\cdot$ L^{-1}) compared with when fat is used (4.7 kcal $\cdot$ L^{-1}).

Carbohydrate fuels for muscular exercise include muscle glycogen and blood glucose. Muscle glycogen is the primary carbohydrate fuel for heavy exercise lasting less than 2 hr, and inadequate muscle glycogen results in premature fatigue (11). As muscle glycogen is depleted during prolonged heavy exercise, blood glucose becomes more important in supplying the carbohydrate fuel. Toward the end of heavy exercise lasting 3 hr or more, blood glucose provides almost all the carbohydrate used by the muscles. Therefore, heavy exercise is limited by the availability of carbohydrate fuels, which must be either stored in abundance before exercise (muscle glycogen) or replaced through ingestion of carbohydrate during exercise (blood glucose) (10).

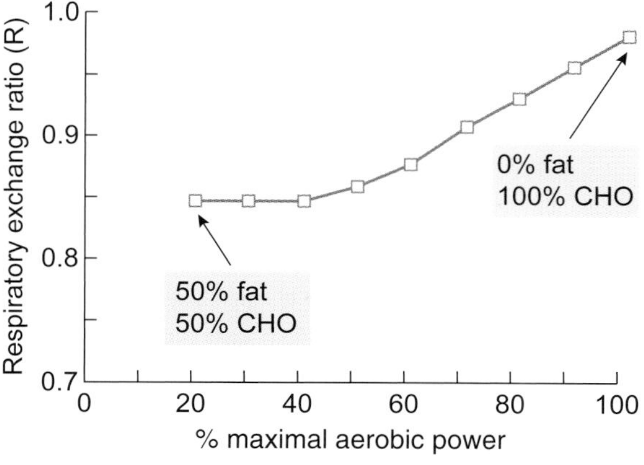

Figure 28.7 Changes in the respiratory exchange ratio with increasing exercise intensity (2).

Effect of Exercise Duration on Fuel Utilization

Figure 28.8 shows how R changes during a 90 min test performed at 65% of the subject's $\dot{V}O_2max$ (50). R decreases over time, indicating a greater reliance on fat as a fuel. The fats are derived from both intramuscular fat stores and adipose tissue, which releases free fatty acids into the blood to be carried to the muscle. Using more fat spares the remaining carbohydrate stores and extends the time to exhaustion.

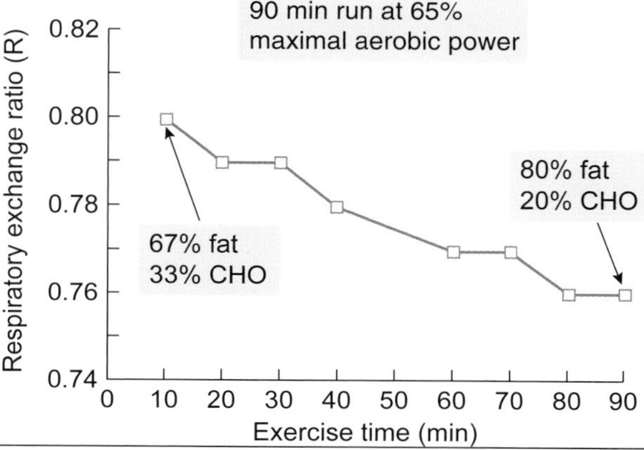

Figure 28.8 Changes in the respiratory exchange ratio during prolonged steady-state exercise (50).

Effect of Diet and Training on Fuel Utilization

The type of fuel used during exercise depends on diet. It has been demonstrated clearly that a diet high in carbohydrate (versus an average diet) increases the muscle glycogen content and extends the time to exhaustion (33). Further, the muscle gains a greater capacity to increase its glycogen store if a person performs strenuous exercise before eating high-carbohydrate meals (33, 61). Finally, during prolonged heavy exercise, carbohydrate drinks help to maintain the blood glucose concentration and extend the time to fatigue (10).

Endurance training increases the number of mitochondria in the muscles involved in the training program. Having more mitochondria increases the ability of the muscle to use fat as a fuel and to process the available carbohydrate aerobically. This ability spares the carbohydrate store and reduces lactate production, both of which favorably influence performance (30).

> **Key Point**
>
> The respiratory exchange ratio (R) tracks fuel use during steady-state exercise. When R = 1.0, 100% of the energy is derived from carbohydrate; when R = 0.7, 100% of the energy is derived from fat. When lactic acid increases in the blood during heavy exercise, the acid is buffered by plasma bicarbonate. This buffering produces CO_2 and invalidates using R as an indicator of fuel use during exercise. As exercise intensity increases, R increases, indicating that carbohydrate plays a bigger role in generating ATP. During prolonged moderately strenuous exercise, R decreases over time, indicating that fat is being used more and carbohydrate is being spared.

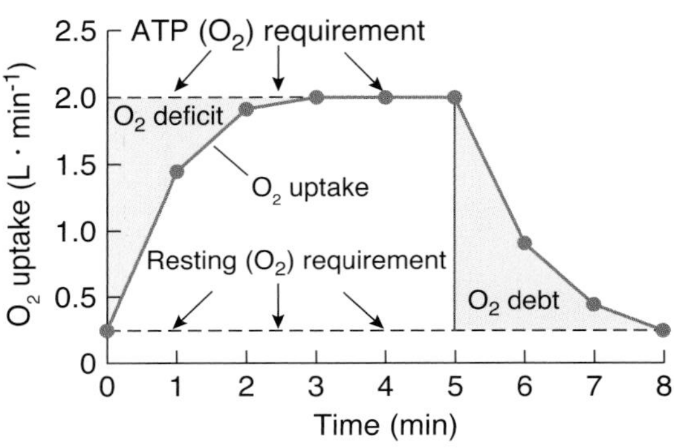

Figure 28.9 Oxygen (O_2) deficit and debt (repayment) during a 5 min run on a treadmill.

Transition From Rest to Steady-State Work

Some readers might mistakenly assume from our discussion up to this point that immediate, short-term, and long-term sources of energy (ATP) are used in distinct activities and do not work together to allow the body to make the transition from rest to exercise. When a person steps onto a treadmill belt moving at a velocity of 200 $m \cdot min^{-1}$ (7.5 $mi \cdot hr^{-1}$), the ATP requirement increases from the low level needed to stand alongside the treadmill to the new level required to run at 200 $m \cdot min^{-1}$. This change in the ATP supply to the muscle must take place in the first step on the treadmill. If this change fails to occur, the person will drift off the back of the treadmill. What energy sources supply ATP during the first minutes of work?

Oxygen Uptake

The cardiovascular and respiratory systems cannot instantaneously increase the delivery of oxygen to the muscles to completely meet the ATP demands of aerobic processes. In the interval between the time a person steps onto the treadmill and the time the cardiovascular and respiratory systems deliver the required oxygen, the immediate and short-term sources of energy supply the needed ATP. The volume of oxygen missing in the first few minutes of work is the **oxygen deficit** (figure 28.9). Creatine phosphate supplies some of the needed ATP, and the anaerobic breakdown of glycogen to lactic acid provides the rest until the oxidative mechanisms meet the ATP requirement. When the uptake of oxygen levels off during submaximal work, the oxygen uptake value represents the **steady-state oxygen requirement** for the activity. At this point, the ATP need of the cell is being met by the aerobic production of ATP in the mitochondria of the muscle on a "pay as you go" basis.

When the individual stops running and steps off the treadmill, the ATP need of the muscles that were involved in the activity suddenly drops toward the resting value. The oxygen uptake decreases quickly at first and then more gradually approaches the resting value. This elevated oxygen uptake during recovery from exercise is the **oxygen debt,** also called *oxygen repayment* or *excess postexercise oxygen consumption* (figure 28.9). In part, the elevated oxygen uptake is used to make additional ATP to bring the CP store of the muscle back to normal (remember that it was depleted somewhat at the onset of work). Some of the extra oxygen taken in during recovery is used to pay the ATP requirement for the higher heart rate (HR) and breathing during recovery (compared with rest). The liver uses a small part of the oxygen repayment to convert some of the lactic acid produced at the onset of work into glucose (49).

If an individual reaches the steady-state oxygen requirement earlier during the first minutes of work, a smaller oxygen deficit is incurred. The body depletes less CP and produces less lactic acid. Endurance training speeds up the kinetics of oxygen transport; that is, it decreases the time needed to reach a steady state of oxygen uptake. People in poor condition, as well as people with cardiovascular or pulmonary disease, take longer to reach the steady-state oxygen requirement. They incur a larger oxygen deficit and must produce more ATP from the immediate and short-term sources of energy when beginning work or transitioning from one intensity to the next (26, 47).

Heart Rate and Pulmonary Ventilation

The link between the cardiorespiratory responses to work and the time it takes to reach the steady-state oxygen requirement should be no surprise. Figure 28.10 shows how HR and pulmonary ventilation typically respond to a submaximal run test. The shape of the curve in each case resembles the curve for oxygen uptake described earlier.

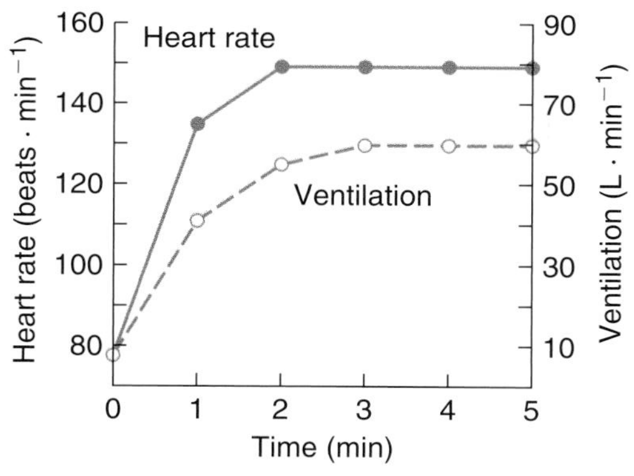

Figure 28.10 Response of heart rate and pulmonary ventilation during a 5 min run on a treadmill.

In addition, the muscle contributes to the lag in the oxygen uptake at the onset of work. An untrained muscle has relatively few mitochondria available to produce ATP aerobically and relatively few capillaries per muscle fiber to bring the oxygen-enriched arterial blood to those mitochondria. Following endurance training, both of these factors increase so that the muscle can produce more ATP aerobically at the onset of work. In addition, less lactic acid is produced at the onset of work and the blood lactic acid concentration drops for a fixed submaximal work rate (26, 30, 47).

Key Point

At the onset of submaximal exercise, $\dot{V}O_2$ does not increase immediately (oxygen deficit), and some of the ATP must be supplied anaerobically by CP and glycolysis. At the end of exercise, $\dot{V}O_2$ remains elevated for some time to replenish CP stores, support the energy cost of the elevated HR and breathing, and synthesize glucose from lactic acid. Training reduces the oxygen deficit because it creates a more rapid increase in $\dot{V}O_2$ at the onset of work, allowing the steady-state oxygen requirement to be reached more quickly.

Graded Exercise Test

Oxygen consumption and cardiorespiratory fitness are clearly linked, because oxygen delivery to tissue depends on lung and heart function. One of the most common tests used to evaluate cardiorespiratory function is a graded exercise test (GXT), in which an individual exercises at progressively increasing work rates until she reaches her maximum work tolerance. During the test the individual may be monitored for cardiovascular variables (ECG, HR, BP), respiratory variables (pulmonary ventilation, respiratory frequency), and metabolic variables (oxygen uptake, blood lactic acid level). The way a person responds to the GXT reveals cardiorespiratory function and the capacity for prolonged work.

Oxygen Uptake and Maximal Aerobic Power

Oxygen uptake, measured as described earlier, is expressed per kilogram of body weight to facilitate comparisons between people or between tests for the same person over time. The $\dot{V}O_2$ value in liters per minute is simply multiplied by 1,000 to convert the $\dot{V}O_2$ to ml · min^{-1}; that value is divided by the subject's body weight in kilograms to yield a value expressed in milliliters per kilogram per minute.

$$\dot{V}O_2 = 2.4\ \text{L} \cdot \text{min}^{-1} \cdot 1{,}000\ \text{ml} \cdot \text{L}^{-1}$$
$$\dot{V}O_2 = 2{,}400\ \text{ml} \cdot \text{min}^{-1}$$

For a 60 kg subject,

$$\dot{V}O_2 = 2{,}400\ \text{ml} \cdot \text{min}^{-1} \div 60\ \text{kg} = 40\ \text{ml} \cdot \text{kg}^{-1} \cdot \text{min}^{-1}.$$

Figure 28.11 shows a GXT conducted on a treadmill in which the speed is constant at 3 mi · hr^{-1} (4.8 km · hr^{-1}) and the grade changes 3% every 3 min. With each stage of a GXT, the oxygen uptake increases to meet the ATP demand of the work rate. Also, the individual incurs a small oxygen deficit at each stage as the cardiovascular system tries to adjust to the new demand of the increased work rate.

Apparently healthy individuals reach the steady-state oxygen requirement by 1.5 min or so of each stage of the

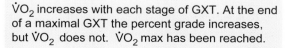

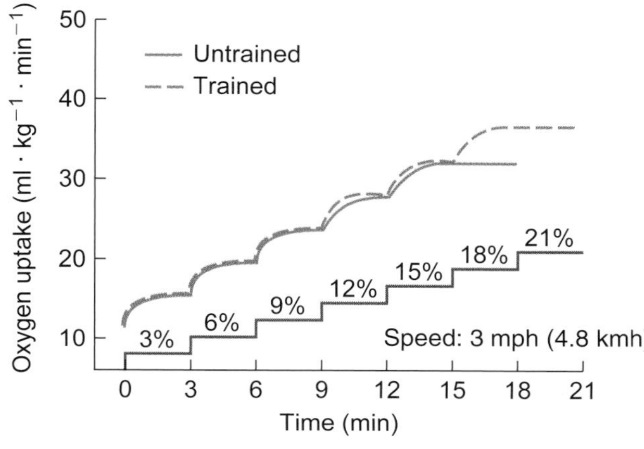

Figure 28.11 Oxygen uptake responses to a GXT (38).

test up to moderately heavy work (44, 45). People who have low cardiorespiratory fitness or who have cardiovascular and pulmonary diseases may not be able to reach the expected values in the same amount of time and might incur larger oxygen deficits with each stage of the test. For these individuals, the oxygen uptake measured at various stages of the test is lower than expected because they do not reach the expected steady-state demands of the test at each stage.

Toward the end of a GXT, a point is reached at which the work rate changes (i.e., the grade on the treadmill increases) but the oxygen uptake does not. In effect, the cardiovascular system has reached its limits for transporting oxygen to the muscle. This point is called **maximal aerobic power,** or **maximal oxygen uptake ($\dot{V}O_2$max).** A complete leveling off in the oxygen consumption is not seen in all cases because it requires the individual to work one stage past the actual point at which $\dot{V}O_2$max is reached. This requires the subject to be highly motivated. In some GXT protocols, the plateau in oxygen uptake is judged against the criterion of less than 2.1 ml · kg^{-1} · min^{-1} increase in $\dot{V}O_2$ from one stage to the next (62). Other criteria for having achieved $\dot{V}O_2$max include an R greater than 1.15 (34) and a blood lactate concentration greater than 8 mmol · L^{-1}, about 8 times the resting value (1). These and other criteria have been used alone and in combination to increase the likelihood that the individual has really achieved $\dot{V}O_2$max (32). Participation in a 10 to 20 wk endurance training program increases $\dot{V}O_2$max. If trained people retake the GXT, they reach the steady state sooner at light to moderate work rates and then go one or more stages further into the test, at which time the greater $\dot{V}O_2$max is measured.

Maximal aerobic power is the greatest rate at which the body (primarily muscle) can produce ATP aerobically. It is also the upper limit at which the cardiovascular system can deliver oxygen-enriched blood to the muscles. Thus, maximal aerobic power is not only a good index of cardiorespiratory fitness; it is also a good predictor of performance capability in aerobic events such as distance running, cycling, cross-country skiing, and swimming (4, 5). In the apparently healthy person, maximal aerobic power is the quantitative limit at which the cardiovascular system can deliver oxygen to tissues. This usual interpretation must be tempered by the mode of exercise (test type) used to impose the work rate on the subject.

Test Type

For the average person, the highest value for maximal aerobic power is measured when the subject completes a GXT involving uphill running. A GXT conducted at a walking speed usually results in a $\dot{V}O_2$max value 4% to 6% below the graded running value, and a test on a cycle ergometer may yield a value 10% to 12% lower than the graded running value (20, 42, 43). Last, if a subject works to exhaustion using an arm ergometer, then the highest oxygen uptake value is less than 70% of that measured with the legs (23). Knowing these variations in maximal aerobic power is helpful in making recommendations about the intensity of different exercises needed to achieve the target HR. At any given submaximal work rate, most physiological responses (HR, BP, and blood lactic acid) are greater for arm work than for leg work (23, 60). Maximal aerobic power is influenced by more than the type of test used in its measurement. Other factors include endurance training, heredity, sex, age, altitude, pollution, and cardiovascular and pulmonary disease.

Training and Heredity

Typically, endurance training increases $\dot{V}O_2$max by 5% to 25%, with the magnitude of the change depending primarily on the initial level of fitness. A person with a low $\dot{V}O_2$max sees the largest percent change from training. Eventually, a point is reached where further training does not increase $\dot{V}O_2$max. Approximately 40% of the extremely high values of maximal aerobic power found in elite cross-country skiers and distance runners relate to a genetic predisposition for having a superior cardiovascular system (6). Because typical endurance programs may increase $\dot{V}O_2$max by only 20% or so, it is unrealistic to expect a person with a $\dot{V}O_2$max of 40 ml · kg^{-1} · min^{-1} to increase to 80 ml · kg^{-1} · min^{-1}, a value measured in some elite cross-country skiers and distance runners (56). On the other hand, those who do severe interval training can achieve gains of 44% in $\dot{V}O_2$max (25).

Sex and Age

Women's $\dot{V}O_2$max values are about 15% lower than men's; that difference exists across ages 20 to 60. The primary reasons for the gender difference relate to differences in percent body fat and in hemoglobin levels (see later discussion). The 15% difference between men and women is an average, and $\dot{V}O_2$max values overlap considerably in these populations (2). In most people, aging gradually but systematically reduces $\dot{V}O_2$max by 1% each year. The $\dot{V}O_2$max of a given person is influenced by physical activity and percent body fat. Those who remain active and maintain body weight (which is not the usual case) have higher $\dot{V}O_2$max values across the age span. In fact, endurance training implemented in middle-aged people gives the appearance of reversing the aging effect because it elevates $\dot{V}O_2$max to a level consistent with that of a younger, sedentary individual (35-37).

Altitude and Pollution

$\dot{V}O_2$max decreases with increasing altitude. At 7,400 ft (2,300 m), $\dot{V}O_2$max is only 88% of the sea-level value.

This decrease in $\dot{V}O_2max$ is attributable primarily to the reduction in arterial oxygen content that occurs as the oxygen pressure in the air decreases with increasing altitude. When the arterial oxygen content is lower, the heart must pump more blood per minute to meet the oxygen needs of any task. As a result, the HR response is higher at submaximal intensities performed at greater altitudes (31).

Carbon monoxide, produced from the burning of fossil fuel as well as from cigarette smoke, binds readily to hemoglobin and can decrease oxygen transport to muscles. The critical concentration of carbon monoxide in blood needed to decrease $\dot{V}O_2max$ is about 4%. After that, $\dot{V}O_2max$ decreases approximately 1% for every 1% increase in the carbon monoxide concentration in the blood (51).

Key Point

Maximal oxygen uptake, $\dot{V}O_2max$, is the greatest rate at which O_2 can be delivered to working muscles during dynamic exercise. $\dot{V}O_2max$ is influenced by heredity and training, decreases about 1% per year with age, and is about 15% lower in women compared with men of the same age. $\dot{V}O_2max$ is lower at high altitudes, and carbon monoxide in the blood decreases $\dot{V}O_2max$ because it binds to hemoglobin and limits oxygen transport. Cardiovascular and pulmonary diseases lower $\dot{V}O_2max$; however, individuals with cardiovascular disease can attain large improvements in $\dot{V}O_2max$ through endurance training.

Cardiovascular and Pulmonary Diseases

Cardiovascular and pulmonary diseases decrease $\dot{V}O_2max$ by diminishing the delivery of oxygen from the air to the blood and reducing the capacity of the heart to deliver blood to the muscles. Patients with cardiovascular disease have some of the lowest $\dot{V}O_2max$ (functional capacity) values, but they also experience the largest percent changes in $\dot{V}O_2max$ from endurance training. Table 28.1 shows common values for $\dot{V}O_2max$ in a variety of populations (2, 22, 64).

Blood Lactate and Pulmonary Ventilation

Muscle produces lactic acid, which is released into the blood. Figure 28.12 shows that during a GXT, blood lactate concentration changes little or not at all at the lower work rates; lactate is metabolized as fast as it is produced (7). As the GXT increases in intensity, a work rate is reached at which the blood lactate concentration suddenly increases. This work rate is referred to as the **lactate threshold.** It is also called the *anaerobic threshold,* but because several conditions other than a lack of oxygen (hypoxia) at the muscle cell can result in lactate being produced and released into the blood, *lactate threshold* is the preferred term. Endurance training increases the number of mitochondria in the trained muscles, facilitating the aerobic metabolism of carbohydrate and the use of more fat as fuel. As a result, when the subject retakes the GXT following training, less lactate is produced and the lactate threshold occurs at a later stage of the test. The lactate threshold is a good indicator of endurance performance and has been used to predict performance in endurance races (4, 5).

Pulmonary ventilation is the volume of air inhaled or exhaled per minute and is calculated by

Table 28.1 Maximal Aerobic Power in Healthy and Diseased Populations

	$\dot{V}O_2max$ ($ml \cdot kg^{-1} \cdot min^{-1}$)	
Population	**Men**	**Women**
Cross-country skiers	82	68
Distance runners	79	68
College students	45	38
Middle-aged adults	35	30
Patients with postmyocardial infarction	22	18
Patients with severe pulmonary disease	13	13

Data compiled from Åstrand and Rodahl, 1986; Fox, Bowers, and Foss, 1993; Wilmore and Costill, 1999; the Fort Sanders Cardiac Rehabilitation Program; and J.T. Daniels (personal communication).

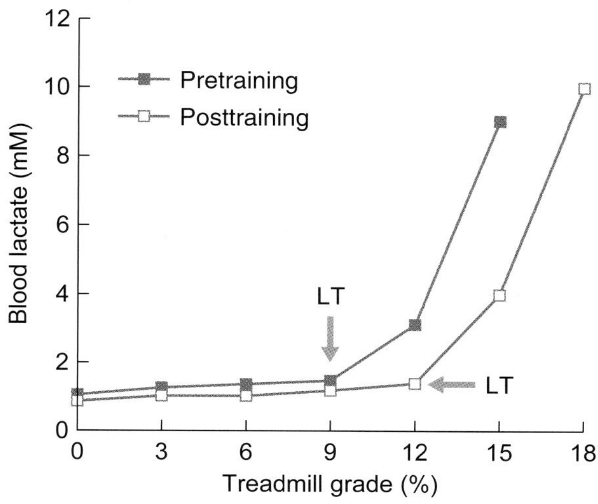

Figure 28.12 Training causes the lactate threshold (LT) to occur at a higher exercise intensity (19).

multiplying the frequency *(f)* of breathing by the tidal volume *(TV)*, the volume of air moved in one breath. For example,

$$\text{ventilation } (L \cdot min^{-1}) = TV\,(L \cdot breath^{-1}) \cdot f\,(breaths \cdot min^{-1}), \text{ and}$$

$$30\ (L \cdot min^{-1}) = 1.5\ L \cdot breath^{-1} \cdot 20\ breaths \cdot min^{-1}.$$

Pulmonary ventilation increases linearly with work rate until 50% to 80% of $\dot{V}O_2max$, at which point a relative **hyperventilation** results (see figure 28.13). The inflection point in the pulmonary ventilation response is the **ventilatory threshold.** The ventilatory threshold has been used as a noninvasive indicator of the lactate threshold and as a predictor of performance (17, 48). The increase in pulmonary ventilation is mediated by changes in the frequency of breathing (from about 10-12 breaths $\cdot$ min^{-1} at rest to 40-50 breaths $\cdot$ min^{-1} during maximal work) and in the tidal volume (from 0.5 L $\cdot$ breath^{-1} at rest to 2-3 L $\cdot$ breath^{-1} in maximal work). Endurance training lowers pulmonary ventilation during submaximal work; the ventilatory threshold occurs later into the GXT. The maximal value for pulmonary ventilation tends to change in the direction of $\dot{V}O_2max$.

Key Point

The points at which the blood lactic acid concentration and the pulmonary ventilation increase suddenly during a GXT are called the *lactate* and *ventilatory thresholds,* respectively. The lactate and ventilatory thresholds are good predictors of performance in endurance events (e.g., 10K runs, marathons).

Heart Rate

Once the HR reaches about 110 beats $\cdot$ min^{-1}, it increases linearly with work rate during a GXT until near-maximal efforts. Figure 28.14 shows how training influences the subject's HR response at the same work rates. The lower HR at submaximal work rates is a beneficial effect because it decreases the oxygen needed by the heart muscle. Maximal HR shows no change or is slightly reduced as a result of endurance training.

Stroke Volume

The volume of blood pumped by the heart per beat (ml $\cdot$ beat^{-1}) is called the *stroke volume (SV).* For individuals doing work in the upright position (cycling, walking), SV increases in the early stages of the GXT until about 40% $\dot{V}O_2max$ is reached and then levels off (see figure 28.15) (2). Consequently, when $\dot{V}O_2max$ is greater than 40%, HR is the sole factor responsible for the increased flow of blood from the heart to the working muscles. This is what makes the HR a good indicator of the metabolic rate during exercise; it is linearly related to exercise intensity from light exercise to heavy exercise. One of the primary effects of endurance training is an increase in SV at rest and during work; this increase is caused, in part, by a larger volume of the ventricle (19). This allows a greater **end-diastolic volume,** the volume of blood in the heart just before contraction. So, following endurance training, even if the same fraction of blood in the ventricle is pumped per beat **(ejection fraction),** the heart pumps more blood per minute at the same HR.

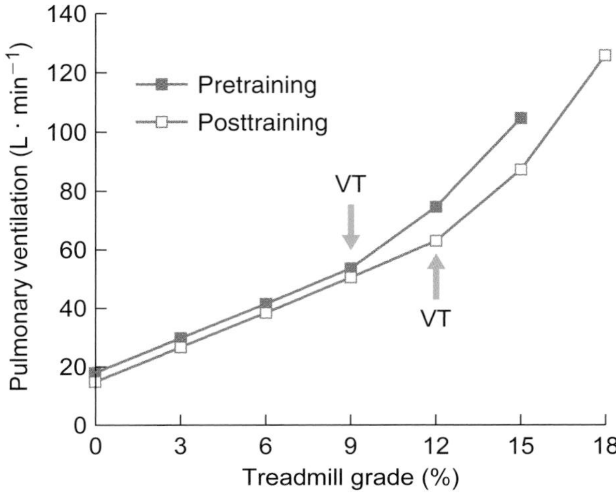

Figure 28.13 Following training, the ventilatory threshold (VT) occurs later in the GXT.

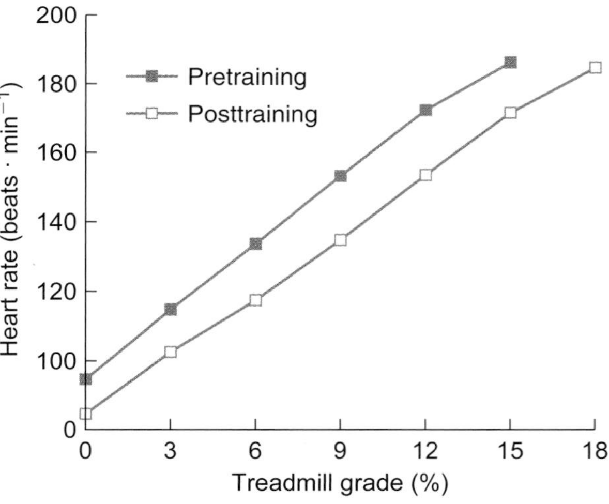

Figure 28.14 Training reduces the HR response to submaximal exercise (19).

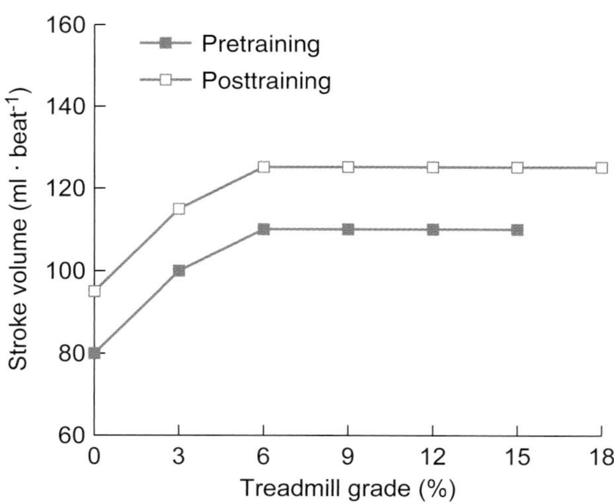

Figure 28.15 Stroke volume increases with training due to a larger volume of the ventricle (19).

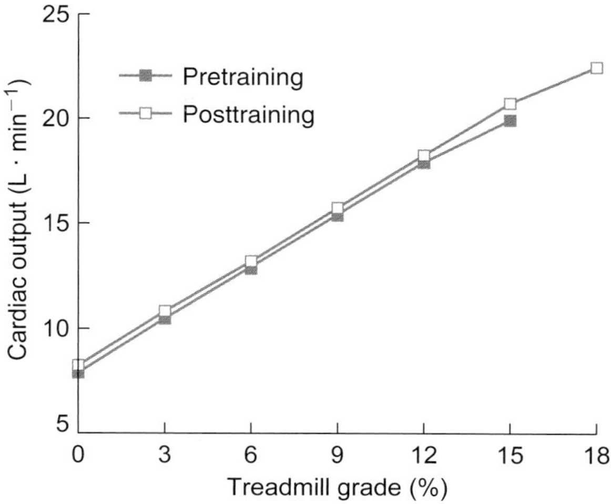

Figure 28.16 Maximal cardiac output increases following training (19).

Cardiac Output

Cardiac output (Q) is the volume of blood pumped by the heart per minute and is calculated by multiplying the HR (beats · min $^{-1}$) by the SV (ml · beat^{-1}).

$$\text{Cardiac output} = \text{HR} \cdot \text{SV}$$
$$= 60 \text{ beats} \cdot \text{min}^{-1} \cdot 80 \text{ ml} \cdot \text{beat}^{-1}$$
$$= 4{,}800 \text{ ml} \cdot \text{min}^{-1}, \text{ or } 4.8 \text{ L} \cdot \text{min}^{-1}$$

Cardiac output increases linearly with work rate. Generally, the cardiac output response to light and moderate work is not affected by endurance training. What changes is how the cardiac output is achieved: with a lower HR and a higher SV.

The maximal cardiac output (highest value reached in a GXT) is the most important cardiovascular variable determining maximal aerobic power because the oxygen-enriched blood (carrying about 0.2 L of O_2 per liter of blood) must be delivered to the muscle for the mitochondria to use. If a person's maximal cardiac output is 10 L · min $^{-1}$, only 2 L of O_2 would leave the heart each minute (i.e., 0.2 L of O_2 per liter of blood times a cardiac output of 10 L · min^{-1} = 2 L of O_2 · min $^{-1}$). A person with a maximal cardiac output of 30 L· min^{-1} would deliver 6 L of O_2 per minute to the tissues. Endurance training increases the maximal cardiac output and thus the delivery of oxygen to the muscles (see figure 28.16). This increase in maximal cardiac output is matched by greater capillary numbers in the muscle to allow the blood to move slowly enough through the muscle to maintain the time needed for oxygen to diffuse from the blood to the mitochondria (57). The increase in maximal cardiac output accounts for 50% of the increase in maximal oxygen uptake that occurs in previously sedentary individuals who engage in endurance training (54).

In the normal population, SV is the major variable influencing maximal cardiac output. Differences in maximal cardiac output and maximal aerobic power that exist between females and males, between trained and untrained individuals, and between the world-class endurance athlete and the average person can be explained largely by the differences in maximal stroke volume. This is shown in table 28.2, where $\dot{V}O_2$max varies by a factor of 3 among three distinct groups, while maximal HR stays almost the same for all three groups. Clearly, maximal SV is the primary factor related to the differences in $\dot{V}O_2$max that exist among individuals.

Oxygen Extraction

Two factors determine the oxygen uptake at any time: the volume of blood delivered to the tissues per minute (cardiac output) and the volume of oxygen extracted from each liter of blood. Oxygen extraction is calculated by subtracting the oxygen content of mixed venous blood (as it returns to the heart) from the oxygen content of the arterial blood. This is called the **arteriovenous oxygen difference,** or the *$(a - \bar{v})O_2$ difference.*

$$\dot{V}O_2 = \text{cardiac output} \cdot (a - \bar{v})O_2 \text{ difference.}$$

At rest, cardiac output = 5 L · min^{-1},
arterial oxygen content = 200 ml of $O_2 \cdot L^{-1}$, and
mixed venous oxygen content = 150 ml of $O_2 \cdot L^{-1}$.

$$\dot{V}O_2 = 5 \text{ L} \cdot \text{min}^{-1} \cdot (200 - 150 \text{ ml of } O_2 \cdot L^{-1})$$
$$\dot{V}O_2 = 5 \text{ L} \cdot \text{min}^{-1} \cdot 50 \text{ ml of } O_2 \cdot L^{-1}$$
$$\dot{V}O_2 = 250 \text{ ml} \cdot \text{min}^{-1}.$$

The $(a - \bar{v})O_2$ difference reflects the ability of the muscle to extract oxygen, and it increases with exercise

Table 28.2 Maximal Values of $\dot{V}O_2$max, Heart Rate, Stroke Volume, and Arteriovenous $(a - \bar{v})$ Oxygen Difference in Three Groups With Very Low, Normal, and High Maximal $\dot{V}O_2$max

Group	$\dot{V}O_2$max ($L \cdot min^{-1}$)	=	Heart rate ($beats \cdot min^{-1}$)	×	Stroke volume ($ml \cdot beats^{-1}$)	×	$(a - \bar{v})$ oxygen difference ($ml \cdot min^{-1}$)
Mitral stenosis	1.60	=	190	×	50	×	170
Sedentary	3.20	=	200	×	100	×	160
Athlete	5.20	=	190	×	160	×	170

Adapted, by permission, from L. Rowell, 1969, "Circulation," *Medicine and Science in Sports and Exercise* 1: 15-22.

intensity. The ability of a tissue to extract oxygen is a function of the capillary-to-muscle fiber ratio and the number of mitochondria in the muscle fiber. Endurance training increases all of these factors (see figure 28.17), thus increasing the maximal capacity to extract oxygen in the last stage of the GXT (57). This increase in the $(a - \bar{v})O_2$ difference accounts for about 50% of the increase in $\dot{V}O_2$max that occurs with endurance training in previously sedentary individuals (54).

Blood Pressure

Blood pressure (BP) is dependent on the balance between the cardiac output and the resistance the blood vessels offer to blood flow (total peripheral resistance). The resistance to blood flow is altered by the constriction or dilation of **arterioles,** which are blood vessels located between the artery and the capillary.

$$BP = \text{cardiac output} \cdot \text{total peripheral resistance}$$

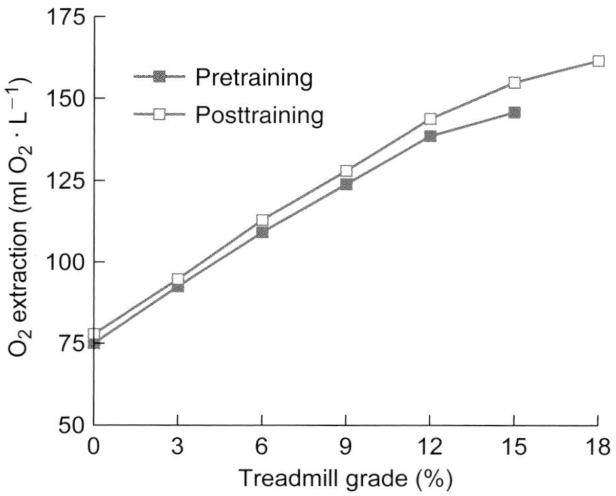

Figure 28.17 Following training, maximal O_2 extraction increases due to greater capillary and mitochondrial density in the trained muscles (19).

BP is sensed by **baroreceptors** in the arch of the aorta and in the carotid arteries. When BP changes, the baroreceptors send signals to the cardiovascular control center in the brain, which in turn alters cardiac output or the diameter of arterioles. For example, if a person who has been lying supine suddenly stands, blood pools in the lower extremities, SV decreases, and BP drops. If BP is not restored, less blood flows to the brain and the person might faint. The baroreceptors monitor this decrease in BP, and the cardiovascular control center simultaneously increases the HR and reduces the diameter of the arterioles (to increase total peripheral resistance) to try to return BP to normal. During exercise, the arterioles dilate in the active muscle to increase blood flow and meet metabolic demands. This dilation is matched with a constriction of arterioles in the liver, kidneys, and gastrointestinal tract and an increase in HR and SV, as already mentioned. These coordinated changes maintain BP and direct most of the cardiac output to the working muscles.

BP is monitored at each stage of a GXT. Figure 28.18 shows how **systolic blood pressure (SBP)** increases with each stage until maximum work tolerance is reached. At

Key Point

During acute exercise, HR increases linearly with work rate once the HR reaches 110 beats · min⁻¹. During exercise in the upright position, SV increases until an intensity of about 40% $\dot{V}O_2$max is reached. Cardiac output (HR · SV) increases linearly with work rate. Endurance training reduces HR and increases SV at rest and during submaximal work; in addition, maximal cardiac output is greater, because SV increases with no change or a slight decrease in maximal HR. Variations in $\dot{V}O_2$max across the population are attributed primarily to differences in maximal SV. Fifty percent of the increase in $\dot{V}O_2$max attributable to endurance training is a result of an increase in maximal SV; the other 50% is attributable to an increase in oxygen extraction.

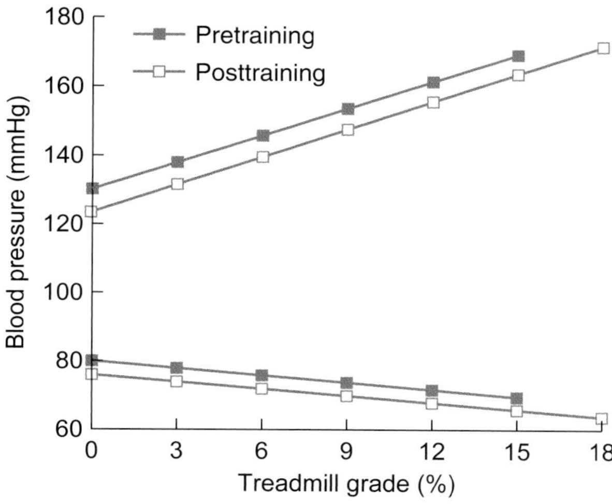

Figure 28.18 Systolic BP increases until maximum work tolerance is reached. Diastolic BP remains steady or decreases.

that point, SBP might decrease. A fall in SBP with an increase in work rate is used as an indicator of maximal cardiovascular function and can aid in determining the end point for an exercise test. **Diastolic blood pressure (DBP)** tends to remain the same or decrease during a GXT. An increase in DBP toward the end of the test is another indicator that an individual has reached the limits of his functional capacity. Endurance training reduces the BP responses at fixed submaximal work rates.

Two factors that determine the oxygen demand (work) of the heart during aerobic exercise are the HR and the SBP. The product of these two variables is called the **rate–pressure product,** or the **double product,** and is proportional to the myocardial oxygen demand (i.e., the volume of oxygen the heart muscle needs each minute to function properly). Factors that decrease the HR and BP responses to work increase the chance that the coronary blood supply to the heart muscle will adequately meet the oxygen demands of the heart. Endurance training decreases the HR and BP responses to fixed submaximal work and protects against any diminished blood supply (ischemia) to the myocardium. Drugs are also used to lower HR and BP to try to reduce the work of the heart (see chapter 24).

When a person does the same rate of work with the arms as with the legs, the HR and BP responses are considerably higher during the arm work. This is shown in figure 28.19, in which the rate–pressure product is plotted for various levels of arm and leg work. Given that the load on the heart and the potential for fatigue are greater for arm work, a fitness professional should choose activities that use the large muscle groups of the legs; such activities result in lower HR, BP, and perception of fatigue (23, 60).

Key Point

SBP increases with each stage of a GXT, whereas DBP remains the same or decreases. The work of the heart is proportional to the product of the HR and the SBP. Training lowers both, making it easier for the coronary arteries to meet the oxygen demand of the heart. HR and BP are higher during arm work compared with leg work at the same work rate.

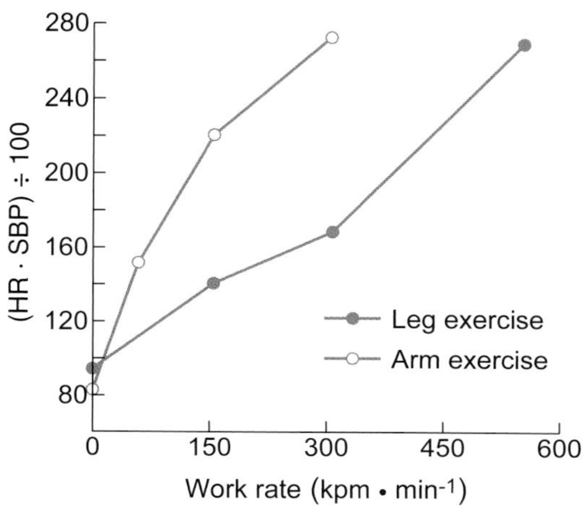

Figure 28.19 Rate–pressure product at rest and during arm and leg exercise.

Adapted from *American Heart Journal*, Vol. 94, J. Schwade, C.G. Blomqvist and W. Shapiro, "A comparison of the response in arm and leg work in patients with ischemic heart disease," pp. 203-208, Copyright 1977, with permission from Elsevier.

Effects of Endurance Training and Detraining on Physiological Responses

Many observations have been made about the effects of endurance training on various physiological responses to exercise. In this section we show how some of these effects interrelate.

- Endurance training increases the number of mitochondria and capillaries in muscle, causing all active fibers to become more oxidative. This effect is manifested by the increase in the type IIa fibers and decrease in type IIx fibers. These changes boost the endurance capacity of the muscle by allowing fat to be used for a greater percentage of energy production, sparing the muscle glycogen store and reducing lactate production. The lactate threshold shifts to the right, and performance times in endurance events improve.

- Endurance training decreases the time it takes to achieve a steady state in submaximal exercise. This reduces the oxygen deficit and reliance on CP and anaerobic glycolysis for energy.
- Endurance training enlarges the volume of the ventricle. This accommodates an increase in the end-diastolic volume, such that more blood is pumped out per beat. The increased SV is accompanied by a decrease in HR during submaximal work, so the cardiac output remains the same. The heart works less to meet the oxygen needs of the tissues.
- Maximal aerobic power increases with endurance training, the increase being inversely related to the initial $\dot{V}O_2$max. In formerly sedentary individuals, about 50% of the increase in $\dot{V}O_2$max results from greater maximal cardiac output, a change brought about by an increase in maximal SV, given that maximal HR either remains the same or decreases slightly. The other 50% of the increase in $\dot{V}O_2$max is attributable to an increase in oxygen extraction at the muscle, shown by an increase in the $(a - \bar{v})O_2$ difference. This occurs because of higher numbers of capillaries and mitochondria in the trained muscles.

Transfer of Training

The training effects that have been discussed are observed only when the trained muscles are the muscles used in the exercise test. Although this may appear obvious for the decrease in blood lactate attributable to, in part, the greater numbers of mitochondria in the trained muscles, it is also linked to the changes that occur in the HR response to submaximal work following the training program. Figure 28.20 shows the results of repeated submaximal exercise tests conducted on individuals who trained only one leg on a cycle ergometer for 13 days. The HR response to a fixed submaximal work rate performed by the trained leg decreased as expected. At the end of the 13 days of training, the untrained leg was subjected to the same exercise test. The HR responded as if a training effect had not occurred. This indicates that part of the reason the HR response to submaximal exercise decreases following training is because of feedback from the trained muscles to the cardiovascular control center that, in turn, reduces sympathetic stimulation to the heart (9, 54). This finding has important implications for evaluating the effects of a training program. The expected training responses (lower lactate production, lower HR, more fat use) are linked to testing the same muscle groups that were involved in the training. The probability of the training effect carrying over to another activity depends on the degree to which the new activity uses the muscles that are already trained.

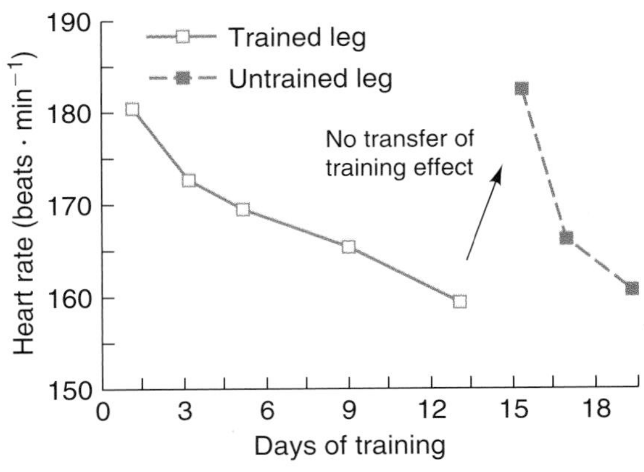

Figure 28.20 Lack of transfer of training effect (9).

Detraining

How fast is a training effect lost? A number of investigations have explored this question by having subjects either reduce or completely cease training. Maximal oxygen uptake usually is used as the principal measure to evaluate changes attributable to detraining, but an individual's response to a submaximal work rate also has been used to track these changes.

Ceasing Training

The following study used subjects who had trained for 10 ± 3 yr and agreed to cease training for 84 days (15). They were tested on days 12, 21, 56, and 84 of detraining. Figure 28.21 shows how their $\dot{V}O_2$max decreased 7% within the first 12 days. Remember that $\dot{V}O_2$max = cardiac output · $(a - \bar{v})O_2$ difference. The decrease in $\dot{V}O_2$max was attributable entirely to a drop in maximal cardiac output because the maximal oxygen extraction, or $(a - \bar{v})O_2$ difference, was unchanged.

In turn, the lower maximal cardiac output was attributable entirely to a decrease in maximal SV because maximal HR actually increased during detraining. A subsequent study showed that the reduced SV was caused by a reduction in plasma volume that occurred in the first 12 days of no training (13). In contrast, the drop in $\dot{V}O_2$max between days 21 and 84 was attributable to a decrease in the $(a - \bar{v})O_2$ difference because maximal cardiac output was unchanged (see figure 28.21). This lower oxygen extraction appeared to result from smaller numbers of mitochondria in the muscle, given that the number of capillaries surrounding each muscle fiber was unchanged (12).

The same subjects also completed a standard (fixed work rate) submaximal exercise test during the 84 days of no training (14). Figure 28.22 shows that HR and

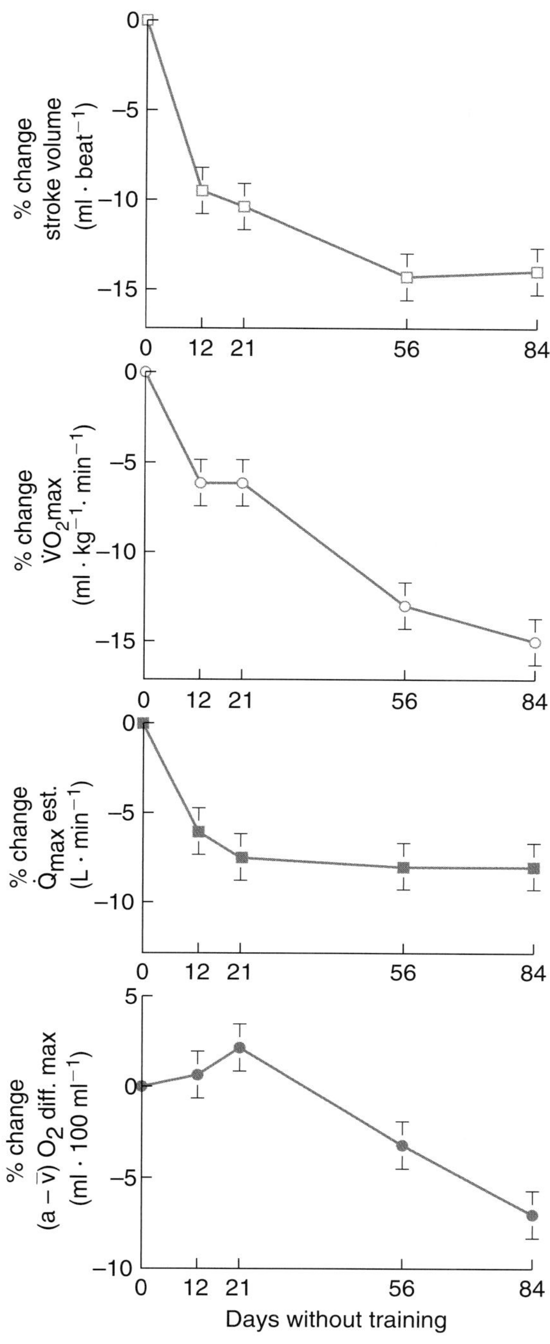

Figure 28.21 Effects of detraining on physiological responses during exercise. $\dot{V}O_2max$ = maximal oxygen uptake; $\dot{Q}_{max}$ est. = maximal cardiac output; $(a-\bar{v})O_2$ diff. max = maximal arteriovenous oxygen difference.

Adapted from E.F. Coyle, 1984, "Time course of loss of adaptations after stopping prolonged intense endurance training," *Journal of Applied Physiology* 57: 1861. Used with permission.

blood lactic acid responses to this work test increased throughout detraining. The higher responses relate to the fact that the same work rate required a greater percentage of $\dot{V}O_2max$ because the latter variable decreased

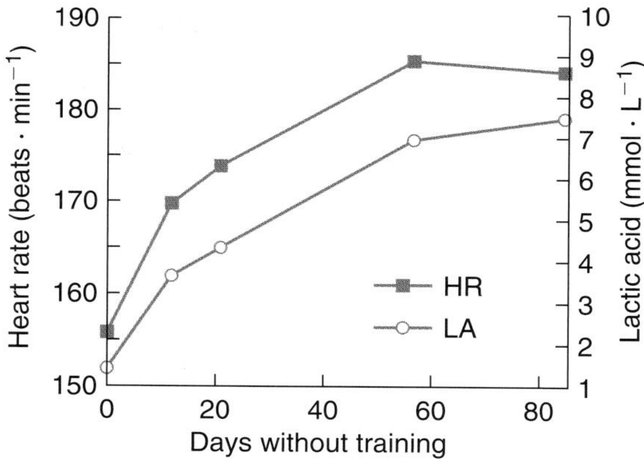

Figure 28.22 Changes in the HR and blood lactic acid (LA) responses to a standard exercise test taken during 84 days of detraining (14).

throughout the detraining. The magnitude of change in HR and blood lactic acid responses to this submaximal work, however, makes them very sensitive indicators of the training state of an individual.

Reduced Training

To evaluate the effect of reducing training, Hickson and colleagues (27-29) trained subjects for 10 wk to increase $\dot{V}O_2max$. The training program was conducted 40 min per day, 6 days per week. Three days involved running at near-maximum intensity for 40 min; the other 3 days required six 5 min bouts at near-maximum intensity on a cycle ergometer, with a 2 min rest between work bouts. Subjects expended about 600 kcal on each day of exercise, or 3,600 kcal each week. At the end of this 10 wk program, the subjects were divided into groups that trained at either a one-third or a two-thirds reduction in the previous frequency (4 and 2 day per wk, respectively), duration (26 and 13 min per day, respectively), or intensity (a one-third or two-thirds reduction in work done or distance run per 40 min session). Data collected on the maximal treadmill tests showed that cutting duration from 40 to 26 or 13 min or frequency from 6 to 4 or 2 days per week did not affect $\dot{V}O_2max$. In contrast, $\dot{V}O_2max$ clearly fell when the intensity of training was reduced by either one third or two thirds. What is interesting is that the subjects were able to maintain $\dot{V}O_2max$ when the total exercise per week was cut from 3,600 to 1,200 kcal in the group whose exercise frequency and duration were reduced by two thirds, but they were not able to maintain $\dot{V}O_2max$ when the intensity was reduced, even though the subjects were still expending about 1,200 kcal · wk^{-1}. This shows that exercise intensity is critical in maintaining $\dot{V}O_2max$

Key Point

Endurance training increases the ability of a muscle to use fat as a fuel and to spare carbohydrate, decreases the time it takes to achieve a steady state during submaximal work, increases the size of the ventricle, and increases $\dot{V}O_2$max by increasing SV and oxygen extraction. Endurance training effects (lower HR, lower blood lactate) do not transfer when untrained muscles are used to perform the work. Maximal oxygen uptake decreases when training stops. The initial decrease is caused by a decrease in SV and, later, in oxygen extraction. Maximal oxygen uptake can be maintained by doing intense exercise, even when cutting exercise duration and frequency.

and confirms that it takes less exercise to maintain than to achieve a specific level of $\dot{V}O_2$max.

Cardiovascular Responses to Exercise for Females and Males

Generally, prepubescent boys and girls differ little in $\dot{V}O_2$max or in their cardiovascular responses to submaximal exercise. During puberty, differences between girls and boys appear because of the female's higher percentage of body fat, lower hemoglobin concentration, and smaller heart size relative to body weight (2). The two latter factors also affect a woman's cardiovascular responses to submaximal work. For example, if an 80 kg male walks on a 10% grade on a treadmill at 3 mi · hr^{-1}(4.8 km · hr^{-1}), his $\dot{V}O_2$ is 2.07 L · min^{-1}, or 25.9 ml · kg^{-1} · min^{-1}.

His HR might be 140 beats · min^{-1}. If he carries a backpack weighing 15 kg, his $\dot{V}O_2$ expressed per kilogram does not change (25.9 ml · kg^{-1} · min^{-1}), but his total oxygen requirement increases 389 ml · min^{-1} (i.e., 15 kg · 25.9 ml · kg^{-1} · min^{-1}). His HR obviously is higher with this load than without it, even though the $\dot{V}O_2$ expressed per kilogram of body weight is the same. Likewise, performance in the 12 min run test to evaluate maximal aerobic power decreased by 89 m when body weight was experimentally increased to simulate a 5% gain in body fat (16). When a woman walks on a treadmill at a given grade and speed, her HR is higher than a comparable male's HR because of the additional fat weight she carries. Her lower hemoglobin concentration and smaller heart size also elevate the HR at the same oxygen uptake expressed per unit of body weight.

The differences between males and females in the cardiovascular response to submaximal work become more exaggerated when work is done on a cycle ergometer where a given work rate demands a similar $\dot{V}O_2$ in liters per minute, independent of sex or training. As previously mentioned, the average female has less hemoglobin and a smaller heart volume than the average male has. To deliver the same volume of oxygen to the muscles, the woman must have a higher HR to compensate for the smaller SV and must have a slightly higher cardiac output to compensate for the lower hemoglobin concentration (2). These differences between women and men in the cardiovascular responses to cycle ergometry are shown in figure 28.23.

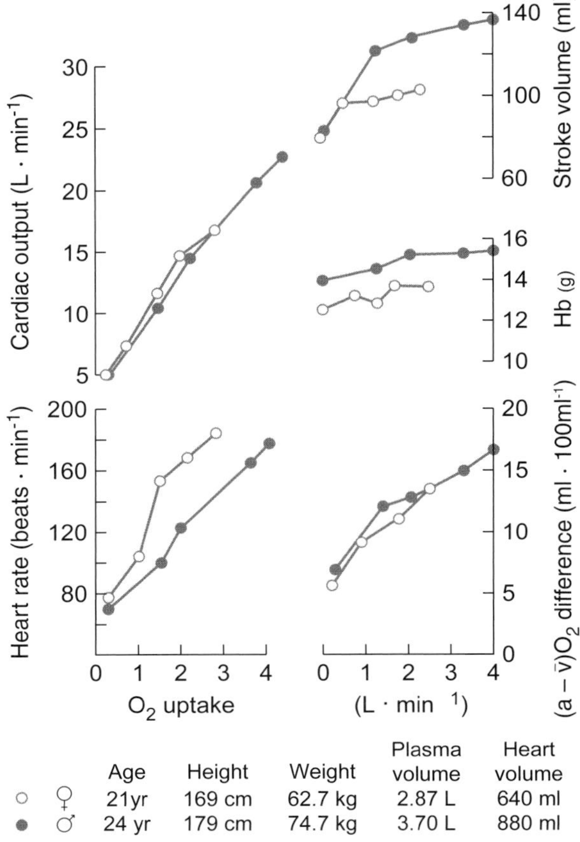

Figure 28.23 The cardiovascular responses of well-trained men and women to cycle ergometry exercise. Hb = hemoglobin.

Reprinted from P.-O. Astrand and K. Rodahl, 1986, *Textbook of work physiology*, 3rd ed. (New York, NY: McGraw-Hill), 200, with permission of the McGraw-Hill Companies.

Key Point

At the same work rate, or $\dot{V}O_2$, women respond with a higher HR to compensate for a lower SV. The cardiac output is slightly higher to compensate for the lower hemoglobin level (and oxygen content) of the arterial blood.

Cardiovascular Responses to Isometric Exercise and Weightlifting

Most endurance exercise programs use dynamic activities involving large muscle masses to place loads on the cardiorespiratory system. The previous summary of the physiological responses to a GXT indicates that the cardiovascular load is rather proportional to the exercise intensity. But this is not necessarily the case for resistance training, in which a person can have a disproportionately high cardiovascular load relative to the exercise intensity. In the previous discussion of cardiovascular responses to a GXT, the HR and SBP responses progressively increased with each stage of the test. Figure 28.24 shows the HR and BP responses to an isometric exercise test (sustained handgrip) at only 30% maximal voluntary contraction strength and to a treadmill test at two exercise intensities. The most impressive change during the sustained handgrip is in BP; the SBP and DBP increase over time, and the magnitude of the SBP exceeds 220 mmHg. This kind of exercise additionally loads the heart and is not recommended for older adults or people with heart disease (39).

Dynamic, heavy-resistance exercises can also cause extreme BP responses. Figure 28.25 shows the peak BP response achieved during exercise at 95% to 100% of the maximum weight that could be lifted one time (1RM). Both DBP and SBP are elevated, with average values exceeding 300/200 mmHg for the two-leg leg press done to fatigue. The elevation in pressure was believed to be caused by the compression of the arteries by the muscles, a reflex response attributable to the static component associated with near-maximal dynamic lifts, and by the Valsalva maneuver, which can independently elevate BP (40). Another study reported peak values of about 190/140 mmHg for exercises of 50%, 70%, and 80% of 1RM done to fatigue in untrained lifters. Bodybuilders responded with lower pressures, indicating a cardiovascular adaptation to resistance training (21).

Key Point

Isometric exercise and heavy resistance exercise elicit very high BP responses compared with dynamic endurance exercise. Both SBP and DBP increase with isometric and dynamic resistance training.

Regulating Body Temperature

Under resting conditions, the body's core temperature is 37 °C, and heat production and heat loss are balanced.

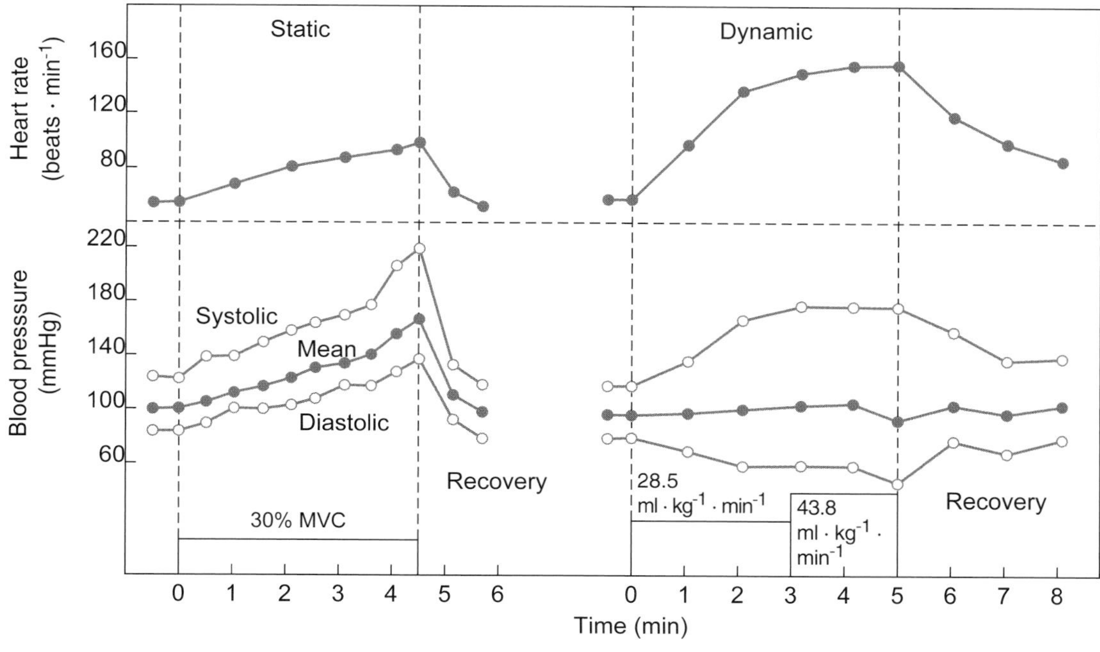

Figure 28.24 Comparison of the heart rate and blood pressure responses to a fatiguing, sustained handgrip at 30% of maximal voluntary contraction strength (30% MVC) and to an exhausting treadmill test.

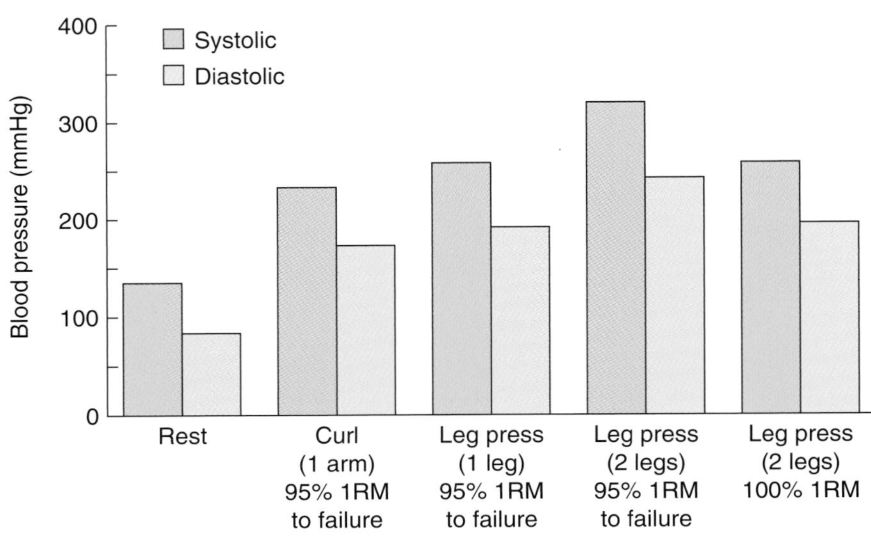

Figure 28.25 Blood pressure responses during weightlifting (40). RM = repetition maximum.

Mechanisms of heat production include the basal metabolic rate, shivering, work, and exercise. During exercise, the mechanical efficiency is about 20% or less, which means that 80% or more of the energy production ($\dot{V}O_2$) is converted to heat. For example, if you are working on a cycle ergometer at a rate requiring a $\dot{V}O_2$ of 2.0 L · min^{-1}, your energy production is about 10 kcal · min^{-1}. At 0% efficiency, 2 kcal · min^{-1} are used to do work, and 8 kcal · min^{-1} are converted to heat. If most of this added heat is not lost, core temperature might quickly rise to dangerous levels. How does the body lose excess heat?

Heat-Loss Mechanisms

The body loses heat by four processes. In **radiation,** heat is transferred from the surface of one object to the surface of another, with no physical contact between the objects. Heat loss depends on the temperature gradient, that is, the temperature difference between the surfaces of the objects. When a person is seated at rest in a comfortable environment (21-22 °C), about 60% of body heat is lost through radiation to cooler objects. **Conduction** is the transfer of heat from one object to another by direct contact, and, like radiation, conduction depends on a temperature gradient. A person sitting on a cold marble bench loses body heat by conduction. **Convection** is a special case of conduction in which heat is transferred to air (or water) molecules, which become lighter and rise away from the body to be replaced by cold air (or water). Heat loss can be enhanced by increasing the movement of the air (or water) over the surface of the body. For example, a fan stimulates heat loss by placing more cold air molecules into contact with the skin. All of these heat-loss mechanisms can be heat-gain mechanisms as well. We gain heat from the sun by radiation across 93 million mi (150 million km) of space, and we gain heat by conduction when we sit on hot sand at the beach. Similarly, if a fan were to place more hot air (warmer than skin temperature) into contact with the skin, we would gain, not lose, heat. Heat gained from the environment adds to that generated by exercise and puts an additional strain on heat-loss mechanisms.

The fourth heat-loss mechanism is the evaporation of sweat. **Sweating** is the process of producing a watery solution over the surface of the body. **Evaporation** is a process in which liquid water converts to a gas. This conversion requires about 580 kcal of heat per liter of sweat evaporated. The heat for this comes from the body and, thus, the body is cooled. At rest, about 25% of heat loss is caused by evaporation, but during exercise evaporation becomes the primary mechanism for heat loss.

Evaporation depends on the **water vapor pressure gradient** between the skin and the air and does not directly depend on temperature. The water vapor pressure of the air relates to the **relative humidity** and the **saturation pressure** at that air temperature. For example, the relative humidity can be 90% in winter, but because the saturation pressure of cold air is low, on such a day the water vapor pressure of the air is also low, and you can see water vapor rising from your body following exercise. In warm temperatures, however, the relative humidity is a good indicator of the water vapor pressure of the air. If the water vapor pressure of the air is too high, sweat will not evaporate, and sweat that does not evaporate does not cool the body (49).

Body Temperature Response to Exercise

Figure 28.26 shows that during exercise in a comfortable environment, the core temperature increases proportionally to the relative intensity (% $\dot{V}O_2$max) of the exercise and then levels off (59). The gain in body heat that occurs early in exercise triggers the heat-loss mechanisms discussed in the preceding section. After 10 to 20 min, heat loss equals heat production, and the core temperature remains steady (24). What are the most important heat-loss mechanisms during exercise?

Heat Loss During Exercise

Exercise intensity and environmental temperature influence which heat-loss mechanism is primarily responsible for maintaining a steady core temperature during exercise. When a person participates in progressively difficult

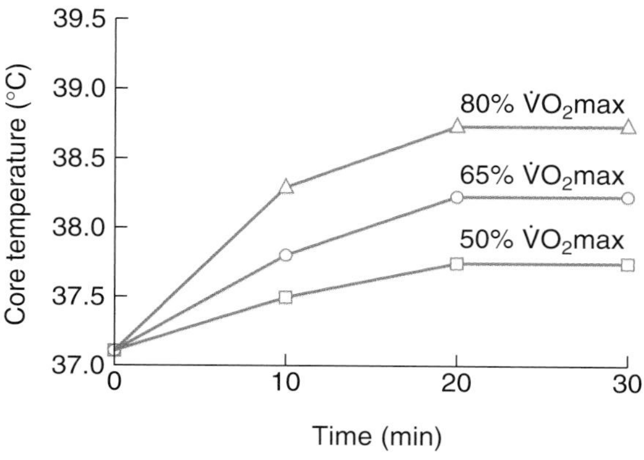

Figure 28.26 Core temperature increases over time as exercise intensity increases (2).

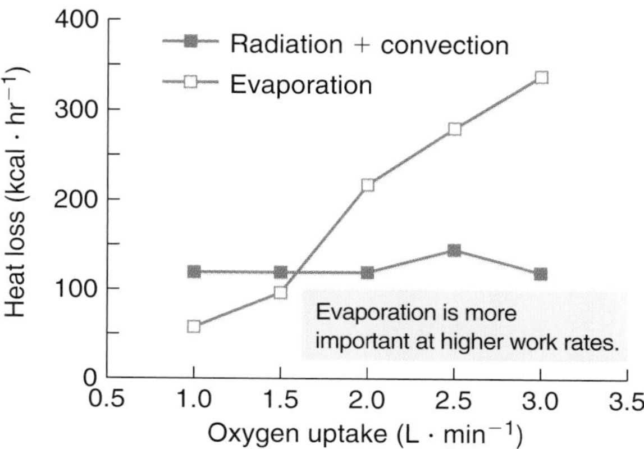

Figure 28.27 Importance of evaporation to the relative work rate (59). Evaporation is more important at higher work rates.

exercise tests in an environment that allows heat loss by all four mechanisms, the contribution that convection and radiation make to overall heat loss is modest. Because the temperature gradient between the skin and the room does not alter much during exercise, the rate of heat loss is relatively constant. To compensate for this, evaporation picks up when heat losses by convection and radiation plateau, and evaporation is responsible for most of the heat loss in heavy exercise (figure 28.27).

When a person performs steady-state exercise in a warmer environment, the role that evaporation plays becomes even more important. Figure 28.28 shows that as environmental temperature increases, the gradient for heat loss by convection and radiation decreases, and, with it, the rate of heat loss by these processes also decreases. As a result, evaporation must compensate to maintain core temperature.

In strenuous exercise or hot environments, evaporation is the most important process for losing heat and maintaining body temperature in a safe range. It should be no surprise, then, that factors affecting sweat production (such as dehydration) or sweat evaporation (such as impermeable clothing) are causes for concern. Chapter 10 provides the specifics on how to deal with heat and humidity when prescribing exercise, and chapter 25 discusses how to prevent and treat heat-related disorders.

Key Point

Heat can be lost from the body by radiation and convection when a temperature gradient exists between the skin and the environment; however, evaporation is the primary mechanism of heat loss during high-intensity exercise or during exercise in a hot environment. Body temperature increases proportionally during submaximal exercise. Acclimatization to heat can be achieved in 7 to 12 days of training in a hot and humid environment and improves one's ability to exercise safely.

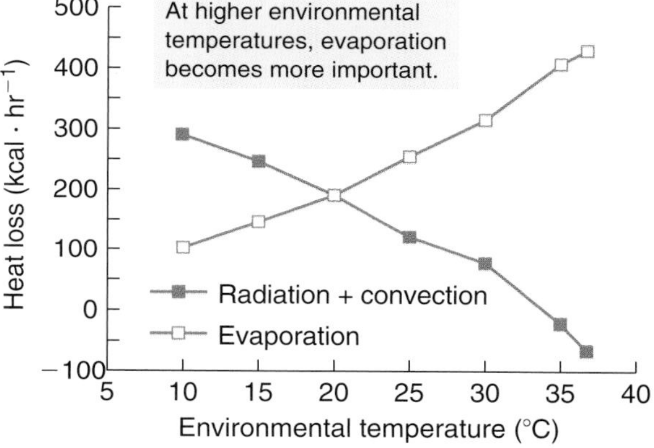

Figure 28.28 Importance of evaporation as a heat-loss mechanism during exercise as environmental temperature increases (2). At higher environmental temperatures, evaporation becomes more important.

Training in a hot and humid environment for as few as 7 to 12 days results in specific adaptations that improve heat tolerance and, as a result, lower the trained individual's body temperature during submaximal exercise (24). Adaptations that improve heat tolerance include the following:

- Increase in plasma volume
- Earlier onset of sweating
- Higher sweat rate
- Reduction in salt loss through sweat
- Reduced blood flow to the skin

Case Studies

You can check your answers by referring to pages 476 and 477 in appendix A.

1. A female competitive distance runner took a GXT on a motor-driven treadmill in which the speed of the run increased 0.5 mi · hr^{-1} (0.8 km · hr^{-1}) each minute, with the test starting at 5 mi · hr^{-1} (8 km · hr^{-1}). Blood samples for lactic acid determination were obtained each minute, and the lactate threshold was found to occur at the 8 mi · hr^{-1} (13 km · hr^{-1}) stage of the test. Unfortunately, no one at the testing center knew what this meant relative to performance, and she has come to you for help. What would you tell her?
2. A client with whom you have been working retakes a maximal GXT following 10 wk of endurance training and finds that his HR is lower at each stage of the test. He is bothered by this because he thought his heart would be stronger and beat more times per minute. How would you help him understand what happened?
3. A female client is bothered by the fact that elite women runners who train as hard as elite male runners don't achieve the same performance times in distance races. She wants to know why and has come to you for the answer. How would you respond?

Appendix A

Case Study Answers

Chapter 1

1. You might respond by admitting that there are risks related to exercise, with 7 deaths occurring each year for every 100,000 exercisers. However, more people die while sleeping or after eating and yet few people advocate the cessation of those activities. In addition, deterioration of the cardiovascular system through sedentary living causes a much higher risk of major health problems than being active causes. Finally, exercise-related risks can be minimized by starting very slowly and gradually increasing the amount and intensity of work done during exercise.
2. You might state that the CDC recommendations were aimed at individuals who are currently sedentary and not individuals who are habitually active and involved in strenuous exercise. In addition, you might indicate that participation in more strenuous exercise is associated with other health-related benefits (increases in cardiorespiratory fitness [$\dot{V}O_2$max]) that cannot be realized with moderate exercise.

Chapter 2

1. You would help Fred see that his goals are primarily health related at this time. After engaging in moderate-intensity exercise, he may want to add fitness goals to his list. Susan, on the other hand, has already reached her health and fitness goals—she now has performance goals in mind. You would help her analyze the various underlying factors and skills needed to compete in soccer and would suggest training to help her improve in these areas.

Chapter 3

1a. Tom's primary risk factors for CHD include hypertension, dyslipidemia, type 2 diabetes, and physical inactivity. Thus, he would be classified as high risk because he appears to have Type 2 diabetes. Although Tom's BP and cholesterol appear to be within their recommended ranges, he is taking medication to control both. Therefore, he meets the CHD risk factor threshold for both.

1b. Yes, according to the AHA and ACSM guidelines for physician consent, the fitness professional should contact his physician to obtain medical clearance because he was classified as high risk. Although Tom has seen his physician recently it was not necessarily to inquire if he should begin exercising regularly. Contacting the physician ensures that they are aware of Tom's plans to pursue regular physical activity and provides the fitness professional with consent from a medical authority. It would also be prudent to ask if Tom's physician has informed him that he may have diabetes.

2. Although she is 65 yr old, she did not indicate any risk factors on her PAR-Q, has had a recent physician-administered exam, and participates regularly in moderate-intensity exercise. Thus, she is classified as moderate risk and does not need physician consent before participation in moderate-intensity physical activities. She should be instructed to alert the instructor if she experiences any abnormal responses to exercise, to begin with a light weight such as 3 to 5 lb (1.4-2.3 kg) dumbbells, and to expect some mild soreness for 1 to 2 days after class participation.
3. Initially, ask Barbara to confirm that she has not been diagnosed with high blood pressure and is

not taking medication to control it. If she does take medication to manage her blood pressure, make certain she has taken it within the last 24 hr. Next, inquire if she has eaten, consumed caffeine, smoked, or performed physical activity within the last hour. If she answers these questions to your satisfaction, it is likely her elevated HR and BP may be attributed to anxiety regarding the fitness assessment. You may want to review the procedures for the fitness tests, reassure her of their safety, and remind her she can stop any test at any time if she desires to do so. You may also want discuss activities she enjoys for a couple of minutes in order to help her relax. Next, reassess her HR and BP. If they are within normal values, continue with the fitness tests. Be certain to reassure her throughout each test. If HR and BP remain high, then you may ask her to make a second appointment when it is convenient to her schedule.

Chapter 4

1. $3.5 \text{ mi} \cdot \text{hr}^{-1} \cdot 26.8 \text{m} \cdot \text{min}^{-1} = 93.8 \text{m} \cdot \text{min}^{-1}$

$$93.8 \text{m} \cdot \text{min}^{-1}\left(\frac{0.1 \text{ml} \cdot \text{kg}^{-1} \cdot \text{min}^{-1}}{\text{m} \cdot \text{min}^{-1}}\right) +$$
$$3.5 \text{ml} \cdot \text{kg}^{-1} \cdot \text{min}^{-1} = 12.9 \text{ml} \cdot \text{kg}^{-1} \cdot \text{min}^{-1}$$
$$12.9 \text{ml} \cdot \text{kg}^{-1} \cdot \text{min}^{-1} \cdot 75 \text{kg} =$$
$$968 \text{ml} \cdot \text{min}^{-1}, \text{or } 0.97 \text{L} \cdot \text{min}^{-1}$$
$$0.97 \text{L} \cdot \text{min}^{-1} \cdot 5 \text{kcal} \cdot \text{L}^{-1} = 4.85 \text{kcal} \cdot \text{min}^{-1}$$
$$4.85 \text{kcal} \cdot \text{min}^{-1} \cdot 30 \text{min} = 146 \text{kcal}$$

2. $100 \text{ W} = 600 \text{ kpm} \cdot \text{min}^{-1}$

$$\dot{V}O_2 = \frac{(600 \text{ kpm} \cdot \text{min}^{-1} \cdot 1.8 \text{ ml } O_2 \cdot \text{min}^{-1})}{60 \text{ kg} + 7 \text{ ml} \cdot \text{kg}^{-1} \cdot \text{min}^{-1}}$$
$$25 \text{ ml} \cdot \text{kg}^{-1} \cdot \text{min}^{-1} =$$
$$18 \text{ ml} \cdot \text{kg}^{-1} \cdot \text{min}^{-1} + 7 \text{ ml} \cdot \text{kg}^{-1} \cdot \text{min}^{-1}$$

3. $3 \text{ mi} \cdot 1{,}610 \text{ m} \cdot \text{mi}^{-1} = 4{,}830 \text{ m} \div 24 \text{ min} = 201 \text{ m} \cdot \text{min}^{-1}$

$$201 \text{ m} \cdot \text{min}^{-1}\left(\frac{0.2 \text{ ml} \cdot \text{kg}^{-1} \cdot \text{min}^{-1}}{\text{m} \cdot \text{min}^{-1}}\right) +$$
$$3.5 \text{ ml} \cdot \text{kg}^{-1} \cdot \text{min}^{-1} = 43.7 \text{ ml} \cdot \text{kg}^{-1} \cdot \text{min}^{-1}$$
$$43.7 \text{ ml} \cdot \text{kg}^{-1} \cdot \text{min}^{-1} \cdot 70 \text{ kg} =$$
$$3{,}059 \text{ ml} \cdot \text{min}^{-1}, \text{or } 3.06 \text{ L} \cdot \text{min}^{-1}$$
$$3.06 \text{ L} \cdot \text{min}^{-1} \cdot 5 \text{ kcal} \cdot \text{L}^{-1} =$$
$$15.3 \text{ kcal} \cdot \text{min}^{-1} \cdot 24 \text{ min} = 367 \text{ kcal}$$

4. $12 \text{ METs} = 12 \text{ kcal} \cdot \text{kg}^{-1} \cdot \text{hr}^{-1} \cdot 70\% =$

$$8.4 \text{ kcal} \cdot \text{kg}^{-1} \cdot \text{hr}^{-1}$$

5. You might indicate that the cost of jogging 1 m · min^{-1} (0.2 ml · kg^{-1} · min^{-1}) is about twice that for walking (0.1 ml · kg^{-1} · min^{-1}) due to the extra energy needed to propel the body off the ground and absorb the force of impact on each step. You might provide a summary table he can use describing the caloric cost of walking and running 1 mi (1.6 km).

Chapter 5

1. Requiring sedentary middle-aged participants to take a maximal, unmonitored test at the beginning of their fitness program is inappropriate. You might suggest the club replace the 1.5 mi run with the 1 mi walk test, which should be used after the participants have demonstrated that they can comfortably walk 1 mi (1.6 km).
2. His estimated $\dot{V}O_2max$ = 37.8 ml · kg^{-1} · min^{-1}. His level of cardiorespiratory fitness is adequate for most activities and just short of being "good" for his age group.
3. The heart rate response of 100 beats · min^{-1} at the work rate of 300 kgm · min^{-1} should be ignored. The heart rate values are extrapolated to 170 beats · min^{-1}, and the vertical line dropped from that point indicates a work rate of about 1,050 kgm · min^{-1},

$$\dot{V}O_2 = \frac{(1050 \text{ kpm} \cdot \text{min}^{-1} \cdot 1.8 \text{ ml } O_2 \cdot \text{kpm}^{-1})}{81.7 \text{ kg} + 7 \text{ ml} \cdot \text{kg}^{-1} \cdot \text{min}^{-1}}$$
$$= \frac{30.1 \text{ ml} \cdot \text{kg}^{-1} \cdot \text{min}^{-1}}{3.5 \text{ ml} \cdot \text{kg}^{-1} \cdot \text{min}^{-1}} = 8.6 \text{ METs}$$

4. The graph should ignore the heart rate value of 96 beats · min^{-1}. The line is extrapolated to 190 beats · min^{-1}, and the vertical line dropped from that point indicates a value of about 16.75% grade, which equals a $\dot{V}O_2$ of about 35.6 ml · kg · min^{-1}. This is 10.2 METs, or 1.94 L · min^{-1}.
5. The reference point for the scale is the zero point established when the free-swinging pendulum stops (with the cycle on a flat surface). All scale values are relative to this zero, and if the zero is off, all scale readings are off. If the pendulum does not rest at zero when no weight is attached, the entire scale is off by the amount the zero value is off by. For example, if the scale reads 0.25 kg when no weight is attached, each scale value shifts 0.25 kg upward when known weights are attached.

Chapter 6

1a. BMI = 34.5 kg · m^{-2}; WHR = 1.02; %BF = 33.75%. Mr. Jackson's BMI is in the obese range. Both his waist circumference and WHR indicate abdominal obesity. His %BF is also well above the recommended range. Clearly Mr. Jackson's health would benefit from a successful weight loss program.

1b. Target goal = 159 ÷ (1 – 0.3) = 227 lb. At 227 lb (103 kg), Mr. Jackson will still be classified in the obese category; however, if he finds success in achieving this initial goal, he may be encouraged to continue with his attempts to lose weight.

Chapter 7

1. This athlete weighs 86.4 kg. The ACSM, ADA, and Dietitians of Canada position statement (4) suggests that such an athlete may benefit from ingesting 1.2 to 1.4 g of protein for each kilogram of body weight. This athlete is consuming approximately 525 kcal of protein each day (3,500 kcal · 0.15 = 525 kcal). This amount roughly equals 131 g of protein (525 kcal ÷ 4 kcal · g^{-1} = 131.25 g). This is approximately 1.5 g · kg^{-1} (131.25 g ÷ 86.4 kg = 1.52 g · kg^{-1}). Additional protein intake appears unwarranted.

Chapter 9

1. The sacral angle should be at least 80° (a book or a board on edge placed against the sacrum would be snug if the angle were 90°). Next examine the curvature of the spine; it should be smooth with no evident flatness or hypermobility in any one particular area. Arm–leg length discrepancy might also be a factor (e.g., long arms in relation to legs).
2. Most false positives in the Thomas test result when the individual being tested brings the thigh too close to the chest. This can result in excessive posterior rotation of the pelvis which, in turn, can make it appear that the hip flexors are tight.

Chapter 10

1. If a person has a normal response to a GXT, HR and systolic blood pressure increase with each stage of the test, whereas the diastolic pressure remains the same or decreases slightly. In addition, the ECG shows no significant S-T segment depression or elevation, and no significant arrhythmias. In these cases it can be assumed that the last load achieved on the test represents the true functional capacity (max METs). The GXT presented in case study 10.1 is representative of such a test.

   Paul has normal resting BP and a negative family history for CHD. Risk factors include a relatively high percentage of body fat, sedentary lifestyle, and a poor blood lipid profile. Based on these findings, a THR range of 158 to 177 beats · min^{-1} was calculated (60%-80% $\dot{V}O_2max$ as measured during the maximal GXT); this HR range corresponds to work rates equal to 6.3 to 8.4 METs. Initially, he will work at or below the lower end of the calculated THR range, with the emphasis on the duration of activity. As he becomes more active he will be able to work within the THR range, depending, of course, on his interests. He was referred for nutritional counseling to improve his blood lipid profile. Paul has an estimated HRmax of 174 beats · min^{-1}; his measured HR was 24 beats · min^{-1} higher. Given the inherent biological variation in the estimated HRmax, use the measured values when they are available.
2. Mary's maximal work rate was estimated to be 750 kpm · min^{-1} by extrapolating the relationship between HR and work rate to the predicted maximal heart rate (see chapter 5). This is equivalent to a $\dot{V}O_2max$ of 29 ml · kg^{-1} · min^{-1}, or 8.3 METs.

   Her blood chemistry values and BP are normal. Her family history is negative for CHD. Her HR response to the test is normal and indicates poor cardiorespiratory fitness. The low maximal aerobic power is related to the sedentary lifestyle, the cigarette smoking (carbon monoxide), and the 30% BF. She was encouraged to participate in a smoking-cessation program and was given the names of two local professional groups.

   The recommended exercise program emphasized the low end of the THR zone (70% HRmax: 127 beats · min^{-1}) with long duration. She preferred a walking program because of the freedom it gave her schedule. She was given the walking program in chapter 14 and was asked to record her HR response to each of the exercise sessions.

   A body fatness goal of 22% resulted in a target body weight of 121 lb (55 kg). She did not feel the need for dietary counseling at this time, but she agreed to record her food intake for 10 days to determine the patterns of eating behavior that would be beneficial to change (see chapters 7 and 11). She made an appointment for a meeting with the fitness professional in 2 wk to discuss the progress with her program.

Chapter 11

1. Convert weight and height to metric units: 160 lb = 72.6 kg; 5 ft 5 in. = 1.65 m.
2. Since the client does not currently perform any exercise or physical activity, *PA* = 1.12.
3. Use the following equation to calculate the client's daily calorie need:

   EER = 354 – 6.91 (52) + 1.12[9.36 (72.6) + 726 (1.65)] = 2,098 kcal
4. In order to lose 1 lb (0.5 kg) each week, a caloric deficit of 3,500 kcal · wk^{-1} (or 500 kcal · day^{-1})

is needed. The subject has added 200 kcal · day^{-1} in physical activity, so an additional 300 kcal should be cut from the diet. This would lead to a recommendation of consuming approximately 1,800 kcal · day^{-1}.

Chapter 12

1. While any reasonable resistance training program can increase muscle strength during the first few months of training, more advanced programs are needed following the initial adaptation stage. This member has become stale because he has performed the same resistance training program for 4 mo. Although there are many different ways to modify a resistance training program, it would be appropriate to increase his training volume, training intensity, and, time permitting, his training frequency. It would also be beneficial to replace a few weight machine exercises with free weight exercises that require more balance and coordination. Advising this member to follow a nonlinear periodized training program with light (12RM-15RM), moderate (8RM-10RM), and heavy (4 RM-6RM) training days throughout the week would promote additional strength gains and prevent boredom. Although all exercises do not need to be performed for the same number of sets, 1 set of each exercise on the light training day, 2 sets on the moderate training day, and 3 sets on the heavy training day (with adequate recovery between sets) would be appropriate.
2. With appropriate guidance and supervision, resistance training can offer observable health value to seniors at an assisted-living home. However, established guidelines need to be followed to ensure safe and effective programming. All seniors should undergo a preparticipation health screening to identify coexisting medical conditions that may limit or prevent participation in a resistance training program. Seniors should begin resistance training with minimal resistance during the first 8 wk of training to allow for favorable changes in connective tissue. As a general recommendation, seniors should perform 1 set of 10 to 15 repetitions on a variety of exercises and should be encouraged to maintain proper breathing patterns while exercising. In addition, fitness professionals should carefully monitor the performance of each exercise to ensure that each repetition is performed in a controlled manner within a pain-free ROM. Since weight machines are not available, exercises should be performed while sitting in a chair. Once seniors can perform each exercise correctly and gain confidence in their abilities to resistance train, additional exercises can be performed in the standing position, which requires more balance. In addition to light dumbbells and elastic bands, items such as 16 oz cans of vegetables can also be used as resistance. The following exercises would be appropriate for this population: leg extension (without resistance), seated elastic band chest press, seated elastic band row (with middle of cord secured to immovable object), seated dumbbell (or vegetable can) lateral raise, seated dumbbell (or vegetable can) curl, and seated dumbbell overhead triceps extension. At the end of the session seniors should perform static stretching exercises for the major muscle groups.

Chapter 13

1. Although it is possible that this exercise might be appropriate for some individuals with well-developed abdominal musculature, it is not an appropriate exercise to give the masses since the quality of the movement is so critical. The individual with extremely well-developed abdominal muscles may be able to perform this exercise and keep her low back in contact with the exercise surface throughout its execution; however, the individual with weaker abdominals or tight hip flexors will invariably anteriorly tilt the pelvis, and the resulting lumbar lordosis places the lumbar vertebra in a potentially compromising position. Undoubtedly the physical therapists who use this activity use it only as a test on a one-to-one basis; this enables them to immediately stop the activity if they believe it is compromising to any individual.
2. It is good that the exercise leader emphasizes the importance of not doing ballistic stretches even from the sitting position; however, there are other factors that she should also consider. This maneuver is a fair exercise for improving hamstring extensibility. However, if the individual has extremely tight hamstrings (i.e., if the sacrum should be less than 80° to 90° with the exercise surface in the sit and reach), the forward stretching from this position could potentially stretch the tissues of the low back instead of the hamstrings. Therefore, for the individual with fairly tight hamstrings the sit-and-reach exercise may be contraindicated; the standing toe touch could be worse because of the effect of gravity on the moment arm of force.
3. Although isometric exercises have become less popular as a strength development activity in most applications (joint injury would be an exception), they can be used most appropriately for strengthening trunk musculature, assuming the exerciser

does not have high BP. The oblique curl could be particularly advantageous since the internal and external oblique muscles play an important role in stabilizing the spine. This factor may decrease the likelihood of having low-back problems; for the individual who is symptomatic, developing these muscles in this way may enable him to better maintain his neutral spine and avoid postures which exacerbate his condition.

Chapter 14

1. Topics to address include
   - paying attention to signs and symptoms that indicate problems and instructions to act on them with a visit to the physician,
   - proper shoes,
   - clothing appropriate for the season and site (e.g., safety, surface, lighting),
   - buddy system, where possible, to encourage participation, and
   - alternate walking location for poor weather (shopping mall).
2. Before beginning an aerobic dance class, the participant should be able to walk 2 mi a day at a brisk pace without discomfort. The appropriate transition from a walking program would be into a low-intensity, low-impact aerobics class. The participant should stay at the low end of the THR zone during this transition and increase the intensity of the class only after these low-intensity, low-impact sessions can be comfortably completed.

Chapter 15

1. Refer the parent to the recommendations for resistance training in children, explaining that the emphasis should be on proper form, supervision, and endurance at this age. After puberty, he can include resistance training with fewer repetitions.
2. Acknowledge that reading and math are very important. The school needs to provide a good foundation in these areas, but it cannot possibly do it all—some reading and math work will need to be done at home and in the community. Including physical activity (through physical education and recess) is essential for the health of the children. Basic health is a prerequisite for other learning. In the same way that the school cannot provide all the necessary math and reading, the school cannot provide all the recommended physical activity, but it can provide a foundation that can be supplemented in the home and community.

Chapter 16

1. You should begin by finding out when he had his last physical and what his physician told him about his arthritis. A submaximal cycle ergometer test should be carried out to obtain some baseline measures (HR, RPE) to use as reference points for subsequent follow-ups. Establish a THR zone for him (50%-70% of HRR), and verify that this elicits an RPE of about 10 to 13. Have him begin his exercise program at 50% HRR, performing work–relief intervals (5 min on, 1 min off) to determine if he can do a series of these intervals with little or no joint discomfort. The goal is for 30 min of continuous activity as long as the discomfort is little or nothing. Increase the work interval to 10 min in the second week. If joint discomfort is a problem, stay with intervals within his tolerance. Intensity can be increased after he has achieved 30 min of total exercise time. Introduce him to a variety of weight-supported exercise modes (cycle, rower, water aerobics) that he should be able to use with less joint discomfort than what he experienced with jogging. Workouts should be done 3 to 4 times each week and include regular warm-up and flexibility activities.

Chapter 17

1. This client will benefit from both weight-bearing aerobic activity and resistance training. To increase her aerobic fitness, protect her against chronic disease, and load her bones, a walking program is appropriate. She should gradually progress to a 30 min brisk walk on most, preferably all, days of the week. Additionally, she should engage in resistance training 2 to 3 days each week. The program should include upper- and lower-body exercises and focus on areas at high risk for osteoporotic fractures (hip, spine, wrist). Three sets of approximately 70% of 1RM (8-12 reps) are appropriate. Suggested exercises include the standing toe raise, leg press, leg extension, leg curl, back extension (use care to avoid hyperextension), bench press, shoulder press, biceps curl, triceps extension, and wrist curl. Additionally, the client should consume adequate amounts of calcium and vitamin D (see chapter 7).

Chapter 18

1. Since John is a 46-yr-old male with typical effort-induced angina and an elevated total cholesterol/HDL ratio over 5.0 (signifying increased risk), he has a high likelihood of CHD. A reasonable next step would be to refer him for a GXT in the presence of a physician, to see if signs or symptoms of

CHD occur. If they do, a more definitive diagnostic test such as coronary angiography might be recommended.

2. Jane's GXT results indicated that her maximal aerobic capacity was 7 METs; therefore, prescribing exercise at about 60% of this value, or around 4 METs, would be appropriate. Appropriate exercises would be treadmill walking, stationary cycling, and arm cranking. Realize that her maximal heart rate is low because she is taking a beta-blocker. Thus, exercise could be prescribed on the basis of RPE (e.g., a target rating of somewhat hard on the Borg RPE scale). Light resistance exercises using dumbbells and elastic bands, as tolerated, would also be acceptable. The resistance should be selected so as to allow her to perform 12 to 15 repetitions with good form.

Chapter 19

1a. Because Marsha is hypertensive, has extreme (class III) obesity, is inactive, has a strong family history of cardiovascular disease and diabetes, and has not undergone a medical examination in several years, medical clearance before beginning an exercise program is recommended. The medical examination should be used to reveal any underlying medical conditions that would make it unsafe for Marsha to engage in moderate or vigorous exercise.

1b. In addition to height and weight, measurement of waist and hip circumference is recommended. In addition to BMI calculations and examination of abdominal adiposity, an estimate of body fat percentage could be useful, but only if methods are chosen that are both reliable and accurate for obese individuals (see chapter 6). Cardiovascular fitness could be assessed with either a treadmill or a cycle ergometer protocol. Standard flexibility and strength tests could be used.

1c. A conversation with Marsha is crucial to determine her goals and interests. To increase adherence, close attention should be paid to her willingness to engage in a variety of activities. Attempts should be made to increase lifestyle activity and structured exercise. Assuming that Marsha is willing to invest 3 day · wk^{-1} for 1 hr in structured exercise and is willing to exercise on her own on other days, the following program would target a weight loss of 2 lb · wk^{-1} (0.9 kg · wk^{-1}).

- Exercise 6 day · wk^{-1} and try to expend 300 kcal of energy on each of these days. The structured exercise should focus on improving cardiovascular endurance, strength, and flexibility. On 3 day · wk^{-1} Marsha could walk on her own (preferably with an exercise partner) for 1 hr (could be divided into shorter sessions). This increase in activity will increase her caloric expenditure by approximately 1,800 kcal · wk^{-1}.
- She should target an energy intake that is approximately 745 kcal below her estimated calorie need. Using the formula in chapter 11, Marsha's daily energy need is approximately 2,480 kcal. Targeting her daily caloric intake to approximately 1,735 kcal · day^{-1} will result in a caloric deficit of 5,200 kcal · wk^{-1} from caloric restriction.
- The combination of caloric restriction (5,200 kcal · wk^{-1}) and energy expenditure (1,800 kcal · wk^{-1}) will result in a weight loss of approximately 2 lb (0.9 kg) each week. Weekly weigh-ins and consultation with the fitness professional are recommended in order to adjust the program as needed.

Chapter 20

1. Mr. Conner has both type 2 diabetes and metabolic syndrome. Because of his medical issues and his history of inactivity, a supervised program is recommended during the initial phase of his exercise program. He has medical approval to begin exercise, so programming can proceed. The overall exercise objective is to have Mr. Conner engage in regular exercise to improve his fitness and assist with his weight loss and glucose control. Dietary restriction of approximately 500 kcal below daily caloric need and caloric expenditure averaging 250 kcal · day^{-1} will lead to weight loss of approximately 18 lb (8.2 kg) during the 3 mo program.

   Initially, supervised aerobic activity (walking, cycling, etc.) for 30 min on 3 day · wk^{-1} is recommended. The intensity should be low to moderate as his body acclimates to exercise. If there are no problems during the first 2 wk, he can be educated on the signs of hypoglycemia and then encouraged to walk without supervision. Gradually build his aerobic exercise to 45 to 60 min of moderate-intensity activity on 5 or more days a week.

   Resistance training (moderate intensity) should be performed 3 day · wk^{-1} under supervision. He should complete 2 sets of 10 to 15 repetitions of the following exercises: leg press, leg extension, leg curl, bench press, shoulder press, row, biceps curl, and triceps extension. His focus is to engage the large muscle groups of the upper and lower body in order to assist with glucose control.

Chapter 21

1. Find out if she has worked with her physician and is currently not experiencing problems with her medication. In addition, ask if she carries a bronchodilator with her to class, and determine that she knows how to use it at the onset of wheezing. Lastly, pay special attention to her during the early phases of the class.
2. The patient likely has emphysema and possibly bronchitis, two forms of chronic obstructive pulmonary disease (COPD) that commonly result from cigarette smoking. This is shown by his reduced ability to exhale air quickly (FEV_1). The logical course of treatment is a program to help him stop smoking, followed by a pulmonary rehabilitation program to help him regain his ability to exercise so that he can carry out functional activities of daily living.
3. The patient has a limited ability to exercise, but intermittent treadmill walking (with treadmill level), cycle ergometry, and rowing would be suitable. Arm exercises with very light weights or stretch cords for upper-body conditioning are also appropriate. During physical training his oxygen saturation, ECG, and symptoms of dyspnea should be closely monitored. Supplemental oxygen will help increase his oxygen saturation, maintaining it above 90%.

Chapter 22

1. Dana is in the preparation stage and has low exercise self-efficacy. She has had a bad experience with exercise in the past, so you want to educate her about what to expect at the beginning of an exercise program and make sure the prescription is appropriate for her fitness level. Use the fitness evaluation to give her a realistic idea of her current fitness level and how much progress she can expect based on a sensible prescription. In setting goals with her, find out what *she* wants to achieve and activities she might enjoy. Brainstorm about her barriers to exercise and how to counter them. Identify supports and ways she could reward herself during the program. Target her low exercise self-efficacy with a beginners' exercise class where she would have social support. Make sure she gets individual attention and encouragement, especially during the first few weeks. A behavioral contract with Mike doing something she wants him to do when she meets short-term goals could provide incentives and support that she will need to keep her program going.
2. Jack is in the action stage and is especially susceptible to relapse. You could make a point of walking with Jack the next time he comes in to provide support and education about relapse prevention. Extra work at the end of the term is a high-risk situation for him; he is discouraged and at risk of relapse. Talk with him about setting short-term goals that can be readjusted during exams. Help him to make the goals realistic and reachable. He might want to take walk breaks for 10 to 15 min during the days he can't get to the facility. Point out that these breaks will help him stay on track and give him a way to manage stress at work. Praise him for how far he has come and for continuing even though he is very busy. Help him see that the high-risk situation is time limited, and brainstorm about ways he can reward himself for the walking he can do. Recruit veteran walkers to provide support and encouragement.

Chapter 23

1. Explain to her what Hatha yoga is and describe its attributes. Check with local Hatha yoga resources and refer her to a yoga teacher who specializes in restorative yoga. Explain to your client that this form of Hatha yoga progresses through a variety of yoga poses while utilizing props, blankets, and bolsters to ease the stress of each pose. Gradually these props are withdrawn as her flexibility and strength improve and she can progress to a more vigorous style of yoga such as Iyengar yoga.
2. You could refer him to an experienced and certified Alexander teacher for 2 to 4 sessions. The Alexander teacher will observe the subject running, perhaps sprinting, and will observe posture, movement mechanics and breathing pattern. She will particularly stress a more efficient alignment of the runner's head, neck, shoulders, and spine. The Alexander teacher will help the runner relearn more efficient alignment, movement, and breathing patterns, which will be particularly useful during the more stressful segments of a race.

Chapter 24

1a. HR = 1500 ÷ 12 = 125 beats · min^{-1}

P-R interval duration = 0.12 sec

QRS complex duration = 0.08 sec

Q-T interval duration = 0.32 sec

1b. Sinus tachycardia—Fast heart rate over 100 beats · min^{-1}.

1c. Common causes of sinus tachycardia are anxiety, nervousness, caffeine, or low fitness.

2a. Atrial fibrillation—Jagged baseline with irregularly spaced PVCs.

2b. Ventricular rate = 6 cardiac cycles in a 6 sec strip · 10 = 60 beats · min^{-1}.

3a. Trigeminy—Every third heartbeat is a PVC.

3b. Gradually decrease treadmill speed and grade, and notify the physician.

4. Because the person was on Inderal (a nonselective β-blocker) at the time of his exercise test, his heart rate would have been suppressed. Now that he is no longer taking the medication, his previously calculated target HR will be too low. The exercise intensity should be adjusted upward.

5. Isordil contains nitroglycerin and is used to reduce the chance of having an angina attack. The drug relaxes vascular smooth muscle and might cause pooling of blood in the extremities. This pooling could decrease blood pressure and result in symptoms of dizziness.

Chapter 25

1a. Suspect insulin shock.

1b. Ask the following questions: What happened? Are you a diabetic? Have you taken your insulin today? Have you eaten?

1c. Check her medical-alert tag. If insulin shock is still suspected, administer sugar (orange juice, candy, sugar granules). If she is unconscious or her recovery is slow (greater than 1-2 min), refer to a physician.

2a. Suspect heatstroke.

2b. Implement EMS—call 911. This is a medical emergency. Cool quickly, starting at the head and working down. Expose as much skin surface as possible. Monitor vital signs. Treat cramps by stretching and by applying ice, direct pressure, and gentle massage. Treat for shock. Wrap in cold, wet sheets for transport.

2c. Emergency plans and materials should include

- access to cooling agents, such as water, ice, ice towels, and a cool environment;
- access to a phone, with knowledge of EMS and emergency phone numbers;
- knowledge of roles in emergency: person in charge, person who assists person in charge, person responsible for making emergency phone call, person who meets and directs the emergency vehicle to the injured; and
- knowledge of rules to move person if necessary.

Chapter 26

The following steps should be followed for each employee's evaluation:

1. Review the employees' job descriptions for pertinent professional responsibilities they perform on a regular basis.
2. Determine how each responsibility can be quantified (satisfactory or nonsatisfactory or graded on a scale from 1 to 5).
3. Evaluate their performance for each responsibility either through direct observation or via conversations with the fitness director.
4. During a confidential meeting, share your evaluation with each employee, including specific examples that support exemplary or substandard performance. The employee should be permitted to add comment to the evaluation before it is forwarded to the wellness director.

Your evaluation should utilize the following resources:

1. How the fitness facility's objectives help achieve the organization's mission statement.
2. Specific examples of how these objectives are currently attained.
3. Predetermined quality assessment measures (e.g., health and fitness outcomes, revenue generated) that provide additional support for the program's efficacy.
4. Possible solutions for programs which are not performing as projected.
5. Positive customer service examples that directly relate to the exercise facility's programming.

Chapter 27

1. Explain to the exerciser that the hip and knee extensor muscles that are used to push against the weights are also working to control the descent. The press requires concentric contraction; the return requires eccentric contraction. Both kinds of contractions lead to increases in strength.
2. When she's doing the wrist curls with her palms down (radioulnar pronated position), the wrist extensors are the contracting muscles; when her palms are up (supinated position), the wrist flexors are the working muscles. The wrist flexors are usually stronger than the wrist extensors.

   The explanation is different for the pull-ups. The elbow flexor muscles are working regardless of the radioulnar joint position. However, when the palms are facing away (pronation), the distal tendon of the biceps brachii muscle is wrapped around the radius bone and therefore this muscle cannot exert as much force as when the palms are facing toward the body (supinated position).
3. He should make a conscious effort to maintain a backward pelvic tilt. He should also keep his arms in

front of his head instead of by his ears and his knees slightly flexed to help him maintain the backward tilt.

Chapter 28

1. The lactate threshold is the point during a graded exercise test when the blood lactic acid concentration suddenly increases. The lactate threshold has been used to indicate performance, in that the speed at which it occurs closely relates to the speed that can be maintained in distance runs (10K or marathon). As she improves her training, the lactate threshold occurs later into the GXT, indicating that she can maintain a faster pace in distance runs.
2. You need to confirm your client's feeling that the heart is stronger after training and, as a result, can pump more blood out per beat (increased stroke volume). As a result, the heart does not have to beat as many times to deliver the same amount of oxygen to the tissues. This is a more efficient way for the heart to pump blood, and in fact, the heart does not have to work as hard at this lower rate.
3. You might begin by briefly stating that running speed in distance races relates to the amount of oxygen the runner can deliver to the muscles. When more oxygen can be delivered, the running speed is faster. The elite female distance runner differs from the elite male distance runner in three ways that have a bearing on this issue: Her heart size is smaller and she cannot pump as much oxygen-rich blood to the muscle per minute; the oxygen content of her blood is lower due to the lower hemoglobin concentration; and she is also carrying relatively more body fat, which negatively affects sustained running speed, even at the same level of fitness.

Appendix B

Calculation of Oxygen Uptake and Carbon Dioxide Production

Calculation of Oxygen Consumption ($\dot{V}O_2$)

The air we breathe is composed of 20.93% oxygen (O_2), 0.03% carbon dioxide (CO_2), and the balance, 79.04%, nitrogen (N_2). When we exhale, the fraction of the air represented by O_2 is decreased and the fraction represented by CO_2 is increased. To calculate the volume of O_2 used by the body ($\dot{V}O_2$), we simply subtract the number of liters of O_2 exhaled from the number of liters of O_2 inhaled. Equation 1 summarizes these words.

(1) Oxygen consumption =
[Volume of O_2 inhaled] – [Volume of O_2 exhaled].

Now, using VO_2 to mean volume of *oxygen* used, V_I to mean volume of *air* inhaled, V_E to mean volume of *air* exhaled, F_{IO_2} to mean fraction of oxygen in inhaled air, and F_{EO_2} to mean fraction of oxygen in exhaled air, equation 1 can be written.

$$(2)\ VO_2 = [V_I \cdot F_{IO_2}] - [V_E \cdot F_{EO_2}].$$

You know that $F_{IO_2} = 0.2093$, and F_{EO_2} will be determined on an oxygen analyzer. Consequently, you are left with only two unknowns; the volume of air (liters) inhaled (V_I) and the volume of air (liters) exhaled (V_E). It appears that you must measure both volumes, but fortunately, this is not necessary. It was determined years ago that N_2 is neither used nor produced by the body. Consequently, the number of liters of N_2 inhaled must equal the number of liters of N_2 exhaled. Equation 3 states this equality using the symbols mentioned earlier.

$$(3)\ V_I \cdot F_{IN_2} = V_E \cdot F_{EN_2}.$$

This is a very important relationship because it permits you to calculate V_E when V_I is known or vice versa. Using equation 3, here are two formulas, one giving V_E when V_I is known and one giving V_I when V_E is known.

$$V_I = \frac{V_E \cdot F_{EN_2}}{F_{IN_2}},\ V_E = \frac{V_I \cdot F_{IN_2}}{F_{EN_2}}.$$

Now that you know how to do this, you need only one other piece to the puzzle to calculate $\dot{V}O_2$. The value for F_{IN_2} is constant (0.7904), so we must determine F_{EN_2}. When the expired gas sample is analyzed you will obtain a value for F_{EO_2} and F_{ECO_2} but not F_{EN_2}. However, since all the gas fractions must add up to 1.0000, you can calculate F_{EN_2} in the same way we calculated F_{IN_2}: 1.0000 – .0003 (CO_2) – .2093 (O_2) = .7904.

Problem: Calculate F_{EN_2} when F_{EO_2} = .1600 and F_{ECO_2} = .0450.

Answer: F_{EN_2} = 1.0000 – .1600 – .0450 = .7950.

The following problem shows how these equations are used. Given that V_I equals 100 L, F_{EO_2} = .1600, and F_{ECO_2} = .0450, calculate V_E.

$$V_E \cdot F_{EN_2} = V_I \cdot F_{IN_2}\text{, so } V_E = \frac{V_I \cdot F_{IN_2}}{F_{EN_2}}.$$

$$F_{IN_2} = .7904 \text{ and}$$

$$F_{EN_2} = 1.0000 - .1600 - .0450 = .7950$$

$$V_E = 100\text{ L} \cdot \frac{.7904}{.7950} = 99.4\text{ L}.$$

At this point, the equation for VO_2 can be rewritten, using V_I, V_E, F_{IO_2}, and F_{EO_2}.

$$VO_2 = V_I \cdot F_{IO_2} - V_E \cdot F_{EO_2}.$$

Assuming that you measure only V_I, this formula is rewritten:

$$VO_2 = V_I \cdot F_{IO_2} - \frac{V_I \cdot F_{IN_2}}{F_{EN_2}} \cdot F_{EO_2}.$$

V_I can be factored out of this equation, so

$$VO_2 = V_I \left[F_{IO_2} - \frac{F_{IN_2}}{F_{EN_2}} \cdot F_{EO_2} \right].$$

We will repeat the last two steps assuming that V_E is the volume that is measured and then factor out V_E.

$$VO_2 = \frac{V_E \cdot F_{EN_2}}{F_{IN_2}} \cdot F_{IO_2} - V_E \cdot F_{EO_2}$$

$$= V_E \left[\frac{F_{EN_2}}{F_{IN_2}} \cdot F_{IO_2} - F_{EO_2} \right].$$

At this point you know how to calculate VO_2. If you ever get stuck, always go back to the formula:

$VO_2 = V_I \cdot F_{IO_2} - V_E \cdot F_{EO_2}$ and simply substitute for V_E or V_I, depending on what was measured.

Some comments:

1. You must always match the volume measurement with the F_{EO_2} and F_{ECO_2} values measured in that expired volume. If you measure V_I for 2 min, you must have a single 2 min bag of expired gas to get F_{EO_2} and F_{ECO_2} values. If you measure a 30 sec volume your expired bag must be collected over those 30 sec.
2. VO_2 and VCO_2 are usually expressed in liters per minute: the *rate* at which O_2 is used or CO_2 is produced per minute. To signify this *rate*, we write $\dot{V}O_2$ (read *Vee dot*). You would convert 30 sec or 2 min volumes to 1 min values before calculating $\dot{V}O_2$.

Sample problem:

$\dot{V}_I = 100\text{ L} \cdot \text{min}^{-1}$, $F_{EO_2} = .1600$, and $F_{ECO_2} = .0450$.

Calculate $\dot{V}O_2$.

$$\dot{V}O_2 = V_I \cdot F_{IO_2} - \dot{V}_E \cdot F_{EO_2}\text{, and}$$

$$\dot{V}_E = \frac{\dot{V}_I \cdot F_{IN_2}}{F_{EN_2}}.$$

$$\dot{V}O_2 = \dot{V}_I \cdot F_{IO_2} - \frac{\dot{V}_I \cdot F_{IN_2}}{F_{EN_2}} \cdot F_{EO_2}$$

$$= \dot{V}_I \left[F_{IO_2} - \frac{F_{IN_2}}{F_{EN_2}} \cdot F_{EO_2} \right].$$

$$F_{EN_2} = 1{,}0000 - .1600 - .0450 = .7950.$$

$$\dot{V}O_2 = 100\text{ L} \cdot \text{min}^{-1} \left[.2093 - \frac{.7904}{.7950} \cdot .1600 \right]$$

$$= 5.02\text{ L} \cdot \text{min}^{-1}.$$

The volume (let's assume that $\dot{V}_E$ was measured) used in the above equations was measured at room temperature (23 °C) and at the barometric pressure of that moment (740 mmHg). The environmental conditions under which the volume was measured are called *ambient conditions*. If this volume of gas were transported to 10,000 ft (3,050 m) above sea level, where the barometric pressure is lower, the volume would increase because of the reduced pressure. The volume of a gas varies inversely with pressure (at a constant temperature). Another factor influencing the volume of a gas is the temperature. If that volume, measured at 23 °C, were placed in a refrigerator at 0 °C, the volume of gas would decrease. The volume of gas varies directly with the temperature (at constant pressure).

Since the volume ($\dot{V}_E$) is influenced by both pressure and temperature, the value measured as O_2 used ($\dot{V}O_2$) might reflect changes in pressure or temperature rather than a change in workload, training, and so on. Consequently, it would be convenient to express $\dot{V}_E$ in such a way as to make measurements comparable when they are obtained under different environmental conditions. This is done by standardizing the temperature, barometric pressure, and water vapor pressure at which the volume is expressed. By convention, volumes are expressed at Standard Temperature and Pressure, Dry (STPD): 273 K (equals 0 °C), 760 mmHg pressure (sea level), and with no water vapor pressure. When $\dot{V}O_2$ is expressed at STPD, you can calculate the number of molecules of oxygen actually used by the body because *at STPD 1 mol of oxygen equals 22.4 L*.

Let's make the correction to STPD one step at a time. Let's assume that a volume ($\dot{V}_E$) was measured at 740 mmHg and 23 °C and equaled 100 L · min^{-1}. This *expired* volume is *always* saturated with water vapor.

To correct for temperature you use 273 K as the standard (0 °C).

$$\text{Volume} \cdot \frac{273 \text{ K}}{273 \text{ K} + {}^\circ\text{C}} = \frac{273 \text{ K}}{273 + 23}.$$

$$100 \text{ L} \cdot \text{min}^{-1} \cdot \frac{273 \text{ K}}{296 \text{ K}} = 92.23 \text{ L} \cdot \text{min}^{-1}.$$

When we correct for pressure we must remove the effect of water vapor pressure because the gas volume is adjusted on the basis of the standard pressure (760 mmHg), which is a dry pressure.

To correct the volume to the standard 760 mmHg pressure (dry), use

$$\text{Volume} \cdot \frac{\text{barometric pressure} - \text{water vapor pressure}}{760 \text{ mmHg (dry)}}.$$

Water vapor pressure is dependent on two things: the temperature and the relative humidity. In expired gas the gas volume is saturated (100% relative humidity). Consequently, you can obtain a value for water vapor pressure directly from the table below.

Going back to our pressure correction,

$$92.23 \text{ L} \cdot \text{min}^{-1} \cdot \frac{740 - 21.1}{\text{k}760} = 87.24 \text{ L} \cdot \text{min}^{-1}(\text{STPD}).$$

To combine the temperature and pressure correction,

$$100 \text{ L} \cdot \text{min}^{-1} \cdot \frac{273 \text{ K}}{273 \text{ K} + 23} \cdot \frac{740 - 21.1}{760} = 87.24 \text{ L} \cdot \text{min}^{-1}(\text{STPD}).$$

Temperature (°C)	Saturation water vapor pressure (mmHg)
18	15.5
19	16.5
20	17.5
21	18.7
22	19.8
23	21.1
24	22.4
25	23.8
26	25.2
27	26.7

A special note must be made here. If you are using an inspired (inhaled) volume ($\dot{V}_I$), you are rarely dealing with a gas saturated with water vapor. Consequently, when you correct for pressure you must find how much water vapor is in the inspired air. You do this by finding the relative humidity of the air. You then multiply this value by the water vapor pressure valve for saturated air at whatever the temperature is. To clarify, if your volume in the above example was $\dot{V}_I$ and had a relative humidity of 50%, the pressure correction woud have been

$$\text{volume} \cdot \frac{740 - (.50 \cdot 21.1 \text{ mmHg})}{760 \text{ mmHg}}.$$

While this may seem like a minor point, it is critical to the accurate measurement of $\dot{V}O_2$ that the proper water vapor correction be used. When you calculate $\dot{V}O_2$ you usually find the STPD factor first since you will be multiplying this factor by each volume measured.

Problem: Given $\dot{V}_I$ = 100 L · min^{-1}, FEO_2 = .1700, and $FECO_2$ = .0385. The temperature = 20 °C, barometric pressure = 740 mmHg, and the relative humidity = 30%.

Answer:

$$\text{STPD factor} = \frac{740 \text{ mmHg} - (.30)\ 17.5 \text{ mmHg}}{760} \cdot \frac{273 \text{ K}}{273 \text{ K} + 20\ {}^\circ\text{C}} = .900.$$

$$100 \text{ L} \cdot \text{min}^{-1} \cdot .900 = 90 \text{ L} \cdot \text{min}^{-1} \text{ STPD}.$$

$$\dot{V}O_2 = \dot{V}_{I_{STPD}} \left[F_{IO_2} - \frac{F_{IN_2}}{F_{EN_2}} \cdot F_{EO_2} \right].$$

$$\dot{V}O_2 = 90 \text{ L} \cdot \text{min}^{-1} \left[.2093 - \frac{.7904}{.7915} \cdot .1700 \right]$$

$$\dot{V}O_2 = 3.56 \text{ L} \cdot \text{min}^{-1}.$$

Carbon Dioxide Production ($\dot{V}CO_2$)

When O_2 is used, CO_2 is produced. The ratio of CO_2 production ($\dot{V}CO_2$) to O_2 consumption ($\dot{V}O_2$) is an important measurement in metabolism. This ratio ($\dot{V}CO_2 \div \dot{V}O_2$) is called the *respiratory exchange ratio* and is abbreviated as *R*.

How do we measure $\dot{V}CO_2$max? We start at the same step as for $\dot{V}O_2$:

$$\dot{V}CO_2 = \text{liters of } CO_2 \text{ expired} - \text{liters of } CO_2 \text{ inspired}$$
$$= \dot{V}_E \cdot F_{ECO_2} - \dot{V}_I \cdot F_{ICO_2}.$$

The steps to follow are the same as those for measuring $\dot{V}O_2$. Always use an STPD volume in your calculations. The following is the equation to use when $\dot{V}_I$ is measured:

$$\dot{V}CO_2 = \dot{V}_{I_{STPD}} \left[\frac{F_{IN_2}}{F_{EN_2}} \cdot F_{ECO_2} - \dot{V}_I \cdot F_{ICO_2} \right].$$

The following steps summarize the calculations for $\dot{V}CO_2$ and R for the previous problem.

$$\dot{V}CO_2 = 90 \cdot \text{L} \cdot \text{min}^{-1} \left[\frac{.7904}{.7915} \cdot .0385 - .0003 \right]$$
$$= 3.43 \text{ L} \cdot \text{min}^{-1}.$$

$$R = \dot{V}CO_2 + \dot{V}O_2 = 3.43 \text{ L} \cdot \text{min}^{-1} + 3.56 \text{ L} \cdot \text{min}^{-1}$$

$$R = 96.$$

Appendix C

Energy Costs of Various Physical Activities

METS	Specific activity	Examples
8.5	bicycling,	bicycling, BMX or mountain
4.0	bicycling,	bicycling, <10 mph, leisure, to work or for pleasure (Taylor Code 115)
8.0	bicycling,	bicycling, general
6.0	bicycling,	bicycling, 10-11.9 mph, leisure, slow, light effort
8.0	bicycling,	bicycling, 12-13.9 mph, leisure, moderate effort
10.0	bicycling,	bicycling, 14-15.9 mph, racing or leisure, fast, vigorous effort
12.0	bicycling,	bicycling, 16-19 mph, racing/not drafting or > 19 mph drafting, very fast, racing general
16.0	bicycling,	bicycling, >20 mph, racing, not drafting
5.0	bicycling,	unicycling
7.0	conditioning exercise,	bicycling, stationary, general
3.0	conditioning exercise,	bicycling, stationary, 50 watts, very light effort
5.5	conditioning exercise,	bicycling, stationary, 100 watts, light effort
7.0	conditioning exercise,	bicycling, stationary, 150 watts, moderate effort
10.5	conditioning exercise,	bicycling, stationary, 200 watts, vigorous effort
12.5	conditioning exercise,	bicycling, stationary, 250 watts, very vigorous effort
8.0	conditioning exercise,	calisthenics (e.g. pushups, sit ups, pull ups, jumping jacks), heavy, vigorous effort
3.5	conditioning exercise,	calisthenics, home exercise, light or moderate effort, general (example: back exercises), going up & down from floor (Taylor Code 150)
8.0	conditioning exercise,	circuit training, including some aerobic movement with minimal rest, general
6.0	conditioning exercise,	weight lifting (free weight, Nautilus or universal-type), power lifting or body building, vigorous effort (Taylor Code 210)
5.5	conditioning exercise,	health club exercise, general (Taylor Code 160)
9.0	conditioning exercise,	stair-treadmill ergometer, general
7.0	conditioning exercise,	rowing, stationary ergometer, general
3.5	conditioning exercise,	rowing, stationary, 50 watts, light effort
7.0	conditioning exercise,	rowing, stationary, 100 watts, moderate effort

(continued)

METS	Specific activity	Examples
8.5	conditioning exercise,	rowing, stationary, 150 watts, vigorous effort
12.0	conditioning exercise,	rowing, stationary, 200 watts, very vigorous effort
7.0	conditioning exercise,	ski machine, general
6.0	conditioning exercise,	Slimnastics, Jazzercise
2.5	conditioning exercise,	stretching, Hatha yoga
2.5	conditioning exercise,	mild stretching
6.0	conditioning exercise,	teaching aerobic exercise class
4.0	conditioning exercise,	water aerobics, water calisthenics
3.0	conditioning exercise,	weight lifting (free, Nautilus or universal-type), light or moderate effort, light workout, general
1.0	conditioning exercise,	whirlpool, sitting
4.8	dancing,	ballet or modern, twist, jazz, tap, jitterbug
6.5	dancing,	aerobic, general
8.5	dancing,	aerobic, step, with 6-8 inch step
10.0	dancing,	aerobic, step, with 10-12 inch step
5.0	dancing,	aerobic, low impact
7.0	dancing,	aerobic, high impact
4.5	dancing,	general, Greek, Middle Eastern, hula, flamenco, belly, swing
5.5	dancing,	ballroom, fast (Taylor Code 125)
4.5	dancing,	ballroom, fast (disco, folk, square), line dancing, Irish step dancing, polka, contra, country
3.0	dancing,	ballroom, slow (e.g. waltz, foxtrot, slow dancing), samba, tango, 19th C, mambo, chacha
5.5	dancing,	Anishinaabe Jingle Dancing or other traditional American Indian dancing
3.0	fishing and hunting,	fishing, general
4.0	fishing and hunting,	digging worms, with shovel
4.0	fishing and hunting,	fishing from river bank and walking
2.5	fishing and hunting,	fishing from boat, sitting
3.5	fishing and hunting,	fishing from river bank, standing (Taylor Code 660)
6.0	fishing and hunting,	fishing in stream, in waders (Taylor Code 670)
2.0	fishing and hunting,	fishing, ice, sitting
2.5	fishing and hunting,	hunting, bow and arrow or crossbow
6.0	fishing and hunting,	hunting, deer, elk, large game (Taylor Code 170)
2.5	fishing and hunting,	hunting, duck, wading
5.0	fishing and hunting,	hunting, general
6.0	fishing and hunting,	hunting, pheasants or grouse (Taylor Code 680)
5.0	fishing and hunting,	hunting, rabbit, squirrel, prairie chick, raccoon, small game (Taylor Code 690)
2.5	fishing and hunting,	pistol shooting or trap shooting, standing
3.3	home activities,	carpet sweeping, sweeping floors
3.0	home activities,	cleaning, heavy or major (e.g. wash car, wash windows, clean garage), vigorous effort
3.5	home activities,	mopping
2.5	home activities,	multiple household tasks all at once, light effort
3.5	home activities,	multiple household tasks all at once, moderate effort
4.0	home activities,	multiple household tasks all at once, vigorous effort
3.0	home activities,	cleaning, house or cabin, general
2.5	home activities,	cleaning, light (dusting, straightening up, changing linen, carrying out trash)
2.3	home activities,	wash dishes–standing or in general (not broken into stand/walk components)
2.5	home activities,	wash dishes; clearing dishes from table–walking
3.5	home activities,	vacuuming
6.0	home activities,	butchering animals
2.0	home activities,	cooking or food preparation–standing or sitting or in general (not broken into stand/walk components), manual appliances

METS	Specific activity	Examples
2.5	home activities,	serving food, setting table–implied walking or standing
2.5	home activities,	cooking or food preparation–walking
2.5	home activities,	feeding animals
2.5	home activities,	putting away groceries (e.g. carrying groceries, shopping without a grocery cart), carrying packages
7.5	home activities,	carrying groceries upstairs
3.0	home activities,	cooking Indian bread on an outside stove
2.3	home activities,	food shopping with or without a grocery cart, standing or walking
2.3	home activities,	non-food shopping, standing or walking
2.3	home activities,	ironing
1.5	home activities,	sitting–knitting, sewing, light wrapping (presents)
2.0	home activities,	implied standing–laundry, fold or hang clothes, put clothes in
2.3	home activities,	implied walking–putting away clothes, gathering clothes to pack, putting away laundry
2.0	home activities,	making bed
5.0	home activities,	maple syruping/sugar bushing (including carrying buckets, carrying wood)
6.0	home activities,	moving furniture, household items, carrying boxes
3.8	home activities,	scrubbing floors, on hands and knees, scrubbing bathroom, bathtub
4.0	home activities,	sweeping garage, sidewalk or outside of house
3.5	home activities,	standing–packing/unpacking boxes, occasional lifting of household items light–moderate effort
3.0	home activities,	implied walking–putting away household items–moderate effort
2.5	home activities,	watering plants
2.5	home activities,	building a fire inside
9.0	home activities,	moving household items upstairs, carrying boxes or furniture
2.0	home activities,	standing–light (pump gas, change light bulb, etc.)
3.0	home activities,	walking–light, non-cleaning (readying to leave, shut/lock doors, close windows, etc.)
2.5	home activities,	sitting–playing with child(ren)–light, only active periods
2.8	home activities,	standing–playing with child(ren)–light, only active periods
4.0	home activities,	walk/run–playing with child(ren)–moderate, only active periods
5.0	home activities,	walk/run–playing with child(ren)–vigorous, only active periods
3.0	home activities,	carrying small children
2.5	home activities,	child care: sitting/kneeling–dressing, bathing, grooming, feeding, occasional lifting of child–light effort, general
3.0	home activities,	child care: standing–dressing, bathing, grooming, feeding, occasional lifting of child–light effort
4.0	home activities,	elder care, disabled adult, only active periods
1.5	home activities,	reclining with baby
2.5	home activities,	sit, playing with animals, light, only active periods
2.8	home activities,	stand, playing with animals, light, only active periods
2.8	home activities,	walk/run, playing with animals, light, only active periods
4.0	home activities,	walk/run, playing with animals, moderate, only active periods
5.0	home activities,	walk/run, playing with animals, vigorous, only active periods
3.5	home activities,	standing–bathing dog
3.0	home repair,	airplane repair
4.0	home repair,	automobile body work
3.0	home repair,	automobile repair
3.0	home repair,	carpentry, general, workshop (Taylor Code 620)
6.0	home repair,	carpentry, outside house, installing rain gutters, building a fence, (Taylor Code 640)
4.5	home repair,	carpentry, finishing or refinishing cabinets or furniture
7.5	home repair,	carpentry, sawing hardwood
5.0	home repair,	caulking, chinking log cabin

(continued)

METS	Specific activity	Examples
4.5	home repair,	caulking, except log cabin
5.0	home repair,	cleaning gutters
5.0	home repair,	excavating garage
5.0	home repair,	hanging storm windows
4.5	home repair,	laying or removing carpet
4.5	home repair,	laying tile or linoleum, repairing appliances
5.0	home repair,	painting, outside home (Taylor Code 650)
3.0	home repair,	painting, papering, plastering, scraping, inside house, hanging sheet rock, remodeling
4.5	home repair,	painting, (Taylor Code 630)
3.0	home repair,	put on and removal of tarp–sailboat
6.0	home repair,	roofing
4.5	home repair,	sanding floors with a power sander
4.5	home repair,	scraping and painting sailboat or powerboat
5.0	home repair,	spreading dirt with a shovel
4.5	home repair,	washing and waxing hull of sailboat, car, powerboat, airplane
4.5	home repair,	washing fence, painting fence
3.0	home repair,	wiring, plumbing
1.0	inactivity,	lying quietly and watching television
1.0	quiet inactivity,	lying quietly, doing nothing, lying in bed awake, listening to music (not talking or reading)
1.0	quiet inactivity,	sitting quietly and watching television
1.0	quiet inactivity,	sitting quietly, sitting smoking, listening to music (not talking or reading), watching a movie in a theater
0.9	quiet inactivity,	sleeping
1.2	quiet inactivity,	standing quietly (standing in a line)
1.0	quiet inactivity,	reclining–writing
1.0	light inactivity,	reclining–talking or talking on phone
1.0	light inactivity,	reclining–reading
1.0	light inactivity,	meditating
5.0	light lawn and garden,	carrying, loading or stacking wood, loading/unloading or carrying lumber
6.0	lawn and garden,	chopping wood, splitting logs
5.0	lawn and garden,	clearing land, hauling branches, wheelbarrow chores
5.0	lawn and garden,	digging sandbox
5.0	lawn and garden,	digging, spading, filling garden, composting, (Taylor Code 590)
6.0	lawn and garden,	gardening with heavy power tools, tilling a garden, chain saw
5.0	lawn and garden,	laying crushed rock
5.0	lawn and garden,	laying sod
5.5	lawn and garden,	mowing lawn, general
2.5	lawn and garden,	mowing lawn, riding mower (Taylor Code 550)
6.0	lawn and garden,	mowing lawn, walk, hand mower (Taylor Code 570)
5.5	lawn and garden,	mowing lawn, walk, power mower
4.5	lawn and garden,	mowing lawn, power mower (Taylor Code 590)
4.5	lawn and garden,	operating snow blower, walking
4.5	lawn and garden,	planting seedlings, shrubs
4.5	lawn and garden,	planting trees
4.3	lawn and garden,	raking lawn
4.0	lawn and garden,	raking lawn (Taylor Code 600)
4.0	lawn and garden,	raking roof with snow rake
3.0	lawn and garden,	riding snow blower
4.0	lawn and garden,	sacking grass, leaves

METS	Specific activity	Examples
6.0	lawn and garden,	shoveling snow, by hand (Taylor Code 610)
4.5	lawn and garden,	trimming shrubs or trees, manual cutter
3.5	lawn and garden,	trimming shrubs or trees, power cutter, using leaf blower, edger
2.5	lawn and garden,	walking, applying fertilizer or seeding a lawn
1.5	lawn and garden,	watering lawn or garden, standing or walking
4.5	lawn and garden,	weeding, cultivating garden (Taylor Code 580)
4.0	lawn and garden,	gardening, general
3.0	lawn and garden,	picking fruit off trees, picking fruits/vegetables, moderate effort
3.0	lawn and garden,	implied walking/standing–picking up yard, light, picking flowers or vegetables
3.0	lawn and garden,	walking, gathering gardening tools
1.5	miscellaneous,	sitting–card playing, playing board games
2.3	miscellaneous,	standing–drawing (writing), casino gambling, duplicating machine
1.3	miscellaneous,	sitting–reading, book, newspaper, etc.
1.8	miscellaneous,	sitting–writing, desk work, typing
1.8	miscellaneous,	standing–talking or talking on the phone
1.5	miscellaneous,	sitting–talking or talking on the phone
1.8	miscellaneous,	sitting–studying, general, including reading or writing
1.8	miscellaneous,	sitting–in class, general, including note-taking or class discussion
1.8	miscellaneous,	standing–reading
2.0	miscellaneous,	standing–miscellaneous
1.5	miscellaneous,	sitting–arts and crafts, light effort
2.0	miscellaneous,	sitting–arts and crafts, moderate effort
1.8	miscellaneous,	standing–arts and crafts, light effort
3.0	miscellaneous,	standing–arts and crafts, moderate effort
3.5	miscellaneous,	standing–arts and crafts, vigorous effort
1.5	miscellaneous,	retreat/family reunion activities involving sitting, relaxing, talking, eating
2.0	miscellaneous,	touring/traveling/vacation involving walking and riding
2.5	miscellaneous,	camping involving standing, walking, sitting, light-to-moderate effort
1.5	miscellaneous,	sitting at a sporting event, spectator
1.8	music playing,	accordion
2.0	music playing,	cello
2.5	music playing,	conducting
4.0	music playing,	drums
2.0	music playing,	flute (sitting)
2.0	music playing,	horn
2.5	music playing,	piano or organ
3.5	music playing,	trombone
2.5	music playing,	trumpet
2.5	music playing,	violin
2.0	music playing,	woodwind
2.0	music playing,	guitar, classical, folk (sitting)
3.0	music playing,	guitar, rock and roll band (standing)
4.0	music playing,	marching band, playing an instrument, baton twirling (walking)
3.5	music playing,	marching band, drum major (walking)
4.0	occupation,	bakery, general, moderate effort
2.5	occupation,	bakery, light effort
2.3	occupation,	bookbinding
6.0	occupation,	building road (including hauling debris, driving heavy machinery)
2.0	occupation,	building road, directing traffic (standing)

(continued)

METS	Specific activity	Examples
3.5	occupation,	carpentry, general
8.0	occupation,	carrying heavy loads, such as bricks
8.0	occupation,	carrying moderate loads up stairs, moving boxes (16-40 lbs)
2.5	occupation,	chambermaid, making bed (nursing)
6.5	occupation,	coal mining, drilling coal, rock
6.5	occupation,	coal mining, erecting supports
6.0	occupation,	coal mining, general
7.0	occupation,	coal mining, shoveling coal
5.5	occupation,	construction, outside, remodeling
3.0	occupation,	custodial work–buffing the floor with electric buffer
2.5	occupation,	custodial work–cleaning sink and toilet, light effort
2.5	occupation,	custodial work–dusting, light effort
4.0	occupation,	custodial work–feathering arena floor, moderate effort
3.5	occupation,	custodial work–general cleaning, moderate effort
3.5	occupation,	custodial work–mopping, moderate effort
3.0	occupation,	custodial work–take out trash, moderate effort
2.5	occupation,	custodial work–vacuuming, light effort
3.0	occupation,	custodial work–vacuuming, moderate effort
3.5	occupation,	electrical work, plumbing
8.0	occupation,	farming, baling hay, cleaning barn, poultry work, vigorous effort
3.5	occupation,	farming, chasing cattle, non-strenuous (walking), moderate effort
4.0	occupation,	farming, chasing cattle or other livestock on horseback, moderate effort
2.0	occupation,	farming, chasing cattle or other livestock, driving, light effort
2.5	occupation,	farming, driving harvester, cutting hay, irrigation work
2.5	occupation,	farming, driving tractor
4.0	occupation,	farming, feeding small animals
4.5	occupation,	farming, feeding cattle, horses
4.5	occupation,	farming, hauling water for animals, general hauling water
6.0	occupation,	farming, taking care of animals (grooming, brushing, shearing sheep, assisting with birthing, medical care, branding)
8.0	occupation,	farming, forking straw bales, cleaning corral or barn, vigorous effort
3.0	occupation,	farming, milking by hand, moderate effort
1.5	occupation,	farming, milking by machine, light effort
5.5	occupation,	farming, shoveling grain, moderate effort
12.0	occupation,	fire fighter, general
11.0	occupation,	fire fighter, climbing ladder with full gear
8.0	occupation,	fire fighter, hauling hoses on ground
17.0	occupation,	forestry, ax chopping, fast
5.0	occupation,	forestry, ax chopping, slow
7.0	occupation,	forestry, barking trees
11.0	occupation,	forestry, carrying logs
8.0	occupation,	forestry, felling trees
8.0	occupation,	forestry, general
5.0	occupation,	forestry, hoeing
6.0	occupation,	forestry, planting by hand
7.0	occupation,	forestry, sawing by hand
4.5	occupation,	forestry, sawing, power
9.0	occupation,	forestry, trimming trees
4.0	occupation,	forestry, weeding

METS	Specific activity	Examples
4.5	occupation,	furriery
6.0	occupation,	horse grooming
8.0	occupation,	horse racing, galloping
6.5	occupation,	horse racing, trotting
2.6	occupation,	horse racing, walking
3.5	occupation,	locksmith
2.5	occupation,	machine tooling, machining, working sheet metal
3.0	occupation,	machine tooling, operating lathe
5.0	occupation,	machine tooling, operating punch press
4.0	occupation,	machine tooling, tapping and drilling
3.0	occupation,	machine tooling, welding
7.0	occupation,	masonry, concrete
4.0	occupation,	masseur, masseuse (standing)
7.5	occupation,	moving, pushing heavy objects, 75 lbs or more (desks, moving van work)
12.0	occupation,	skindiving or SCUBA diving as a frogman (Navy Seal)
2.5	occupation,	operating heavy duty equipment/automated, not driving
4.5	occupation,	orange grove work
2.3	occupation,	printing (standing)
2.5	occupation,	police, directing traffic (standing)
2.0	occupation,	police, driving a squad car (sitting)
1.3	occupation,	police, riding in a squad car (sitting)
4.0	occupation,	police, making an arrest (standing)
2.5	occupation,	shoe repair, general
8.5	occupation,	shoveling, digging ditches
9.0	occupation,	shoveling, heavy (more than 16 lbs/min)
6.0	occupation,	shoveling, light (less than 10 lbs/min)
7.0	occupation,	shoveling, moderate (10 to 15 lbs/min)
1.5	occupation,	sitting–light office work, general (chemistry lab work, light use of hand tools, watch repair or micro-assembly, light assembly/repair), sitting, reading, driving at work
1.5	occupation,	sitting–meetings, general, or with talking involved, eating at a business meeting
2.5	occupation,	sitting; moderate (heavy levers, riding mower/forklift, crane operation), teaching stretching or yoga
2.3	occupation,	standing; light (bartending, store clerk, assembling, filing, duplicating, putting up a Christmas tree), standing and talking at work, changing clothes when teaching physical education
3.0	occupation,	standing; light/moderate (assemble/repair heavy parts, welding, stocking, auto repair, pack boxes for moving, etc.), patient care (as in nursing)
4.0	occupation,	lifting items continuously, 10-20 lbs, with limited walking or resting
3.5	occupation,	standing; moderate (assembling at fast rate, intermittent, lifting 50 lbs, hitch/twisting ropes)
4.0	occupation,	standing; moderate/heavy (lifting more than 50 lbs, masonry, painting, paper hanging)
5.0	occupation,	steel mill, fettling
5.5	occupation,	steel mill, forging
8.0	occupation,	steel mill, hand rolling
8.0	occupation,	steel mill, merchant mill rolling
11.0	occupation,	steel mill, removing slag
7.5	occupation,	steel mill, tending furnace
5.5	occupation,	steel mill, tipping molds
8.0	occupation,	steel mill, working in general
2.5	occupation,	tailoring, cutting
2.5	occupation,	tailoring, general
2.0	occupation,	tailoring, hand sewing

(continued)

METS	Specific activity	Examples
2.5	occupation,	tailoring, machine sewing
4.0	occupation,	tailoring, pressing
3.5	occupation,	tailoring, weaving
6.5	occupation,	truck driving, loading and unloading truck (standing)
1.5	occupation,	typing, electric, manual or computer
6.0	occupation,	using heavy power tools such as pneumatic tools (jackhammers, drills, etc.)
8.0	occupation,	using heavy tools (not power) such as shovel, pick, tunnel bar, spade
2.0	occupation,	walking on job, less than 2.0 mph (in office or lab area), very slow
3.3	occupation,	walking on job, 3.0 mph, in office, moderate speed, not carrying anything
3.8	occupation,	walking on job, 3.5 mph, in office, brisk speed, not carrying anything
3.0	occupation,	walking, 2.5 mph, slowly and carrying light objects less than 25 lbs
3.0	occupation,	walking, gathering things at work, ready to leave
4.0	occupation,	walking, 3.0 mph, moderately and carrying light objects less than 25 lbs
4.0	occupation,	walking, pushing a wheelchair
4.5	occupation,	walking, 3.5 mph, briskly and carrying objects less than 25 lbs
5.0	occupation,	walking or walk downstairs or standing, carrying objects about 25 to 49 lbs
6.5	occupation,	walking or walk downstairs or standing, carrying objects about 50 to 74 lbs
7.5	occupation,	walking or walk downstairs or standing, carrying objects about 75 to 99 lbs
8.5	occupation,	walking or walk downstairs or standing, carrying objects about 100 lbs or more
3.0	occupation,	working in scene shop, theater actor, backstage employee
4.0	occupation,	teach physical education, exercise, sports classes (non-sport play)
6.5	occupation,	teach physical education, exercise, sports classes (participate in the class)
6.0	running,	jog/walk combination (jogging component of less than 10 min) (Taylor Code 180)
7.0	running,	jogging, general
8.0	running,	jogging, in place
4.5	running,	jogging on a mini-tramp
8.0	running,	running, 5 mph (12 min/mile)
9.0	running,	running, 5.2 mph (11.5 min/mile)
10.0	running,	running, 6 mph (10 min/mile)
11.0	running,	running, 6.7 mph (9 min/mile)
11.5	running,	running, 7 mph (8.5 min/mile)
12.5	running,	running, 7.5 mph (8 min/mile)
13.5	running,	running, 8 mph (7.5 min/mile)
14.0	running,	running, 8.6 mph (7 min/mile)
15.0	running,	running, 9 mph (6.5 min/mile)
16.0	running,	running, 10 mph (6 min/mile)
18.0	running,	running, 10.9 mph (5.5 min/mile)
9.0	running,	running, cross country
8.0	running,	running (Taylor Code 200)
15.0	running,	running, stairs, up
10.0	running,	running, on a track, team practice
8.0	running,	running, training, pushing a wheelchair
2.0	self care,	standing–getting ready for bed, in general
1.0	self care,	sitting on toilet
1.5	self care,	bathing (sitting)
2.0	self care,	dressing, undressing (standing or sitting)
1.5	self care,	eating (sitting)
2.0	self care,	talking and eating or eating only (standing)
1.0	self care,	taking medication, sitting or standing

METS	Specific activity	Examples
2.0	self care,	grooming (washing, shaving, brushing teeth, urinating, washing hands, putting on make-up), sitting or standing
2.5	self care,	hairstyling
1.0	self care,	having hair or nails done by someone else, sitting
2.0	self care,	showering, toweling off (standing)
1.5	sexual activity,	active, vigorous effort
1.3	sexual activity,	general, moderate effort
1.0	sexual activity,	passive, light effort, kissing, hugging
3.5	sports,	archery (non-hunting)
7.0	sports,	badminton, competitive (Taylor Code 450)
4.5	sports,	badminton, social singles and doubles, general
8.0	sports,	basketball, game (Taylor Code 490)
6.0	sports,	basketball, non-game, general (Taylor Code 480)
7.0	sports,	basketball, officiating (Taylor Code 500)
4.5	sports,	basketball, shooting baskets
6.5	sports,	basketball, wheelchair
2.5	sports,	billiards
3.0	sports,	bowling (Taylor Code 390)
12.0	sports,	boxing, in ring, general
6.0	sports,	boxing, punching bag
9.0	sports,	boxing, sparring
7.0	sports,	broomball
5.0	sports,	children's games (hopscotch, 4-square, dodge ball, playground apparatus, t-ball, tetherball, marbles, jacks, race games)
4.0	sports,	coaching: football, soccer, basketball, baseball, swimming, etc.
5.0	sports,	cricket (batting, bowling)
2.5	sports,	croquet
4.0	sports,	curling
2.5	sports,	darts, wall or lawn
6.0	sports,	drag racing, pushing or driving a car
6.0	sports,	fencing
9.0	sports,	football, competitive
8.0	sports,	football, touch, flag, general (Taylor Code 510)
2.5	sports,	football or baseball, playing catch
3.0	sports,	Frisbee playing, general
8.0	sports,	Frisbee, ultimate
4.5	sports,	golf, general
4.5	sports,	golf, walking and carrying clubs
3.0	sports,	golf, miniature, driving range
4.3	sports,	golf, walking and pulling clubs
3.5	sports,	golf, using power cart (Taylor Code 070)
4.0	sports,	gymnastics, general
4.0	sports,	hacky sack
12.0	sports,	handball, general (Taylor Code 520)
8.0	sports,	handball, team
3.5	sports,	hang gliding
8.0	sports,	hockey, field
8.0	sports,	hockey, ice
4.0	sports,	horseback riding, general

(continued)

METS	Specific activity	Examples
3.5	sports,	horseback riding, saddling horse, grooming horse
6.5	sports,	horseback riding, trotting
2.5	sports,	horseback riding, walking
3.0	sports,	horseshoe pitching, quoits
12.0	sports,	jai alai
10.0	sports,	judo, jujitsu, karate, kick boxing, tae kwan do
4.0	sports,	juggling
7.0	sports,	kickball
8.0	sports,	lacrosse
4.0	sports,	motor-cross
9.0	sports,	orienteering
10.0	sports,	paddleball, competitive
6.0	sports,	paddleball, casual, general (Taylor Code 460)
8.0	sports,	polo
10.0	sports,	racquetball, competitive
7.0	sports,	racquetball, casual, general (Taylor Code 470)
11.0	sports,	rock climbing, ascending rock
8.0	sports,	rock climbing, rappelling
12.0	sports,	rope jumping, fast
10.0	sports,	rope jumping, moderate, general
8.0	sports,	rope jumping, slow
10.0	sports,	rugby
3.0	sports,	shuffleboard, lawn bowling
5.0	sports,	skateboarding
7.0	sports,	skating, roller (Taylor Code 360)
12.5	sports,	roller blading (in-line skating)
3.5	sports,	sky diving
10.0	sports,	soccer, competitive
7.0	sports,	soccer, casual, general (Taylor Code 540)
5.0	sports,	softball or baseball, fast or slow pitch, general (Taylor Code 440)
4.0	sports,	softball, officiating
6.0	sports,	softball, pitching
12.0	sports,	squash (Taylor Code 530)
4.0	sports,	table tennis, ping pong (Taylor Code 410)
4.0	sports,	tai chi
7.0	sports,	tennis, general
6.0	sports,	tennis, doubles (Taylor Code 430)
5.0	sports,	tennis, doubles
8.0	sports,	tennis, singles (Taylor Code 420)
3.5	sports,	trampoline
4.0	sports,	volleyball (Taylor Code 400)
8.0	sports,	volleyball, competitive, in gymnasium
3.0	sports,	volleyball, non-competitive, 6-9 member team, general
8.0	sports,	volleyball, beach
6.0	sports,	wrestling (one match = 5 min)
7.0	sports,	wallyball, general
4.0	sports,	track and field (shot, discus, hammer throw)
6.0	sports,	track and field (high jump, long jump, triple jump, javelin, pole vault)
10.0	sports,	track and field (steeplechase, hurdles)

METS	Specific activity	Examples
2.0	transportation,	automobile or light truck (not a semi) driving
1.0	transportation,	riding in a car or truck
1.0	transportation,	riding in a bus
2.0	transportation,	flying airplane
2.5	transportation,	motor scooter, motorcycle
6.0	transportation,	pushing plane in and out of hangar
3.0	transportation,	driving heavy truck, tractor, bus
7.0	walking,	backpacking (Taylor Code 050)
3.5	walking,	carrying infant or 15 lb load (e.g., suitcase), level ground or downstairs
9.0	walking,	carrying load upstairs, general
5.0	walking,	carrying 1 to 15 lb load, upstairs
6.0	walking,	carrying 16 to 24 lb load, upstairs
8.0	walking,	carrying 25 to 49 lb load, upstairs
10.0	walking,	carrying 50 to 74 lb load, upstairs
12.0	walking,	carrying 74+ lb load, upstairs
3.0	walking,	loading or unloading a car
7.0	walking,	climbing hills with 0 to 9 lb load
7.5	walking,	climbing hills with 10 to 20 lb load
8.0	walking,	climbing hills with 21 to 42 lb load
9.0	walking,	climbing hills with 42+ lb load
3.0	walking,	downstairs
6.0	walking,	hiking, cross country (Taylor Code 040)
2.5	walking,	bird watching
6.5	walking,	marching, rapidly, military
2.5	walking,	pushing or pulling stroller with child or walking with children
4.0	walking,	pushing a wheelchair, non-occupational setting
6.5	walking,	race walking
8.0	walking,	rock or mountain climbing (Taylor Code 060)
8.0	walking,	up stairs, using or climbing up ladder (Taylor Code 030)
5.0	walking,	using crutches
2.0	walking,	walking, household
2.0	walking,	walking, less than 2.0 mph, level ground, strolling, very slow
2.5	walking,	walking, 2.0 mph, level, slow pace, firm surface
3.5	walking,	walking for pleasure (Taylor Code 010)
2.5	walking,	walking from house to car or bus, from car or bus to go places, from car or bus to and from the worksite
2.5	walking,	walking to neighbor's house or family's house for social reasons
3.0	walking,	walking the dog
3.0	walking,	walking, 2.5 mph, firm surface
2.8	walking,	walking, 2.5 mph, downhill
3.3	walking,	walking, 3.0 mph, level, moderate pace, firm surface
3.8	walking,	walking, 3.5 mph, level, brisk, firm surface, walking for exercise
6.0	walking,	walking, 3.5 mph, uphill
5.0	walking,	walking, 4.0 mph, level, firm surface, very brisk pace
6.3	walking,	walking, 4.5 mph, level, firm surface, very, very brisk
8.0	walking,	walking, 5.0 mph
3.5	walking,	walking, for pleasure, work break
5.0	walking,	walking, grass track
4.0	walking,	walking, to work or class (Taylor Code 015)

(continued)

METS	Specific activity	Examples
2.5	walking,	walking to and from an outhouse
2.5	water activities,	boating, power
4.0	water activities,	canoeing, on camping trip (Taylor Code 270)
3.3	water activities,	canoeing, harvesting wild rice, knocking rice off the stalks
7.0	water activities,	canoeing, portaging
3.0	water activities,	canoeing, rowing, 2.0-3.9 mph, light effort
7.0	water activities,	canoeing, rowing, 4.0-5.9 mph, moderate effort
12.0	water activities,	canoeing, rowing, >6 mph, vigorous effort
3.5	water activities,	canoeing, rowing, for pleasure, general (Taylor Code 250)
12.0	water activities,	canoeing, rowing, in competition, or crew or sculling (Taylor Code 260)
3.0	water activities,	diving, springboard or platform
5.0	water activities,	kayaking
4.0	water activities,	paddle boat
3.0	water activities,	sailing, boat and board sailing, windsurfing, ice sailing, general (Taylor Code 235)
5.0	water activities,	sailing, in competition
3.0	water activities,	sailing, Sunfish/Laser/Hobby Cat, Keel boats, ocean sailing, yachting
6.0	water activities,	skiing, water (Taylor Code 220)
7.0	water activities,	skimobiling
16.0	water activities,	skindiving, fast
12.5	water activities,	skindiving, moderate
7.0	water activities,	skindiving, scuba diving, general (Taylor Code 310)
5.0	water activities,	snorkeling (Taylor Code 320)
3.0	water activities,	surfing, body or board
10.0	water activities,	swimming laps, freestyle, fast, vigorous effort
7.0	water activities,	swimming laps, freestyle, slow, moderate or light effort
7.0	water activities,	swimming, backstroke, general
10.0	water activities,	swimming, breaststroke, general
11.0	water activities,	swimming, butterfly, general
11.0	water activities,	swimming, crawl, fast (75 yards/min), vigorous effort
8.0	water activities,	swimming, crawl, slow (50 yards/min), moderate or light effort
6.0	water activities,	swimming, lake, ocean, river (Taylor Codes 280, 295)
6.0	water activities,	swimming, leisurely, not lap swimming, general
8.0	water activities,	swimming, sidestroke, general
8.0	water activities,	swimming, synchronized
10.0	water activities,	swimming, treading water, fast vigorous effort
4.0	water activities,	swimming, treading water, moderate effort, general
4.0	water activities,	water aerobics, water calisthenics
10.0	water activities,	water polo
3.0	water activities,	water volleyball
8.0	water activities,	water jogging
5.0	water activities,	whitewater rafting, kayaking, or canoeing
6.0	winter activities,	moving ice house (set up/drill holes, etc.)
5.5	winter activities,	skating, ice, 9 mph or less
7.0	winter activities,	skating, ice, general (Taylor Code 360)
9.0	winter activities,	skating, ice, rapidly, more than 9 mph
15.0	winter activities,	skating, speed, competitive
7.0	winter activities,	ski jumping (climb up carrying skis)
7.0	winter activities,	skiing, general
7.0	winter activities,	skiing, cross country, 2.5 mph, slow or light effort, ski walking

METS	Specific activity	Examples
8.0	winter activities,	skiing, cross country, 4.0-4.9 mph, moderate speed and effort, general
9.0	winter activities,	skiing, cross country, 5.0-7.9 mph, brisk speed, vigorous effort
14.0	winter activities,	skiing, cross country, >8.0 mph, racing
16.5	winter activities,	skiing, cross country, hard snow, uphill, maximum, snow mountaineering
5.0	winter activities,	skiing, downhill, light effort
6.0	winter activities,	skiing, downhill, moderate effort, general
8.0	winter activities,	skiing, downhill, vigorous effort, racing
7.0	winter activities,	sledding, tobogganing, bobsledding, luge (Taylor Code 370)
8.0	winter activities,	snow shoeing
3.5	winter activities,	snowmobiling
1.0	religious activities,	sitting in church, in service, attending a ceremony, sitting quietly
2.5	religious activities,	sitting, playing an instrument at church
1.5	religious activities,	sitting in church, talking or singing, attending a ceremony, sitting, active participation
1.3	religious activities,	sitting, reading religious materials at home
1.2	religious activities,	standing in church (quietly), attending a ceremony, standing quietly
2.0	religious activities,	standing, singing in church, attending a ceremony, standing, active participation
1.0	religious activities,	kneeling in church/at home (praying)
1.8	religious activities,	standing, talking in church
2.0	religious activities,	walking in church
2.0	religious activities,	walking, less than 2.0 mph–very slow
3.3	religious activities,	walking, 3.0 mph, moderate speed, not carrying anything
3.8	religious activities,	walking, 3.5 mph, brisk speed, not carrying anything
2.0	religious activities,	walk/stand combination for religious purposes, usher
5.0	religious activities,	praise with dance or run, spiritual dancing in church
2.5	religious activities,	serving food at church
2.0	religious activities,	preparing food at church
2.3	religious activities,	washing dishes/cleaning kitchen at church
1.5	religious activities,	eating at church
2.0	religious activities,	eating/talking at church or standing eating, American Indian Feast days
3.0	religious activities,	cleaning church
5.0	religious activities,	general yard work at church
2.5	religious activities,	standing–moderate (lifting 50 lbs., assembling at fast rate)
4.0	religious activities,	standing–moderate/heavy work
1.5	religious activities,	typing, electric, manual, or computer
1.5	volunteer activities,	sitting–meeting, general, or with talking involved
1.5	volunteer activities,	sitting–light office work, in general
2.5	volunteer activities,	sitting–moderate work
2.3	volunteer activities,	standing–light work (filing, talking, assembling)
2.5	volunteer activities,	sitting, child care, only active periods
3.0	volunteer activities,	standing, child care, only active periods
4.0	volunteer activities,	walk/run play with children, moderate, only active periods
5.0	volunteer activities,	walk/run play with children, vigorous, only active periods
3.0	volunteer activities,	standing–light/moderate work (pack boxes, assemble/repair, set up chairs/furniture)
3.5	volunteer activities,	standing–moderate (lifting 50 lbs., assembling at fast rate)
4.0	volunteer activities,	standing–moderate/heavy work
1.5	volunteer activities,	typing, electric, manual, or computer
2.0	volunteer activities,	walking, less than 2.0 mph, very slow
3.3	volunteer activities,	walking, 3.0 mph, moderate speed, not carrying anything
3.8	volunteer activities,	walking, 3.5 mph, brisk speed, not carrying anything

(continued)

METS	Specific activity	Examples
3.0	volunteer activities,	walking, 2.5 mph slowly and carrying objects less than 25 lbs
4.0	volunteer activities,	walking, 3.0 mph moderately and carrying objects less than 25 lbs, pushing something
4.5	volunteer activities,	walking, 3.5 mph, briskly and carrying objects less than 25 lbs
3.0	volunteer activities,	walk/stand combination, for volunteer purposes

Adapted, by permission, from B.E. Ainsworth, W.L. Haskell, M.C. Whitt, M.L. Irwin, A.M. Swartz, S.J. Strath, W.L. O'Brien, D.R. Bassett, K.H. Scmitz, Jr., P.O. Emplaincourt, D.R. Jacobs, Jr., and A.S. Leon, 2000, "Compendium of physical activities: An update of activity codes and MET intensities," *Medicine and Science in Sports and Exercise* 32(9): S498-S516. Additional values from H.J. Montoye, H.C.G. Kemper, W.H.M. Saris and R.A. Washburn, 1996, *Measuring physical activity and energy expenditure* (Champaign, IL: Human Kinetics).

Appendix D

Common Medications

Table D.1 Generic and Brand Names of Common Drugs by Class

Generic name	Brand name*
β-Blockers	
Acebutolol**	Sectral**
Atenolol	Tenormin
Betaxolol	Kerlone
Bisoprolol	Zebeta
Esmolol	Brevibloc
Metoprolol	Lopressor SR, Toprol XL
Nadolol	Corgard
Penbutolol**	Levatol**
Pindolol**	Visken**
Propranolol	Inderal
Sotalol	Betapace
Timolol	Blocadren
**β-Blockers with intrinsic sympathomimetic activity.	
β-Blockers in Combination With Diuretics	
Atenolol + chlorthalidone	Tenoretic
Bisoprolol + hydrochlorothiazide	Ziac
Propranolol LA + hydrochlorothiazide	Inderide
Metoprolol + hydrochlorothiazide	Lopressor HCT
Nadolol + bendroflumethiazide	Corzide
Timolol + hydrochlorothiazide	Timolide
α- and β-Adrenergic Blocking Agents	
Carvedilol	Coreg
Labetalol	Normodyne, Trandate
α_1-Adrenergic Blocking Agents	
Doxazosin	Cardura
Prazosin	Minipress, Minizide
Terazosin	Hytrin

(continued)

Table D.1 Generic and Brand Names of Common Drugs by Class *(continued)*

Generic name	Brand name*
Central α_2-Agonists and Other Centrally Acting Drugs	
Clonidine	Catapres, Catapres-TTS (patch)
Guanfacine	Tenex
Methyldopa	Aldomet
Reserpine	Serpasil
Central α_2-Agonists in Combination With Diuretics	
Methyldopa + hydrochlorothiazide	Aldoril
Reserpine + chlorothiazide	Diupres
Reserpine + hydrochlorothiazide	Hydropres
Nitrates and Nitroglycerin	
Amyl nitrite	Amyl nitrite
Isosorbice mononitrate	Ismo, Monoket, Imdur
Isosorbice dinitrate	Isordil, Sorbitrate, Dilatrate
Nitroglycerin, sublingual	Nitrostat, NitroQuick
Nitroglycerin, translingual	Nitrolingual
Nitroglycerin, transmucosal	Nitrogard
Nitroglycerin, sustained release	Nitrong, Nitrocine, Nitroglyn, Nitro-Bid
Nitroglycerin, transdermal	Minitran, Nitro-Dur, Transderm-Nitro, Deponit, Nitrodisc, Nitro-Derm
Nitroglycerin, topical	Nitro-Bid, Nitrol
Calcium Channel Blockers (Nondihydropyridines)	
Diltiazem Extended Release	Cardizem CD, Cardizem LA, Dilacor XR, Tiazac
Verapamil Immediate Release	Calan, Isoptin
Verapamil Long Acting	Calan SR, Isoptin SR
Verapamil-Coer	Covera HS, Verelan PM
Calcium Channel Blockers (Dihydropyridines)	
Amlodipine	Norvasc
Felodipine	Plendil
Isradipine	DynaCirc CR
Nicardipine Sustained Release	Cardene SR
Nifedipine Long-Acting	Adalat, Procardia XL
Nimodipine	Nimotop
Nisoldipine	Sular
Cardiac Glycosides	
Digoxin	Lanoxin, Lanoxicaps
Direct Peripheral Vasodilators	
Hydralazine	Apresoline
Minoxidil	Loniten

Generic name	Brand name*
Angiotensin-Converting Enzyme (ACE) Inhibitors	
Benazepril	Lotensin
Captopril	Capoten
Cilazapril	Inhibace
Enalapril	Vasotec
Fosinopril	Monopril
Lisinopril	Zestril, Prinivil
Moexipril	Univasc
Perindopril	Aceon
Quinapril	Accupril
Ramipril	Altace
Trandolapril	Mavik
ACE Inhibitors in Combination With Diuretic	
Benazepril + hydrochlorothiazide	Lotensin HCT
Captopril + hydrochlorothiazide	Capozide
Enalapril + hydrochlorothiazide	Vaseretic
Lisinopril + hydrochlorothiazide	Prinzide, Zestoretic
Moexipril + hydrochlorothiazide	Uniretic
Quinapril + hydrochlorothiazide	Accuretic
ACE Inhibitors in Combination With Calcium Channel Blockers	
Benazepril + Amlodipine	Lotrel
Enalapril + felodipine	Lexxel
Trandolapril + verapamil	Tarka
Angiotensin II Receptor Antagonists	
Candesartan	Atacand
Eprosartan	Tevetan
Irbesartan	Avapro
Losartan	Cozaar
Olmesartan	Benicar
Telmisartan	Micardis
Valsartan	Diovan
Angiotensin II Receptor Antagonists in Combination With Diuretics	
Candesartan + hydrochlorothiazide	Atacand HCT
Eprosartan + hydrochlorothiazide	Teveten HCT
Irbesartan + hydrochlorothiazide	Avalide
Losartan + hydrochlorothiazide	Hyzaar
Temisartan + hydrochlorothiazide	Micardis HCT
Valsartan + hydrochlorothiazide	Diovan HCT
Diuretics	
Thiazides	
Chlorothiazide	Diuril
Hydrochlorothiazide (HCTZ)	Microzide, HydroDiuril, Oretic
Polythiazide	Renese
Indapamide	Lozol
Metolazone	Mykron, Zaroxolyn

(continued)

Table D.1 Generic and Brand Names of Common Drugs by Class *(continued)*

Generic name	Brand name*
Diuretics *(continued)*	
"Loop" Diuretics	
Bumetanide	Bumex
Ethacrynic Acid	Edecrin
Furosemide	Lasix
Torsemide	Demadex
Potassium-Sparing Diuretics	
Amiloride	Midamor
Triamterene	Dyrenium
Aldosterone Receptor Blockers	
Eplerenone	Inspra
Spironolactone	Aldactone
Diuretic Combined With Diuretic	
Triamterene + hydrochlorothiazide	Dyazide, Maxzide
Amiloride + hydrochlorothiazide	Moduretic
Antiarrhythmic Agents	
Class I	
IA	
Disopyramide	Norpace
Moricixine	Ethmozine
Procainamide	Pronestyl, Procan SR
Quinidine	Quinora, Quinidex, Quinaglute, Quinalan, Cardioquin
Class I	
IB	
Lidocaine	Xylocaine, Xylocard
Mexiletine	Mexitil
Phenytoin	Dilantin
Tocainide	Tonocard
IC	
Flecainide	Tambocor
Propafenone	Rythmol
Class II	
β-Blockers	see page 500
Class III	
Amiodarone	Cordarone, Pacerone
Bretylium	Bretylol
Sotalol	Betapace
Dofetilide	Tikosyn
Class IV	
Calcium channel blockers	see page 500

Generic name	Brand name*
Antilipemic Agents	
Bile Acid Sequestrants	
Cholestyramine	Questran, Cholybar, Prevalite
Colesevelam	Welchol
Colestipol	Colestid
Fibric Acid Derivatives	
Clofibrate	Atromid
Gemfibrozil	Lopid
Fenofibrate	Tricor, Lofibra
HMG-CoA Reductase Inhibitors	
Atorvastatin	Lipitor
Fluvastatin	Lescol
Lovastatin	Mevacor
Pravastatin	Pravachol
Simvastatin	Zocor
Rosuvastatin	Crestor
Lovastatin + Niacin	Advicor
Nicotinic Acid	
Niacin	Niaspan, Nicobid, Slo-Niacin
Cholesterol Absorption Inhibitor	
Ezetimibe	Zeta
Ezetimibe + Simvastatin	Vytorin
Blood Modifiers (Anticoagulant or Antiplatelet)	
Clopidogrel	Plavix
Dipyridamole	Persantine
Pentoxifylline	Trental
Ticlopidine	Ticlid
Cilostazol	Pletal
Warfarin	Coumadin
Respiratory Agents	
Steroidal Antiinflammatory Agents	
Flunisolide	AeroBid
Triamcinolone	Azmacort
Beclomethasone	Beclovent, Qvar
Fluticasone	Flovent
Fluticasone and salmeterol (β_2-receptor agonist)	Advair Diskus
Budesonide	Pulmicort
Bronchodilators	
Anticholinergics (Acetylcholine Receptor Antagonist)	
Ipratropium	Atrovent
Anticholinergics With Sympathomimetics (β_2-Receptor Agonists)	
Ipratropium and Albuterol	Combivent

(continued)

• Table D.1 Generic and Brand Names of Common Drugs by Class *(continued)* •

Generic name			Brand name*	
Respiratory Agents *(continued)*				
Sympathomimetics (β_2-Receptor Agonists)				
Salmeterol			Serevent	
Metaproterenol			Alupent	
Terbutaline			Brethine	
Pirbuterol			Maxair	
Albuterol			Proventil, Ventolin	
Salmeterol and Fluticasone (steroid)			Advair	
Xanthine Derivatives				
Theophylline			Theo-Dur, Uniphyl	
Leukotriene Antagonists and Formation Inhibitors				
Zafirlukast			Accolate	
Montelukast			Singulair	
Zileuton			Zyflo	
Mast Cell Stabilizers				
Cromolyn Inhaled			Intal	
Nedocromil			Tilade	
Omalizumab			Xolair	
Antidiabetic Agents				
Biguanides (Decrease hepatic glucose production and intestinal glucose absorption)				
Metformin			Glucophage, Riomet	
Metformin and Glyburide			Glucovance	
Glucosidase Inhibitors (Inhibit intestinal glucose absorption)				
Miglitol			Glyset	
Insulins				
Rapid-acting	**Intermediate-acting**	**Intermediate- and rapid-acting combination**		**Long-acting**
Humalog	Humulin L	Humalog Mix		Humulin U
Humulin R	Humulin N	Humalog 50/50		Lantus Injection
Novolin R	Iletin II Lente	Humalog 70/30		
Iletin II R	Iletin II NPH	Novolin 70/30		
	Novolin L			
	Nivalin N			
Meglitinides (Stimulate pancreatic islet β cells)				
Nateglinide			Starlix	
Repaglinide			Prandin, Gluconorm	
Sulfonylureas (Stimulate pancreatic islet β cells)				
Glyburide			DiaBeta, Glynase, Micronase	
Gilpizide			Glucotrol	
Gliclazide			Diamicron	
Glimepiride			Amaryl	
Tolazamide			Tolinase	
Tolbutamide			Orinase	
Chlorpropamide			Diabinese	

Generic name	Brand name*
	Antidiabetic Agents *(continued)*
Thiazolidinediones (Increase insulin sensitivity)	
Pioglitazone	Actos
Rosiglitazone	Avandia
	Obesity Management
Appetite Suppressants	
Sibutramine	Meridia
Lipase Inhibitors	
Orlistat	Xenical

*Represent selected brands; these are not necessarily all inclusive.

Reprinted, by permission, from American College of Sports Medicine (ACSM), 2006, *ACSM's guidelines for exercise testing and prescription*, 7th ed. (Philadelphia, PA: Lippincott, Williams & Wilkins), 255-266.

• Table D.2 Effects of Medications on Heart Rate, Blood Pressure, the Electrocardiogram (ECG), and Exercise Capacity •

Medications	Heart rate	Blood pressure	ECG	Exercise capacity
I. β-Blockers (including carvedilol and labetalol	↓* (R and E)	↓ (R and E)	↓ HR* (R) ↓ Ischemia⁺ (E)	↑ in patients with angina; ↓ or ↔ in patients without angina
II. Nitrates	↑ (R) ↑ or ↔ (E)	↓ (R) ↓ or ↔ (E)	↑ HR (R) ↑ or ↔ HR (E) ↓ ischemia⁺ (E)	↑ in patients with angina; ↔ in patients without angina; ↑ or ↔ in patients with congestive heart failure (CHF)
III. Calcium channel blockers				
Amlodipine, Felodipine, Isradipine, Nicardipine, Nifedipine, Nimodipine, Nisoldipine	↑ or ↔ (R and E)	↓ (R and E)	↑ or ↔ HR (R and E) ↓ ischemia⁺ (E)	↑ in patients with angina; ↔ in patients without angina
Diltiazem, Verapamil	↓ (R and E)		↓ HR (R and E) ↓ ischemia⁺ (E)	
IV. Digitalis	↓ in patients with atrial fibrillation and possibly CHF Not significantly altered in patients with sinus rhythm	↔ (R and E)	May produce nonspecific ST-T wave changes (R) May produce ST segment depression (E)	Improved only in patients with atrial fibrillation or in patients with CHF
V. Diuretics	↔ (R and E)	↔ or ↓ (R and E)	↔ or PVCs (R) May cause PVCs and "false positive" test results if hypokalemia occurs May cause PVCs if hypomagnesemia occurs (E)	↔, except possibly in patients with CHF
VI. Vasodilators, nonadrenergic	↑ or ↔ (R and E)	↓ (R and E)	↑ or ↔ HR (R and E)	↔, except ↑ or ↔ in patients with CHF
ACE inhibitors and Angiotensin II receptor blockers	↔ (R and E)	↓ (R and E)	↔ (R and E)	↔, except ↑ or ↔ in patients with CHF
α-Adrenergic blockers	↔ (R and E)	↓ (R and E)	↔ (R and E)	↔
Antiadrenergic agents without selective blockade	↓ or ↔ (R and E)	↓ (R and E)	↓ or ↔ HR (R and E)	↔

*β-Blockers with ISA lower resting HR only slightly.

Medications	Heart rate	Blood pressure	ECG	Exercise capacity
VII. Antiarrhythmic agents	All antiarrhythmic agents may cause new or worsened arrhythmias (proarrythmic effect)			
Class I				
Quinidine Disopyramide	↑ or ↔ (R and E)	↓ or ↔ (R) ↔ (E)	↑ or ↔ HR (R) May prolong QRS and QT intervals (R) Quinidine may result in "false-negative" test results (E)	↔
Procainamide	↔ (R and E)	↔ (R and E)	May prolong QRS and QT intervals (R) May result in "false-positive" test results (E)	↔
Phenytoin Tocainide Mexiletine	↔ (R and E)	↔ (R and E)	↔ (R and E)	↔
Moricizine	↔ (R and E)	↔ (R and E)	May prolong QRS and QT intervals (R) ↔ (E)	↔
Propafenone	↓ (R) ↓ or ↔ (E)	↔ (R and E)	↓ HR (R) ↓ or ↔ HR (E)	↔
Class II				
β-Blockers (see I.)				
Class III				
Amiodarone Sotalol	↓ (R and E)	↔ (R and E)	↓ HR (R) ↔ (E)	↔
Class IV				
Calcium channel blockers (see III.)				
VIII. Bronchodilators	↔ (R and E)	↔ (R and E)	↔ (R and E)	Bronchodilators ↑ exercise capacity in patients limited by bronchospasm
Anticholinergic agents Xanthine derivatives	↑ or ↔ (R and E)	↔	↑ or ↔ HR May produce PVCs (R and E)	
Sympathomimetic agents	↑ or ↔ (R and E)	↑, ↔, or ↓ (R and E)	↑ or ↔ (R and E)	↔
Cromolyn sodium	↔ (R and E)	↔ (R and E)	↔ (R and E)	↔
Steroidal Anti-inflammatory Agents	↔ (R and E)	↔ (R and E)	↔ (R and E)	↔
IX. Antilipemic agents	Clofibrate may provoke arrhythmias, angina in patients with prior myocardial infarction Nicotinic acid may ↓ BP All other hyperlipidemic agents have no effect on HR, BP, and ECG			↔

(continued)

• Table D.2 Effects of Medications on Heart Rate, Blood Pressure, the Electrocardiogram (ECG), and Exercise Capacity *(continued)* •

Medications	Heart rate	Blood pressure	ECG	Exercise capacity
X. Psychotropic medications				
Minor tranquilizers	May ↓ HR and BP by controlling anxiety; no other effects			
Antidepressants	↑ or ↔ (R and E)	↓ or ↔ (R and E)	Variable (R) May result in "false-positive" test results (E)	
Major tranquilizers	↑ or ↔ (R and E)	↓ or ↔ (R and E)	Variable (R) May result in "false-positive" or "false-negative" test results (E)	
Lithium	↔ (R and E)	↔ (R and E)	May result in T wave changes and arrhythmias (R and E)	
XI. Nicotine	↑ or ↔ (R and E)	↑ (R and E)	↑ or ↔ HR May provoke ischemia, arrthythmias (R and E)	↔, except ↓ or ↔ in patients with angina
XII. Antihistamines	↔ (R and E)	↔ (R and E)	↔ (R and E)	↔
XIII. Cold medications with sympathomimetic agents	Effects similar to those described in sympathomimetic agents, although magnitude of effects is usually smaller			↔
XIV. Thyroid medications Only levothyroxine	↑ (R and E)	↑ (R and E)	↑ HR May provoke arrhythmias ↑ ischemia (R and E)	↔, unless angina worsened
XV. Alcohol	↔ (R and E)	Chronic use may have role in ↑ BP (R and E)	May provoke arrhythmias (R and E)	↔
XVI. Hypoglycemic agents Insulin and oral agents	↔ (R and E)	↔ (R and E)	↔ (R and E)	↔
XVII. Blood Modifiers (Anticoagulants and Antiplatelets)	↔ (R and E)	↔ (R and E)	↔ (R and E)	↔
XVIII. Pentoxifylline	↔ (R and E)	↔ (R and E)	↔ (R and E)	↑ or ↔ in patients limited by intermittent claudication
XIX. Antigout medications	↔ (R and E)	↔ (R and E)	↔ (R and E)	↔
XX. Caffeine	Variable effects depending on previous use Variable effects on exercise capacity May provoke arrhythmias			
XXI. Anorexiants/diet pills	↑ or ↔ (R and E)	↑ or ↔ (R and E)	↑ or ↔ HR (R and E)	

*β-Blockers with ISA lower resting HR only slightly.

+May prevent or delay myocardial ischemia.

Abbreviations: PVCs = premature ventricular contractions; ↑ = increase; ↔ = no effect; ↓ = decrease; R = rest; E = exercise; HR = heart rate.

Reprinted, by permission, from American College of Sports Medicine (ACSM), 2006, *ACSM's guidelines for exercise testing and prescription* (Philadelphia, PA: Lippincott, Williams & Wilkins), 255-266.

Appendix E

Evaluating Fitness

This appendix provides a foundation for the areas of fitness evaluation covered in part II, allowing you to better explain what fitness test scores really mean. In part II, we examined the evaluation of energy cost, cardiorespiratory fitness, body composition and nutrition, muscular strength and endurance, and flexibility and low-back function.

The first step toward fitness testing is to choose your fitness tests wisely. You must consider the following factors in your selection:

- **Reliability:** Can I get consistent results with this test?
- **Objectivity:** Do different test administrators get the same results on this test?
- **Validity:** Does the test measure the characteristic I'm interested in evaluating?

Although a test can be reliable and objective and still not be valid, tests that are unreliable or lack objectivity cannot be valid. Once the consistency of the test is ensured, there are ways to determine whether the test measures what it is supposed to measure. For example, do experts agree that the test is valid? Does the test compare favorably with an established test (a standard) in the same area?

The fitness tests recommended in this book have been shown to be reliable and objective when carefully administered by trained professionals. There also is evidence that the tests in this book are valid (experts recommend them or the tests compare favorably with valid tests).

Fitness professionals can do several things to maximize accuracy (i.e., minimize error) in testing:

- Properly prepare the person being tested.
- Organize the testing session.
- Attend to details.

Fitness testing has many uses in a fitness setting, from prescribing exercise to refining programs. Fitness professionals must know how to interpret test scores and provide feedback to all program participants.

You can help participants evaluate their fitness test scores by doing the following (3, 4):

- Emphasize health status rather than comparison with others.
- Emphasize change rather than current status.
- Provide specific recommendations based on the test data and your understanding of the participant.

One common approach to evaluating test scores is to compare the fitness participant with people of the same gender and similar age (i.e., use percentiles). Much of the way the individual compares with others is based on heredity and early experience. There are limits to how much people can change even with great effort. It is unfortunate that many people in fitness programs try to use the performance model of being number one. The emphasis should not be on who can run the fastest or who has the lowest cholesterol but on helping all people understand, obtain, and maintain cardiorespiratory fitness, healthy body composition, and low-back function.

The current edition of the *ACSM's Guidelines for Exercise Testing and Prescription* (1) uses percentiles for evaluation of fitness tests. We understand that much more research is needed before health criteria can be finalized; however, we think that attempting to set health criteria is better, even with its limitations, than relying on percentiles. For example, a person could weigh significantly more now than in 1980 and be at the same percentile because the whole population gained weight. In addition, a person could gain fat and lose muscle with age and stay at the same percentile.

• Fitness Test Standards for Ages 6 Through 70 •

Test item		6-9 yr	10-12 yr	13-15 yr	16-30 yr	31-50 yr	51-70 yr
1 mi (1.6 km) run in min							
Males	Good	14	12	11	10	10	10
	Borderline	16	14	13	12	12	12
	Needs work	≥18	≥16	≥15	≥14	≥14	≥14
Females	Good	14	12	13	12	12	12
	Borderline	16	14	15	14	14	14
	Needs work	≥18	≥16	≥17	≥16	≥16	≥16
Percent body fat (%)							
Males	Good	7-18	7-18	7-18	7-18	7-18	7-18
	Borderline	22	22	22	22	22	22
	Needs work	>25	>25	>25	>25	>25	>25
Females	Good	7-18	7-18	16-25	16-25	16-25	16-25
	Borderline	22	22	27	27	27	27
	Needs work	>25	>25	>30	>30	>30	>30
Curl-ups (#)							
	Good	≥20	≥25	≥30	≥35	≥35	≥35
	Borderline	12	10	22	25	25	25
	Needs work	≤5	≤10	≤13	≤15	≤15	≤15
Sit and reach (in./cm)[a]							
	Good	12/30.5	12/30.5	12/30.5	12/30.5	12/30.5	12/30.5
	Borderline	8/20.3	8/20.3	8/20.3	8/20.3	8/20.3	8/20.3
	Needs work	≤6/15.2	≤6/15.2	≤6/15.2	≤6/15.2	≤6/15.2	≤6/15.2
Modified pull-ups (#)							
	Good	≥10	≥12	≥15	≥15	≥15	≥15
	Borderline	6	8	10	10	10	10
	Needs work	≤2	≤4	≤5	≤5	≤5	≤5

[a]The feet touch the base of the box at 9 in. (22.9 cm). A score of 9 (22.9) indicates the person can touch her feet.

Individuals over 70 yr should be encouraged to do the walk test (see chapter 5) and strive to monitor the other fitness components.

Adapted from Corbin and Lindsey, 2002; Cooper Institute for Aerobics Research, 1992; President's Council on Physical Fitness and Sports, 2001; Franks, 1989 (pp. 42-47).

We have set fitness standards based on what is needed for good health. Although performance decreases with age, the minimal fitness standards are the same for adults of all ages. More research is needed so that we can refine these standards; as we find out more about the relationship between test scores and positive health, some of these standards may need to be modified.

The most important question for a fitness participant is not what her health status is at this moment in life, but what it will be 6 mo, 2 yr, or 20 yr from now. In this way, the person is encouraged to deal with her current status (compared to health standards) so that she can set reasonable, desirable, and achievable goals for the next testing time.

Test results can also help people meet specific goals. It may be that the health standards are not appropriate or reasonable for an individual. For example, the standards for running the mile cannot be used for people who swim for their fitness workouts or for people who use wheelchairs. However, individual goals for covering a certain distance in the water or in a wheelchair can be established. Or, the fitness professional may want to set intermediary goals for a person who is very unfit. For example, a person who can only walk a quarter of a mile without stopping would be discouraged by discussing the standards for running 1 mi. The initial goal for that person may be to work up to being able to walk 1 mi without stopping. As indicated in chapter 22, it is important to set goals and subgoals to help people begin and continue healthy behaviors.

Fitness and lifestyle behaviors (e.g., getting adequate exercise, nutrition, and rest; avoiding substance abuse;

coping with stress) and fitness test scores are interrelated. The fitness leader should emphasize fitness *behaviors*. It is more important for people to begin and continue regular physical activity than to reach a certain level on a graded exercise test. Likewise, it is more important for people to develop healthy eating habits than to have a certain percentage of body fat. By emphasizing healthy behaviors, fitness professionals can recognize people for their effort, and in the long run recognizing effort is the best way to improve fitness test scores.

Overemphasizing test scores can discourage some participants. Two good examples of programs that recognize fitness behaviors are the Canadian *Active Living Challenge* (2) and the President's Council on Physical Fitness and Sports' *Presidential Sports Award* programs (7). Both programs award people who do various physical activities for a certain number of hours, thus rewarding the behavior rather than the fitness test result.

Many people have one or more disabilities resulting in mild to severe limitations regarding physical activity and assessment. It is beyond the scope of this book to recommend specific activities and tests to deal with each possible condition (8). The fitness professional can, however, apply the following general principles:

- Almost all individuals with disabilities can benefit from regular physical activity.
- Most of these individuals can participate in a variety of activities with simple adaptations.
- Individuals with disabilities can gain motivation from periodic assessment.
- The same types of fitness tests can be used with simple adaptations.
- Adaptations of activities and assessments are often simply commonsense adjustments made by the fitness professional and the participant.
- Experts in adapted physical education and special education can provide additional assistance.

Analyzing test scores from different fitness classes can help the fitness professional decide what revisions need to be made in the overall fitness program. How many people drop out of various classes? What kind of changes in cardiorespiratory fitness, body fatness, and low-back function are being made? How many injuries relate to the various classes? The answers to such questions help you evaluate, revise, and improve your fitness programs. You might consider your programs to be improving steadily rather than having reached perfection. This improvement can result from program evaluation.

Another use of test scores is to educate the public and to get positive attention for your program. What percentage of the participants stay with the program long enough to make important fitness gains? What is the total amount of fat lost by participants over a year? How many miles have the participants run during the year? Careful testing, record keeping, and analysis can provide helpful information about your program to the public.

Glossary

β-adrenergic blocking medications (β-blockers)—Drugs that block receptors that respond to catecholamines (epinephrine and norepinephrine); they slow HR.

β-adrenergic receptors—Receptors in the heart and lungs that respond to catecholamines (epinephrine and norepinephrine).

A band—Portion of the sarcomere composed of myosin and actin; the length of the A band remains constant during muscle shortening.

abduction—Movement of a bone laterally away from the anatomical position.

Acceptable Macronutrient Distribution Range (AMDR)—The percentages of calories from carbohydrates, fats, and proteins thought to promote good health.

actin—The thin contractile filament of the sarcomere to which myosin binds to release the energy in the activated cross bridges, leading to sarcomere shortening.

adduction—The return back to the anatomical position from the abducted position.

Adequate Intake (AI)—The amount of a nutrient considered adequate although insufficient data exist to establish an RDA.

adipose tissue—Tissue composed of fat cells.

aerobic energy—When oxygen is used to help supply energy (ATP) to a person who is working.

agility—Ability to start, stop, and move the body quickly in different directions.

agonist—A muscle that is very effective in causing a certain joint movement; also called the *prime mover.*

air displacement plethysmography—Method of body composition assessment that estimates body density from body volume and body weight.

airway obstruction—Blockage of the airway that can be caused by a foreign object. Swelling is secondary to direct trauma or allergic reaction.

alcohol—Ethanol; a depressant that may affect the response to an exercise test.

amenorrhea—A cessation of menses.

amino acids—Nitrogen-containing building blocks for proteins that can be used for energy.

amortization phase—Time between the eccentric and concentric phases of a muscle action.

amphiarthrodial joint—A joint that allows only slight movement in all directions; also called the *cartilaginous joint.*

anaerobic energy—Energy (ATP) supplied without oxygen. Creatine phosphate and glycolysis supply ATP without using oxygen.

android-type obesity—Obesity in which there is a disproportionate amount of fat in the trunk and abdomen.

aneurysm—A spindle-shaped or saclike bulging of the wall of a blood-filled vein, artery, or ventricle.

angina pectoris—Severe cardiac pain that may radiate to the jaw, arms, or legs. Angina is caused by myocardial ischemia, which can be induced by exercise in susceptible individuals.

angular momentum—The quantity of rotation. Angular momentum is the product of the rotational inertia and the angular velocity.

anorexia nervosa—An eating disorder in which a preoccupation with body weight leads to self-starvation.

antagonist—A muscle that causes movement at a joint in a direction opposite to that of the joint's agonist (prime mover).

antiarrhythmics—Drugs that reduce the number of arrhythmias.

anticoagulant—A drug that delays blood clotting.

antihistamines—Drugs that relieve allergy symptoms, thus making it easier to breathe.

antihypertensives—Drugs that lower blood pressure.

antioxidant vitamins—Substances that attach to free radicals and diminish their effects. Antioxidants are touted to be effective in decreasing the risk of cardiovascular disease and cancer.

aortic valve—Heart valve located between the aorta and the left ventricle.

apnea—Temporary cessation of breathing; often caused by an excess amount of oxygen or too little carbon dioxide in the brain.

aponeuroses—Broad, flat, tendinous sheaths attaching muscles to one another.

arterioles—Blood vessels between the artery and the capillary that are involved in the regulation of blood flow and blood pressure.

arteriosclerosis—An arterial disease characterized by the hardening and thickening of vessel walls.

arteriovenous oxygen difference—volume of oxygen extraction; calculated by subtracting the oxygen content of mixed venous blood (as it returns to the heart) from the oxygen content of the arterial blood.

arthritis—Inflammation of a joint.

articular capsule—A ligamentous structure that encloses a diarthrodial joint.

articular cartilage—Cartilage which covers bone surfaces that articulate (meet or come into contact) with other bone surfaces.

atherosclerosis—A form of arteriosclerosis in which fatty substances are deposited in the inner walls of the arteries.

atrial fibrillation—The atrial rate is 400 to 700 beats $\cdot$ min^{-1}, whereas the ventricle's rate is 60 to 160 beats $\cdot$ min^{-1}; P waves cannot be seen on the ECG.

atrial flutter—The atrial rate is 200 to 350 beats $\cdot$ min^{-1}, whereas the ventricular rate is 60 to 160 beats $\cdot$ min^{-1}; ECG shows a sawtooth pattern between QRS complexes.

atrioventricular (AV) node—The origin of the bundle of His in the right atrium of the heart. Normal electrical activity of the heart passes through the AV node before depolarization of the ventricles.

atrophy—A reduction in muscle fiber size.

avascular—Without a blood supply.

balance—Ability to maintain a certain posture or to move without falling.

ballistic movement—A rapid movement with three phases: an initial concentric action by agonist muscles to begin movement, a coasting phase, and a deceleration by the eccentric action of the antagonist muscles.

bariatric surgery—A surgical procedure designed to help with weight loss. These surgeries alter the gastrointestinal system to restrict food intake and nutrient uptake.

baroreceptors—Receptors that monitor arterial BP.

behavioral contracts—Written, signed, public agreements to engage in specific goal-directed activities. Contracts include a designated time frame and clear consequences of meeting and not meeting the agreed upon objectives.

bench stepping—A graded exercise test that can be used for both submaximal and maximal testing to evaluate cardiorespiratory function. The height of the bench and the number of steps per minute determine the intensity of the effort. Bench stepping is also a very popular conditioning exercise.

beta-carotene—A precursor of vitamin A and an important antioxidant.

binge eating disorder—An eating disorder characterized by consuming large amounts of food in a short time.

bioelectrical impedance analysis (BIA)—Method of body composition assessment based on the electrical conductivity of various tissues in the body.

black-globe temperature (Tg)—A measure of radiant heat energy; a measurement taken in the sunlight to evaluate the potential to gain or lose heat by radiation.

body composition—Description of the tissues that make up the body. It typically refers to the relative percentages of fat and nonfat tissues in the body.

body fat distribution (fat patterning)—Pattern of fat accumulation that often is inherited.

body mass index (BMI)—Measure of the relationship between height and weight; calculated by dividing the weight in kilograms by height in meters squared.

bodybuilding—A competitive sport in which the primary goal is to enhance muscular size, symmetry, and definition.

bone mineral density (BMD)—Amount of bone mineral per unit area. Typically measured with DXA and used for clinical diagnosis of osteoporosis.

bradycardia—Slow HR, below 60 beats $\cdot$ min^{-1} at rest. Bradycardia is healthy if it is the result of physical conditioning.

bronchodilators—Drugs that dilate the bronchioles, providing relief from an asthma attack.

budget—A financial plan including estimated income and expenditure.

bulimia nervosa—An eating disorder characterized by consuming large amounts of food followed by food purging.

bundle branch—Bundle of nerve fibers between both ventricles of the heart; conducts impulses.

bundle of His—Conduction pathway that connects the AV node with bundle branches in the ventricles.

bursae—Fibrous sacs lined with synovial membrane that contain a small quantity of synovial fluid. Bursae are found between tendon and bone, between skin and bone, and between muscle and muscle. Their function is to facilitate movement without friction between these surfaces.

calcium channel blockers—Medications that act by blocking the entry of calcium into the cell; used to treat angina, arrhythmias, and hypertension.

caloric equivalent of oxygen—Approximately 5 kcal of energy is produced per liter of oxygen consumed (5 kcal $\cdot$ L^{-1}).

carbohydrate loading—Increasing carbohydrate intake and decreasing activity in the days preceding competition.

carbohydrate—An essential nutrient composed of carbon, hydrogen, and oxygen that is an energy source for the body.

carbon monoxide (CO)—A pollutant derived from the incomplete combustion of fossil fuels; binds to hemoglobin to reduce oxygen transport and thus reduce maximal aerobic power.

cardiac output (Q)—the volume of blood pumped by the heart per minute; is calculated by multiplying the HR (beats $\cdot$ min^{-1}) by the SV (ml $\cdot$ beat^{-1}).

cardiopulmonary resuscitation (CPR)—Established procedures to restore breathing and blood circulation.

cardiorespiratory function—The ability of the circulatory and respiratory systems to supply fuel during sustained physical activity.

cholesterol—A fatty substance in which carbon, hydrogen, and oxygen atoms are arranged in rings, which may be deposited in the arterial walls, contributing to atherosclerosis.

chronic obstructive pulmonary diseases—Diseases that cause flow obstruction of air in the airways of the lung.

claudication—Interference with the blood supply to the legs, often resulting in limping.

closed-circuit spirometry—The subject breathes 100% oxygen from a spirometer while carbon dioxide is absorbed; the decrease in the volume of oxygen in the spirometer is proportional to the oxygen consumption.

communication—Interaction, often verbal, to share information and emotions.

compartment syndrome—Increased pressure within a muscular compartment that compromises blood flow and nerve supply.

complex carbohydrates—Polysaccharides formed by combining three or more sugar molecules. Polysaccharides include starches and fiber and are found in high numbers in rice, pasta, and whole grain breads.

concentric—A type of muscle action that occurs when the muscle shortens.

concentric action—A shortening of the muscle; causes movement at the joint.

concreteness—Being specific about events and ideas; not abstract.

conduction—Heat-exchange mechanism in which heat is lost from warmer to cooler objects in direct contact with each other.

confrontation—Point out incongruities or inconsistencies between what a person says and does that are observable facts.

convection—Special case of conduction related to heat loss. Heat is transferred to air or water in direct contact with the skin; warm air or water is less dense and rises, carrying heat away from the body.

coordination—Ability to perform a task integrating movements of the body and different parts of the body.

coronary angiography—A diagnostic procedure where a flexible guide wire is inserted into a coronary artery, and a catheter is then passed over it. A radiographic contrast dye is then injected into the artery to allow any potential blockages to be seen.

coronary arteries—Blood vessels that supply the heart muscle.

coronary artery bypass graft (CABG)—Procedure in which arteries or veins are sutured above and below a blocked coronary artery to restore adequate blood flow to that portion of the myocardium.

coronary artery thrombosis—Occlusion of a coronary artery by a blood clot.

coronary heart disease (CHD)—Atherosclerosis of the coronary arteries. Also called *coronary artery disease (CAD).*

creatine phosphate (CP)—A high-energy phosphate compound that represents the primary immediate anaerobic source of ATP at the onset of exercise. CP is important in all-out activities lasting a few seconds.

creeping obesity—Slow accumulation of adipose tissue with aging.

criterion method—Method used as the gold standard, or the method against which other methods are compared.

cross bridge—Part of myosin filament that binds to actin, releasing energy that results in shortening of the sarcomere.

cycle ergometer—A one-wheeled stationary cycle with adjustable resistance used as a work task for exercise testing or conditioning.

daily caloric need—Number of calories needed to maintain current body weight. This number is composed of resting metabolic rate, calories for activity, and the thermic effect of food.

Daily Values (DVs)—Indicate the percentage of daily recommended levels of nutrients that are contained in a food. DVs are based on a calorie intake of 2,000 kcal $\cdot$ day^{-1}.

decongestants—Drugs that reduce nasal and bronchial congestion and dry out the airways.

diabetes mellitus—Group of metabolic diseases characterized by high blood glucose concentrations.

diaphysis—The shaft of a long bone.

diarthrodial joint—A freely moving joint characterized by its synovial membrane and capsular ligament; also called a *synovial joint.*

diastolic blood pressure (DBP)—The pressure blood exerts on the vessel walls during the resting portion of the cardiac cycle, measured in millimeters of mercury by a sphygmomanometer.

dietary fiber—Substances found in plants that cannot be broken down by the human digestive system.

Dietary Reference Intake (DRI)—Set of values used to evaluate dietary intake.

digitalis—A drug that augments the contraction of the heart muscle and slows the rate of conduction of cardiac impulses through the AV node.

direct calorimetry—A method of measuring the metabolic rate using a closed chamber in which a subject's heat loss is picked up by water flowing through the walls of a chamber; the gain in temperature of the water plus that lost in evaporation determines the metabolic rate.

disc—Located between vertebrae; acts as a shock absorber and frequently is involved in low-back pain.

disordered eating—Unhealthy eating pattern that can in some cases be a precursor to eating disorders.

diuretics—Drugs that increase urine production, thereby ridding the body of excess fluid.

dose—The quantity (intensity, frequency, and duration) of exercise needed to bring about a response (e.g., lower resting blood pressure).

double product—See rate presure product.

dry-bulb temperature (Tdb)—The temperature of the air measured in the shade by an ordinary thermometer.

duration—The length of time for a fitness workout. Guidelines often include 20 to 60 min of aerobic work at THR; however, the total work accomplished (e.g., distance covered) should be emphasized.

dynamic testing—Strength assessment that involves movement of the body (e.g., a push-up) or an external load (e.g., a bench press).

dyspnea—Difficult or labored breathing beyond what is expected for the intensity of work. The exercise test or activity should be stopped.

eating disorders—Clinical eating patterns that result in severe negative health consequences.

eccentric—A type of muscle action that occurs when the muscle lengthens.

eccentric action—Lengthening of the muscle during its action; controls speed of movement caused by another force.

ectopic focus—An irritated portion of the myocardium or electrical conducting system; gives rise to extra heart beats that do not originate from the sinoatrial (SA) node.

effect—The desired response resulting from exercise training (e.g., lower resting blood pressure).

ejection fraction—The fraction of the end-diastolic volume ejected per beat (stroke volume divided by end-diastolic volume).

elasticity—Ability of ligaments and tendons to lengthen passively and return to their resting length.

electrocardiogram (ECG)—Graphic recording of the electrical activity of the heart. The ECG is obtained with the electrocardiograph.

electrolytes—Particles that in solution convey an electrical charge. Most electrolyte drinks are diluted solutions of glucose, salt, and other minerals, with artificial flavoring. Other than sodium, the minerals provided by an electrolyte solution do not provide much benefit.

embolism—Sudden obstruction of a blood vessel by a solid body such as a clot carried in the bloodstream.

emergency medical system (EMS)—A system designed to handle medical emergencies; 911 or other community emergency numbers.

emergency procedure—Plan of action to follow in emergency situations.

empathy—Identification with the thoughts or feelings of another person and the effective communication that the other person's feelings are understood.

end-diastolic volume—The volume of blood in the heart just before ventricular contraction; a measure of the stretch of the ventricle.

endothelial cells—cells that form the interior lining of the blood vessels, heart, and lymphatic vessels.

end-ROM—Point at which further movement may stretch ligaments or other soft-tissue structures such as discs.

epimysium—The connective tissue sheath surrounding a muscle.

epiphyseal plates—The sites of ossification in long bones.

epiphyses—The ends of long bones.

ergogenic aids—Substances taken in hopes of improving athletic performance.

essential amino acids—The eight amino acids that the body cannot synthesize and therefore must be ingested.

essential fat—The minimum amount of body fat needed for good health.

evaporation—Conversion of water from the liquid to the gaseous state by means of heat, as in evaporation of sweat; results in the loss of 580 kcal for each liter of sweat evaporated.

Exercise Specialist—A person certified by the ACSM to work in exercise rehabilitation settings with populations who are at high-risk or have a medical condition (e.g., cardiac and diabetic).

exercise-induced asthma—A reactive airway disease in which exercise tends to cause the bronchioles to constrict.

exercise tests—A series of tests which evaluate prospective exercise participants' current level of fitness and commonly include cardiovascular, muscular strength, and endurance, body composition, and flexibility.

extension—Increasing the angle at a joint, such as straightening the elbow.

facet joint—Junction of the superior and inferior articular processes of the vertebrae.

fasciculi—Bundles of muscle fibers surrounded by perimysium.

fat mass (FM)—The mass of the fat tissues in the body.

fat-free mass (FFM)—Weight of the nonfat tissues of the body.

fats—Non-water-soluble substances composed of hydrogen, oxygen, and carbon that serve a variety of functions in the body including energy production.

female athlete triad—A condition sometimes observed in female athletes that is characterized by disordered eating, amenorrhea, and osteoporosis.

first-degree AV block—The delayed transmission of impulses from atria to ventricles (in excess of 0.20 sec).

flexibility—The ability to move a joint through its full range of motion without discomfort or pain.

flexion—Anterior or posterior movement that brings two bones together.

Food Guide Pyramid—the United States Department of Agriculture's approach to recommending healthy eating and exercise. The pyramid contains recommendations for grains, fruits, vegetables, milk, meat and beans, oils, discretionary calories, and physical activity.

force arm (FA)—Perpendicular distance from the axis of rotation to the direction of the application of the force causing movement.

forced expiratory volume in 1 sec (FEV_1)—The maximal amount of air that can be forcibly exhaled in 1 sec, as measured by spirometry; this variable is used to diagnose chronic obstructive pulmonary disease. A person who can expel less than 75% of her VC in 1 sec should be referred to a physician.

free radicals—Molecules or fragments of molecules formed during metabolic processes that are highly reactive and can damage cellular components.

functional capacity—Maximal oxygen uptake, expressed in milliliters of oxygen per kilogram of body weight per minute, or in METs.

functional curve—Spinal curve (e.g., lordotic curve) that can be removed by assuming a different posture.

genuineness—Being authentic and sincere in a relationship with another person.

glucose—A simple sugar that is a vital energy source in the human body.

glycemic index—A rating system used to indicate how rapidly a food causes blood glucose to rise.

glycogen—The storage form of carbohydrates in the human body.

glycolysis—The metabolic pathway producing ATP from the anaerobic breakdown of glucose. This short-term source of ATP is important in all-out activities lasting less than 2 min.

goal setting—Goals are desired tasks to accomplish in a specific amount of time. Goals provide direction and foster persistence in the search for task strategies. Effective goal setting includes establishing objectives that can be measured, concretely defined, and practically achieved.

good nutrition—A diet in which foods are eaten in the proper quantities and with the needed distribution of nutrients to maintain good health in the present and in the future.

graded exercise test (GXT)—A multistage test that determines a person's physiological responses to different intensities of exercise and the person's maximal aerobic power.

gynoid-type obesity—Obesity in which there is a disproportionate amount of fat in the hips and thighs.

H zone—The middle area of the sarcomere that contains only myosin.

Health/Fitness Instructor—A person who is certified by the ACSM as qualified in exercise testing, prescription, and leadership in preventive programs.

health—Being alive with no major health problem. Also called *apparently healthy.*

heart rate (HR)—The number of heartbeats per minute.

Heimlich maneuver—Procedure used to dislodge material caught in the respiratory passage that is blocking the airway.

hemorrhage—The escape of a large amount of blood from a vessel.

hepatitis B (HBV)—A type of hepatitis (viral infection of the liver) that is transmitted by sexual or blood-to-blood contact.

high-density lipoprotein cholesterol (HDL-C)—This form of cholesterol protects against the development of CHD, in that it helps transport cholesterol to the liver, where it is eliminated. Thus, low levels of HDL-C are related to a high risk of CHD.

high-risk situation—An event, thought, or interaction that challenges an individual's perceived ability to maintain a desired behavioral change.

human immunodeficiency virus (HIV)—A virus that destroys the body's ability to fight infection; this virus causes AIDS.

hydrostatic weighing—Method of assessing body composition based on Archimedes' principle; also called *underwater weighing*. Hydrostatic weighing is often used as the criterion method for assessing %BF.

hyperextension—A continuation of extension past the anatomical position.

hyperglycemia—Blood glucose concentrations above normal (fasting plasma glucose of 110 mg $\cdot$ dl^{-1}).

hypertension—High blood pressure. Normally systolic blood pressure exceeds 140 mmHg or diastolic blood pressure exceeds 90 mmHg in someone who has hypertension.

hyperthermia—An elevation of the core temperature; if unchecked it can lead to heat exhaustion or heatstroke and death.

hypertrophy—An enlargement in muscle fiber size.

hyperventilation—A level of ventilation beyond that needed to maintain the arterial carbon dioxide level; can be initiated by a sudden increase in the hydrogen ion concentration attributable to lactic acid production during a progressive exercise test.

hypotension—Low blood pressure.

hypothermia—Below-normal body temperature.

hypoxemia—Abnormally low oxygen content in the arterial blood but not total anoxia.

I band—An area of the sarcomere that is bisected by the Z line and is composed of actin; the I band decreases during muscle shortening as the actin slides over the myosin.

impaired fasting glucose—A fasting blood glucose level between 100-125 mg/dL and commonly considered a precursor to the development of diabetes.

impaired glucose tolerance (IGT)—A condition in which the body does not normally process glucose; often an intermediate step before development of type 2 diabetes.

indirect calorimetry—Estimating energy production on the basis of oxygen consumption.

informed consent—A procedure used to obtain a person's voluntary permission to participate in a program. Informed consent requires a description of the procedures to be used as well as the potential benefits and risks and written consent of the participant.

insulin resistance—A condition in which the body's insulin receptors no longer respond normally to insulin.

intensity—A measure of the effort experienced in a workout, usually expressed as a percentage of maximal HR or oxygen consumption.

intercalated disks—Special junctions between adjacent cardiac muscle cells that allow electrical impulses to pass from cell to cell into both ventricles (see bundle of His).

intracoronary stent—A device placed within the lumen of the artery to keep the artery open.

iron-deficiency anemia—A condition characterized by a decreased amount of hemoglobin in red blood cells and a resultant decrease in the ability of the blood to transport oxygen.

isokinetic testing—The assessment of maximal muscle tension throughout a range of joint motion at a constant angular velocity (e.g., 60° $\cdot$ sec^{-1}).

isometric action—A muscle action in which the muscle length is unchanged; the muscle exerts a force that counteracts an opposing force. Isometric action is also called *static action.*

isometric—A type of muscle action in which the muscle length remains constant and no movement occurs.

J point—On an ECG, the point at which the S wave ends and the S-T segment begins.

joint cavity—The space between bones enclosed by the synovial membrane and articular cartilage.

kyphotic—Describes the condition of kyphosis, a convex curvature of the spine (e.g., the thoracic curve).

lactate threshold—The point during a GXT at which the blood lactate concentration suddenly increases; a good indicator of the highest sustainable work rate. Also called the *anaerobic threshold.*

leadership—The ability to influence and motivate people in a group to make decisions and to act on those decisions.

lean body mass—Term often used synonymously with *fat-free mass.*

liability—Legal responsibility.

ligament—The connective tissue that attaches bone to bone.

lipoproteins—Large molecules responsible for transporting fats in the blood.

local muscular endurance—The ability of a muscle or muscle group to perform repeated contractions against a submaximal resistance.

lordotic curve—Describes the condition of lordosis; a forward, concave curve of the lumbar spine when the spine is viewed from the side.

low-back problems—Strong discomfort in the low-back area, often caused by lack of muscular endurance and flexibility in the midtrunk region or improper posture or lifting.

low-density lipoprotein cholesterol (LDL-C)—The form of cholesterol that is responsible for the buildup of plaque in the inner walls of the arteries (atherosclerosis). Thus, high levels of LDL-C are related to a high risk of CHD.

lumbosacral area—Area encompassing the lumbar vertebrae and the sacrum.

lumen—the open space inside of a structure such as an artery or intestine.

macrocycle—A phase of training that lasts about 1 year.

malnutrition—A diet in which there is an underconsumption, overconsumption, or unbalanced consumption of nutrients that leads to disease or increased susceptibility to disease.

maximal aerobic power or **maximal oxygen uptake** (**$\dot{V}O_2$max**)—The maximal rate at which oxygen can be used by the body during maximal work; related directly to the maximal capacity of the heart to deliver blood to the muscles. Expressed in $L \cdot min^{-1}$ or $ml \cdot kg^{-1} \cdot min^{-1}$.

maximum voluntary contraction (MVC)—Maximum amount of force that can be elicited during a single repetition.

menisci—Partial, semilunar-shaped disks between the femur and the tibia at the knee.

mesocycle—A phase of training that lasts for several months.

microcycle—A phase of training that lasts about 1 wk.

mindful exercise—Low-to-moderate physical activity performed with a meditative, proprioceptive, or sensory awareness component.

minerals—Inorganic atoms or ions that serve a variety of functions in the human body.

mitochondria—Cellular organelles responsible for generating energy (ATP) through aerobic metabolism.

mitral valve—Heart valve located between the left atrium and left ventricle.

Mobitz type I AV block—On an ECG, the P-R interval progressively increases until the P wave is not followed by a QRS complex. The site of the block is within the AV node.

Mobitz type II AV block—On an ECG, a constant P-R interval with some but not all P waves followed by QRS. The site of the block is the bundle of His.

monounsaturated fatty acids—Fats that have a single double bond between carbon atoms in the fatty acid chain. Examples are olive and canola oil.

motion segment—Fundamental unit of the lumbar spine; made up of two vertebrae and their intervening disc.

motor unit—The functional unit of muscular action that includes a motor nerve and the muscle fibers that its branches innervate.

muscle fiber—Muscle cell. Contains myofibrils that are composed of sarcomeres; uses chemical energy of ATP to generate tension, which, when greater than the resistance, results in movement.

muscle group—A group of specific muscles that are responsible for the same action at the same joint.

muscular endurance—The ability of the muscle to perform repetitive contractions over a prolonged time.

muscular fitness—Describes the integrated status of muscular strength and muscular endurance.

muscular strength—The ability of the muscle to generate the maximum amount of force.

myocardial infarction (MI)—Death of a section of heart tissue in which the blood supply has been cut off; commonly called a *heart attack.*

myocardial ischemia—A lack of blood flow to the heart tissue.

myocardium—The middle layer of the heart wall; involuntary, striated muscle innervated by autonomic nerves.

myofibril—Component inside muscle fibers that is composed of a long string of sarcomeres.

myosin—The thick contractile filament in sarcomeres that can bind actin and split ATP to generate cross-bridge movement and develop tension.

My Pyramid—the United States Department of Agriculture's individualized recommendations for food intake and exercise based on age, sex, and current activity patterns. The pyramid contains recommendations for grains, fruits, vegetables, milk, meat and beans, oils, discretionary calories, and physical activity.

negative caloric balance—When less energy is consumed than is expended, which decreases body weight.

negligence—The failure to provide reasonable care or the care required by the circumstances. The fitness professional, program, or both are legally liable for injury that results from this failure.

nicotine gum—Gum containing nicotine that is used for smoking cessation. Nicotine is absorbed through the oral mucosa, providing sufficient plasma nicotine concentrations to curb the craving to smoke.

nitrates—A class of medications used to treat angina pectoris, or chest pain.

nutrient density—The amount of essential nutrients in a food compared with the calories it contains.

nutrient—A substance that the body requires for the maintenance, growth, and repair of tissues.

obesity—Condition in which a person has an excessive accumulation of fat tissue; also may be classified by the relationship between weight and height.

oligomenorrhea—Irregular menses.

open-circuit spirometry—Measuring oxygen consumption by inhaling room air while collecting and analyzing the expired air.

oral antiglycemic agents—Medications used to treat non-insulin-dependent diabetes mellitus; they stimulate the pancreas to secrete more insulin.

ossification—The replacement of cartilage by bone.

osteoarthritis—Most common form of arthritis (90%-95% of all cases); affects joints whose articular cartilage is damaged or injured.

osteopenia—When bone has been lost but has not yet reached osteoporotic levels.

osteoporosis—A disease characterized by a decrease in the total amount of bone mineral and a decrease in the strength of the remaining bone.

overload—To place greater than usual demands on some part of the body (e.g., picking up more weight than usual overloads the muscle involved). Chronic overloading leads to increased function.

overweight—Condition in which a person is above the recommended weight-to-height range but is below obesity levels.

oxygen consumption (**$\dot{V}O_2$**)—The rate at which oxygen is used during a specific intensity of an activity; oxygen uptake.

oxygen debt—The amount of oxygen used during recovery from work that exceeds the amount needed for rest. Also called *oxygen repayment* and *excess postexercise oxygen consumption.*

oxygen deficit—The difference between the steady-state oxygen requirement of a physical activity and the measured oxygen uptake during the first minutes of work.

ozone—An active form of oxygen formed in reaction to UV light and as an emission from internal combustion engines; exposure can decrease lung function.

P wave—On an ECG, a small positive deflection preceding a QRS complex, indicating atrial depolarization. The P wave is normally less than 0.12 sec in duration, with an amplitude of 0.25 mV or less.

pars interarticularis—The part of the vertebra between its upper elements (superior articular process and transverse process) and its lower elements (inferior articular process and spinous process).

percent body fat (%BF)—Percentage of the total weight composed of fat tissue; calculated by dividing fat mass by total weight and multiplying by 100.

percentage of HRR (%HRR)—The HRR is calculated by subtracting resting HR from maximal HR. The %HRR is a percentage of the difference between resting and maximal HR and is calculated by subtracting resting HR from the exercise HR, dividing by the HRR, and multiplying by 100%.

percentage of maximal HR (%HRmax)—HR expressed as a simple percentage of the maximal HR.

percentage of maximal oxygen uptake (%$\dot{V}O_2$max)—Ratio of submaximal oxygen uptake to maximal oxygen uptake, multiplied by 100%.

percentage of oxygen uptake reserve (%$\dot{V}O_2$R)—$\dot{V}O_2$R is calculated by subtracting 1 MET (3.5 ml · kg^{-1} · min^{-1}) from the subject's $\dot{V}O_2$max. The %$\dot{V}O_2$R is a percentage of the difference between resting $\dot{V}O_2$ and $\dot{V}O_2$max and is calculated by subtracting 1 MET from the measured oxygen uptake, dividing by the subject's $\dot{V}O_2$R, and multiplying by 100%.

percutaneous transluminal coronary angioplasty (PTCA)—A surgical procedure in which a flexible guide wire is inserted into a partially blocked coronary artery, and then a catheter with an inflatable balloon near the tip is passed over the guide wire. The balloon is then inflated, then subsequently deflated and removed, to open the coronary artery.

performance—The ability to perform a task or sport at a desired level. Also called *motor fitness* or *skill-related fitness.*

perimysium—The connective tissue surrounding fasciculi within a muscle.

periodization—A process of varying the training stimulus to promote long-term fitness gains and to avoid overtraining.

periosteum—The connective tissue surrounding all bone surfaces except the articulating surfaces.

personal trainer—fitness professional who designs and delivers individualized exercise programs (usually one-on-one), primarily with healthy individuals.

phospholipids—Fatty compounds that are essential constituents of cell membranes.

physical fitness—A set of attributes that people have or achieve relating to their ability to perform physical activity.

polyunsaturated fatty acids—Fats that have two or more double bonds between carbon atoms in the fatty acid chain. Examples are fish, corn, soybean, and peanut oils.

positive caloric balance—When more calories are consumed than are expended, resulting in weight gain.

positron emission tomography (PET)—A scanning technique that involves infusing the blood with radionuclides. The photons emitted by destruction of positrons are used to generate color images that correspond to blood flow and uptake of substances in various tissues, such as the heart.

postpubescent—After puberty changes.

power—Ability to exert muscular strength quickly.

powerlifting—A competitive sport in which athletes attempt to lift maximal amounts of weight in the squat, deadlift, and bench press exercises.

P-R interval—The time interval between the beginning of the P wave and the QRS complex. The upper normal limit is 0.2 sec. This segment is normally used as the isoelectric baseline.

P-R segment—Forms the isoelectric line, or baseline, from which S-T segment deviations are measured.

prediabetes—A condition in which an individual has impaired fasting glucose or impaired glucose tolerance. Without treatment, prediabetes typically evolves into type 2 diabetes.

premature atrial contraction—On an ECG, the rhythm is irregular and the R-R interval is short; the origin of the beat is somewhere other than the SA node.

premature junctional contraction (PJC)—On an ECG, the ectopic pacemaker in the AV junctional area causes a QRS complex; frequently seen with inverted P waves.

premature ventricular contraction (PVC)—Wide, bizarrely shaped QRS complex originating from an ectopic focus in the His-Purkinje system. The QRS interval lasts longer than 0.12 sec, and the T wave is usually in the opposite direction.

prepubescent—Children who have not yet reached puberty.

pressure points—The points where to apply pressure over major arteries to control bleeding.

prevalence—The percentage of a population that has a particular characteristic. For example, obesity prevalence is calculated by dividing the number of people classified as obese by the total number of people.

PRICE—The suggested treatment for minor sprains and strains: protection, rest, ice, compression, and elevation.

primary amenorrhea—The absence of menarche (i.e., first menses) in girls age 16 or older.

principle of reversibility—A corollary to the principle of overload; loss of a training effect with disuse.

proteins—Nutrients composed of amino acids that serve a variety of functions in the human body.

pubescent—During change from child to adult.

pulmonary function testing—Procedures used to test the capacity of the respiratory system to move air into or out of the lungs.

pulmonary valve—A set of three crescent-shaped flaps at the opening of the pulmonary artery; also called the *semilunar valves.*

pulmonary ventilation—The number of liters of air inhaled or exhaled per minute.

pulse oximeter—Device used to measure the percent saturation of hemoglobin in the arterial blood.

Purkinje fibers—The fibers found beneath the endocardium of the heart; the impulse-conducting network of the heart.

Q wave—The initial negative deflection of the QRS complex on an ECG.

QRS complex—The largest complex on an ECG, indicating a depolarization of the left ventricle and normally lasting less than 0.1 sec.

Q-T interval—The time interval from the beginning of the QRS complex to the end of the T wave. The Q-T interval reflects the electrical systole of the cardiac cycle.

R wave—The positive deflection of the QRS complex in the ECG.

radiation—The process of heat exchange from the surface of one object to the surface of another object that depends on a temperature gradient but does not require direct contact between objects, for example, heat loss from the sun to the earth.

rate–pressure product—The product of HR and SBP; indicative of the oxygen requirement of the heart during exercise. Training lowers the rate–pressure product at rest and during submaximal work. Also called the *double product.*

rating of perceived exertion (RPE)—A scale, by Borg, used to quantify the subjective feeling of physical effort. The original scale was from 6 to 20; the revised scale is from 0 to 10.

Recommended Dietary Allowance (RDA)—The amount of a nutrient found to be adequate for approximately 97% of the population.

recruitment—Stimulation of additional motor units to increase the strength of a muscle action.

Registered Clinical Exercise Physiologist—A person with a MS degree in exercise science (or equivalent) who possesses good clinical experience in the use of exercise in rehabilitation.

reinforcement—Positive reinforcement involves adding something positive to increase the frequency of the target behavior. Negative reinforcement also increases the frequency of the desired behavior, but it is the removal of something negative, like losing weight because of a regular walking program. Reinforcement can be administered by oneself (self-reinforcement) or by other people (social reinforcement).

relapse prevention—Way to identify and deal successfully with high-risk situations by educating the client about the relapse process and using a variety of strategies to foster an effective coping response.

relative humidity—A measure of the relative wetness of the air; the ratio of the amount of water vapor in the air to the maximum the air can hold at that temperature times 100%. High relative humidity in a warm environment helps determine the potential for losing heat by evaporation.

relative leanness—The relative amounts of body weight that are fat and nonfat. Also called *body composition.*

repetition maximum (RM)—The maximum amount of weight that can be lifted for a predetermined number of repetitions with proper exercise technique. For example, a 5RM is the most weight that can be lifted five but not six times.

1-repetition maximum (1RM)—The heaviest weight that can be lifted only once using good form.

repetition—One complete movement of an exercise, which typically consists of a concentric (lifting) and eccentric (lowering) phase.

rescue breathing—Artificial respiration; used to promote oxygenation of blood in an unconscious person who is not breathing.

resistance arm (RA)—Perpendicular distance from the axis of rotation to the direction of the application of the force resisting movement.

resistance force (R)—The opposing force that is resisting another force.

resistance training—A method of exercise designed to enhance musculoskeletal strength, power, and local muscular endurance. Resistance training encompasses a wide range of training modalities including weight machines, free weights, medicine balls, elastic cords, and body weight.

respect—Objective, nonjudgmental regard for another person's values, beliefs, rights, and property.

respiratory quotient (RQ) or **respiratory exchange ratio (R)**—The ratio of the volume of carbon dioxide produced to the volume of oxygen used during a given time ($\dot{V}O_2CO_2 \div \dot{V}O_2$).

respiratory shock—A condition in which the lungs are unable to supply enough oxygen to the circulating blood.

resting metabolic rate (RMR)—Number of calories needed to sustain the body under normal resting conditions.

restrictive lung diseases—Diseases that restrict a person's ability to expand the lungs.

rheumatoid arthritis—Debilitating arthritis of unknown cause that can affect few or many joints (pauciarticular and polyarticular, respectively).

risk factor—A characteristic, sign, symptom, or test score that is associated with increased probability of developing a health problem. For example, people with hypertension have increased risk of developing coronary heart disease.

rotation—The movement of a bone around its longitudinal axis.

rotational inertia—Reluctance to rotate; proportional to the mass and distribution of the mass around the axis.

R-R interval—The time interval from the peak of the QRS of one cardiac cycle to the peak of the QRS of the next cycle.

S wave—The first negative wave (preceded by Q or R waves) of the QRS complex in the ECG.

salt tablets—Supplements that generally are not recommended as a means to increase salt in the diet; if used, they must be taken with large amounts of water.

sarcomeres—The basic units of muscle contraction. They contain actin and myosin; tension develops as the myosin cross bridges pull the actin toward the center of the sarcomere.

sarcoplasmic reticulum (SR)—The network of membranes that surround the myofibril; stores calcium needed for muscle contraction.

saturation pressure—Water vapor pressure that exists at a particular temperature when the air is saturated with water.

sciatic nerve—Nerve originating in the sacral area; it is involved in low-back problems that can result in loss of feeling and control in the legs.

scoliosis—An abnormal lateral curvature of the spine.

secondary amenorrhea—A lack of menses for 3 or more consecutive months occurring in females after menarche.

secondary prevention—Steps taken to prevent the recurrence of a heart attack.

second-degree AV block—On an ECG, some but not all P waves precede the QRS complex and result in ventricular depolarization.

set—A group of repetitions performed without stopping.

simple sugars—Monosaccharides and disaccharides, such as glucose, fructose, and sucrose. These carbohydrates provide the majority of calories in candy, soft drinks, and fruit drinks.

sinoatrial (SA) node—A mass of tissue in the right atrium of the heart, near the vena cava, that initiates the heartbeat.

sinus arrhythmia—A normal variant in sinus rhythm in which the R-R interval varies by more than 10% per beat.

sinus bradycardia—Normal heart rhythm and sequence, with a slow HR (below 60 beats $\cdot$ min^{-1} at rest). Sinus bradycardia may indicate a high level of fitness or a mental illness such as depression.

sinus rhythm—The normal timing and sequence of the cardiac events, with the sinus node as a pacemaker; resting rate is between 60 and 100 beats $\cdot$ min^{-1}.

sinus tachycardia—The normal heart rhythm and sequence, with a fast HR (above 100 beats $\cdot$ min^{-1} at rest). Sinus tachycardia may indicate illness or stress.

sliding-filament theory—The theory that muscular tension is generated when the actin in the sarcomere slides over the myosin because of the action of the myosin cross bridges.

specificity—The principle that states that training effects derived from an exercise program are specific to the exercise done (endurance versus strength training) and the muscle fiber types involved.

speed—The ability to move the whole body quickly.

sphygmomanometer—A blood pressure measurement system.

spondylolisthesis—Condition in which the vertebral body and transverse processes slip anteriorly (forward) on the vertebral body below; it is common for L5 to slip over L4.

spondylolysis—A stress fracture in the pars interarticularis.

spot reduction—The myth that exercise emphasizing a particular body part will cause that area to lose fat faster than the rest of the body loses it.

S-T segment—The part of the ECG between the end of the QRS complex and the beginning of the T wave. Depression below (or elevation above) the isoelectric line indicates ischemia.

S-T segment depression—When the S-T segment of the ECG is depressed below the baseline; may signify myocardial ischemia.

S-T segment elevation—When the S-T segment of the ECG is elevated above the baseline; may signify the early (acute) stages of a myocardial infarction.

stability—The ease with which balance is maintained.

standard deviation (SD)—A measure of the deviation from the mean (average) value generalized to the population. One SD above and below the mean includes about 68% of the population, 2 SD includes about 95%, and 3 SD includes about 99% of the population. For example, if the mean $\dot{V}O_2max$ = 25 ml $\cdot$ kg^{-1} $\cdot$ min^{-1} and SD = 3 ml $\cdot$ kg^{-1} $\cdot$ min^{-1}, then you would expect 68% of the population to have $\dot{V}O_2max$ values between 22 (25 – 3) and 28 (25 + 3) ml $\cdot$ kg^{-1} $\cdot$ min^{-1}, 95% of the population to be between 19 and 31 ml $\cdot$ kg^{-1} $\cdot$ min^{-1}, and almost all the population to be between 16 and 34 ml $\cdot$ kg^{-1} $\cdot$ min^{-1}. A special term called the *standard error of estimate (SEE)* is used to indicate the standard deviation of any estimate derived for a prediction formula.

steady-state oxygen requirement—When the oxygen uptake levels off during submaximal work, so that the oxygen uptake value represents the steady-state oxygen (ATP) requirement for the activity.

strength—The maximal force a muscle or muscle group can generate at a specified velocity.

strength training—See *resistance training*.

stroke—A vascular accident (embolism, hemorrhage, or thrombosis) in the brain, often resulting in sudden loss of body function.

structural curve—Curve that cannot be removed in normal movement because of chronically shortened musculotendinous units or ligaments.

submaximal—Less than maximal (e.g., an exercise that can be performed with less than maximal effort).

sulfur dioxide (SO_2)—A pollutant that can cause bronchoconstriction in people with asthma.

summation—The additive effect of force generated during higher rates of stimulation when the muscle fiber does not completely relax between stimuli.

sweating—The process of moisture coming through the pores of the skin from the sweat glands, usually as a result of heat, exertion, or emotion.

synarthrodial joint—Immovable joint.

synovial membrane—The inner lining of the joint capsule; secretes synovial fluid into the joint cavity.

systolic blood pressure (SBP)—The pressure exerted on the vessel walls during ventricular contraction, measured in millimeters of mercury by a sphygmomanometer.

T wave—On an ECG, the wave that follows the QRS complex and represents ventricular repolarization.

tachycardia—HR greater than 100 beats $\cdot$ min^{-1} at rest. Tachycardia may be seen in deconditioned people or people who are apprehensive about a situation (e.g., an exercise test).

tachypnea—Excessively rapid breathing that may be a sign of overexertion, shock, or hyperventilation.

talocrural joint—Ankle joint.

target heart rate (THR)—The heart rate recommended for fitness workouts.

tendon—A band of tough, inelastic, fibrous connective tissue that attaches muscle to bone.

tetanus—Increase in skeletal muscle tension in response to very high-stimulation frequencies. The resulting contractions fuse together into a smooth, sustained, high-tension contraction.

thermic effect of food—The energy needed to digest, absorb, transport, and store the food that is eaten.

third-degree AV block—On an ECG, the QRS appears independently, the P-R interval varies with no regular pattern, and HR is less than 45 beats $\cdot$ min^{-1}.

threshold—The minimum level needed for a desired effect; often used to refer to the minimum level of exercise intensity needed for improving cardiorespiratory function.

thrombosis—A blood clot in a blood vessel.

Tolerable Upper Intake Level (UL)—The highest intake of a nutrient believed to pose no health risk.

torque (T)—The effect produced by a force causing rotation; the product of the force and length of the force arm.

total cholesterol—The sum of all forms of cholesterol in the bloodstream. Because LDL-C is usually the primary factor in the total amount, a high level of total cholesterol is also a risk factor for CHD.

total fitness—Optimal quality of life, including social, mental, spiritual, and physical components. Also called *wellness* or *positive health.*

total work—The amount of work accomplished during a workout.

tranquilizers—Medications that bring tranquility by calming, soothing, quieting, or pacifying.

trans fats (trans fatty acids)—Hydrogenated fats created to be solid at room temperature and to be used in cooking. Consuming these fats lowers high-density lipid cholesterol (HDL-C) and raises low-density lipid cholesterol (LDL-C).

transfer of angular momentum—Angular momentum can be transferred from one body segment to another by stabilizing the initial moving part at a joint.

transtheoretical model—A general model of intentional behavior change in which behavior change is seen as a dynamic process that occurs through a series of interrelated stages. Basic concepts emphasize the individual's motivational readiness to change, the cognitive and behavioral strategies for changing behavior, self-efficacy, and the evaluation of the pros and cons of the new behavior.

transverse tubule—Connects the sarcolemma (muscle membrane) to the sarcoplasmic reticulum; action potentials move down the transverse tubule to cause the sarcoplasmic reticulum to release calcium to initiate muscle contraction.

treadmill—A machine with a moving belt that can be adjusted for speed and grade, allowing a person to walk or run in place. Treadmills are used extensively for exercise testing and training.

tricuspid valve—A valve located between the right atrium and right ventricle of the heart.

triglycerides—The primary storage form of fat in the human body.

tropomyosin—A protein (part of the thin filament) that regulates muscle contraction; works with troponin.

troponin—A protein (part of the thin filament) that can bind the calcium released from the sarcoplasmic reticulum; works with tropomyosin to allow the myosin cross bridge to interact with actin and initiate cross-bridge movement.

two-compartment model—Model that divides the body into fat and fat-free component parts.

type 1 diabetes—Type of diabetes mellitus in which insulin is not produced. It is caused by damage to the beta-cells of the pancreas.

type 2 diabetes—Type of diabetes mellitus in which the insulin receptors lose their sensitivity to insulin.

type I or **slow oxidative fiber**—A muscle fiber that contracts slowly and generates a small amount of tension with most of the energy coming from aerobic processes; active in light-to-moderate activities and possesses great endurance.

type IIa or **fast oxidative glycolytic fiber**—A muscle that contracts quickly, can produce energy aerobically, and generates great tension; adds to type I fiber's tension as exercise intensity increases.

type IIx or **fast glycolytic fiber**—A muscle fiber that contracts quickly and generates great tension; produces energy by anaerobic metabolism and fatigues quickly.

universal precaution—Safety measures taken to prevent exposure to blood or other body fluids.

ventilatory threshold—The intensity of work at which the rate of ventilation increases sharply during a GXT.

ventricular fibrillation—The heart contracts in an unorganized, quivering manner, with no discernible P waves or QRS complexes on the ECG; requires immediate emergency attention.

ventricular tachycardia—An extremely dangerous condition in which three or more consecutive premature ventricular contractions occur. Ventricular tachycardia may degenerate into ventricular fibrillation.

vital capacity (VC)—The greatest amount of air that can be exhaled after a maximal inspiration. A person whose VC is less than 75% of the value predicted for his age, sex, and height should be referred to a physician for further testing.

vitamins—Organic substances essential to the normal functioning of the human body. They may be subdivided into fat soluble and water soluble.

waist-to-hip ratio (WHR)—Waist circumference divided by hip circumference; often used as an indicator of android-type obesity.

water vapor pressure gradient—The gradient between the water vapor pressure on the skin and the water vapor pressure in the air.

weightlifting—A competitive sport in which athletes attempt to lift maximal amounts of weight in the snatch and the clean and jerk exercises.

wellness—Positive health that is more than simply being free from illness.

wet-bulb globe temperature (WBGT)—Heat stress index that considers dry-bulb, wet-bulb, and black-globe temperatures.

wet-bulb temperature (Twb)—Air temperature measured with a thermometer whose bulb is surrounded by a wet wick; an indication of the ability to evaporate moisture from the skin.

windchill index—The temperature equivalent, under calm air conditions, attributable to a combination of temperature and wind velocity.

Z line—Connective tissue elements that mark the beginning and end of the sarcomere.

References

Chapter 1

1. American College of Sports Medicine. 1978. The recommended quality and quantity of exercise for developing and maintaining fitness in healthy adults. *Medicine and Science in Sports and Exercise* 10: vii-x.
2. American College of Sports Medicine. 1998. The recommended quantity and quality of exercise for developing and maintaining cardiorespiratory and muscular fitness in healthy adults. *Medicine and Science in Sports and Exercise* 30:975-991.
3. American College of Sports Medicine. 2006. *ACSM's guidelines for exercise testing and prescription.* 7th ed. Philadelphia: Lippincott Williams & Wilkins.
4. American Heart Association. 1992. Statement on exercise. *Circulation, Internal Medicine* 103:994-995.
5. Anderson, R.N., and B.L. Smith. 2005. Deaths: Leading causes for 2002. *National vital statistics reports* 53(no. 17). Hyattsville, MD: National Center for Health Statistics.
6. Åstrand, P-O., and K. Rodahl. 1986. *Textbook of work physiology.* 3rd ed. New York: McGraw-Hill.
7. Blair, S.N., H.W. Kohl III, R.S. Paffenbarger Jr., D.G. Clark, K.H. Cooper, and L.W. Gibbons. 1989. Physical fitness and all-cause mortality. *Journal of the American Medical Association* 262:2395-2401.
8. Bouchard, C., and L. Perusse. 1994. Heredity, activity level, fitness, and health. In *Physical activity, fitness, and health,* ed. C. Bouchard, R.J. Shephard, and T. Stephens, 106-118. Champaign, IL: Human Kinetics.
9. Caspersen, C.J., K.E. Powell, and G.M. Christensen. 1985. Physical activity, exercise, and physical fitness: Definition and distinctions for health-related research. *Public Health Reports* 100:126-131.
10. Centers for Disease Control and Prevention. 2003. Prevalence of physical activity, including lifestyle activities among adults—United States, 2000-2001. *Morbidity and Mortality Weekly* 52:764-769.
11. Chodzko-Zajko, W.J. 1998. Physical activity and aging: Implications for health and quality of life in older persons. *PCPFS Research Digest* 3(4).
12. Corbin, C.B., R.P. Pangrazi, and G.C. LaMasurier. 2004. Physical activity for children: Current patterns and guidelines. *PCPFS Research Digest* 5(2).
13. Fagard, R.H., and C.M. Tipton. 1994. Physical activity, fitness, and hypertension. In *Physical activity, fitness, and health,* ed. C. Bouchard, R.J. Shephard, and T. Stephens, 633-655. Champaign, IL: Human Kinetics.
14. Franks, B.D. 1997. Personalizing physical activity prescription. *PCPFS Research Digest* 2(9).
15. Gordon, N.F. 1998. Conceptual basis for coronary artery disease risk factor assessment. In *ACSM's resource manual for guidelines for exercise testing and prescription,* 3rd ed. Ed. J.L. Roitman, pp. 3-12. Philadelphia: Lippincott Williams & Wilkins.
16. Haskell, W.L. 1984. The influence of exercise on the concentrations of triglyceride and cholesterol in human plasma. *Exercise and Sport Sciences Reviews* 12:205-244.
17. Haskell, W.L. 1996. Historical background, terminology, evolution of recommendations and measurement. In *Surgeon General's report: Physical activity and health,* ed. S. Blair, pp. 11-57. Washington, DC: U.S. Department of Health and Human Services.
18. Haskell, W.L. 1996. Personal communication.
19. Howley, E.T., D.R. Bassett Jr., and D.L. Thompson. 2005. Get them moving: Balancing weight with physical activity, part II. *ACSM's Health and Fitness Journal* 9:19-23.
20. Jones, W.H.S., trans. 1953. *Regimen (Hippocrates).* Cambridge, MA: Harvard University Press.
21. Kesaniemi, Y.A., E. Danforth Jr., M.D. Jensen, P.G. Kopelman, P. Lefebvre, and B.A. Reeder. 2001. Dose-response issues concerning physical activity and health: An evidence-based symposium. *Medicine and Science in Sports and Exercise* 33: S351-S358.
22. Kohl, H.W., and J.D. McKenzie. 1994. Physical activity, fitness, and stroke. In *Physical activity, fitness, and health,* ed. C. Bouchard, R.J. Shephard, and T. Stephens, 609-621. Champaign, IL: Human Kinetics.
23. Kriska, A. 1997. Physical activity and the prevention of type II diabetes. *PCPFS Research Digest* 2(10).
24. Landers, D.M. 1997. The influence of exercise on mental health. *PCPFS Research Digest* 2(12).
25. Lee, I.M. 1995. Physical activity and cancer. *PCPFS Research Digest* 2(2).
26. Moore, S. 1994. Physical activity, fitness, and atherosclerosis. In *Physical activity, fitness, and health,* ed. C. Bouchard, R.J. Shephard, and T. Stephens, 570-578. Champaign, IL: Human Kinetics.
27. Mokdad, A.H., J.S. Marks, D.F. Stroup, and J.L. Gerberding. 2004. Actual causes of death in the United States, 2000. *Journal of the American Medical Association* 291:1238-1245.
28. Mokdad, A.H., J.S. Marks, D.F. Stroup, and J.L. Gerberding. 2005. Correction: Actual causes of death in the United States, 2000. *Journal of the American Medical Association* 293:293-294.
29. National Institutes of Health. 1996. *Physical activity and cardiovascular health.* Rockville, VA: Author.
30. Paffenbarger, R.S., R.T. Hyde, and A.L. Wing. 1986. Physical activity, all-cause mortality, and longevity of college alumni. *New England Journal of Medicine* 314:605-613.
31. Pate, R.R., M. Pratt, S.N. Blair, W.L. Haskell, C.A. Marcera, and C. Bouchard. 1995. Physical activity and public health: A recommendation from the Centers for Disease Control and Prevention and the American College of Sports Medicine. *Journal of the American Medical Association* 273:402-407.
32. Plowman, S.A. 1993. Physical fitness and healthy low back function. *PCPFS Research Digest* 1(3).
33. Seaman, J.A. 1999. Physical activity and fitness for persons with disabilities. *PCPFS Research Digest* 3(5).
34. Shaw, J.M., and C. Snow-Harter. 1995. Osteoporosis and physical activity. *PCPFS Research Digest* 2(3).
35. Shephard, R. 1996. Exercise, independence, and quality of life in the elderly. *Quest* 48:354-365.
36. Spirduso, W.W., and D.L. Cronin. 2001. Exercise dose–response effects on quality of life and independent living in older adults. *Medicine and Science in Sports and Exercise* 33(Suppl. 6): S598-S608.
37. Strong, W.B., R.M. Malina, C.J.R. Blimkie, S.R. Daniles, R.K. Dishman, B. Gutin, A.C. Hergenroeder, A. Must, P.A. Nixon, J.M.

Pivarnik, T. Rowland, S. Trost, and F. Trudeau. 2005. Evidenced-based physical activity for school-age youth. *Journal of Pediatrics* 146:732-737.

38. Thompson, P.D., and M.C. Fahrenbach. 1994. Risks of exercising: Cardiovascular including sudden cardiac death. In *Physical activity, fitness, and health,* ed. C. Bouchard, R.J. Shephard, and T. Stephens, 1019-1028. Champaign, IL: Human Kinetics.
39. U.S. Department of Agriculture and U.S. Department of Health and Human Services. 2005. *Dietary guidelines for Americans 2005.* Washington, DC: U.S. Government Printing Office.
40. U.S. Department of Health and Human Services. 1991. *Healthy people 2000: National health promotion and disease prevention objectives.* PHS 91-50212. Washington, DC: Author.
41. U.S. Department of Health and Human Services. 1996. *Surgeon General's report on physical activity and health.* Washington, DC: Author.
42. U.S. Department of Health and Human Services. 2000. *Healthy people 2010: National health promotion and disease prevention objectives.* Washington, DC: Author.
43. Welk, G.J., and S.N. Blair. 2000. Physical activity protects against the health risks of obesity. *PCPFS Research Digest* 3(12).
44. Whipp, B.J., and R. Casaburi. 1994. Physical activity, fitness, and chronic lung disease. In *Physical activity, fitness, and health,* ed. C. Bouchard, R.J. Shephard, and T. Stephens, 749-761. Champaign, IL: Human Kinetics.

Chapter 2

1. Caspersen, C.J., K.E. Powell, and G.M. Christensen. 1985. Physical activity, exercise, and physical fitness: Definition and distinctions for health-related research. *Public Health Reports* 100:126-131.
2. Corbin, C.B., R.P. Pangrazi, and B.D. Franks. 2000. Definitions: Health, fitness, and physical activity. *PCPFS Research Digest* 3(9).
3. U.S. Department of Health and Human Services. 2000. *Healthy people 2010: National health promotion and disease prevention objectives.* Washington, DC: Author.

Chapter 3

1. American College of Sports Medicine. 2006. *ACSM's guidelines for exercise testing and prescription.* 7th ed. Philadelphia: Lippincott Williams & Wilkins.
2. American College of Sports Medicine. 2006. ACSM 's resource manual for guidelines for exercise testing and prescription (5th ed.). Philadelphia: Lippincott Williams & Wilkins.
3. American College of Sports Medicine. 2007. ACSM 's health/fitness facility standards and guidelines (3rd ed.). Champaign, IL: Lippincott Williams & Wilkins.
4. American College of Sports Medicine and American Heart Association. 1998. ACSM/AHA joint position statement: Recommendations for cardiovascular screening, staffing, and emergency policies at health/fitness facilities. *Medicine and Science in Sports and Exercise* 30(6):1009-1018.
5. American Heart Association Science Advisory. 1997. Guide to primary prevention of cardiovascular diseases: A statement for healthcare professionals from the task force on risk reduction. *Circulation* 95:2-4.
6. Balady, G., B. Chaitman, D. Driscoll, C. Foster, E. Froelicher, N. Gordon, R. Pate, J. Rippe, and T. Bazzarre. 1998 American Heart Association and American College of Sports Medicine Joint Scientific Statement: Recommendations for cardiovascular screening, staffing, and emergency policies at health/fitness facilities. *Medicine and Science in Sports and Exercise* 30(96): 1009-1018.
7. Canadian Fitness Safety Standards and Recommended Guidelines. 2005. Ontario association of sport and end exercise sciences. www.csep.ca/forms.asp.
8. Cardinal B., J. Esters, and M. Cardinal. 1996. Evaluation of the revised physical activity readiness questionnaire in older adults. *Medicine and Science in Sports and Exercise* 28(5):468-472.
9. Expert Panel on Detection, Evaluation, and Treatment of High Blood Cholesterol in Adults. 2001. Executive summary of the third report of the National Cholesterol Education Program (NCEP)(Adult Treatment Panel III). *Journal of the American Medical Association* 285(19):2486-2497.
10. Fletcher, G., G. Balady, S. Blair, J. Blumenthal, C. Caspersen, B. Chaitman, S. Epstein, E. Froelicher, V. Froelicher, I . Pina, and M. Pollock. 1996. Statement on exercise: Benefits and recommendations for physical activity programs for all Americans. *Circulation* 94:857-862.
11. Fletcher, G., G. Balady, V. Froelicher, L. Hartley, W. Haskell, and M. Pollock. 1995. Exercise standards: A statement from the American Heart Association. *Circulation* 91:580-615.
12. Franke, W. 2005. Covering all bases: Working with new clients. *ACSM's Health and Fitness Journal* 9(2):13-17.
13. Gibbons, R., G. Balady, J. Bricker, B. Chaitman, G. Fletcher, V. Froelicher, D. Mark et al. ACC/AHA 2002 guideline update to exercise testing: Summary article. 2002. A report of the American College of Cardiology/American Heart Association task force on practice guidelines (Committee to update the 1997 exercise testing guidelines). *Journal of the American College of Cardiology* 40(8):1531-1540.
14. Goodyear, L., and B. Kahn. 1998. Exercise, glucose transport, and insulin sensitivity. *Annual Reviews in Medicine* 49:235-261.
15. Grundy, S., R. Pasternak, P. Greenland, S. Smith Jr., and V. Fuster. (1999). Assessment of cardiovascular risk by use of multiple-risk-factor assessment equations: A statement for healthcare professionals from the American Heart Association and the American College of Cardiology. *Circulation* 100:1481-1492.
16. Painter, P., and W.H. Haskell. 1998. Decision making in programming exercise. In *Resource manual for guidelines for exercise testing and prescription,* ed. S.N. Blair, P. Painter, R.R. Pate, L.K. Smith, and C.B. Taylor, pp. 256-262. Philadelphia: Lea & Febiger.
17. *Health Insurance Portability and Accountability Act, Subtitle F Section 1171 4(a).* August 21, 1996. Public law 104-191, 104th Cong.

Chapter 4

1. Ainsworth, B.E., W.L. Haskell, M.C. Whitt, M.I. Irwin, A.M. Swartz, S.J. Strath, W.L. O'Brien, D.R. Bassett Jr., K.H. Schmitz, P.O. Emplaincourt, D.R. Jacobs Jr., and A.S. Leon. 2000. Compendium of physical activities: An update of activity codes and MET intensities. *Medicine and Science in Sports and Exercise* 32:S498-S516.
2. American College of Sports Medicine. 1980. *Guidelines for graded exercise testing and exercise prescription.* 2nd ed. Philadelphia: Lea & Febiger.
3. American College of Sports Medicine. 2006. *ACSM's guidelines for exercise testing and prescription.* 7th ed. Baltimore: Lippincott Williams & Wilkins.
4. Åstrand, P-O. 1979. *Work tests with the bicycle ergometer.* Verberg, Sweden: Monark-Crescent AB.
5. Åstrand, P-O., and K. Rodahl. 1986. *Textbook of work physiology.* 3rd ed. New York: McGraw-Hill.
6. Balke, B. 1963. A simple field test for assessment of physical fitness. In *Civil Aeromedical Research Institute report,* 63-66. Oklahoma City: Civil Aeromedical Research Institute.

7. Balke, B., and R.W. Ware. 1959. An experimental study of "physical fitness" of Air Force personnel. *Armed Forces Medical Journal* 10:675-688.
8. Bassett Jr., D.R., M.D. Giese, F.J. Nagle, A. Ward, D.M. Raab, and B. Balke. 1985. Aerobic requirements of overground versus treadmill running. *Medicine and Science in Sports and Exercise* 17:477-481.
9. Bransford, D.R., and E.T. Howley. 1977. The oxygen cost of running in trained and untrained men and women. *Medicine and Science in Sports* 9:41-44.
10. Bubb, W.J., A.D. Martin, and E.T. Howley. 1985. Predicting oxygen uptake during level walking at speeds of 80 to 130 meters per minute. *Journal of Cardiac Rehabilitation* 5(10): 462-465.
11. Daniels, J.T. 1985. A physiologist's view of running economy. *Medicine and Science in Sports and Exercise* 17:332-338.
12. Dill, D.B. 1965. Oxygen cost of horizontal and grade walking and running on the treadmill. *Journal of Applied Physiology* 20:19-22.
13. Franklin, B.A. 1985. Exercise testing, training, and arm ergometry. *Sports Medicine* 2:100-119.
14. Haskell, W.L., W. Savin, N. Oldridge, and R. DeBusk. 1982. Factors influencing estimated oxygen uptake during exercise testing soon after myocardial infarction. *American Journal of Cardiology* 50:299-304.
15. Holmer, I. 1979. Physiology of swimming man. *Exercise and Sport Sciences Reviews* 7:87-123.
16. Howley, E.T., and M.E. Glover. 1974. The caloric costs of running and walking 1 mile for men and women. *Medicine and Science in Sports* 6:235-237.
17. Howley, E.T., and D. Martin. 1978. Oxygen uptake and heart-rate responses measured during rope skipping. *Tennessee Journal of Health, Physical Education and Recreation* 16:7-8.
18. Knoebel, L.K. 1984. Energy metabolism. In *Physiology.* 5th ed. Ed. E. Selkurt, 635-650. Boston: Little, Brown.
19. Margaria, R., P. Cerretelli, P. Aghemo, and J. Sassi. 1963. Energy cost of running. *Journal of Applied Physiology* 18:367-370.
20. Montoye, H.J., T. Ayen, F. Nagle, and E.T. Howley. 1986. The oxygen requirement for horizontal and grade walking on a motor-driven treadmill. *Medicine and Science in Sports and Exercise* 17:640-645.
21. Nagle, F.J., B. Balke, G. Baptista, J. Alleyia, and E. Howley. 1971. Compatibility of progressive treadmill, bicycle, and step tests based on oxygen-uptake responses. *Medicine and Science in Sport* 3:149-154.
22. Nagle, F.J., B. Balke, and J.P. Naughton. 1965. Gradational step tests for assessing work capacity. *Journal of Applied Physiology* 20:745-748.
23. Sharkey, B.J. 1990. *Physiology of fitness.* 3rd ed. Champaign, IL: Human Kinetics.
24. Williford, H.N., M. Scharff-Olson, and D.L. Blessing. 1989. The physiological effects of aerobic dance—A review. *Sports Medicine* 8:335-345.

Chapter 5

1. American College of Sports Medicine. 2006. *ACSM's guidelines for exercise testing and prescription.* 7th ed. Philadelphia: Lippincott Williams & Wilkins.
2. American College of Sports Medicine. 2006. *ACSM's resource manual for guidelines for exercise testing and prescription.* 5th ed. Baltimore: Lippincott Williams & Wilkins.
3. Åstrand, I. 1960. Aerobic work capacity in men and women with special reference to age. *Acta Physiologica Scandinavica* 49(Suppl. 169): 1-92.
4. Åstrand, P-O. 1979. *Work tests with the bicycle ergometer.* Varberg, Sweden: Monark-Crescent AB.
5. Åstrand, P-O. 1984. Principles of ergometry and their implications in sport practice. *International Journal of Sports Medicine* 5:102-105.
6. Åstrand, P-O., and I. Rhyming. 1954. A nomogram for calculation of aerobic capacity (physical fitness) from pulse rate during submaximal work. *Journal of Applied Physiology* 7:218-221.
7. Åstrand, P-O., and B. Saltin. 1961. Maximal oxygen uptake and heart rate in various types of muscular activity. *Journal of Applied Physiology* 16:977-981.
8. Balke, B. 1963. A simple field test for assessment of physical fitness. In *Civil Aeromedical Research Institute report,* 63-66. Oklahoma City: Civil Aeromedical Research Institute.
9. Balke, B. 1970. *Advanced exercise procedures for evaluation of the cardiovascular system* (Monograph). Milton, WI: Burdick.
10. Baum, W.A. 1961. Sphygmomanometers, principles and precepts. New York: Baum.
11. Blair, S.N., H.W. Kohl III, R.S. Paffenbarger Jr., D.G. Clark, K.H. Cooper, and L.W. Gibbons. 1989. Physical fitness and all-cause mortality. *Journal of the American Medical Association* 262:2395-2401.
12. Borg, G. 1998. *Borg's perceived exertion and pain scales.* Champaign, IL: Human Kinetics.
13. Bransford, D.R., and E.T. Howley. 1977. The oxygen cost of running in trained and untrained men and women. *Medicine and Science in Sports* 9:41-44.
14. Bruce, R.A. 1972. Multistage treadmill test of submaximal and maximal exercise. In *Exercise testing and training of apparently healthy individuals: A handbook for physicians,* ed. American Heart Association, 32-34. New York: American Heart Association.
15. Cooper, K.H. 1977. *The aerobics way.* New York: Bantam Books.
16. Cooper Institute for Aerobics Research. 1999. *FITNESSGRAM test administration manual.* Champaign, IL: Human Kinetics.
17. Daniels, J.T. 1985. A physiologist's view of running economy. *Medicine and Science in Sports and Exercise* 17:332-338.
18. Daniels, J., N. Oldridge, F. Nagle, and B. White. 1978. Differences and changes in $\dot{V}O_2$ among young runners 10-18 years of age. *Medicine and Science in Sports* 10:200-203.
19. Ellestad, M. 1994. *Stress testing: Principles and practice.* Philadelphia: Davis.
20. Franks, B.D. 1979. Methodology of the exercise ECG test. In *Exercise electrocardiography: Practical approach,* ed. E.K. Chung, 46-61. Baltimore: Williams & Wilkins.
21. Frohlich, E.D., C. Grim, D.R. Labarthe, M.H. Maxwell, D. Perloff, and W.H. Weidman. 1988. Recommendations for human blood-pressure determination by sphygmomanometers. *Circulation* 77:501A-514A.
22. Golding, L.A. 2000. *YMCA fitness testing and assessment manual.* 4th edition. Champaign, IL: Human Kinetics.
23. Hagberg, J.M., J.P. Mullin, M.D. Giese, and E. Spitznagel. 1981. Effect of pedaling rate on submaximal exercise responses of competitive cyclists. *Journal of Applied Physiology* 51:447-451.
24. Howley, E.T. 1988. The exercise testing laboratory. In *Resource manual for guidelines for exercise testing and prescription,* ed. S.N. Blair, P. Painter, R.R. Pate, L.K. Smith, and C.B. Taylor, 406-413. Philadelphia: Lea & Febiger.
25. Kline, G.M., J.P. Porcari, R. Hintermeister, P.S. Freedson, A. Ward, R.F. McCarron, J. Ross, and J.M. Rippe. 1987. Estimation of $\dot{V}O_2$max from a 1-mile track walk, gender, age, and body weight. *Medicine and Science in Sports and Exercise* 19:253-259.

26. Maritz, J.S., J.F. Morrison, J. Peter, N.B. Strydom, and C.H. Wyndham. 1961. A practical method of estimating an individual's maximal oxygen uptake. *Ergonomics* 4:97-122.

27. McArdle, W.D., F.I. Katch, and G.S. Pechar. 1973. Comparison of continuous and discontinuous treadmill and bicycle tests for max $\dot{V}O_2$. *Medicine and Science in Sports* 5(3):156-160.

28. Montoye, H.J., and T. Ayen. 1986. Body-size adjustment for oxygen requirement in treadmill walking. *Research Quarterly for Exercise and Sport* 57:82-84.

29. Montoye, H.J., T. Ayen, F. Nagle, and E.T. Howley. 1986. The oxygen requirement for horizontal and grade walking on a motor-driven treadmill. *Medicine and Science in Sports and Exercise* 17:640-645.

30. Naughton, J.P., and R. Haider. 1973. Methods of exercise testing. In *Exercise testing and exercise training in coronary heart disease,* ed. J.P. Naughton, H.R. Hellerstein, and L.C. Mohler, 79-91. New York: Academic Press.

31. Oldridge, N.B., W.L. Haskell, and P. Single. 1981. Carotid palpation, coronary heart disease, and exercise rehabilitation. *Medicine and Science in Sports and Exercise* 13:6-8.

32. Pollock, M.L., and J.H. Wilmore. 1990. *Exercise in health and disease.* 2nd ed. Philadelphia: Saunders.

33. President's Council on Physical Fitness and Sports. 2002. *President's Challenge Physical Activity and Fitness Award Program.* Washington, DC: Author.

34. Shephard, R.J. 1970. Computer programs for solution of the Åstrand nomogram and the calculation of body surface area. *Journal of Sports Medicine and Physical Fitness* 10:206-210.

Chapter 6

1. American College of Sports Medicine. 2006. *ACSM's guidelines for exercise testing and prescription.* Baltimore, MD: Lippincott Williams & Wilkins.

2. Cataldo, D., and V.H. Heyward. 2000. Pinch an inch: A comparison of several high-quality and plastic skinfold calipers. *ACSM's Health and Fitness Journal* 4:12-16.

3. Dempster, P., and S. Aitkens. 1995. A new air displacement method for the determination of human body composition. *Medicine and Science in Sports and Exercise* 27:1692-1697.

4. Fields, D., M. Goran, and M. McCrory. 2002. Body composition assessment via air-displacement plethysmography in adults and children: A review. *American Journal of Clinical Nutrition* 75:453-467.

5. Flegal, K.M., M.D. Carroll, C.L. Ogden, and C.L. Johnson. 2002. Prevalence and trends in obesity among US adults, 1999-2000. *Journal of the American Medical Association,* 288:1723-1727.

6. Flegal, K.M., B.I. Graubard, D.F. Williamson, and M.H. Gail. 2005. Excess deaths associated with underweight, overweight, and obesity. *Journal of the American Medical Association* 293:1861-1867.

7. Folsom, A., L. Kushi, K. Anderson, P. Mink, J. Olson, C-P. Hong, T. Sellers, D. Lazovich, and R. Prineas. 2000. Associations of general and abdominal obesity with multiple health outcomes in older women. *Archives of Internal Medicine* 160:2117-2128.

8. Goldman, H.I., and M.R. Becklake. 1959. Respiratory function tests. *American Review of Tuberculosis and Pulmonary Disease* 79:457-467.

9. Hedley, A.A., C.L. Ogden, C.L. Johnson, M.D. Carroll, L.R. Curtin, and K.M. Flegal. 2004. Prevalence of overweight and obesity among U.S. children, adolescents, and adults, 1999-2002. *Journal of the American Medical Association* 291:2847-2850.

10. Heymsfield, S.B., S. Lichtman, R.N. Baumgartner, J. Wang, Y. Kamen, A. Aliprantis, N. Richard, and J. Pierson. 1990. Body composition of humans: Comparison of two improved four-compartment models that differ in expense, technical complexity, and radiation exposure. *American Journal of Clinical Nutrition* 52:52-58.

11. Heyward, V.H., and D.R. Wagner. 2004. *Applied body composition assessment.* Champaign, IL: Human Kinetics.

12. Hu, G., J. Tuomilehto, K. Silventoinen, N. Barengo, and P. Jousilahti. 2004. Joint effects of physical activity, body mass index, waist circumference and waist-to-hip ratio with the risk of cardiovascular disease among Finnish men and women. *European Heart Journal* 25:2212-2219.

13. Jackson, A.S., and M.L. Pollock. 1978. Generalized equations for predicting body density of men. *British Journal of Nutrition* 40:497-504.

14. Jackson, A.S., and M.L. Pollock. 1985. Practical assessment of body composition. *Physician and Sportsmedicine* 13:76-90.

15. Jackson, A.S., M.L. Pollock, and A. Ward. 1980. Generalized equations for predicting body density of women. *Medicine and Science in Sports and Exercise* 12:175-182.

16. Janssen, I., P.T. Katzmarzyk, and R. Ross. 2004. Waist circumference and not body mass index explains obesity-related health risk. *American Journal of Clinical Nutrition* 79:379-384.

17. Kaminsky, L.A., and G. Dwyer. 2006. Body composition. In *ACSM's resource manual for guidelines for exercise testing and prescription,* ed. L.A. Kaminsky, 195-205. Baltimore: Lippincott Williams & Wilkins.

18. Kohrt, W.M. 1995. Body composition by DXA: Tried and true? *Medicine and Science in Sports and Exercise* 27:1349-1353.

19. Lohman, T.G. 1986. Applicability of body composition techniques and constants for children and youth. In *Exercise and Sports Science Reviews,* ed. K.B. Pandolf, 325-357. New York: Macmillan.

20. Lohman, T.G. 1992. *Advances in body composition assessment.* Champaign, IL: Human Kinetics.

21. Lohman, T.G., L. Houtkooper, and S.B. Going. 1997. Body fat measurement goes high-tech: Not all are created equal. *ACSM's Health and Fitness Journal* 1:30-35.

22. Lohman, T.G., A.F. Roche, and R. Martorell. 1988. *Anthropometric standardization reference manual.* Champaign, IL: Human Kinetics.

23. Mark, D.H. 2005. Deaths attributable to obesity. *Journal of the American Medical Association* 293:1918-1919.

24. McCrory, M.A., T.D. Gomez, E.M. Bernauer, and P.A. Mole. 1995. Evaluation of a new air displacement plethysmograph for measuring human body composition. *Medicine and Science in Sports and Exercise* 27:1686-1691.

25. Mokdad, A.H., J.S. Marks, D.F. Stroup, and J.L. Gerberding. 2004. Actual causes of death in the United States, 2000 [published correction appears in *JAMA* 2005; 293:298]. *Journal of the American Medical Association* 291:1238-1245.

26. National Heart, Lung, and Blood Institute. 1998. *Clinical guidelines on the identification, evaluation, and treatment of overweight and obesity in adults* (NIH Publication No. 98-4083). Bethesda, MD: National Institutes of Health—National Heart, Lung, and Blood Institute.

27. National Institutes of Health. 1994. *Bioelectrical impedance analysis in body composition measurement: NIH Technology Assessment Conference statement.* Bethesda, MD: National Institutes of Health.

28. Schutte, J.E., E.M. Townsend, J. Hugg, R.F. Shoup, R.M. Malina, and C.G. Blomqvist. 1984. Density of lean body mass is greater in Blacks than in Whites. *Journal of Applied Physiology: Respiratory, Environmental, and Exercise Physiology* 56:1647-1649.

29. Siri, W.E. 1961. Body composition from fluid spaces and density: Analysis of methods. In *Techniques for Measuring Body Composition,* ed. J. Brozek and A. Henschel, 223-244. Washington, DC: National Academy of Sciences.

30. Weltman, A., S. Levine, R.L. Seip, and Z.V. Tran. 1988. Accurate assessment of body composition in obese females. *American Journal of Clinical Nutrition* 48:1179-1183.

31. Weltman, A., R.L. Seip, and Z.V. Tran. 1987. Practical assessment of body composition in obese males. *Human Biology* 59:523-536.

32. Wilmore, J. 1969. A simplified method for determination of residual volume. *Journal of Applied Physiology* 27:96-100.

Chapter 7

1. American College of Sports Medicine. 1996. Position stand on exercise and fluid replacement. *Medicine and Science in Sports and Exercise* 28: i-vii.

2. American College of Sports Medicine. 1997. Position stand on the female athlete triad. *Medicine and Science in Sports and Exercise* 29(5): i-ix.

3. American College of Sports Medicine. 2000. The physiological and health effects of oral creatine supplementation. *Medicine and Science in Sports and Exercise* 32(3): 706-717.

4. American College of Sports Medicine, American Dietetic Association, and Dietitians of Canada. 2000. Nutrition and athletic performance. *Medicine and Science in Sports and Exercise* 32(12): 2130-2145.

5. American Diabetes Association. 2004. Nutrition principles and recommendations in diabetes. *Diabetes Care* 27 (Suppl. 1): S36-S46.

6. American Dietetic Association and Canadian Dietetic Association. 1993. Nutrition for physical fitness and athletic performance for adults. *Journal of the American Dietetic Association* 93: 691-696.

7. American Dietetic Association. 1997. Health implications of dietary fiber—Position of the ADA. *Journal of the American Dietetic Association* 97: 1157-1159.

8. Berning, J.R. 1995. Nutritional concerns of recreational endurance athletes with an emphasis on swimming. In *Nutrition for the recreational athlete,* ed. C.G.R. Jackson, 55-68. Boca Raton, FL: CRC Press.

9. Brodney-Folse, S., and R.A. Carpenter. 2006. Assessment of dietary intake. In *ACSM's resource manual for guidelines for exercise testing and prescription.* 5th ed. Ed. L. Kaminsky, 165-178. Baltimore: Lippincott Williams & Wilkins.

10. Casa, D.J., L.E. Armstrong, S.K. Hillman, S.J. Montain, R.V. Reiff, B.S.E. Rich, W.O. Roberts, and J.A. Stone. 2000. National Athletic Trainers' Association position statement: Fluid replacement for athletes. *Journal of Athletic Training* 35(2): 212-224.

11. Driskell, J.A. 2000. *Sports nutrition.* Boca Raton, FL: CRC Press.

12. Durstine, J.L., and W.L. Haskell. 1994. Effects of exercise training on plasma lipids and lipoproteins. *Exercise and Sport Sciences Reviews* 22: 477-521.

13. Expert Panel on Detection, Evaluation, and Treatment of High Blood Cholesterol in Adults. 2001. Executive Summary of the Third Report of the National Cholesterol Education Program (NCEP) Expert Panel on detection, evaluation, and treatment of high blood cholesterol in adults (Adult Treatment Panel III). *Journal of the American Medical Association* 285(19): 2486-2497.

14. Food and Nutrition Board, Institute of Medicine. 2000. *Dietary reference intakes: Applications in dietary assessment.* Washington, DC: National Academy Press.

15. Food and Nutrition Board, Institute of Medicine. 2001. *Dietary reference intakes for vitamin A, vitamin K, arsenic, boron, chromium, copper, iodine, iron, manganese, molybdenum, nickel, silicon, vanadium, and zinc.* Washington, DC: National Academy Press.

16. Food and Nutrition Board, Institute of Medicine. 2002. *Dietary reference intakes for energy, carbohydrate, fiber, fat, fatty acids, cholesterol, protein, and amino acids.* Washington, DC: National Academies Press.

17. Food and Nutrition Board, Institute of Medicine. 2004. *Dietary reference intakes for water, potassium, sodium, chloride, and sulfate.* Washington, DC: National Academies Press.

18. Krenkel, J., S. St. Jeor, and D. Kulick. 2006. Relationship of nutrition to chronic disease. In *ACSM's resource manual for guidelines for exercise testing and prescription.* 5th ed. Ed. L. Kaminsky, 146-164. Baltimore: Lippincott Williams & Wilkins.

19. Messina, V., V. Melina, and A.R. Mangels. 2003. A new food guide for North American vegetarians. *Canadian Journal of Dietetic Practice and Research* 64:82-86.

20. Morris, K.L., and M.B. Zemel. 1999. Glycemic index, cardiovascular disease, and obesity. *Nutrition Reviews* 57(9): 273-276.

21. National Institutes of Health. 2000. *Osteoporosis prevention, diagnosis, and therapy: NIH Consensus Development Conference statement.* Bethesda, MD: Author.

22. Ruud, J.S., and I. Wolinsky. 1995. Nutritional concerns of recreational strength athletes. In *Nutrition for the recreational athlete,* ed. C.G.R. Jackson, 55-68. Boca Raton, FL: CRC Press.

23. U.S. Department of Health and Human Services and U.S. Department of Agriculture. 2005. *Dietary guidelines for Americans, 2005.* 6th ed. Washington, DC: U.S. Government Printing Office.

24. Walberg-Rankin, J. 1997. Glycemic index and exercise metabolism. *Gatorade Sports Science Institute: Sports Science Exchange* 10(1): 1-7.

25. Westerterp, K.R. 2000. The assessment of energy and nutrient intake in humans. In *Physical activity and obesity,* ed. C. Bouchard, 133-149. Champaign, IL: Human Kinetics.

26. Williams, M.H. 1998. Nutritional ergogenics and sports performance. *PCPFS Physical Activity and Fitness Research Digest* 3(2): 1-14.

Chapter 8

1. American Association of Cardiovascular and Pulmonary Rehabilitation. 1999. *Guidelines for cardiac rehabilitation and secondary prevention programs.* 3rd ed. Champaign, IL: Human Kinetics.

2. American College of Sports Medicine. 1998. ACSM position stand on exercise and physical activity for older adults. *Medicine and Science in Sports and Exercise* 30:992-1008.

3. American College of Sports Medicine. 1998. ACSM position stand: The recommended quantity and quality of exercise for developing and maintaining cardiorespiratory and muscular fitness, and flexibility in healthy adults. *Medicine and Science in Sports and Exercise* 30:875-991.

4. American College of Sports Medicine. 2006. *ACSM's guidelines for exercise testing and prescription.* 7th ed. Baltimore: Lippincott Williams & Wilkins.

5. Bohannon, R.W. 1990. Muscle strength testing with handheld dynamometers. In *Muscle strength testing: Instrumented and non-instrumented systems,* ed. L.R. Amundsen, 69-112. New York: Churchill Livingstone.

6. Bohannon, R.W. 1995. Sit to stand test for measuring performance of lower extremity muscles. *Perceptual and Motor Skills* 80:163-166.

7. Borg, G. 1982. Psychophysical bases of perceived exertion. *Medicine and Science in Sports and Exercise* 14:377-381.

8. Government of Canada, Fitness and Amateur Sport. 1986. *Canadian Standardized Test of Fitness operations manual.* 3rd ed. Ottawa: Author.

9. Csuka, M., and D.J. McCarty. 1985. Simple method for measurement of lower extremity muscle strength. *Journal of the American Medical Association* 78:77-81.

10. Diener, M.H., L.A. Golding, and D. Diener. 1995. Validity and reliability of a one-minute half sit-up test of abdominal muscle strength and endurance. *Sports Medicine Training and Rehabilitation* 6:105-119.

11. Faigenbaum, A., G. Skrinar, W. Cesare, W. Kraemer, and H. Thomas. 1990. Physiologic and symptomatic responses of cardiac patients to resistance exercise. *Archives of Physical Medicine and Rehabilitation* 71:395-398.

12. Faulkner, R.A., E.S. Springings, A. McQuarrie, R.D. Bell. 1989. A partial curl-up protocol for adults based on an analysis of two procedures. *Canadian Journal of Sports Science* 14:135-141.

13. Featherstone, J.F., R. Holly, and E. Amsterdam. 1993. Physiologic responses to weight lifting in coronary artery disease. *American Journal of Cardiology* 71:287-292.

14. Fletcher, G.F., G. Balady, V.F. Froelicher, L.H. Hartley, W.L. Haskell, and M.L. Pollock. 1995. Exercise standards: A statement for healthcare professionals from the American Heart Association. *Circulation* 91:580-615.

15. Golding, L.A., C.R. Myers, and W.E. Sinning. 1989. *The Y's way to physical fitness.* 3rd ed. Champaign, IL: Human Kinetics.

16. Graves, J.E., M.L. Pollock, and C.X. Bryant. 2001. Assessment of muscular strength and endurance. In *ACSM's resource manual for guidelines for exercise testing and prescription.* 4th ed. Ed. J.L. Roitman, 376-380. Baltimore: Williams & Wilkins.

17. Guralnik, J.M., E.M. Simosick, L. Ferrucci, R.J. Glynn, L.F. Berkman, D.G. Blazer, P.A. Scherr, and R.B. Wallace. 1994. A short physical performance battery assessing lower extremity function: Association with self reported disability and prediction of mortality and nursing home admission. *Journal of Gerontology* 49:M85-M94.

18. Haslam, K.A., S.N. McCartney, R.S. McKelvie, and J.D. MacDougall. 1988. Direct measurements of arterial blood pressure during formal weightlifting in cardiac patients. *Journal of Cardiopulmonary Rehabilitation* 8:213-225.

19. Jackson, A.W., J.R. Morrow, P.A. Brill, and H.W. Kohl. 1998. Relations of sit-up and sit-and-reach to low back pain in adults. *Journal of Orthopaedic and Sports Physical Therapy* 27:22-26.

20. Jones, C.J., R.E. Rikli, and B.C. Beam. 1999. A 30-s chair-stand test as a measure of lower body strength in community residing older adults. *Research Quarterly for Exercise and Sports* 70:113-119.

21. Kraemer, W., and A. Fry. 1995. Strength testing development and evaluation of methodology. In *Physiological assessments of human fitness,* ed. P.J. Maud and C. Foster, 115-138. Champaign, IL: Human Kinetics.

22. Lawrence, R., and A.M. Jette. 1996. Disentangling the disablement process. *Journals of Gerontology. YES Series B, Psychological Sciences and Social Sciences* 51b: 5173-5182.

23. McMurdo, M., and L. Rennie. 1993. A controlled trial of exercise by residents of old people's homes. *Age and Aging* 22:11-15.

24. Federal Interagency Forum on Aging Related Statistics. 2000. *Older Americans 2000: Key indicators of well-being.* Hyattsville, MD: Author.

25. Pollock, M., and W. Evans. 1999. Resistance training for health and disease. *Medicine and Science in Sports and Exercise* 31:10-11.

26. Pollock, M.L., B.A. Franklin, G.J. Balady, L. Bernard, M.D. Chaitman, J.L. Fleg, B. Fletcher, M. Limacher, I.L. Pina, R.A. Stein, M. Williams, and T. Bazzarre. 2000. Resistance exercise in individuals with and without cardiovascular disease benefits, rationale, safety, and prescription. *Circulation* 101:828-833.

27. Rikli, R.E., and C.J. Jones. 1999. Development and validation of a functional fitness test for community residing older adults. *Journal of Aging and Physical Activity* 7:129-161.

28. Rikli, R.E., and C.J. Jones. 2001. *Senior fitness test manual.* Champaign, IL: Human Kinetics.

29. Wenger, N.K., E.S. Froelicher, L.K. Smith, P.A. Ades, K. Berra, J.A. Blumenthal, C.M. Cerro, A.M. Dattilo, D. Davis, R.F. DeBusk, J.P. Drozda, B.J. Fletcher, B.A. Franklin, H. Gaston, P. Greenland, P.E. McBride, C.G.A. McGregor, N.B. Oldridge, J.C. Piscarella, and F.J. Rogers. 1995. *Cardiac rehabilitation as secondary prevention. Clinical practice guideline* (AHCPR publication no. 96-0672). Rockville, MD: U.S. Department of Health and Human Services, Public Health Service, Agency for Health Care Policy and Research and the National Heart, Lung, and Blood Institute.

Chapter 9

1. Beattie, P.F. 2004. Structure and function of the bones and joints of the lumbar spine. In *Kinesiology—The mechanics and pathomechanics of human movement,* ed. C.A. Oatis, 539-562. Philadelphia: Lippincott Williams & Wilkins.

2. Biering-Sorensen, F. 1984. Physical measurements as risk indicators for low-back trouble over a one-year period. *Spine* 9(2): 106-119.

3. Cady, L.D., D.P. Bischoff, E.R. O'Connell, P.C. Thomas, and J.H. Allan. 1979. Strength and fitness and subsequent back injuries in firefighters. *Journal of Occupational Medicine* 21(4):269-272.

4. Cailliet, R. 1988. *Low back pain syndrome.* Philadelphia: Davis.

5. Cooper Institute for Aerobics Research. 1992. *The Prudential FITNESSGRAM.* Dallas: Author.

6. Gracovetsky, S. 1988. *The spinal engine.* New York: Springer-Verlag.

7. Hopkins, D.R., and W.W.K. Hoeger. 1992. A comparison of the sit-and-reach test and the modified sit-and-reach test in the measurement of flexibility for males. *Journal of Applied Sport Science Research* 6:7-10.

8. Hui, S.S., and P.Y. Yuen. 2000. Validity of the modified backsaver sit-and-reach test: A comparison with other protocols. *Medicine and Science in Sports and Exercise* 32(9):1655-1659.

9. Imrie, D., and L. Barbuto. 1988. *The back power program.* Toronto: Stoddart.

10. Kendall, F.P., E.K. McCreary, P.G. Provance. 1993. *Muscles: Testing and function.* 4th ed. Baltimore: Williams & Wilkins.

11. Lee, R. 2002. Measurement of movements of the lumbar spine. *Physiotherapy Theory and Practice* 18:159-164.

12. Liemohn, W., S.B. Martin, and G. Pariser. 1997. The effect of ankle posture on sit-and-reach test performance in young adults. *Journal of Strength and Conditioning Research* 11:239-241.

13. Liemohn, W., M. Miller, T. Haydu, S. Ostrowski, S. Miles, and S. Riggs. 2000. An examination of a passive and an active back extension range of motion (ROM) tests. *Medicine and Science in Sports and Exercise* 32(5):S307.

14. Liemohn, W., G.L. Sharpe, J.F. Wasserman. 1994. Lumbosacral movement in the sit-and-reach and in Cailliet's protective-hamstring stretch. *Spine* 19:2127-2130.

15. Magnusson, S.P., E.B. Simonsen, P. Aagaard, G.W. Gleim, M.P. McHugh, and M. Kjaer. 1995. Viscoelastic response to repeated static stretching in the human hamstring muscle. *Scandinavian Journal of Medicine and Science in Sports* 5:342-347.

16. Martin, S.B., A.W. Jackson, J.R. Morrow, W. Liemohn. 1998. The rationale for the sit and reach test revisited. *Measurement in Physical Education and Exercise Science* 2(2):85-92.

17. McGill, S. 2004. *Ultimate back fitness and performance.* Waterloo, ON: Wabuno.

18. McHugh, M.P., I.J. Kremenic, M.B. Fox, and G.W. Gleim. 1998. The role of mechanical and neural restraints to joint range of motion during passive stretch. *Medicine and Science in Sports and Exercise* 30(6): 928-932.

19. McKenzie, R. 1981. *The lumbar spine—Mechanical diagnosis and therapy.* Waikanae, New Zealand: Spinal.

20. Nachemson, A. 1975. Towards a better understanding of low-back pain: A review of the mechanics of the lumbar disc. *Rheumatology Rehabilitation* 14:129-143.

21. Pope, M.H., T. Bevins, D.G. Wilder, and J.W. Frymoyer. 1985. The relationship between anthropometric, postural, muscular, and mobility characteristics of males ages 18-55. *Spine* 10:644-648.

22. Saal, J.S., and J.A. Saal. 1991. Strength training and flexibility. In *Conservative care of low back pain,* ed. A.H. White and R. Anderson, 65-77. Baltimore: Williams & Wilkins.

23. Williams, R., J. Binkley, R. Bloch, C.H. Goldsmith, and T. Minuk. 1993. Reliability of the modified-modified Schober and double inclinometer methods for measuring lumbar flexion and extension. *Physical Therapy* 73:26-37.

24. Zuhosky, J.P., and J.L. Young. 2001. Functional physical assessment for low back injuries in the athlete. In *Exercise prescription and the back,* ed. W. Liemohn, 67-88. New York: McGraw-Hill Medical.

Chapter 10

1. American College of Sports Medicine. 1996. Heat and cold illnesses during distance running. *Medicine and Science in Sports and Exercise* 28:i-x.

2. American College of Sports Medicine. 1998. The recommended quantity and quality of exercise for developing and maintaining cardiorespiratory and muscular fitness, and flexibility in healthy adults. *Medicine and Science of Sports and Exercise* 30(6): 975-991.

3. American College of Sports Medicine. 2006. *ACSM's guidelines for exercise testing and prescription.* 7th ed. Philadelphia: Lippincott Williams & Wilkins.

4. American College of Sports Medicine. 2006. *ACSM's resource manual for guidelines for exercise testing and prescription.* 5th ed. Philadelphia: Lippincott Williams & Wilkins.

5. Bernard, T.E. 2001. Environmental considerations: Heat and cold. In *ACSM's resource manual for guidelines for exercise testing and prescription.* 4th ed. Ed. J.L. Roitman, 209-216. Baltimore: Lippincott Williams & Wilkins.

6. Blair, S.N., H.W. Kohl III, R.S. Paffenbarger Jr., D.G. Clark, K.H. Cooper, and L.W. Gibbons. 1989. Physical fitness and all-cause mortality. *Journal of the American Medical Association* 262:2395-2401.

7. Borg, G. 1998. *Borg's perceived exertion and pain scales.* Champaign, IL: Human Kinetics.

8. Burton, A.C., and O.G. Edholm. 1955. *Man in a cold environment.* London: Edward Arnold.

9. Buskirk, E.R., and D.E. Bass. 1974. Climate and exercise. In *Science and medicine of exercise and sport,* ed. W.R. Johnson and E.R. Buskirk, 190-205. New York: Harper & Row.

10. Campbell, M.E., Q. Li, S.E. Gingrich, R.G. Macfarlane, and S. Cheng. 2005. Should people be physically active outdoors on smog alert days? *Canadian Journal of Public Health* 96:24-28.

11. Dehn, M.M., and C.B. Mullins. 1977. Physiologic effects and importance of exercise in patients with coronary artery disease. *Cardiovascular Medicine* 2:365.

12. Dionne, F.T., L. Turcotte, M.-C. Thibault, M.R. Boulay, J.S. Skinner, and C. Bouchard. 1991. Mitochondrial DNA sequence polymorphism, $\dot{V}O_2$max, and response to endurance training. *Medicine and Science in Sports and Exercise* 23:177-185.

13. Dodd, S., S.K. Powers, T. Callender, and E. Brooks. 1984. Blood lactate disappearance at various intensities of recovery exercise. *Journal of Applied Physiology* 57:1462-1465.

14. Dose-response issues concerning physical activity and health: An evidence-based symposium (Suppl.). 2001. *Medicine and Science in Sports and Exercise* 33(6).

15. Drinkwater, B.L., J.E. Denton, I.C. Kupprat, T.S. Talag, and S.M. Horvath. 1976. Aerobic power as a factor in women's response to work within hot environments. *Journal of Applied Physiology* 41:815-821.

16. Folinsbee, L.J. 1990. Discussion: Exercise and the environment. In *Exercise, fitness, and health,* ed. C. Bouchard, R.J. Shephard, T. Stephens, J.R. Sutton, and B.D. McPherson, 179-183. Champaign, IL: Human Kinetics.

17. Frampton, M.W., M.J. Utell, W. Zareba, G. Oberdorster, C. Cox, L.S. Huang, P.E. Morrow, F.E. Lee, D. Chalupa, L.M. Frasier, D.M. Speers, and J. Stewart. 2004. Effects of exposure to ultrafine carbon particles in healthy subjects and subjects with asthma. *Research Report—Health Effects Institute* 126:1-63.

18. Gisolfi, G.V., and J. Cohen. 1979. Relationships among training, heat acclimation, and heat tolerance in men and women: The controversy revisited. *Medicine and Science in Sports and Exercise* 11:56-59.

19. Goodman, L.S., and A. Gilman, eds. 1975. *The pharmacological basis of therapeutics.* New York: Macmillan.

20. Grover, R., J. Reeves, E. Grover, and J. Leathers. 1967. Muscular exercise in young men native to 3,100 m altitude. *Journal of Applied Physiology* 22:555-564.

21. Hanson, P.G., and S.W. Zimmerman. 1979. Exertional heatstroke in novice runners. *Journal of the American Medical Association* 242:154-157.

22. Hardy, J.D., and P. Bard. 1974. Body temperature regulation. In vol. 2 of *Medical physiology.* 13th ed. Ed. V.B. Mountcastle, 1305-1342. St. Louis: Mosby.

23. Hart, L.E., and J.R. Sutton. 1987. Environmental considerations for exercise. *Cardiology Clinics* 5:245-258.

24. Haskell, W.L. 1978. Design and implementation of cardiac conditioning programs. In *Rehabilitation of the coronary patient,* ed. N.K. Wenger and H.K. Hellerstein, 203-241. New York: Wiley.

25. Haskell, W.L. 1984. The influence of exercise on the concentrations of triglyceride and cholesterol in human plasma. *Exercise and Sport Sciences Reviews* 12:205-244.

26. Haskell, W.L. 1985. Physical activity and health: Need to define the required stimulus. *American Journal of Cardiology* 55:4D-9D.

27. Haskell, W.L. 1994. Dose-response issues from a biological perspective. In *Physical activity, fitness, and health,* ed. C. Bouchard, R.J. Shephard, and T. Stevens, 1030-1039. Champaign, IL: Human Kinetics.

28. Haskell, W.L. 2001. What to look for in assessing responsiveness to exercise in a health context. *Medicine and Science in Sports and Exercise* 33:S454-S458.

29. Hayward, M.G., and W.R. Keatinge. 1981. Roles of subcutaneous fat and thermoregulatory reflexes in determining ability to stabilize body temperature in water. *Journal of Physiology* (London) 320:229-251.

30. Hellerstein, H.K., and B.A. Franklin. 1984. Exercise testing and prescription. In *Rehabilitation of the coronary patient.* 2nd ed. Ed. N.K. Wenger and H.K. Hellerstein, 197-284. New York: Wiley.

31. Holmer, I. 1979. Physiology of swimming man. *Exercise and Sport Sciences Reviews* 7:87-123.

32. Horvath, S.M. 1981. Exercise in a cold environment. *Exercise and Sport Sciences Reviews* 9:221-263.

33. Horvath, S.M., P.R. Raven, T.E. Dahms, and D.J. Gray. 1975. Maximal aerobic capacity of different levels of carboxyhemoglobin. *Journal of Applied Physiology* 38:300-303.

34. Howley, E.T. 1980. Effect of altitude on physical performance. In *Encyclopedia of physical education, fitness, and sports: Training, environment, nutrition, and fitness,* ed. G.A. Stull and T.K. Cureton, 177-187. Salt Lake City: Brighton.

35. Howley, E.T. 2001. Type of activity: Resistance, aerobic and leisure versus occupational physical activity. *Medicine and Science in Sports and Exercise* 33: S364-S369.

36. Hughson, R.L., H.J. Green, M.E. Houston, J.A. Thompson, D.R. MacLean, and J.R. Sutton. 1980. Heat injuries in Canadian mass-participation runs. *Canadian Medical Association Journal* 122:1141-1144.

37. Jennings, G.L., G. Deakin, P. Korner, I. Meredith, B. Kingwell, and L. Nelson. 1991. What is the dose-response relationship between exercise training and blood pressure? *Annals of Medicine* 23:313-318.

38. Karvonen, M.J., E. Kentala, and O. Mustala. 1957. The effects of training heart rate: A longitudinal study. *Annales Medicinae Experimentalis et Biologiae Fenniae* 35:307-315.

39. Kesaniemi, Y.A., E. Danforth Jr., M.D. Jensen, P.G. Kopelman, P. Lefebvre, and B.A. Reeder. 2001. Dose-response issues concerning physical activity and health: An evidence-based symposium. *Medicine and Science in Sports and Exercise* 33: S351-S358.

40. Londeree, B.R., and S.A. Ames. 1976. Trend analysis of the %$\dot{V}O_2$max-HRregression. *Medicine and Science in Sports* 8:122-125.

41. Londeree, B.R., and M.L. Moeschberger. 1982. Effect of age and other factors on maximal heart rate. *Research Quarterly for Exercise and Sport* 53:297-304.

42. McArdle, W.D., J.R. Magel, T.J. Gergley, R.J. Spina, and M.M. Toner. 1984. Thermal adjustment to cold-water exposure in resting men and women. *Journal of Physiology: Respiratory, Environmental and Exercise Physiology* 56:1565-1571.

43. McArdle, W.D., J.R. Magel, R.J. Spina, T.J. Gergley, and M.M. Toner. 1984. Thermal adjustments to cold-water exposure in exercising men and women. *Journal of Applied Physiology* 56:1572-1577.

44. Paffenbarger, R.S., R.T. Hyde, and A.L. Wing. 1986. Physical activity, all-cause mortality, and longevity of college alumni. *New England Journal of Medicine* 314:605-613.

45. Pate, R.R., M. Pratt, S.N. Blair, W.L. Haskell, C.A. Marcera, and C. Bouchard. 1995. Physical activity and public health: A recommendation from the Centers for Disease Control and Prevention and the American College of Sports Medicine. *Journal of the American Medical Association* 273:402-407.

46. Pollock, M.L., L.R. Gettman, C.A. Mileses, M.D. Bah, J.L. Durstine, and R.B. Johnson. 1977. Effects of frequency and duration of training on attrition and incidence of injury. *Medicine and Science in Sports* 9:31-36.

47. Pollock, M.L., and J.H. Wilmore. 1990. *Exercise in health and disease.* 2nd ed. Philadelphia: Saunders.

48. Powers, S.K., and E.T. Howley. 1997. *Exercise physiology.* Madison, WI: Brown & Benchmark.

49. Pugh, L.G.C. 1964. Deaths from exposure in Four Inns Walking Competition, March 14-15, 1964. *Lancet* 1:1210-1212.

50. Pugh, L.G.C., and O.G. Edholm. 1955. The physiology of Channel swimmers. *Lance,* 2:761-768.

51. Raven, P.B. 1980. Effects of air pollution on physical performance. In vol. 2 of *Encyclopedia of physical education: Physical fitness, training, environment and nutrition related to performance,* ed. G.A. Stull and T.K. Cureton, 201-216. Salt Lake City: Brighton.

52. Raven, P.B., B.L. Drinkwater, R.O. Ruhling, N. Bolduan, S. Taguchi, J. Gliner, and S.M. Horvath. 1974. Effect of carbon monoxide and peroxyacetylnitrate on man's maximal aerobic capacity. *Journal of Applied Physiology* 36:288-293.

53. Sawka, M.N., R.P. Francesconi, A.J. Young, and K.B. Pandolf. 1984. Influence of hydration level and body fluids on exercise performance in the heat. *Journal of the American Medical Association* 252(9): 1165-1169.

54. Sawka, M.N., A.J. Young, R.P. Francesconi, S.R. Muza, and K.B. Pandolf. 1985. Thermoregulatory and blood responses during exercise at graded hypohydration levels. *Journal of Applied Physiology* 59:1394-1401.

55. Sharman, J.E., J.R. Cockcroft, and J.S. Coombes. 2004. Cardiovascular implications of exposure to traffic air pollution during exercise. *QJM* 97:637-643.

56. Sharkey, B.J. 1990. *Physiology of fitness.* 3rd ed. Champaign, IL: Human Kinetics.

57. Sutton, J.R. 1990. Exercise and the environment. In *Exercise, fitness, and health,* ed. C. Bouchard, R.J. Shephard, T. Stephens, J.R. Sutton, and B.D. McPherson, 165-178. Champaign, IL: Human Kinetics.

58. Swain, D.P., K.S. Abernathy, C.S. Smith, S.J. Lee, and S.A. Bunn. 1994. Target heart rates for the development of cardiorespiratory fitness. *Medicine and Science in Sports and Exercise* 26:112-116.

59. Swain, D.P., and B.C. Leutholtz. 1997. Heart rate reserve is equivalent to %$\dot{V}O_2$reserve, not to %$\dot{V}O_2$max. *Medicine and Science in Sports and Exercise* 29:410-414.

60. Swain, D.P., B.C. Leutholtz, M.E. King, L.A. Haas, and J.D. Branch. 1998. Relationship between % heart rate reserve and % $\dot{V}O_2$reserve in treadmill exercise. *Medicine and Science in Sports and Exercise* 30:318-321.

61. Swain, D.P., and B.A. Franklin. 2002. $\dot{V}O_2$ reserve and the minimal intensity for improving cardiorespiratory fitness. *Medicine and Science in Sports and Exercise* 34:152-157.

62. Tanaka, H., K.D. Monahan, and D.R. Seals. 2001. Age-predicted maximal heart rate revisited. *Journal of the American College of Cardiology* 37:153-156.

63. United States Department of Health and Human Services. 1996. *Surgeon General's report on physical activity and health.* Washington, DC: Author.

64. United States Department of Health and Human Services. 2000. *Healthy people 2010: National health promotion and disease prevention objectives.* Washington, DC: Author.

65. Zanobetti, A., M.J. Canner, P.H. Stone, J. Schwartz, D. Sher, E. Eagan-Bengston, K.A. Gates, L.H. Hartley, H. Suh, and D.R. Gold. 2004. Ambient pollution and blood pressure in cardiac rehabilitation patients. *Circulation* 110:2184-2189.

Chapter 11

1. American College of Sports Medicine. 2001. Appropriate intervention strategies for weight loss and prevention of weight regain for adults. *Medicine and Science in Sports and Exercise* 33:2145-2156.

2. American College of Sports Medicine. 2006. *ACSM's guidelines for exercise testing and prescription.* Baltimore: Lippincott Williams & Wilkins.

3. American Psychiatric Association. 1994. *Diagnostic and statistical manual of mental disorders.* Washington, DC: American Psychiatric Press.

4. Bassett, D.R., P.L. Schneider, and G.E. Huntington. 2004. Physical activity in an Old Order Amish community. *Medicine and Science in Sports and Exercise* 36:79-85.

5. Beamer, B.A. 2003. Genetic influences on obesity. In *Obesity: Etiology, assessment, treatment and prevention,* ed. R.E. Anderson, 43-56. Champaign, IL: Human Kinetics.

6. Bouchard, C., L. Perusse, C. Leblanc, A. Tremblay, and G. Theriault. 1988. Inheritance of the amount and distribution of human body fat. *International Journal of Obesity* 12:205-215.

7. Cottrell, R.R. 1992. *Weight control.* Guilford, CT: Dushkin.

8. Cunningham, J.J. 1991. Body composition as a determinant of energy expenditure: A synthetic review and a proposed general prediction equation. *American Journal of Clinical Nutrition* 54:963-969.

9. DiPietro, L. 1999. Physical activity in the prevention of obesity: Current evidence and research issues. *Medicine and Science in Sports and Exercise* 31: S542-S546.

10. Flegal, K., M. Carroll, C. Ogden, and C. Johnson. 2002. Prevalence and trends in obesity among US adults, 1999-2000. *Journal of the American Medical Association* 288:1723-1727.

11. Flegal, K.M. 1999. The obesity epidemic in children and adults: Current evidence and research issues. *Medicine and Science in Sports and Exercise* 31:S509-S514.

12. Food and Nutrition Board, Institute of Medicine. 2002. *Dietary reference intakes for energy, carbohydrate, fiber, fat, fatty acids, cholesterol, protein, and amino acids.* Washington, DC: National Academies Press.

13. Grundy, S.M., G. Blackburn, M. Higgins, R. Lauer, M.G. Perri, and D. Ryan. 1999. Physical activity in the prevention and treatment of obesity and its comorbidities: Roundtable consensus statement. *Medicine and Science in Sports and Exercise* 31: S502-S508.

14. Hedley, A.A., C.L. Ogden, C.L. Johnson, M.D. Carroll, L.R. Curtin, and K.M. Flegal. 2004. Prevalence of overweight and obesity among US children, adolescents, and adults, 1999-2002. *Journal of the American Medical Association* 291:2847-2850.

15. Hill, J.O., and E.L. Melanson. 1999. Overview of the determinants of overweight and obesity: Current evidence and research issues. *Medicine and Science in Sports and Exercise* 31: S515-S521.

16. Holden, J.H., L.L. Darga, S.M. Olson, D.C. Stettner, E.A. Ardito, and C.P. Lucas. 1992. Long-term follow-up of patients attending a combination very-low calorie diet and behaviour therapy weight loss programme. *International Journal of Obesity* 16:605-613.

17. Hornbuckle, L.M., D.R. Bassett Jr., and D.L. Thompson. 2005. Pedometer-determined walking and body composition variables in African-American women. *Medicine and Science in Sports and Exercise* 37:1069-1074.

18. Jebb, S.A., and M.S. Moore. 1999. Contribution of a sedentary lifestyle and inactivity to the etiology of overweight and obesity: Current evidence and research issues. *Medicine and Science in Sports and Exercise* 31:S534-S541.

19. Johnson, M.D. 1994. Disordered eating. In *Medical and orthopedic issues of active and athletic women,* ed. R. Agostini, 141-151. Philadelphia: Hanley & Belfus.

20. Krumm, E.M., O.L. Dessieux, P. Andrews, and D.L. Thompson. 2006. The relationship between daily steps and body composition in postmenopausal women. *Journal of Women's Health* 15(2):202-210.

21. Lavery, M.A., and J.W. Loewy. 1993. Identifying predictive variables for long-term weight change after participation in a weight loss program. *Journal of the American Dietetic Association* 93:1017-1024.

22. Lichtman, S.W., K. Pisarska, E.R. Berman, M. Pestone, H. Dowling, E. Offenbacher, H. Weisel, S. Heshka, D.E. Matthews, and S.B. Heymsfield. 1992. Discrepancy between self-reported and actual caloric intake and exercise in obese subjects. *New England Journal of Medicine* 327:1893-1898.

23. Molé, P.A. 1990. Impact of energy intake and exercise on resting metabolic rate. *Sports Medicine* 10:72-87.

24. Montoye, H.J., H.C.G. Kemper, W.H.M. Saris, and R.A. Washburn. 1996. *Measuring physical activity and energy expenditure.* Champaign, IL: Human Kinetics.

25. Must, A., J. Spandano, E.H. Coakley, A.E. Field, G. Colditz, and W.H. Dietz. 1999. The disease burden associated with overweight and obesity. *Journal of the American Medical Association* 282:1523-1529.

26. National Heart, Lung, and Blood Institute. 1998. *Clinical guidelines on the identification, evaluation, and treatment of overweight and obesity in adults* (NIH Publication No. 98-4083). Bethesda, MD: National Institutes of Health—National Heart, Lung, and Blood Institute.

27. Ogden, C.L., C.D. Fryar, M.D. Carroll, and K.M. Flegal. 2004. *Mean body weight, height, and body mass index, United States 1960-2002* (Advance data from vital and health statistics; No. 347). Hyattsville, MD: National Center for Health Statistics.

28. Prentice, A.M., and S.A. Jebb. 2000. Physical activity level and weight control in adults. In *Physical activity and obesity,* ed. C. Bouchard, 247-261. Champaign, IL: Human Kinetics.

29. Salbe, A.D., and E. Ravussin. 2000. The determinants of obesity. In *Physical activity and obesity,* ed. C. Bouchard, 69-102. Champaign, IL: Human Kinetics.

30. Stunkard, A.J., T.I.A. Sørensen, C. Hanis, T.W. Teasdale, R. Charkraborty, W.J. Schull, and F. Schulsinger. 1986. An adoption study of human obesity. *New England Journal of Medicine* 314:193-198.

31. Thompson, D.L., J. Rakow, and S.M. Perdue. 2004. Relationship between accumulated walking and body composition in middle-aged women. *Medicine and Science in Sports and Exercise* 36:911-914.

32. Wadden, T.A., and A.J. Stunkard. 1993. Psychosocial consequences of obesity and dieting: Research and clinical findings. In *Obesity: Theory and therapy,* ed. A.J. Stunkard and T.A. Wadden, 163-177. New York: Raven Press.

33. Welle, S., G.B. Forbes, M. Statt, R.R. Barnard, and J.M. Amatruda. 1992. Energy expenditure under free-living conditions in normal-weight and overweight women. *American Journal of Clinical Nutrition* 55:14-21.

34. Westerterp, K.R. 2000. The assessment of energy and nutrient intake in humans. In *Physical activity and obesity,* ed. C. Bouchard, 133-149. Champaign, IL: Human Kinetics.

35. Williamson, D.F., J. Madans, R.F. Anda, J.C. Kleinman, H.S. Kahn, and T. Byers. 1993. Recreational physical activity and ten-year weight change in a US national cohort. *International Journal of Obesity* 17:279-286.

36. Wing, R.R., and J.O. Hill. 2001. Successful weight loss maintenance. *Annual Review of Nutrition* 21:323-341.

37. Wright, J.D., J. Kennedy-Stephenson, C.Y. Wang, M.A. McDowell, and C.L. Johnson. 2004. Trends in intake of energy and macronutrients—United States, 1971-2000. *Morbidity and Mortality Weekly Report* 53:80-82.

Chapter 12

1. American Academy of Pediatrics. 2001. Strength training for children and adolescents. *Pediatrics* 107:1470-1472.

2. American Association of Cardiovascular and Pulmonary Rehabilitation. 2003. *Guidelines for cardiac rehabilitation and secondary prevention programs.* 4th ed. Champaign, IL: Human Kinetics.

3. American College of Obstetricians and Gynecologists. 2002. Exercise during pregnancy and the postpartum period. *International Journal of Gynecology and Obstetrics* 77:79-81.

4. American College of Sports Medicine. 1997. *ACSM's health/fitness facility standards and guidelines.* 2nd ed. Champaign, IL: Human Kinetics.

5. American College of Sports Medicine. 1998. Exercise and physical activity for older adults. *Medicine and Science in Sports and Exercise* 30:992-1008.

6. American College of Sports Medicine. 2006. *ACSM's guidelines for exercise testing and prescription.* 7th ed. Philadelphia: Lippincott Williams & Wilkins.

7. Baechle, T., and R. Earle. 2000. *Essentials of strength training and conditioning.* 2nd ed. Champaign, IL: Human Kinetics.

8. Baechle, T., and R. Earle. 2006. *Weight training: Steps to success.* 3rd ed. Champaign, IL: Human Kinetics.

9. Bass, S. 2000. The prepubertal years. A uniquely opportune stage of growth when the skeletal is most responsive to exercise? *Sports Medicine* 30(2): 73-78.

10. Beniamini, Y., J. Rubenstein, A. Faigenbaum, A. Lichtenstein, and M. Crim. 1999. High intensity strength training of patients enrolled in an outpatient cardiac rehabilitation program. *Journal of Cardiopulmonary Rehabilitation* 19:8-17.

11. Brown, L. 2000. *Isokinetics in human performance.* Champaign, IL: Human Kinetics.

12. Carpinelli, R., and R. Otto. 1998. Strength training: Single versus multiple sets. *Sports Medicine* 26:73-84.

13. Campos, G., T. Luecke, H. Wendeln, K. Toma, F. Hagerman, T. Murray, K. Ragg, N. Ratamess, W. Kraemer, and R. Staron. 2002. Muscular adaptations in response to three different resistance training regimens: Specificity of repetition maximum training zones. *European Journal of Applied Physiology* 88: 50-60.

14. Chu, D. 1998. *Jumping into plyometrics.* 2nd ed. Champaign, IL: Human Kinetics.

15. Cunningham, C., M. Morris, C. Murphy, J. Wenson. 2002. *Stability ball training.* Monterey, CA: Healthy Learning.

16. Davies, G. 1995. The need for critical thinking in rehabilitation. *Journal of Sport Rehabilitation* 4:1-22.

17. Davies, G., L. Wolfe, M. Mottola, and C. MacKinnon. 2003. Joint SOGC/CSEP clinical practice guideline: Exercise in pregnancy and the postpartum period. *Canadian Journal of Applied Physiology* 28: 329-341.

18. DeLorme, T., and A. Watkins. 1948. Techniques of progressive resistance exercise. *Archives of Physical Medicine and Rehabilitation* 29:263-273.

19. Dempsey, J., C. Butler, and M. Williams. 2005. No need for a pregnant pause: Physical activity may reduce the occurrence of gestational diabetes mellitus and preclampsia. *Exercise and Sport Science Reviews* 33:141-149.

20. Drinkwater, B. 1995. Weight-bearing exercise and bone mass. *Physical Medicine and Rehabilitation Clinics of North America* 6:567-578.

21. Faigenbaum, A. 2001. Strength training and children's health. *Journal of Physical Education, Recreation and Dance* 72:24-30.

22. Faigenbaum, A. 2003. Youth resistance training. *PCPFS Research Digest* 4(3): 1-8.

23. Faigenbaum, A., W. Kraemer, B. Cahill, J. Chandler, J. Dziados, L. Elfrink, E. Forman, M. Gaudiose, L. Micheli, M. Nitka, and S. Roberts. 1996. Youth resistance training: Position statement paper and literature review. *Strength and Conditioning* 18:62-75.

24. Faigenbaum, A., and Westcott, W. 2000. *Strength and power for young athletes.* Champaign, IL: Human Kinetics.

25. Fiatarone, M.A., E.C. Marks, N.D. Ryan, C.N. Meredith, L.A. Lipsitz, and W. Evans. 1990. High-intensity strength training in nonagenarians: Effects on skeletal muscle. *Journal of the American Medical Association* 263:3029-3034.

26. Fiatarone, M., E. O'Neill, N. Ryan, K. Clements, G. Solares, M. Nelson, S. Roberts, J. Kehayias, L. Lipsitz, and W. Evans. 1990. Exercise training and nutritional supplementation for physical frailty in very elderly people. *New England Journal of Medicine* 330:1769-1775.

27. Fleck, S. 1999. Periodized strength training: A critical review. *Journal of Strength and Conditioning Research* 13:82-89.

28. Fleck, S., and W. Kraemer. 2004. *Designing resistance training programs.* 3rd ed. Champaign, IL: Human Kinetics.

29. Fry, A., and W. Kraemer. 1997. Resistance exercise overtraining and overreaching. *Sports Medicine* 23(2):106-129.

30. Garshasbi, A., and S. Zadeh. 2005. The effect of exercise on the intensity of low back pain in pregnant women. *International Journal of Gynecology and Obstetrics* 88: 271-275.

31. Glass, S., and D. Stanton. 2004. Self-selected resistance training intensity in novice weightlifters. *Journal of Strength and Conditioning Research* 18:324-327.

32. Graves, J., M. Pollock, S. Leggett, R. Braith, D. Carpenter, and L. Bishop. 1988. Effect of reduced frequency on muscular strength. *International Journal of Sports Medicine* 9:316-319.

33. Hass, C., L. Garzarella, D. De Hoyos, and M. Pollock. 2000. Single versus multiple sets in long-term recreational weightlifters. *Medicine and Science in Sports and Exercise* 32:235-242.

34. Henwood, T., and D. Taaffe. 2005. Improved physical performance in older adults undertaking a short-term programme of high velocity resistance training. *Gerontology* 51:108-115.

35. Hettinger, R., and E. Muller. 1953. Muskelleistung und muskeltraining (Muscle achievement and muscle training). *ArbeitsPhysiologie* 15:111-126.

36. Hewett, T., G. Myer, and K. Ford. 2005. Reducing knee and anterior cruciate ligament injuries among female athletes. *Journal of Knee Surgery* 18:82-88.

37. Hoeger, W., S. Barette, D. Hale, and D. Hopkins. 1987. Relationship between repetitions and selected percentages on the one repetition maximum. *Journal of Applied Sport Science Research* 1:11-13.

38. Hoffman, J. 2002. *Physiological aspects of sports training and performance.* Champaign, IL: Human Kinetics.

39. Jacobson, B. 1986. A comparison of two progressive weight training techniques on knee extensor strength. *Athletic Training* 21:315-319.

40. Jones, C., C. Christensen, and M. Young. 2000. Weight training injury trends. *Physician and Sportsmedicine* 28:61-72.

41. Kalapotharakos, V., M. Michalopoulos, S. Tokmakidis, G. Godolias, and V. Gourgoulis. 2005. Effects of heavy and moderate resistance training on functional performance in older adults. *Journal of Strength and Conditioning Research* 19: 652-657.

42. Kato, S., and T. Ishiko. 1964. Obstructed growth of children's bones due to excessive labor in remote corners. In *Proceedings of the International Congress of Sports Sciences,* ed. S. Kato, 476. Tokyo: Japanese Union of Sports Sciences.

43. Keeler, L., L. Finkelstein, W. Miller, and B. Fernhall. 2001. Early phase adaptations to traditional speed vs. super slow resistance training on strength and aerobic capacity in sedentary individuals. *Journal of Strength and Conditioning Research* 15:309-314.

44. Kelemen, M.H., K. Stewart, R.E. Gillilan, C.K. Ewart, S.A. Valenti, J.D. Manley, and M.D. Kelemen. 1986. Circuit weight training in cardiac patients. *Journal of the American College of Cardiology* 7:38-42.

45. Kohrt, W., S. Bloomfield, L. Kathleen, M. Nelson, and V. Yingling. 2004. Physical activity and bone health. *Medicine and Science in Sports and Exercise* 36:1985-1996.

46. Komi, P.V. 2000. Stretch-shortening cycle: A powerful model to study normal and fatigued muscle. *Journal of Biomechanics* 33:1197-1206.

47. Kraemer, W., K. Adams, E. Cafarelli, E. Cafarelli, G. Dudley, C. Dooly, M. Feigenbaum, et al. 2002. Progression models in resistance training for healthy adults. *Medicine and Science and Sports and Exercise* 34:364-380.

48. Kraemer, W., and S. Fleck. 1988. Resistance training: Exercise prescription (part 4 of 4). *Physician and Sports Medicine.* 16:69-81.

49. Kraemer, W., B. Noble, B. Culver, and M. Clark. 1987. Physiologic responses to heavy resistance exercise with very short rest periods. *International Journal of Sports Medicine* 8:247-252.

50. Kraemer, W., and N. Ratemess. 2005. Hormonal responses and adaptations to resistance exercise and training. *Sports Medicine* 35:339-361.

51. Kraemer, W., and N. Ratamess. 2004. Fundamentals of resistance training: Progression and exercise prescription. *Medicine and Science in Sports and Exercise* 36:674-688.

52. Kraemer, W., N. Ratemess, and D. French. 2002. Resistance training for health and performance. *Current Sports Medicine Reports* 1:165-171.

53. Kraemer, W., N. Ratamess, A. Fry, T. Triplett-McBride, P. Koziris, J. Bauer, J. Lynch, and S. Fleck. 2000. Influence of resistance training volume and periodization on physiological and performance adaptations in collegiate women tennis players. *American Journal of Sports Medicine* 28(5): 626-632.

54. Kramer, J., M. Stone, H. O'Bryant, M. Conley, R. Johnson, D. Nieman, D. Honeycutt, and T. Hoke. 1997. Effects of single vs. multiple sets of weight training: Impact of volume, intensity and variation. *Journal of Strength and Conditioning Research* 11(3): 143-147.

55. Leon, A., B. Franklin, F. Costa, G. Balady, K. Berra, K. Stewart, P. Thompson, M. Williams, and M. Lauer. 2005. Cardiac rehabilitation and secondary prevention of coronary heart disease. *Circulation* 111:369-376.

56. Lombardi, V. 2000. 1998 U.S. weight training injuries and deaths. *Medicine and Science in Sports and Exercise* 32: S346.

57. Mann, D., and M. Jones. 1999. Guidelines to the implementation of a dynamic stretching program. *Strength and Conditioning Journal* 21:53-55.

58. Marx, J., N. Ratamess, B. Nindl, L. Gotshalk, J. Volek, K. Dohi, J. Bush, A. Gomez, S. Mazzetti, S. Fleck, K. Hakkinen, R. Newton, and W. Kraemer. 2001. Low volume circuit versus high volume periodized resistance training in women. *Medicine and Science in Sports and Exercise* 33:635-643.

59. Mazzette, S., W. Kraemer, J. Volek, N. Duncan, N. Ratamess, A. Gomez, R. Newton, K. Hakkinen, and S. Fleck. 2000. The influence of direct supervision of resistance training on strength performance. *Medicine and Science in Sports and Exercise* 32:1175-1184.

60. Mediate, P., and A. Faigenbaum. 2004. *Medicine ball training for all.* Monterey Bay, CA: Healthy Learning.

61. McCartney, N. 1998. Role of resistance training in heart disease. *Medicine and Science in Sports and Exercise* 30(Suppl. 10): S396-S402.

62. McGee, D., T. Jessee, H. Stone, and D. Blessing. 1992. Leg and hip endurance adaptations to three weight training programs. *Journal of Applied Sport Science Research* 6:92-95.

63. Mikesky, A., C. Gidding, W. Mathews, and W. Gonyea. 1991. Changes in muscle fiber size and composition in response to heavy-resistance exercise. *Medicine and Science in Sports and Exercise* 23:1042-1049.

64. Morris, S., and N. Johnson. 2005. Exercise during pregnancy: A critical appraisal of the literature. *Journal of Reproductive Medicine* 50:181-188.

65. Nelson, M., M. Fiatarone, C. Morganti, I. Trice, R. Greenberg, and W. Evans. 1994. Effects of high intensity strength training on multiple risk factors for osteoporotic fractures. *Journal of the American Medical Association* 272:1909-1914.

66. Pearson, D., A. Faigenbaum, M. Conley, and W. Kraemer. 2000. The National Strength and Conditioning Association's basic guidelines for the resistance training of athletes. *Strength and Conditioning Journal* 22(4): 14-27.

67. Pollock, M., B. Franklin, G. Balady, B. Chaitman, J. Fleg, B. Fletcher, M. Limacher, I. Pina, R. Stein, M. Williams, and T. Bazzarre. 2000. Resistance exercise in individuals with and without cardiovascular disease: Benefits, rationale, safety and prescription. *Circulation* 101(7): 828-833.

68. Potach, D., and D. Chu. 2000. Plyometric training. In *Essentials of strength training and conditioning.* 2nd ed. Ed. T. Baechle and R. Earle, 427-440. Champaign, IL: Human Kinetics.

69. Rhea, M., B. Alavar, L. Brukett, and S. Ball. 2003. A meta-analysis to determine the dose response for strength development. *Medicine and Science in Sports and Exercise* 35:456-464.

70. Rutherford, O.M., and D.D. Jones. 1986. The role of learning and coordination in strength training. *European Journal of Applied Physiology* 55:100-105.

71. Sadres, E., A. Eliakim, N. Constantini, R. Lidor, and B. Falk. 2001. The effect of long-term resistance training on anthropometric measures, muscle strength, and self-concept in pre-pubertal boys. *Pediatric Exercise Science* 13:357-372.

72. Schlicht, J., N. Camaione, and V. Owen. 2001. Effect of intense strength training on standing balance, walking speed, and sit to stand performance in older adults. *Journal of Gerontology* 56A: M281-M286.

73. Schlumberger, A., J. Stec, and D. Schmidtbleicher. 2001. Single- vs. multi-set strength training in women. *Journal of Strength and Conditioning Research* 15:284-289.

74. Sothern, M., J. Loftin, J. Udall, R. Suskind, T. Ewing, S. Tang, and U. Blecker. 2000. Safety, feasibility and efficacy of a resistance training program in preadolescent obese youth. *American Journal of the Medical Sciences* 319(6): 370-375.

75. Starkey, D.B., M.L. Pollock, T. Ishida, Y. Ishida, M. Welsch, W. Bechve, J. Graves, and M. Feigenbaum . 1996. Effect of resistance training volume on strength and muscle thickness. *Medicine and Science in Sports and Exercise* 28:1311-1320.

76. Stewart, K.J, K.L. Turner, A.C. Bacher, J.R. DeRegis, J. Sung, M. Tayback, and P. Ouyang. 2003. Are fitness, activity and fatness associated with health-related quality of life and mood in older persons? *Journal of Cardiopulmonary Rehabilitation* 23:115-121.

77. Stone, M., R. Keith, J. Kearney, S. Fleck, G. Wilson, and N. Triplett. 1991. Overtraining: A review of signs and symptoms. *Journal of Applied Strength and Conditioning Research* 5:35-50.

78. Stone, M.H., H. O'Bryant, and J. Garhammer. 1981. A hypothetical model for strength training. *Journal of Sports Medicine* 21:342-351.

79. Sung, R.Y., C.W Yu, S.K Chang, S.W Mo, K.S. Woo, and C.W. Lam. 2002. Effects of dietary intervention and strength training on blood lipid level in obese children. *Archives of Diseases in Childhood* 86:407-410.

80. Vincent, K., R. Braith, R. Feldman, P. Magyari, R. Cutler, S. Persin, L. Lennon, A. Gabr, B. Lowenthall. 2002. Resistance exercise and physical performance in adults aged 60 to 83. *Journal of the American Geriatric Society* 50:1100-1107.

81. Vincent, S., R. Pangrazi, A. Raustorp, L.Tomson, and T. Cuddihy. 2003. Activity levels and body mass index of children in the United States, Sweden and Australia. *Medicine and Science in Sports and Exercise* 35(8): 1367-1373.

82. Westcott, W., and T. Baechle. 1999. *Strength training for seniors.* Champaign, IL: Human Kinetics.

Chapter 13

1. Axler, C.T., and S.M. McGill. 1997. Low back loads over a variety of abdominal exercises: Searching for the safest abdominal challenge. *Medicine and Science in Sports and Exercise* 29(6): 804-811.
2. Battie, M.C., T. Videman, K. Gill, G.B. Moneta, R. Nyman, J. Kaprio, and M. Koskenvut. 1991. Smoking and lumbar intervertebral disc degeneration: An MRI study of identical twins. *Spine* 16(9): 1015-1021.
3. Biering-Sorensen, F. 1984. Physical measurements as risk indicators for low-back trouble over a one-year period. *Spine* 9(2): 106-119.
4. Bogduk, N. 1998. *Clinical anatomy of the lumbar spine and sacrum.* London: Churchill Livingstone.
5. Borenstein, D.G., and S.W. Wiesel. 1989. *Low back pain—Medical diagnosis and comprehensive management.* Philadelphia: Saunders.
6. Cailliet, R. 1988. *Low back pain syndrome.* Philadelphia: Davis.
7. Crisco, J.J., and M.M. Panjabi. 1991. The intersegmental and multisegmental muscles of the spine: A biomechanical model comparing lateral stabilising potential. *Spine* 16(7): 793-799.
8. Fritz, J.M., and G.E. Hicks. 2001. Exercise protocols for low back pain. In *Exercise prescription and the back,* ed. W. Liemohn, 167-181. New York: McGraw-Hill Medical.
9. Goldby, L.J., A.P. Moore, J. Doust, M.E. Trew. 2006. A randomized controlled trial investigating the efficiency of musculoskeletal physiotherapy on chronic low back disorder. *Spine* 31(10): 1083-1093.
10. Juker, D., S. McGill, P. Kropf, and T. Steffen. 1998. Quantitative intramuscular myoelectric activity of lumbar portions of psoas and the abdominal wall during a wide variety of tasks. *Medicine and Science in Sports and Exercise* 30(2): 301-310.
11. Liemohn, W.P., T.A. Baumgartner, and L.H. Gagnon. 2005. Measuring core stability. *Journal of Strength and Conditioning Research* 19(3): 583-586.
12. Liemohn, W., and L.H. Gagnon. 2001. Efficacy of therapeutic exercise in low back rehabilitation. In *Exercise prescription and the back,* ed. W. Liemohn, 229-240. New York: McGraw-Hill Medical.
13. Liemohn, W., and M. Miller. 2001. Low back pain incidence in sports. In *Exercise prescription and the back*, ed. W. Liemohn, 99-134. New York: McGraw-Hill Medical.
14. Liemohn, W., and G. Pariser. 2002. Core strength: Implications for fitness and low back pain. *ACSM's Health and Fitness Journal* 6(5): 10-16.
15. Luoto, S., M. Heliovaara, H. Hurri, and H. Alaranta. 1995. Static back endurance and the risk of low back pain. *Clinical Biomechanics* 10:323-324.
16. McGill, S. 2004. *Ultimate back fitness and performance.* Waterloo, ON: Wabuno.
17. McGill, S. 2004. Mechanics and pathomechanics of muscles acting on the lumbar spine. In *Kinesiology: The mechanics and pathomechanics of human movement,* ed. C.A. Oatis, 563-575. Philadelphia: Lippincott Williams & Wilkins.
18. Nachemson, A.L., B.J. Andersson, and A.B. Schultz. 1986. Valsalva maneuver biomechanics: Effects on lumbar trunk loads of elevated intraabdominal pressures. *Spine* 11:476-479.
19. Nitz, A.J., and D. Peck. 1986. Comparison of muscle spindle concentrations in large and small human epaxial muscles acting in parallel combinations. *American Journal of Surgery* 52:273-277.
20. O'Sullivan, P.B., L. Twomey, and G.T. Allison. 1997. Dynamic stabilization of the lumbar spine. *Critical Reviews in Physical and Rehabilitation Medicine* 9(3-4): 315-330.
21. Porterfield, J.A., and C. DeRosa. 1998. *Mechanical low back pain—Perspective in functional anatomy.* Philadelphia: Saunders.
22. Sinaki, M., M.P. Lutness, D.M. Ilstrup, C.P. Chu, and R.R. Gramse. 1989. Lumbar spondylolisthesis: Retrospective comparison and three-year follow-up of two conservative treatment programs. *Archives in Physical Medicine and Rehabilitation* 70(8): 594-598.
23. Waddell, G. 1998. *The back pain revolution.* Edinburgh, UK: Churchill Livingstone.
24. White, A.A., and M.M. Panjabbi. 1990. *Clinical biomechanics of the spine.* Philadelphia: Lippincott Williams & Wilkins.
25. Zuhosky, J.P., and J.L. Young. 2001. Functional physical assessment for low back injuries in the athlete. In *Exercise prescription and the back,* ed. W. Liemohn, 67-88. New York: McGraw-Hill Medical.

Chapter 14

1. American College of Sports Medicine. 2006. *ACSM's guidelines for exercise testing and prescription.* 7th ed. Philadelphia: Lippincott Williams & Wilkins.
2. Centers for Disease Control and Prevention. 2003. Prevalence of physical activity, including lifestyle activities among adults—United States, 2000-2001. *Morbidity and Mortality Weekly* 52:764-769.
3. Dishman, R.K. 1990. Determinants of participation in physical activity. In *Exercise, fitness, and health,* ed. C. Bouchard, R.J. Shephard, T. Stephens, J.R. Sutton, and B.D. McPherson , 75-101. Champaign, IL: Human Kinetics.
4. Franklin, B.A., N.B. Oldridge, K.G. Stoedefalke, and W.E. Loechel. 1990. *On the ball.* Carmel, IN: Benchmark Press.
5. Franklin, B.A., N.B. Oldridge, K.G. Stoedefalke, and W.E. Loechel. 2001. *The sport ball exercise handbook.* Monterey, CA: Exercise Science.
6. Franks, B.D., and E.T. Howley. 1998. *Fitness leaders' handbook.* 2nd ed. Champaign, IL: Human Kinetics.
7. Garrick, J.G., and R.K. Requa. 1988. Aerobic dance—A review. *Sports Medicine* 6:169-179.
8. Giese, M.D. 1988. Organization of an exercise session. In *Resource manual guidelines for exercise testing and prescription,* ed. S.N. Blair, P. Painter, R. Pate, L.K. Smith, and C.B. Taylor, 244-247. Philadelphia: Lea & Febiger.
9. Kasser, S.L. 1995. *Inclusive games: Movement fun for everyone.* Champaign, IL: Human Kinetics.
10. Kisselle, J., and K. Mazzeo. 1983. *Aerobic dance.* Englewood, CO: Morton.
11. Londeree, B.R., and M.I. Moeschberger. 1982. Effect of age and other factors on maximal heart rate. *Research Quarterly for Exercise and Sport* 53:297-304.
12. Mazzeo, J.W. 1984. *Shape-up.* Englewood, CO: Morton.
13. McSwegin, P.J., and C.L. Pemberton. 1993. Exercise leadership: Key skills and characteristics. In *ACSM's resource manual for guidelines for exercise testing and prescription.* 2nd ed. Ed. J.L. Durstine, A.C. King, P.L. Painter, J.L. Roitman, L.D. Zwiren, and W.L. Kenney, 319-326. Philadelphia: Lea & Febiger.
14. New Games Foundation. 1976. *The new games book.* Garden City, NY: Dolphin Books.

15. Oldridge, N.B. 1988. Qualities of an exercise leader. In *Resource manual for guidelines for exercise testing and prescription,* ed. S.N. Blair, P. Painter, R.R. Pate, L.K. Smith, and C.B. Taylor, 239-243. Philadelphia: Lea & Febiger.

16. Peters, T.J., and R.H. Waterman. 1982. *In search of excellence.* New York: Warner Books.

17. Sanders, M.E., ed. 1999. *YMCA water fitness for health.* Champaign, IL: Human Kinetics.

18. Seaman, J. 1999. Physical activity and fitness for persons with disabilities. *PCPFS Research Digest* 3(5).

19. Williford, H.N., M. Scharff-Olson, and D.L. Blessing. 1989. The physiological effects of aerobic dance—A review. *Sports Medicine* 8:335-345.

Chapter 15

1. American College of Sports Medicine. 2006. *ACSM's guidelines for exercise testing and prescription.* 7th ed. Philadelphia: Lippincott Williams & Wilkins.

2. Åstrand, P-O. 1952. *Experimental studies of physical working capacity in relation to sex and age.* Copenhagen: Ejnar Munksgaard.

3. Bar-Or, O. 1995. Health benefits of physical activity during childhood and adolescence. *PCPFS Research Digest* 2(4).

4. Bar-Or, O., and R.M. Malina. 1995. Activity, fitness, and health of children and adolescents. In *Child health, nutrition, and physical activity,* ed. L.W.Y. Cheung and J.B. Richmond, 79-123. Champaign, IL: Human Kinetics.

5. Bunker, L.K. 1998. Psycho-physiological contributions of physical activity and sports for girls. *PCPFS Research Digest* 3(1).

6. Centers for Disease Control and Prevention. 1997. Guidelines for school and community programs to promote lifelong physical activity among young people. *Morbidity and Mortality Weekly Report* 44(RR-6): 1-36.

7. Cooper Institute for Aerobic Research. 2005. *FITNESSGRAM: Test administration manual.* 3rd ed. Champaign, IL: Human Kinetics.

8. Corbin, C.B., R.P. Pangrazi, and G.C. LaMasurier. 2004. Physical activity for children: Current patterns and guidelines. *PCPFS Research Digest* 5(2).

9. Cureton, K.J., and G.L. Warren. 1990. Criterion-referenced standards for youth health-related fitness tests: A tutorial. *Research Quarterly for Exercise and Sports* 61:7-19.

10. Fardy, P., and A. Azzollini. 1998. The PATH program. *Active youth: Ideas for implementing CDC physical activity promotion guidelines,* 81-85. Champaign, IL: Human Kinetics.

11. Malina, R.M. 2001. Tracking of physical activity across the lifespan. *PCPFS Research Digest* 3(14).

12. McKenzie, F.D., and J.B. Richmond. 1998. Linking health and learning: An overview of coordinated school health programs. In *Health is academic: A guide to coordinated school health programs,* ed. E. Marx, S. Frelick Wooley, and D. Northrop, 1-14. New York: Teachers College Press.

13. Morrow Jr., J.R., and A.W. Jackson. 1999. Physical activity promotion and school physical education. *PCPFS Research Digest* 3(7).

14. National Association for Sport and Physical Education. 2004. *Physical activity for children: A statement of guidelines for children ages 5-12.* 2nd ed. Reston, VA: Author.

15. National Center for Education in Maternal and Child Health. 2001. *Bright futures in practice: Physical activity.* Arlington, VA: Author.

16. Park, R.S. 1989. *Measurement of physical fitness: A historical perspective.* Washington, DC: ODPHP National Health Information Center.

17. Pate, R. 1998. Physical activity for young people. *PCPFS Research Digest* 3(3).

18. President's Council on Physical Fitness and Sports. 2005. *President's Challenge Physical Activity and Fitness Award Program.* Washington, DC: Author.

19. Robinson, S. 1938. Experimental studies of physical fitness in relation to age. *Arbeitsphysiologie* 10:251-323.

20. Rowland, T.W. 1999. Adolescence: A "risk factor" for physical inactivity. *PCPFS Research Digest* 2(4).

21. Rowland, T.W. 1990. *Exercise and children's health.* Champaign, IL: Human Kinetics.

22. Sallis, J.F. 1994. Influences on physical activity of children, adolescents, and adults or determinants of active living. *PCPFS Research Digest* 1(7).

23. Sallis, J.F., T.L. McKenzie, J.E. Alcaraz, B. Kolody, N. Faucette, and M. Hovell. 1997. The effects of a 2-year physical education program (SPARK) on physical activity and fitness on elementary school students. *American Journal of Public Health* 87:45-50.

24. Sallis, J.F., T.L. McKenzie, B. Kolody, M. Lewis, S. Marshall, and P. Rosegard. 1999. Effects of health-related physical education on academic achievement: Project SPARK. *Research Quarterly for Exercise and Sport* 70:127-134.

25. Sallis, J.F., K. Patrick, and B.L. Long. 1994. An overview of international consensus conference on physical activity guidelines for adolescents. *Pediatric Exercise Science* 6:299-301.

26. Satcher, D. 1998. Opening remarks. *Childhood obesity: Causes and prevention* (CNPP-6). Washington, DC: U.S. Department of Agriculture Center for Nutrition Policy and Promotion.

27. Seefeldt, V.D., and M.E. Ewing. 1997. Youth sports in America: An overview. *PCPFS Research Digest* 2(11).

28. Strong, W.B., R.M. Malina, C.J.R. Blimkie, S.R. Daniles, R.K. Dishman, B. Gutin, A.C. Hergenroeder, A. Must, P.A. Nixon, J.M. Pivarnik, T. Rowland, S. Trost, and F. Trudeau. 2005. Evidenced based physical activity for school-age youth. *J. Pediatrics* 146:732-737.

29. U.S. Department of Agriculture. 1999. *Childhood obesity: Causes and prevention. Symposium proceedings* (CNPP-6). Washington, DC: U.S. Department of Agriculture Center for Nutrition Policy and Promotion.

30. U.S. Department of Health and Human Services. 1996. *Physical activity and health: Report of the Surgeon General.* Atlanta: U.S. Department of Health and Human Services, Centers for Disease Control and Prevention, National Center for Chronic Disease Prevention and Health Promotion.

31. U.S. Department of Health and Human Services. 2000. *Healthy people 2010.* Washington, DC: Author.

32. Weiss, M.R. 2000. Motivating kids in physical activity. *PCPFS Research Digest* 3(11).

33. Zwiren, L.D. 2001. Exercise testing and prescription considerations throughout childhood. In *ACSM's resource manual for guidelines for exercise testing and prescription.* 4th ed. Ed. J.L. Roitman, 520-528. Philadelphia: Lippincott Williams & Wilkins.

Chapter 16

1. American College of Sports Medicine. 1998. Exercise and physical activity for older adults. *Medicine and Science in Sports and Exercise* 30:992-1008.

2. American College of Sports Medicine. 1998. The recommended quantity and quality of exercise for developing and maintaining cardiorespiratory and muscular fitness, and flexibility in healthy adults. *Medicine and Science in Sports and Exercise* 30:975-991.

3. American College of Sports Medicine. 2006. *ACSM's guidelines for exercise testing and prescription.* 7th ed. Baltimore: Lippincott Williams & Wilkins.

4. American Council on Exercise. 1998. *Exercise for the older adult.* Champaign, IL: Human Kinetics.

5. Bloomfield, S.A., and S.S. Smith. 2003. Osteoporosis. In *ACSM's exercise management for persons with chronic diseases and disabilities.* 2nd ed. Eds. J. L. Durstine and G. E. Moore, 222-229. Champaign, IL: Human Kinetics.

6. Chodzko-Zajko, W.J. 1998. Physical activity and aging: Implications for health and quality of life in older persons. *PCPFS Research Digest* 3(4).

7. Criswell, D.S. 2001. Human development and aging. In *ACSM's health and fitness certification review.* Eds. J. L. Roitman and K. W. Bibi, 31-47. Baltimore: Lippincott Williams & Wilkins.

8. Fiatarone, M.A., E.C. Marks, N.D. Ryan, C.N. Meredith, L.A. Lipsitz, and W.J. Evans. 1990. High-intensity strength training in nonagenarians. *Journal of the American Medical Association* 263:3029-3034.

9. Fitzgerald, M.D., H. Tanaka, Z.V. Tran, and D.R. Seals. 1997. Age-related declines in maximal aerobic capacity in regularly exercising vs. sedentary women: A meta-analysis. *Journal of Applied Physiology* 83:160-165.

10. Fitzgerald, P.L. 1985. Exercise for the elderly. *Medical Clinics of North America* 69:189-196.

11. Frontera, W.R., C.N. Meredith, K.P. O'Reilly, and W.J. Evans. 1990. Strength training and determinants of $\dot{V}O_2$max in older men. *Journal of Applied Physiology* 68:329-333.

12. Frontera, W.R., C.N. Meredith, K.P. O'Reilly, H.G. Knuttgen, and W.J. Evans. 1988. Strength conditioning in older men: Skeletal muscle hypertrophy and improved function. *Journal of Applied Physiology* 64:1038-1044.

13. Holloszy, J.O., and W.M. Kohrt. 1995. Exercise. In *Handbook of physiology, section 11: Aging,* ed. E.J. Masoro, 633-666. New York: Oxford Press.

14. Howley, E.T. 2001. Type of activity: Resistance, aerobic and leisure versus occupational physical activity. *Medicine and Science in Sports and Exercise* 33: S364-S369.

15. Kraemer, W.J., S.J. Fleck, and W.J. Evans. 1996. Strength and power training: Physiological mechanisms of adaptations. *Exercise and Sport Sciences Reviews* 24:363-397.

16. Minor, M.A., and D.R. Kay. 2003. Arthritis. In *ACSM's exercise management for persons with chronic diseases and disabilities.* Eds. J. L. Durstine and G. E. Moore 210-216. Champaign, IL: Human Kinetics.

17. Pate, R.R., M. Pratt, S.N. Blair, W.L. Haskell, C.A. Marcera, and C. Bouchard. 1995. Physical activity and public health: A recommendation from the Centers for Disease Control and Prevention and the American College of Sports Medicine. *Journal of the American Medical Association* 273:402-407.

18. Rikli, R.E., and C.J. Jones. 2001. *Senior fitness test manual.* Champaign, IL: Human Kinetics.

19. Rimmer, J.H. 1994. *Fitness and rehabilitation programs for special populations.* Dubuque, IA: Brown & Benchmark.

20. Rogers, M.A., and W.J. Evans. 1993. Changes in skeletal muscle with aging: Effects of exercise training. *Exercise and Sport Sciences Reviews* 21:65-102.

21. Shephard, R.J. 1997. *Aging, physical activity, and health.* Champaign, IL: Human Kinetics.

22. Skinner, J.S. 2005. Aging for exercise testing and exercise prescription. In *Exercise testing and exercise prescription for special cases.* 3rd ed. Ed. J.S. Skinner, 85-99. Baltimore: Lippincott Williams & Wilkins.

23. Spirduso, W.W., K.L. Francis, and P.G. MacRae. 2005. *Physical dimensions of aging.* 2nd ed. Champaign, IL: Human Kinetics.

24. Spirduso, W.W., and D.L. Cronin. 2001. Exercise dose response effects on quality of life and independent living in older adults. *Medicine and Science in Sports and Exercise* 33: S598-S608.

25. U.S. Department of Health and Human Services. 1996. *Physical activity and health: A report of the Surgeon General.* Washington, DC: Author.

26. U.S. Department of Health and Human Services. 2003. *A profile of older Americans: 2003.* Washington, DC: Author.

27. World Health Organization. 1997. *A summary of the physiological benefits of physical activity for older persons.* Geneva, Switzerland: Author.

Chapter 17

1. American College of Sports Medicine. 1995. Position stand on osteoporosis and exercise. *Medicine and Science in Sports and Exercise* 27:i-vii.

2. American College of Sports Medicine. 1997. Position stand on the female athlete triad. *Medicine and Science in Sports and Exercise* 29:i-ix.

3. American College of Sports Medicine. 2004. Physical activity and bone health. *Medicine and Science in Sports and Exercise* 36:1985-1996.

4. American College of Sports Medicine. 2006. *ACSM's guidelines for exercise testing and prescription.* Baltimore: Lippincott Williams & Wilkins.

5. American College of Obstetricians and Gynecologists. 2003. Exercise during pregnancy and the postpartum period. *Clinical Obstetrics and Gynecology* 46:496-499.

6. Artal, R., C. Sherman, and N.A. DiNubile. 1999. Exercise during pregnancy. *The Physician and Sportsmedicine* 27:51-60+.

7. Bloomfield, S.A., and S.S. Smith. 2003. Osteoporosis. In *ACSM's exercise management for persons with chronic diseases and disabilities,* ed. J.L. Durstine and G.E. Moore, 222-229. Champaign, IL: Human Kinetics.

8. Drinkwater, B.L., K. Nilson, C.H. Chesnut, W.J. Bremner, S. Schainholtz, and M.B. Southworth. 1984. Bone mineral content of amenorrheic and eumenorrheic athletes. *New England Journal of Medicine* 311:277-281.

9. Heffernan, A.E. 2000. Exercise and pregnancy in primary care. *The Nurse Practitioner* 25:42, 49, 53-56, 59-60.

10. Hobart, J.A., and D.R. Smucker. 2000. The female athlete triad. *American Family Physician* 61:3357-3364, 3367.

11. Johnson, M.D. 1994. Disordered eating. In *Medical and orthopedic issues of active and athletic women,* ed. R. Agostini, 141-151. Philadelphia: Hanley & Belfus.

12. Khan, K., H. McKay, P. Kannus, D. Bailey, J. Wark, and K. Bennell. 2001. *Physical activity and bone health.* Champaign, IL: Human Kinetics.

13. Metcalfe, L., T. Lohman, S. Going, L. Houtkooper, D. Ferriera, H. Flint-Wagner, T. Guido, J. Martin, J. Wright, and E. Cussler. 2001. Postmenopausal women and exercise for prevention of osteoporosis: The Bone, Estrogen, Strength Training (BEST) study. *ACSM's Health and Fitness Journal* 5:6-14.

14. National Institutes of Health. 2000. Osteoporosis prevention, diagnosis, and therapy. NIH Consensus Development Conference. Bethesda, MD: National Institutes of Health.

15. Nichols, D.L., and E.V. Essery. 2006. Osteoporosis and exercise. In *ACSM's resource manual for guidelines for exercise testing and prescription,* ed. L.A. Kaminsky, 489-499. Baltimore, MD: Lippicott Williams & Wilkins.

16. Smolak, L., S.K. Murnen, and A.E. Ruble. 2000. Female athletes and eating problems: A meta-analysis. *International Journal of Eating Disorders* 27:371-380.

17. U.S. Department of Health and Human Services. 2004. *Bone health and osteoporosis: A report of the Surgeon General*. Rockville, MD: U.S. Department of Health and Human Services, Office of the Surgeon General.

18. Wang, T.W., and B.S. Apgar. 1998. Exercise during pregnancy. *American Family Physician* 57:1846-1852, 1857.

Chapter 18

1. American College of Sports Medicine. 2004. Position stand: Exercise and hypertension. *Medicine and Science in Sports and Exercise* 36(3): 533-553.

2. American College of Sports Medicine. 2006. *ACSM's guidelines for exercise testing and prescription.* 7th ed. Baltimore: Lippincott Williams & Wilkins.

3. American Association for Cardiovascular and Pulmonary Rehabilitation. 2004. *Guidelines for cardiac rehabilitation and secondary prevention programs.* 4th ed. Champaign, IL: Human Kinetics.

4. American Heart Association. 2005. *Heart and stroke statistics—2005 update.* Dallas: American Heart Association.

5. Brubaker, P.H., L.A. Kaminsky, and M.H. Whaley. 2002. *Coronary artery disease: Essentials of prevention and rehabilitation programs.* 83-110. Champaign, IL: Human Kinetics.

6. Clausen, J.P. 1977. Circulatory adjustments to dynamic exercise and physical training in normal subjects and in patients with coronary artery disease. In *Exercise and the heart,* ed. E.H. Sonnenblick and M. Lesch, 39-75. New York: Grune & Stratton.

7. Enos, W., R. Holmes, and J. Beyer. 1953. Coronary disease among United States soldiers killed in action in Korea. *Journal of the American Medical Association* 152:1090-1093.

8. Franklin, B.A. 2003. Myocardial infarction. In *ACSM's exercise management for persons with chronic disease and disability,* ed. J.L. Durstine and G.E. Moore, 24-31. Champaign, IL: Human Kinetics.

9. Franklin, B.A. 2003. Coronary artery bypass grafting and angioplasty. In *ACSM's exercise management for persons with chronic disease and disability,* ed. J.L. Durstine and G.E. Moore, 32-39. Champaign, IL: Human Kinetics.

10. Grines, C.L. 1996. Aggressive intervention for myocardial infarction: Angioplasty, stents, and intra-aortic balloon pumping. *American Journal of Cardiology* 78:29-34.

11. Hagberg, J.M. 1990. Exercise, fitness, and hypertension. In *Physical activity, fitness, and health,* ed. C. Bouchard, R.J. Shephard, and T. Stephens, 993-1005. Champaign, IL: Human Kinetics.

12. Hillegass E.A., and W.C. Temes. 2001. Therapeutic interventions in cardiac rehabilitation and prevention. In *Essentials of cardiopulmonary physical therapy.* 2nd ed. Ed. E.A. Hillegass and H.S. Sadowsky, 676-726. Philadelphia: Saunders.

13. Kaplan, N.M. 1994. *Clinical hypertension.* 6th ed. Baltimore: Williams & Wilkins.

14. Ornish, D., L.W. Scherwitz, and J.H. Billings. 1998. Intensive lifestyle changes for reversal of coronary heart disease. *Journal of the American Medical Association* 280:2001-2007.

15. Paschkow, F.J., and S.A. Harvey. 2001. Diagnosis of coronary artery disease. In *ACSM's resource manual for guidelines for exercise testing and prescription.* 4th ed. Ed. J.L. Roitman, 246-253. Baltimore: Lippincott Williams & Wilkins.

16. Pollock, M.L., and J.H. Wilmore. 1990. *Exercise in health and disease.* 2nd ed. Philadelphia: Saunders.

17. Regensteiner, J.G., and W.G. Hunt. 2001. Exercise in the management of peripheral arterial disease. In *ACSM's resource manual for guidelines for exercise testing and prescription.* 4th ed. Ed. J.L. Roitman, 292-298. Baltimore: Lippincott Williams & Wilkins.

18. Squires, R.W. 2006. Coronary atherosclerosis. In *ACSM's resource manual for guidelines for exercise testing and prescription.* 5th ed. Ed. L.A. Kaminsky, 411-426. Baltimore: Lippincott Williams & Wilkins.

19. Thompson, P.D. 1988. The benefits and risks of exercise training in patients with chronic coronary artery disease. *Journal of the American Medical Association* 259:1537-1540.

20. Wenger, N.K., and J.W. Hurst. 1984. Coronary bypass surgery as a rehabilitative procedure. In *Rehabilitation of the coronary patient,* ed. N.K. Wenger and H.K. Hellerstein, 115-132. New York: Wiley.

Chapter 19

1. American College of Sports Medicine. 2001. Appropriate intervention strategies for weight loss and prevention of weight regain for adults. *Medicine and Science in Sports and Exercise* 33:2145-2156.

2. American College of Sports Medicine. 2006. *ACSM's guidelines for exercise testing and prescription.* Baltimore: Lippincott Williams & Wilkins.

3. Allison, D.B., K.R. Fontaine, J.E. Manson, J. Stevens, and T.B. VanItallie. 1999. Annual deaths attributable to obesity in the United States. *Journal of the American Medical Association* 282:1530-1538.

4. Ball, K., D. Crawford, and N. Owen. 2000. Too fat to exercise? Obesity as a barrier to physical activity. *Australian and New Zealand Journal of Public Health* 24:331-333.

5. Beamer, B.A. 2003. Genetic influences on obesity. In *Obesity: Etiology, assessment, treatment and prevention,* ed. R.E. Anderson, 43-56. Champaign, IL: Human Kinetics.

6. Bouchard, C., L. Perusse, C. Leblanc, A. Tremblay, and G. Theriault. 1988. Inheritance of the amount and distribution of human body fat. *International Journal of Obesity* 12:205-215.

7. DiPietro, L. 1999. Physical activity in the prevention of obesity: Current evidence and research issues. *Medicine and Science in Sports and Exercise* 31:S542-S546.

8. Expert Panel on the Identification, Evaluation and Treatment of Overweight and Obesity in Adults. 1998. Executive summary of the clinical guidelines on the identification, evaluation, and treatment of overweight and obesity in adults. *Archives of Internal Medicine* 158:1855-1867.

9. Flegal, K., M. Carroll, C. Ogden, and C. Johnson. 2002. Prevalence and trends in obesity among US adults, 1999-2000. *Journal of the American Medical Association* 288:1723-1727.

10. Flegal, K.M., B.I. Graubard, D.F. Williamson, and M.H. Gail. 2005. Excess deaths associated with underweight, overweight, and obesity. *Journal of the American Medical Association* 293:1861-1867.

11. Food and Nutrition Board, Institute of Medicine. 2002. *Dietary reference intakes for energy, carbohydrate, fiber, fat, fatty acids, cholesterol, protein, and amino acids.* Washington, DC: National Academies Press.

12. Gortmaker, S., A. Must, A. Sobel, K. Peterson, G.A. Colditz, and W.H. Dietz. 1996. Television viewing as a cause of increasing obesity among children in the United States. *Archives of Pediatric Adolescent Medicine* 150:356-362.

13. Grilo, C.M., and K.D. Brownell. 2001. Interventions for weight management. In *ACSM's resource manual for guidelines for exercise testing and prescription.* 4th ed. Ed. J.L. Roitman, 584-591. Baltimore: Lippincott Williams & Wilkins.

14. Grundy, S.M., G. Blackburn, M. Higgins, R. Lauer, M.G. Perri, and D. Ryan. 1999. Physical activity in the prevention and treatment of obesity and its comorbidities: Roundtable consensus statement. *Medicine and Science in Sports and Exercise* 31: S502-S508.

15. Hedley, A.A., C.L. Ogden, C.L. Johnson, M.D. Carroll, L.R. Curtin, and K.M. Flegal. 2004. Prevalence of overweight and obesity among US children, adolescents, and adults, 1999-2002. *Journal of the American Medical Association* 291:2847-2850.

16. Jakicic, J.M. 2003. Exercise in the treatment of obesity. *Endocrinology and Metabolism Clinics of North America* 32:967-980.

17. Jakicic, J.M. 2003. Exercise strategies for the obese patient. *Primary Care* 30:393-403.

18. Jebb, S.A., and M.S. Moore. 1999. Contribution of a sedentary lifestyle and inactivity to the etiology of overweight and obesity: Current evidence and research issues. *Medicine and Science in Sports and Exercise* 31: S534-S541.

19. Kaminsky, L.A., and G. Dwyer. 2006. Body composition. In *ACSM's resource manual for guidelines for exercise testing and prescription.* 5th ed. Ed. L.A. Kaminsky, 195-205. Baltimore: Lippincott Williams & Wilkins.

20. Khan, L.K., and B.A. Bowman. 1999. Obesity: A major global public health problem. *Annual Review of Nutrition* 19:xiii-xvii.

21. Li, Z., M. Maglione, W. Tu, W. Mojica, D. Arterburn, L.R. Shugarman, L. Hilton, M. Suttorp, V. Solomon, P.G. Shekelle, and S.C. Morton. 2005. Meta-analysis: Pharmacologic treatment of obesity. *Annals of Internal Medicine* 142:532-546.

22. Lohman, T.G., L. Houtkooper, and S.B. Going. 1997. Body fat measurement goes high-tech: Not all are created equal. *ACSM's Health and Fitness Journal* 1:30-35.

23. Maggard, M.A., L.R. Shugarman, M. Suttorp, M. Maglione, H.J. Sugarman, E.H. Livingston, N.T. Nguyen, Z. Li, W. Mojica, L. Hilton, S. Rhodes, S.C. Morton, and P.G. Shekelle. 2005. Meta-analysis: Surgical treatment of obesity. *Annals of Internal Medicine* 142:547-559.

24. National Heart, Lung, and Blood Institute. 1998. *Clinical guidelines on the identification, evaluation, and treatment of overweight and obesity in adults* (NIH Publication No. 98-4083). Bethesda, MD: National Institutes of Health—National Heart, Lung, and Blood Institute.

25. Okosun, I.S., K.M.D. Chandra, A. Boev, J.M. Boltri, S.T. Choi, D.C. Parrish, and G.E.A. Dever. 2004. Abdominal adiposity in U.S. adults: Prevalence and trends, 1960-2000. *Preventive Medicine* 39:197-206.

26. Robinson, T.N. 1998. Does television cause childhood obesity? *Journal of the American Medical Association* 279:959-960.

27. Salbe, A.D., and E. Ravussin. 2000. The determinants of obesity. In *Physical activity and obesity,* ed. C. Bouchard, 69-102. Champaign, IL: Human Kinetics.

28. Saris, W.H.M., S.N. Blair, M.A. van Baak, S.B. Eaton, P.S.W. Davies, L. Di Pietro, M. Fogelholm, A. Rissanen, D. Schoeller, B. Swinburn, A. Tremblay, K.R. Westerterp, and H. Wyatt. 2003. How much physical activity is enough to prevent unhealthy weight gain? Outcome of the IASO 1st Stock Conference and consensus statement. *Obesity Reviews* 4:101-114.

29. Seidell, J.C. 2000. The current epidemic of obesity. In *Physical activity and obesity,* ed. C. Bouchard, 21-30. Champaign, IL: Human Kinetics.

30. Snow, V., P. Barry, N. Fitterman, A. Qaseem, and K. Weiss. 2005. Pharmacologic and surgical management of obesity in primary care: A clinical practice guideline for the American College of Physicians. *Annals of Internal Medicine* 142:525-531.

31. Stubbs, C.O., and A.J. Lee. 2004. The obesity epidemic: Both energy intake and physical activity contribute. *Medical Journal of Australia* 181:489-491.

32. U.S. Department of Health and Human Services. 2001. *The Surgeon General's call to action to prevent and decrease overweight and obesity.* Rockville, MD: U.S. Government Printing Office.

33. Wallace, J.P. 2003. Obesity. In *ACSM's exercise management for persons with chronic diseases and disabilities.* 2nd ed. Ed. J.L. Durstine and G.E. Moore, 149-156. Champaign, IL: Human Kinetics.

34. Welk, G.J., and Blair, S.N. 2000. Physical activity protects against the health risks of obesity. *PCPFS Research Digest* 3:1-7.

35. Wing, R.R. 1999. Physical activity in the treatment of adulthood overweight and obesity: Current evidence and research issues. *Medicine and Science in Sports and Exercise* 31:S547-S552.

36. Wing, R.R., and Hill, J.O. 2001. Successful weight loss maintenance. *Annual Review of Nutrition* 21:323-341.

Chapter 20

1. American College of Sports Medicine. 2000. Exercise and type 2 diabetes. *Medicine and Science in Sports and Exercise* 32:1345-1360.

2. American College of Sports Medicine. 2006. *ACSM's guidelines for exercise testing and prescription.* Baltimore: Lippincott Williams & Wilkins.

3. American Diabetes Association. 2003. Economic costs of diabetes in the U.S. in 2002. *Diabetes Care* 26:917-932.

4. American Diabetes Association. 2004. Physical activity/exercise and diabetes. *Diabetes Care* 27: S58-S62.

5. American Diabetes Association. 2005. Standards of medical care in diabetes. *Diabetes Care* 28: S4-S36.

6. Bassuk, S.S., and J.E. Manson. 2005. Epidemiological evidence for the role of physical activity in reducing risk of type 2 diabetes and cardiovascular disease. *Journal of Applied Physiology* 99:1193-1204.

7. Eriksson, J.G. 1999. Exercise and the treatment of type 2 diabetes mellitus: An update. *Sports Medicine* 27:381-391.

8. Ford, E.S., W.H. Giles, and A.H. Mokdad. 2004. Increasing prevalence of the metabolic syndrome among U.S. adults. *Diabetes Care* 27:2444-2449.

9. Gordon, N.F. 1993. *Diabetes: Your complete exercise guide.* Champaign, IL: Human Kinetics.

10. Grundy, S.M., J.L. Cleeman, S.R. Daniels, K.A. Donato, R.H. Eckel, B.A. Franklin, D.J. Gordon, R.M. Krauss, P.J. Savage, S.C. Smith, J.A. Spertus, and F. Costa. 2005. Diagnosis and management of the metabolic syndrome: An American Heart Association/National Heart, Lung, and Blood Institute Scientific Statement. *Circulation* 112:2735-2752.

11. Hornsby, W.G., and A.L. Albright. 2003. Diabetes. In *ACSM's exercise management for persons with chronic diseases and disabilities,* ed. J.L. Durstine and G.E. Moore, 133-141. Champaign, IL: Human Kinetics.

12. Kriska, A. 2000. Physical activity and the prevention of type 2 diabetes mellitus: How much for how long? *Sports Medicine* 29:147-151.

13. Lampman, R.M., and B.N. Campaigne. 2006. Exercise testing in patients with diabetes. In *ACSM's resource manual for guidelines for exercise testing and prescription,* ed. L.A. Kaminsky, 245-254. Baltimore: Lippincott Williams & Wilkins.

14. U.S. Department of Health and Human Services. 2000. *Healthy people 2010: Understanding and improving health.* Washington, DC: U.S. Government Printing Office.

15. Verity, L.S. 2006. Diabetes mellitus and exercise. In *ACSM's resource manual for guidelines for exercise testing and prescription,* ed. L.A. Kaminsky, 470-479. Baltimore: Lippincott Williams & Wilkins.

Chapter 21

1. American Association of Cardiovascular and Pulmonary Rehabilitation. 2004. *Guidelines for pulmonary rehabilitation programs.* 3rd ed. Champaign, IL: Human Kinetics.
2. American College of Sports Medicine. 2006. *ACSM's guidelines for exercise testing and prescription.* 7th ed. Baltimore: Lippincott Williams & Wilkins.
3. Barr, R.N. 2001. Pulmonary rehabilitation. In *Essentials of cardiopulmonary physical therapy.* 2nd ed. Ed. E.A. Hillegass and H.S. Sadowsky, 727-751. Philadelphia: Saunders.
4. Berman, L.B., and J.R. Sutton. 1986. Exercise and the pulmonary patient. *Journal of Cardiopulmonary Rehabilitation* 6:52-61.
5. Borg, G.A. 1998. *Borg's perceived exertion and pain scales.* Champaign, IL: Human Kinetics.
6. Brubaker, P.H., L.A. Kaminsky, and M.H. Whaley. 2002. *Coronary artery disease: Essentials of prevention and rehabilitation programs.* Champaign, IL: Human Kinetics.
7. Cahalin, L.P., and H.S. Sadowsky. 2001. Pulmonary medications. In *Essentials of cardiopulmonary physical therapy.* 2nd ed. Ed. E.A. Hillegass and H.S. Sadowsky, 587-607. Philadelphia: Saunders.
8. Casaburi, R. 2001. Special considerations for exercise training in chronic lung disease. In *ACSM's resource manual for guidelines for exercise testing and prescription.* 4th ed. Ed. J.L. Roitman, 346-352. Baltimore: Lippincott Williams & Wilkins.
9. Clough, P. 2001. Restrictive lung dysfunction. In *Essentials of cardiopulmonary physical therapy.* 2nd ed. Ed. E.A. Hillegass and H.S. Sadowsky, 183-255. Philadelphia: Saunders.
10. Cooper, C.B. 1995. Determining the role of exercise in patients with chronic pulmonary disease. *Medicine and Science in Sports and Exercise* 27:147-157.
11. Davidson, A.C., R. Leach, R.J.D. George, and D.M. Geddes. 1988. Supplemental oxygen and exercise ability in chronic obstructive airways disease. *Thorax* 43:965-971.
12. Davis, P.B. 1991. Cystic fibrosis: A major cause of obstructive airway disease in the young. In *Chronic obstructive pulmonary disease,* ed. N.S. Cheniack, 297-307. Philadelphia: Saunders.
13. Garritan, S.L. 1994. Chronic obstructive pulmonary disease. In *Essentials of cardiopulmonary physical therapy,* ed. E.A. Hillegass and H.S. Sadowsky, 257-284. Philadelphia: Saunders.
14. Guyton, A.C., and J.E. Hall. 2006. *Textbook of medical physiology.* 11th ed. Philadelphia: Saunders.
15. Hurd, S. 2000. The impact of COPD on lung health worldwide. *Chest* 117:1S-4S.
16. Lacroix, V.J. 1999. Exercise-induced asthma. *The Physician and Sportsmedicine* 27:75-92.
17. Mahler, D.A., and M.B. Horowitz. 1994. Perception of breathlessness during exercise in patients with respiratory disease. *Medicine and Science in Sports and Exercise* 26:1078-1081.
18. Peno-Green, L.A., and C.B. Cooper. 2006. Treatment and rehabilitation of pulmonary diseases. In *ACSM's resource manual for guidelines for exercise testing and prescription.* 4th ed. Ed. M.H. Whaley, 452-469. Baltimore: Lippincott Williams & Wilkins.
19. Rundell, K.W., and D.M. Jenkinson. 2002. Exercise-induced bronchospasm in the elite athlete. *Sports Medicine* 32:583-600.

Chapter 22

1. Adams, J., and M. White. 2003. Are activity promotion interventions based on the transtheoretical model effective? A critical review. *British Journal of Sports Medicine* 37:106-114.
2. Annesi, J.J. 1996. *Enhancing exercise motivation.* Los Angeles: Leisure.
3. Biddle, S., and C.R. Nigg. 2000. Theories of exercise behavior. *International Journal of Sport Psychology* 31:290-304.
4. Buckworth, J. 2000. Exercise determinants and interventions. *International Journal of Sport Psychology* 2:305-320.
5. Croteau, K.A. 2004. A preliminary study on the impact of a pedometer-based intervention on daily steps. *American Journal of Health Promotion* 18:217-220.
6. Dishman, R.K., and J. Buckworth. 1996. Adherence to physical activity. In *Physical activity and mental health,* ed. W.P. Morgan, 63-80. Washington, DC: Taylor & Francis.
7. Ewing, R. 2005. Can the physical environment determine physical activity levels? *Exercise and Sport Sciences Reviews* 33:69-75.
8. Ewing, R., T. Schmid, R. Killingsworth, A. Zlot, and S. Raudenbush. 2003. Relationship between urban sprawl and physical activity, obesity, and morbidity. *American Journal of Health Promotion* 18:47-57.
9. Gabriele, J.M., M.S. Walker, D.L. Gill, K.D. Harber, and E.B. Fisher. 2005. Differentiated roles of social encouragement and social constraint on physical activity behavior. *Annals of Behavioral Medicine* 29:210-215.
10. Hagger, M.S., N.L.D. Chatzisarantis, and S.J.H. Biddle. 2002. A meta-analytic review of the theories of reasoned action and planned behavior in physical activity: Predictive validity and the contribution of additional variables. *Journal of Sport and Exercise Psychology* 24:3-32.
11. Hultquist, C.N, C. Albright, and D.L. Thompson. 2005. Comparison of walking recommendations in previously inactive women. *Medicine and Science in Sports and Exercise* 37:676-683.
12. King, A.C., J.E. Martin, and C. Castro. 2006. Behavioral strategies to enhance physical activity participation. In *ACSM's resource manual for guidelines for exercise testing and prescription,* ed. L.A. Kaminsky and K.A. Bonzheim, 572-580. Philadelphia: Lippincott Williams & Wilkins.
13. King, A.C., D. Stokols, E. Talen, G.S. Brassington, and R. Killingsworth. 2002. Theoretical approaches to the promotion of physical activity: Forging a transdisciplinary paradigm. *American Journal of Preventive Medicine* 23:15-25.
14. Knapp, D.N. 1988. Behavioral management techniques and exercise promotion. In *Exercise adherence,* ed. R.K. Dishman, 203-236. Champaign, IL: Human Kinetics.
15. Kyllo, L.B., and D.M. Landers. 1995. Goal setting in sport and exercise: A research synthesis to resolve the controversy. *Journal of Sport and Exercise Psychology* 17:117-137.
16. Marcus, B., and L. Forsyth. 2003. *Motivating people to be physically active.* Champaign, IL: Human Kinetics.
17. Marcus, B.H., P.M. Dubbert, L.H. Forsyth, T.L. McKenzie, E.J. Stone, A.L. Dunn, and S.N. Blair. 2000. Physical activity behavior change: Issues in adoption and maintenance. *Health Psychology* 19:32-41.
18. Markland, D., and L. Hardy. 1993. The exercise motivation inventory: Preliminary development and validity of a measure of individuals' reasons for participation in regular physical exercise. *Personality and Individual Differences* 15:289-296.
19. Marlatt, G.A., and J.R. Gordon. 1985. *Relapse prevention: Maintenance strategies in the treatment of addictive behaviors.* New York: Guilford Press.

20. Prochaska, J.O., and C.C. DiClemente. 1983. Stages and processes of self-change of smoking: Toward an integrative model of change. *Journal of Consulting and Clinical Psychology* 51:390-395.
21. Prochaska, J.O., and B.H. Marcus. 1994. The transtheoretical model: Applications to exercise. In *Advances in exercise adherence,* ed. R.K. Dishman, 161-180. Champaign, IL: Human Kinetics.
22. Prochaska, J.O., and W.F. Velicer. 1997. The transtheoretical model of behavior change. *American Journal of Health Promotion* 12:38-48.
23. Sonstroem, R.J. 1988. Psychological models. In *Exercise adherence: Its impact on public health,* ed. R.K. Dishman, 125-153. Champaign, IL: Human Kinetics.
24. Southard, D.R., and B.H. Southard. 2001. Health counseling skills. In *ACSM's resource manual for guidelines for exercise testing and prescription,* ed. J.L. Roitman and M. Herridge, 537-540. Baltimore: Williams & Wilkins.
25. Trost, S.G., N. Owen, A. Bauman, J.F. Sallis, and W.J. Brown. 2002. Correlates of adults' participation in physical activity: Review and update. *Medicine and Science in Sports and Exercise* 34:1996-2001.
26. Wallace, J.P., J.S. Raglin, and C.A. Jastremski. 1995. Twelve month adherence of adults who joined a fitness program with a spouse vs without a spouse. *The Journal of Sports Medicine and Physical Fitness* 35:206-213.

Chapter 23

1. Anderson R., and D. Specter. 2000. Introduction to Pilates-based rehabilitation. *Orthopaedic Physical Therapy Clinics of North America* 9:395-410.
2. Cacciatore, T.W., F.B. Horak, and S.M. Henry. 2005. Improvement in automatic postural coordination following Alexander Technique lessons in a person with low back pain. *Physical Therapy* 85:565-578.
3. DiBenedetto, M., K.E. Innes, A. Taylor, P.F. Rodeheaver, J.A. Boxer, H.J. Wright, and D.C. Kerrigan. 2005. Effect of a gentle Iyengar yoga program on gait in the elderly: An exploratory study. *Archives of Physical Medicine and Rehabilitation* 86:1830.
4. IDEA. Fitness Trends 2005. 2005. *IDEA Fitness Manager.* 17:11-12. San Diego: International Dance Exercise Association.
5. Kirkwood, G., H. Rampes, V. Tuffrey, J. Richardson, and K. Pilkington. 2005. Yoga for anxiety: A systematic review of the research evidence. *British Journal of Sports Medicine* 39:884-889.
6. La Forge, R. 1995. Exercise associated mood alterations: A review of interactive neurobiologic mechanisms. *Medicine Exercise and Health.* 4:17-34.
7. Miller, B.S. 1995. *Yoga: Discipline of freedom.* New York: Bantam Books.
8. Murrgesan, R., N. Govindarajulu, and T.K. Bera. 2000. Effect of yogic practices on the management of hypertension. *Indian Journal of Physiological Pharmacology* 44:207-210.
9. Pal, G.K., and S. Velkumary. 2004. Effect of short-term practice of breathing exercises on autonomic functions in normal human volunteers. *Indian Journal of Medical Research* 120:115-121.
10. Prakash, E.S. 2005. Effect of deep breathing at six breaths per minute on the frequency of premature ventricular complexes. *International Journal of Cardiology.* [Online]. Available: *doi:10.1016/j.ijcard.2005.05.075.*
11. Rickover, R.M. 1988. *Fitness without stress: A guide to the Alexander Technique.* Portland, OR: Metamorphous Press.
12. Sancier, K., and D. Holman. 2004. Multifaceted health benefits of qigong. *Journal of Alternative and Complementary Medicine* 10:163-166.
13. Segal, N.A., J. Hein, and J.R. Basford. 2004. The effects of Pilates training on flexibility and body composition: An observational study. *Archives of Physical Medicine and Rehabilitation* 85:1977-1981.
14. Sovik, R. 2000. The science of breathing—The yogic view. In E.A. Mayer and C.B. Sayer (Eds). *Progress in Brain Research* 122:491-505. Elsevier Science BV.
15. Wang, C., J.P. Collet, and J. Lau. 2004. The effect of tai chi on health outcomes in patients with chronic conditions. *Archives of Internal Medicine* 164:493-501.
16. Iyengar, B.K.S. 1977. *Light on Yoga: Yoga Dipika.* New York: Schocken Books.
17. Benson, H., and M.Z. Klipper. 1975. *The Relaxation Response.* William Morrow and Company, Inc.
18. Rosas, D., and C. Rosas. 2005. *The NIA Technique.* New York: Broadway Books.

Chapter 24

1. Ades, P.A., P.G. Gunter, W.L. Meyer, T.C. Gibson, J. Maddalena, and T. Orfeo. 1990. Cardiac and skeletal muscle adaptations to training in systemic hypertension and effect of beta blockade (metoprolol or propranolol). *American Journal of Cardiology* 166(5):591-596.
2. American College of Sports Medicine. 2006. *Guidelines for exercise testing and prescription.* 7th ed. Baltimore: Lippincott Williams & Wilkins.
3. American College of Sports Medicine and American Heart Association. 2002. Joint position statement: Automated external defibrillators in health/fitness facilities. *Medicine and Science in Sports and Exercise* 34(3):561-564.
4. American Hospital Formulary Service. 2001. *Drug information 2001.* Bethesda, MD: American Society of Hospital Pharmacists.
5. Berne, R.M., and M.N. Levy. 2001. *Cardiovascular physiology.* 8th ed. St. Louis: Mosby.
6. Chang, K., and K.F. Hossack. 1982. Effect of diltiazem on heart rate responses and respiratory variables during exercise: Implications for exercise prescription and cardiac rehabilitation. *Journal of Cardiac Rehabilitation* 2:326-332.
7. Conover, M.B. 1996. *Understanding electrocardiography.* 7th ed. St. Louis: Mosby.
8. Donnelly, J.E. 1990. *Living anatomy.* 2nd ed. Champaign, IL: Human Kinetics.
9. Dubin, D. 2000. *Rapid interpretation of EKGs.* 6th ed. Tampa: Cover.
10. Ellestad, M. 1994. *Stress testing: Principles and practice.* Philadelphia: Davis.
11. Hossack, K.F., R.A. Bruce, and L.J. Clark. 1980. Influence of propranolol on exercise prescription of training heart rates. *Cardiology* 65:47-58.
12. Hurst, J.W. 1994. *Diagnostic atlas of the heart.* Philadelphia: Lippincott-Raven.
13. Kannel, W.B., and R.D. Abbot. 1984. Incidence and prognosis of unrecognized myocardial infarction. *New England Journal of Medicine* 311:1144-1147.
14. Kelbaek, H., T. Gjorup, S. Floistrup, O. Hartling, N. Christensen, and J. Godtfredsen. 1985. Acute effects of alcohol on left ventricular function in healthy subjects at rest and during upright exercise. *American Journal of Cardiology* 55: 164-167.
15. Kinderman, W. 1987. Calcium antagonists and exercise performance. *Sports Medicine* 4(3): 177-193.
16. MacGowan, G.A., D. O'Callaghan, and J.H. Horgan. 1992. The effects of verapamil on training in patients with ischemic heart disease. *Chest* 101(2): 411-415.

17. Pavia, L., G. Orlando, J. Myers, M. Maestri, and C. Rusconi. 1995. The effect of beta-blockade therapy on the response to exercise training in postmyocardial infarction patients. *Clinical Cardiology* 18(12):716-720.
18. Stein, E. 2000. *Rapid analysis of electrocardiograms: A self study program.* 3rd ed. Philadelphia: Lea & Febiger.
19. Tesch, P.A. 1985. Exercise performance and beta-blockade. *Sports Medicine* 2(6):389-412.
20. Williams, M.H. 1991. Alcohol, marijuana and beta blockers. In *Perspectives in exercise science and sports medicine: Vol. 4. Ergogenics: Enhancement of performance in exercise and sport,* ed. D.R. Lamb and M.H. Williams, 331-372. Dubuque, IA: Brown & Benchmark.

Chapter 25

1. American Academy of Orthopedic Surgeons. 1977. *Emergency care and transportation of the sick and injured.* 2nd ed. Menasha, WI: Banta.
2. American Academy of Orthopedic Surgeons. 1998. *Emergency care and transportation of the sick and injured.* 7th ed. Sudbury, MA: Jones and Bartlett.
3. American Medical Association. 1966. *Standard nomenclature of athletic injuries.* Chicago: Author.
4. American Heart Association. 2005. *BLS for Healthcare Providers.* Dallas, Texas.
5. American Red Cross. 1993. *Adult CPR.* St. Louis: Mosby.
6. American Red Cross. 1993. *Community CPR.* St. Louis: Mosby.
7. American Red Cross. 1993. *Community first aid and safety.* St. Louis: Mosby.
8. American Red Cross. 1993. *Emergency response.* St. Louis: Mosby.
9. American Red Cross. 1993. *Preventing disease transmission.* St. Louis: Mosby.
10. American Red Cross. 2001. *First aid/CPR/AED program: Participant's booklet.* San Bruno, CA: Author.
11. Arnheim, D.D. 1987. *Essentials of athletic training.* St. Louis: Times Mirror/Mosby.
12. Arnheim, D.D., and W.E. Prentice. 2002. *Essentials of athletic training.* Boston: McGraw-Hill.
13. Arnheim, D.D., and W.E. Prentice. 1993. *Principles of athletic training.* 8th ed. St. Louis: Mosby.
14. Arnheim, D.D. 1989. *Modern principles of athletic training.* St. Louis: Times Mirror/Mosby.
15. Arnheim, D.D., and W.E. Prentice. 1993. *Principles of athletic training.* St. Louis: Mosby.
16. Bloomfield, J., P.A. Fricker, and K.P. Fitch, eds. 1992. *Textbook of science and medicine in sport.* Champaign, IL: Human Kinetics.
17. Booher, J.M., and G.A. Thibadeau. 1994. *Athletic injury assessment.* 3rd ed. St. Louis: Mosby.
18. Burke, E.R., and J.R. Berning. 1996. *Training nutrition: The diet and nutrition guide for peak performance.* Traverse City, MI: Cooper.
19. Department of Labor, Occupational Safety and Health Administration. 1991. Occupational exposure to bloodborne pathogens: Final rule. *Federal Register* [Online], 56(235): 1-36. Available: osha.gov/Publications/Osha3127.pdf [July 10, 2002].
20. Fahey, T.D. 1986. *Athletic training.* Mountain View, CA: Mayfield.
21. Franks, B.D., and E.T. Howley. 1989. *Fitness facts: The healthy living handbook.* Champaign, IL: Human Kinetics.
22. Franks, B.D., and E.T. Howley. 1989. *Fitness leaders' handbook.* Champaign, IL: Human Kinetics.
23. Henderson, J. 1973. *Emergency medical guide.* 3rd ed. St. Louis: Mosby.
24. Hillman, S.K. 2000. *Introduction to athletic training.* Champaign, IL: Human Kinetics.
25. Klafs, C.E., and D.D. Arnheim. 1977. *Modern principles of athletic training.* St. Louis: Mosby.
26. Morris, A.F. 1984. *Sports medicine: Prevention of athletic injuries.* Dubuque, IA: Brown.
27. Nieman, D.C. 1990. *Fitness and sports medicine: An introduction.* Palo Alto, CA: Bull.
28. Pfeiffer, R.P., and B.C. Pfeiffer. 1995. *Concepts of athletic training.* Boston: Jones & Bartlett.
29. Rankin, J.M., and C.D. Ingersoll. 1995. *Athletic training management: Concepts and applications.* St. Louis: Mosby.
30. Rankin, J.M., and C.D. Ingersoll. 2001. *Athletic training management: Concepts and applications.* 2nd ed. Boston: McGraw-Hill.
31. Reid, D. 1992. *Sports injury assessment and rehabilitation.* New York: Churchill Livingstone.
32. Ritter, M.A., and M.J. Albohm. 1987. *Your inquiry: A commonsense guide to sports injuries.* Indianapolis: Benchmark Press.
33. Scribner, K., and E. Burke, eds. 1978. *Relevant topics in athletic training.* New York: Mouvement.
34. Thygerson, A.L. 1987. *First aid and emergency care workbook.* Boston: Jones & Bartlett.
35. Torg, J.S., P.R. Welsh, and R.J. Shepard. 1990. *Current therapy in sports medicine.* St. Louis: Mosby.

Chapter 26

1. Agoglia, J. 2005. The AED agenda. *Fitness Business Pro*, 6(2): 32-33.
2. American College of Sports Medicine. 2006. *ACSM's guidelines for exercise testing and prescription.* 7th ed. Baltimore: Lippincott Williams & Wilkins.
3. American College of Sports Medicine. 2005. *ACSM's resource manual for guidelines for exercise testing and prescription* (5th ed.). Philadelphia: Lippincott Williams & Wilkins.
4. American College of Sports Medicine. 2006. *ACSM's health/fitness facility standards and guidelines* (3rd ed.). Philadelphia: Lippincott Williams & Wilkins.
5. American Heart Association and American College of Sports Medicine Joint Scientific Statement. 2002. Automated external defibrillators in health/fitness facilities. *Circulation* 105(9): 1147-1150.
6. Balady, G. Chaitman, D., Driscoll, C. Foster, E. Froelicher, N. Gordon, R. Pate, J. Rippe, and T. Bazzarre. 1998. American Heart Association and American College of Sports Medicine Joint Scientific Statement: Recommendations for cardiovascular screening, staffing, and emergency policies at health/fitness facilities. *Medicine and Science in Sports and Exercise* 30(96):1009-1018.
7. Brown, S. 2001. *An introduction to exercise science.* Baltimore: Lippincott Williams & Wilkins.
8. Eickhoff-Shemek, J., and F. Forbes. 1999. Waivers are usually worth the effort. *ACSM's Health and Fitness Journal* 3(4):24-30.
9. Eickhoff-Shemek, J., and K. Deja. 2000. Four steps to minimize legal liability in exercise programs. *ACSM's Health and Fitness Journal* 4(4):13-18.
10. Eickhoff-Shemek, J. 2002. Exercise equipment injuries: Who's at fault? *ACSM's Health and Fitness Journal* 6(1):27-30.

11. Herbet, D., and W. Herbert. 2005. Legal considerations. In *ACSM's resource manual for guidelines for exercise testing and prescription.* 5th ed. Ed. L.A. Kaminsky, 658-667. Philadelphia: Lippincott Williams & Wilkins.

12. Morrey, M., S. Finnie, D. Hensrud, and B. Warren. 2002. Screening, staffing, and emergency preparedness at worksite wellness facilities. *Medicine and Science in Sports and Exercise* 34(2):239-244.

13. Newkirk, J. 1999. Budgeting for control. *Fitness Management Magazine* 15(4):34-35.

14. Sattler, T., and C. Doniek. 1998. Planning and preparing a budget. *Fitness Management Magazine* 14(8):30-33.

15. Tharrett, S., and J. Peterson, eds. 1997. *ACSM's health/fitness facility standards and guidelines.* 2nd ed. Champaign, IL: Human Kinetics.

Chapter 27

1. Gowitzke, B.A., and M. Milner. 1988. *Scientific bases of human movement.* 3rd ed. Baltimore: Williams & Wilkins.

2. Gray, H. 1994. *Anatomy of the human body.* Philadelphia: Lea & Febiger.

3. Hall, S.J. 1995. *Basic biomechanics.* 2nd ed. St. Louis: Mosby.

4. Hamill, J., and K. Knutzen. 1995. *Biomechanical basis of human movement.* Baltimore: Williams & Wilkins.

5. Hay, J.G., and J.G. Reid. 1988. *The anatomical and mechanical bases of human motion.* Englewood Cliffs, NJ: Prentice Hall.

6. Kreighbaum, E., and K.M. Barthels. 1996. *Biomechanics.* 4th ed. Minneapolis: Burgess.

7. Luttgens, K., H. Deutsch, and N. Hamilton. 1992. *Kinesiology.* 8th ed. Madison, WI: Brown & Benchmark.

8. Rasch, P.J. 1989. *Kinesiology and applied anatomy.* 7th ed. Philadelphia: Lea & Febiger.

9. Thompson, C.W. 1994. *Manual of structural kinesiology.* St. Louis: Mosby.

Chapter 28

1. Åstrand, P-O. 1952. *Experimental studies of physical working capacity in relation to sex and age.* Copenhagen: Ejnar Munksgaard.

2. Åstrand, P-O., K. Rodahl, H.A. Dahl, and S.B. Strømme. 2003. *Textbook of work physiology.* 4th ed. Champaign, IL: Human Kinetics.

3. Bassett Jr., D.R. 1994. Skeletal muscle characteristics: Relationships to cardiovascular risk factors. *Medicine and Science in Sports and Exercise* 26:957-966.

4. Bassett, D.R., and E.T. Howley. 1997. Maximal oxygen uptake: Classical versus contemporary viewpoints. *Medicine and Science in Sports and Exercise* 29:591-603.

5. Bassett, D.R., and E.T. Howley. 2000. Limiting factors for maximal oxygen uptake and determinants of endurance performance. *Medicine and Science in Sports and Exercise* 32:70-84.

6. Bouchard, C., R. Lesage, G. Lortie, J. Simoneau, P. Hamel, M. Boulay, L. Perusse, G. Theriault, and C. Leblank. 1986. Aerobic performance in brothers, dizygotic and monozygotic twins. *Medicine and Science in Sports and Exercise* 18:639-646.

7. Brooks, G.A. 1985. Anaerobic threshold: Review of the concept, and directions for future research. *Medicine and Science in Sports and Exercise* 17:22-31.

8. Brooks, G.A., T.D. Fahey, and T.P. White. 2005. *Exercise physiology: Human bioenergetics and its application.* 4th ed. Mountain View, CA: Mayfield.

9. Claytor, R.P. 1985. *Selected cardiovascular, sympathoadrenal, and metabolic responses to one-leg exercise training.* Unpublished doctoral dissertation. University of Tennessee at Knoxville.

10. Coggan, A.R., and E.F. Coyle. 1991. Carbohydrate ingestion during prolonged exercise: Effects on metabolism and performance. *Exercise and Sport Sciences Reviews* 19:1-40.

11. Costill, D.L. 1988. Carbohydrates for exercise: Dietary demands of optimal performance. *International Journal of Sports Medicine* 9:1-18.

12. Coyle, E.F. 1988. Detraining and retention of training induced adaptations. In *Resource manual for guidelines for exercise testing and prescription,* ed. S.N. Blair, P. Painter, R.R. Pate, L.K. Smith, and C.B. Taylor, 83-89. Philadelphia: Lea & Febiger.

13. Coyle, E.F., M.K. Hemmert, and A.R. Coggan. 1986. Effects of detraining on cardiovascular responses to exercise: Role of blood volume. *Journal of Applied Physiology* 60:95-99.

14. Coyle, E.F., W.H. Martin III, S.A. Bloomfield, O.H. Lowry, and J.O. Holloszy. 1985. Effects of detraining on responses to submaximal exercise. *Journal of Applied Physiology* 59:853-859.

15. Coyle, E.F., W.H. Martin III, D.R. Sinacore, M.J. Joyner, J.M. Hagberg, and J.O. Holloszy. 1984. Time course of loss of adaptation after stopping prolonged intense endurance training. *Journal of Applied Physiology* 57:1857-1864.

16. Cureton, K.J., P.B. Sparling, B.W. Evans, S.M. Johnson, U.D. Kong, and J.W. Purvis. 1978. Effect of experimental alterations in excess weight on aerobic capacity and distance-running performance. *Medicine and Science in Sports* 10:194-199.

17. Davis, J.H. 1985. Anaerobic threshold: Review of the concept and directions for future research. *Medicine and Science in Sports and Exercise* 17:6-18.

18. Edington, D.W., and V.R. Edgerton. 1976. *The biology of physical activity.* Boston: Houghton Mifflin.

19. Ekblom, B., P-O. Åstrand, B. Saltin, J. Stenberg, and B. Wallstrom. 1968. Effect of training on circulatory response to exercise. *Journal of Applied Physiology* 24:518-528.

20. Faulkner, J.A., D.E. Roberts, R.L. Elk, and J. Conway. 1971. Cardiovascular responses to submaximum and maximum effort cycling and running. *Journal of Applied Physiology* 30:457-461.

21. Fleck, S.J., and L.S. Dean. 1987. Resistance-training experience and the pressor response during resistance exercise. *Journal of Applied Physiology* 63:116-120.

22. Fox, E.L., R.W. Bowers, and M.L. Foss. 1998. *Fox's the physiological basis for exercise and sport.* 6th ed. Dubuque, IA: Brown.

23. Franklin, B.A. 1985. Exercise testing, training, and arm ergometry. *Sports Medicine* 2:100-119.

24. Gisolfi, C., and C.B. Wenger. 1984. Temperature regulation during exercise: Old concepts, new ideas. *Exercise and Sport Sciences Reviews* 12:339-372.

25. Hickson, R.C., H.A. Bomze, and J.O. Holloszy. 1977. Linear increase in aerobic power induced by a strenuous program of endurance exercise. *Journal of Applied Physiology: Respiratory, Environmental and Exercise Physiology* 42:372-376.

26. Hickson, R.C., H.A. Bomze, and J.O. Holloszy. 1978. Faster adjustment of O_2 uptake to the energy requirement of exercise in the trained state. *Journal of Applied Physiology: Respiratory, Environmental and Exercise Physiology* 44:877-881.

27. Hickson, R.C., C. Foster, M.L. Pollock, T.M. Galassi, and S. Rich. 1985. Reduced training intensities and loss of aerobic power, endurance, and cardiac growth. *Journal of Applied Physiology* 58:492-499.

28. Hickson, R.C., C. Kanakis Jr., J.R. Davis, A.M. Moore, and S. Rich. 1982. Reduced training duration effects on aerobic power,

endurance, and cardiac growth. *Journal of Applied Physiology* 53:225-229.

29. Hickson, R.C., and M.A. Rosenkoetter. 1981. Reduced training frequencies and maintenance of increased aerobic power. *Medicine and Science in Sports and Exercise* 13:13-16.
30. Holloszy, J.O., and E.F. Coyle. 1984. Adaptations of skeletal muscle to endurance exercise and their metabolic consequences. *Journal of Applied Physiology: Respiratory, Environmental and Exercise Physiology* 56:831-838.
31. Howley, E.T. 1980. Effect of altitude on physical performance. In *Encyclopedia of physical education, fitness, and sports: Training, environment, nutrition, and fitness,* ed. G.A. Stull and T.K. Cureton, 177-187. Salt Lake City: Brighton.
32. Howley, E.T., D.R. Bassett Jr., and H.G. Welch. 1995. Criteria for maximal oxygen uptake—Review and commentary. *Medicine and Science in Sports and Exercise* 24:1055-1058.
33. Hultman, E. 1967. Physiological role of muscle glycogen in man, with special reference to exercise. *Circulation Research* 20-21(Suppl. 1): 99-114.
34. Issekutz, B., N.C. Birkhead, and K. Rodahl. 1962. The use of respiratory quotients in assessment of aerobic power capacity. *Journal of Applied Physiology* 17:47-50.
35. Kasch, F.W., J.L. Boyer, S.P. VanCamp, L.S. Verity, and J.P. Wallace. 1990. The effects of physical activity and inactivity on aerobic power in older men (a longitudinal study). *The Physician and Sportsmedicine* 18(4): 73-83.
36. Kasch, F.W., J.P. Wallace, and S.P. Van Camp. 1985. Effects of 18 years of endurance exercise on the physical work capacity of older men. *Journal of Cardiopulmonary Rehabilitation* 5:308-312.
37. Kasch, F.W., J.P. Wallace, S.P. Van Camp, and L.S. Verity. 1988. A longitudinal study of cardiovascular stability in active men aged 45 to 65 yrs. *The Physician and Sportsmedicine* 16(1): 117-126.
38. Katch, F.I., and W.D. McArdle. 1977. *Nutrition and weight control.* Boston: Houghton Mifflin.
39. Lind, A.R., and G.W. McNicol. 1967. Muscular factors which determine the cardiovascular responses to sustained and rhythmic exercise. *Canadian Medical Association Journal* 96:706-713.
40. MacDougall, J.D., D. Tuxen, D.G. Sale, J.R. Moroz, and J.R. Sutton. 1985. Arterial blood-pressure response to heavy resistance exercise. *Journal of Applied Physiology* 58:785-790.
41. McArdle, W.D., F.I. Katch, and V.L. Katch. 2006. *Exercise physiology, energy, nutrition, and human performance.* 6th ed. Baltimore: Lippincott Williams & Wilkins.
42. McArdle, W.D., F.I. Katch, and G.S. Pechar. 1973. Comparison of continuous and discontinuous treadmill and bicycle tests for max $\dot{V}O_2$. *Medicine and Science in Sports* 5(3): 156-160.
43. McArdle, W.D., and J.R. Magel. 1970. Physical work capacity and maximum oxygen uptake in treadmill and bicycle exercise. *Medicine and Science in Sports* 2(3):118-123.
44. Montoye, H.J., T. Ayen, F. Nagle, and E.T. Howley. 1986. The oxygen requirement for horizontal and grade walking on a motor-driven treadmill. *Medicine and Science in Sports and Exercise* 17:640-645.
45. Nagle, F.J., B. Balke, G. Baptista, J. Alleyia, and E. Howley. 1971. Compatibility of progressive treadmill, bicycle, and step tests based on oxygen-uptake responses. *Medicine and Science in Sports* 3:149-154.
46. Plowman, S.A., and D.L. Smith. 2003. *Exercise physiology for health, fitness and performance.* 2nd ed. New York: Benjamin Cummings.
47. Powers, S.K., S. Dodd, and R.E. Beadle. 1985. Oxygen-uptake kinetics in trained athletes differing in $\dot{V}O_2$max. *European Journal of Applied Physiology* 54:306-308.
48. Powers, S., S. Dodd, R. Deason, R. Byrd, and T. McKnight. 1983. Ventilatory threshold, running economy, and distance-running performance of trained athletes. *Research Quarterly for Exercise and Sport* 54:179-182.
49. Powers, S.K., and E.T. Howley. 2006. *Exercise physiology.* 6th ed. New York: McGraw-Hill.
50. Powers, S., W. Riley, and E. Howley. 1980. A comparison of fat metabolism in trained men and women during prolonged aerobic work. *Research Quarterly for Exercise and Sport* 52:427-431.
51. Raven, P.B., B.L. Drinkwater, R.O. Ruhling, N. Bolduan, S. Taguchi, J. Gliner, and S.M. Horvath. 1974. Effect of carbon monoxide and peroxyacetyl nitrate on man's maximal aerobic capacity. *Journal of Applied Physiology* 36:288-293.
52. Robergs, R.A., and S.J. Keteyian. 2003. *Fundamentals of exercise physiology: For fitness, performance and health.* 2nd ed. New York: McGraw-Hill.
53. Rowell, L.B. 1969. Circulation. *Medicine and Science in Sports* 1:15-22.
54. Rowell, L.B. 1986. *Human circulation-regulation during physical stress.* New York: Oxford University Press.
55. Sale, D.G. 1987. Influence of exercise and training on motor unit activation. *Exercise and Sport Sciences Reviews* 15:95-151.
56. Saltin, B. 1969. Physiological effects of physical conditioning. *Medicine and Science in Sports* 1:50-56.
57. Saltin, B., and P.D. Gollnick. 1983. Skeletal muscle adaptability: Significance for metabolism and performance. In *Handbook of physiology,* ed. L.D. Peachey, R.H. Adrian, and S.R. Geiger, 555-631. Baltimore: Williams & Wilkins.
58. Saltin, B., J. Henriksson, E. Nygaard, P. Anderson, and E. Jansson. 1977. Fiber types and metabolic potentials of skeletal muscles in sedentary man and endurance runners. *Annals of the New York Academy of Science* 301:3-29.
59. Saltin, B., and L. Hermansen. 1966. Esophageal, rectal, and muscle temperature during exercise. *Journal of Applied Physiology* 21:1757-1762.
60. Schwade, J., C.G. Blomqvist, and W. Shapiro. 1977. A comparison of the response to arm and leg work in patients with ischemic heart disease. *American Heart Journal* 94:203-208.
61. Sherman, W.M. 1983. Carbohydrates, muscle glycogen, and muscle glycogen supercompensation. In *Ergogenic aids in sports,* ed. M.H. Williams, 3-26. Champaign, IL: Human Kinetics.
62. Taylor, H.L., E.R. Buskirk, and A. Henschel. 1955. Maximal oxygen intake as an objective measure of cardiorespiratory performance. *Journal of Applied Physiology* 8:73-80.
63. Vander, A.J., J.H. Sherman, and D.S. Luciano. 1985. *Human physiology.* 4th ed. New York: McGraw-Hill.
64. Wilmore, J.H., and D.L. Costill. 1999. *Physiology of sport and exercise.* 2nd ed. Champaign, IL: Human Kinetics.

Appendix E

1. American College of Sports Medicine. 2006. *ACSM's guidelines for exercise testing and prescription.* 7th ed. Philadelphia: Lippincott Williams & Wilkins.
2. Canadian Association for Health, Physical Education, Recreation and Dance. 1994. *The Canadian active living challenge.* Gloucester, ON: Author.
3. Cooper Institute for Aerobics Research. 1992. *Prudential FITNESSGRAM test administration manual.* Dallas: Author.
4. Corbin, C.B., and R. Lindsey. 2002. *Fitness for life.* 4th ed. Champaign, IL: Human Kinetics.
5. Franks, B.D. 1989. *YMCA youth fitness test.* Champaign, IL: Human Kinetics.

6. President's Council on Physical Fitness and Sports. 2001. *President's challenge physical activity and fitness award program.* Washington, DC: Author.

7. President's Council on Physical Fitness and Sports. 1996. *Presidential sports award.* Washington, DC: Author.

8. Seaman, J.A. 1999. Physical activity and fitness for persons with disabilities. *PCPFS Research Digest* 3(5).

Index

Note: The letters *f* and *t* after page numbers indicate figures and tables, respectively.

U

V

W

Y

Z

About the Authors

Edward T. Howley, PhD, is a professor in the department of exercise, sport, and leisure studies at the University of Tennessee at Knoxville. Dr. Howley, who teaches an undergraduate course in fitness testing and prescription and undergraduate and graduate courses in exercise physiology, has been teaching and conducting research in the field for the past 35 years. He served as president of the American College of Sports Medicine (ACSM) in 2002-03 and helped develop and deliver ACSM certification programs.

Besides the previous editions of this book, Dr. Howley has authored another book, four book chapters, and 45 research articles dealing with exercise physiology, fitness testing, and prescription. He currently serves as editor in chief of *ACSM's Health and Fitness Journal*. He is a fellow in the American Academy of Kinesiology and Physical Education and is chair (2006-2007) of the Science Board of the President's Council for Physical Fitness and Sports. His research interests include exercise metabolism, obesity, and the effects of training. He has received several outstanding teacher awards. In his leisure time, Dr. Howley enjoys playing golf, biking, and swimming.

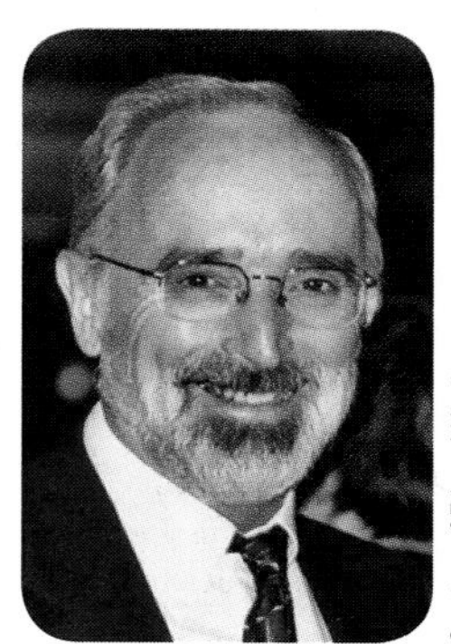
Courtesy of Edward Howley.

B. Don Franks, PhD, is a professor emeritus who has conducted research and taught physical activity, fitness, and health for 40 years. Dr. Franks, who earned his PhD from the University of Illinois under fitness pioneer T.K. Cureton, has received several honor and teaching awards and has been active for 40 years in the American Alliance for Health, Physical Education, Recreation and Dance (AAHPERD); the American Academy of Kinesiology and Physical Education (AAKPE); and the American College of Sports Medicine. He is past president of AAKPE and the AAHPERD Research Consortium. Dr. Franks enjoys playing racquetball and golf and skiing.

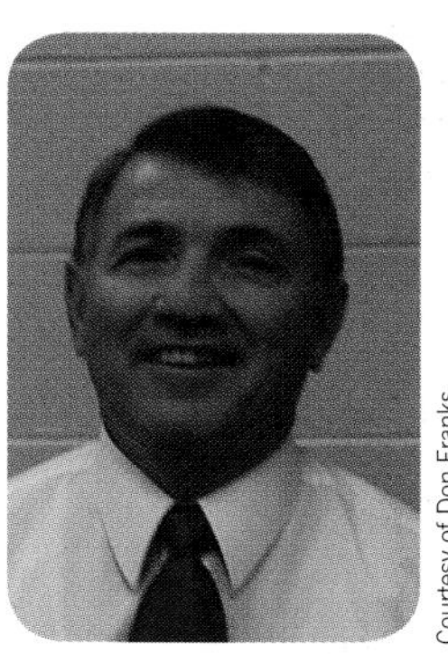
Courtesy of Don Franks.

About the Contributors

David R. Bassett Jr. is a professor in the department of exercise, sport, and leisure studies at the University of Tennessee in Knoxville. He is a fellow of the American College of Sports Medicine and a certified exercise specialist. He is also a frequent reviewer for several scientific journals. Dr. Bassett teaches courses in exercise physiology, clinical exercise physiology, and fitness testing and exercise prescription. His primary research focus is on objective methods of measuring physical activity, including pedometers, accelerometers, and heart rate monitors. He has also studied physical activity levels and obesity rates in Amish youth and adults in an effort to assess the effect of modern technology on these variables. In his spare time he enjoys hiking, bicycling, and running.

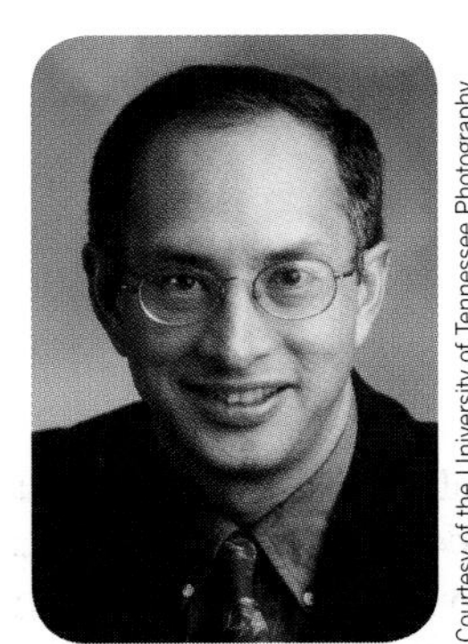

Courtesy of the University of Tennessee Photography Services.

Janet Buckworth, PhD, FACSM, is an associate professor of exercise science at The Ohio State University and part of the Health and Exercise Behavior Research Group. Her research areas are exercise adherence and the psychobiology of exercise and mental health. Dr. Buckworth directed a campus wellness program before earning her PhD in exercise psychology at the University of Georgia. She received funding from the National Institutes of Health to study exercise adherence in college students and coauthored *Exercise Psychology*, published in 2002, with Dr. Rod Dishman. Dr. Buckworth is a fellow of the American College of Sports Medicine.

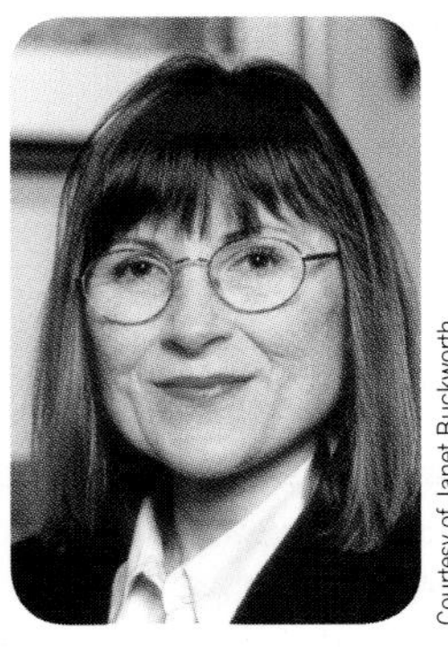

Courtesy of Janet Buckworth.

Sue Carver, ATC, MPT, CMT, is currently co-owner and practicing clinician at A World of Difference Therapy Services, an outpatient physical therapy clinic in Little Rock, Arkansas. She has been a licensed physical therapist since 1987 and has been practicing in Little Rock since 1989. She received her National Athletic Trainers certification in 1978. She served as the women's athletic trainer at the University of Tennessee at Knoxville from 1978 to 1982. In 1984 Ms. Carver was a volunteer athletic trainer at the U.S. Olympic Training Center in Colorado Springs. She was selected to work at the National Sports Festival VI in Baton Rouge in 1985 and the U.S. Olympic Track and Field Trials in Indianapolis in 1988. She was a volunteer trainer for track and field at the 1996 Summer Olympic Games in Atlanta.

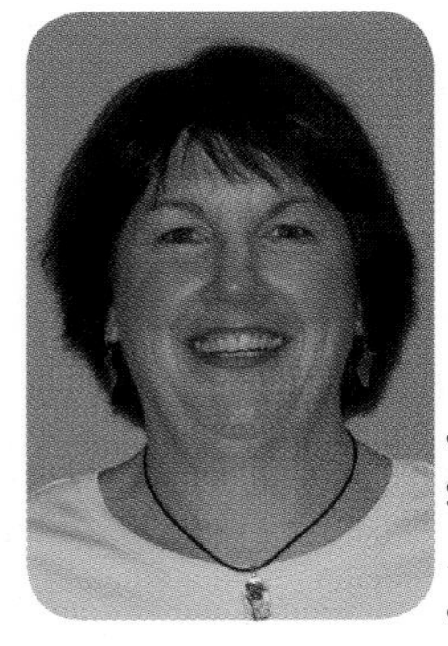

Courtesy of Sue Carver.

Avery D. Faigenbaum, EdD, CSCS, FACSM, is an associate professor in the department of health and exercise science at the College of New Jersey at Ewing, New Jersey. He is a leading researcher and practitioner in strength and conditioning and has coauthored five books and more than 100 articles on youth fitness and resistance training. He is a fellow of the American College of Sports Medicine and has served as vice president of the National Strength and Conditioning Association.

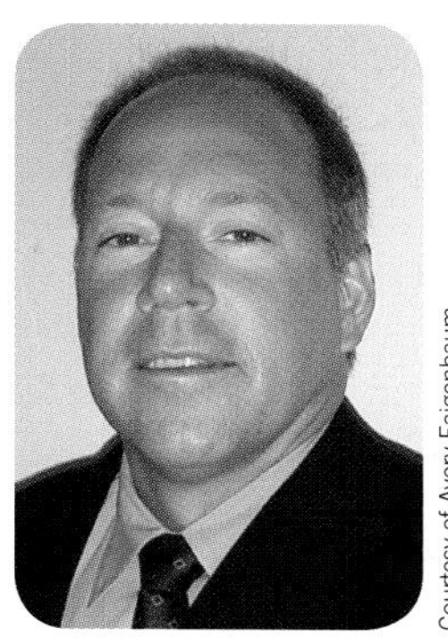
Courtesy of Avery Faigenbaum.

Ralph La Forge, MS, is a physiologist and managing director of the Duke lipid disorder and disease management training program at Duke University Medical Center, Division of Endocrinology, Metabolism and Nutrition. He has worked for 29 years in clinical cardiology and endocrinology and as an instructor of exercise physiology and psychobiology at the University of California at San Diego. He is currently a faculty member of the Center for Complementary Medicine and Alternative Therapies at the University of North Carolina at Chapel Hill.

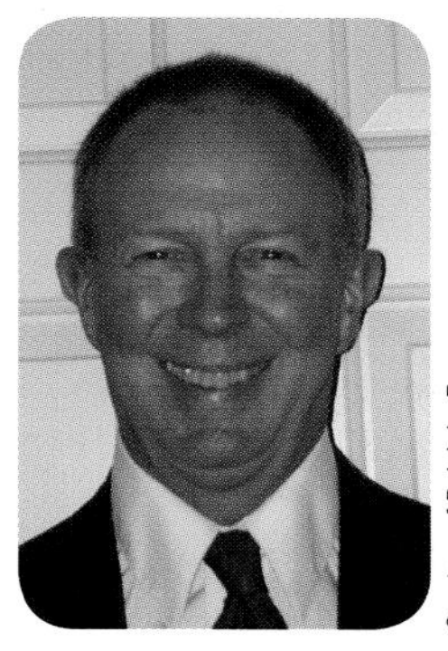
Courtesy of Ralph La Forge.

Jean Lewis received her doctorate in education (physical education with an emphasis in exercise physiology) from the University of Tennessee at Knoxville, where she is now a professor emeritus. She was involved in the establishment of undergraduate major concentrations in physical fitness and exercise physiology and has also developed courses in applied anatomy, applied kinesiology, and weight control, fitness, and exercise. Dr. Lewis was known for innovative teaching methods, which helped physical education majors understand how to apply kinesiological concepts. Recently retired, she misses the students and teaching, but is enjoying working in her garden and workshop.

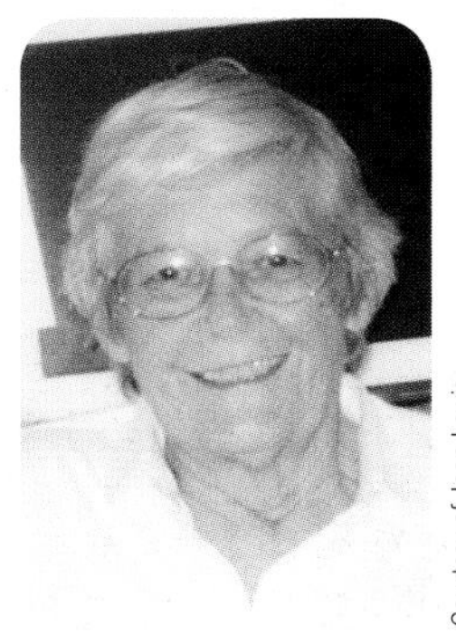
Courtesy of Jean Lewis.

Wendell Liemohn received his BA from Wartburg College in Waverly, Iowa, and his MA from the University of Iowa at Iowa City. After coaching and teaching on the collegiate level, he returned to the University of Iowa and completed his PhD. He was on the faculty of Indiana University for 7 years, where his research centered on psychomotor functioning in special populations. In 1978 he accepted a position as professor at the University of Tennessee. At Tennessee he started the graduate specialization in biomechanics and sports medicine. He is a former president of the Research Consortium for AAHPERD and is a fellow of ACSM and in the American Academy of Kinesiology and Physical Education. His research in sports medicine relates to flexibility and low-back functioning, and he authored the book *Exercise Prescription and the Back* (McGraw-Hill Medical Publishing, 2000). He retired from teaching in January 2005; however, he is still doing research on core stability.

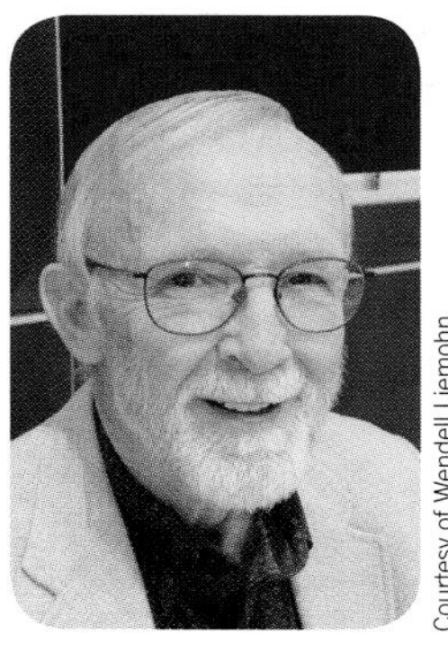
Courtesy of Wendell Liemohn.

Kyle J. McInnis, ScD, is professor and chair in the department of exercise and health sciences at the University of Massachusetts in Boston. Dr. McInnis is an experienced researcher and practitioner in the area of health/fitness and chronic disease prevention. He is a Fellow of the American College of Sports Medicine (ACSM) and a senior co-editor of the *ACSM's Health and Fitness Facilities Standards and Guidelines, Fourth Edition.* He resides in New Hampshire with his wife, Susan, and their three children, Brendan, Riley, and Shane.

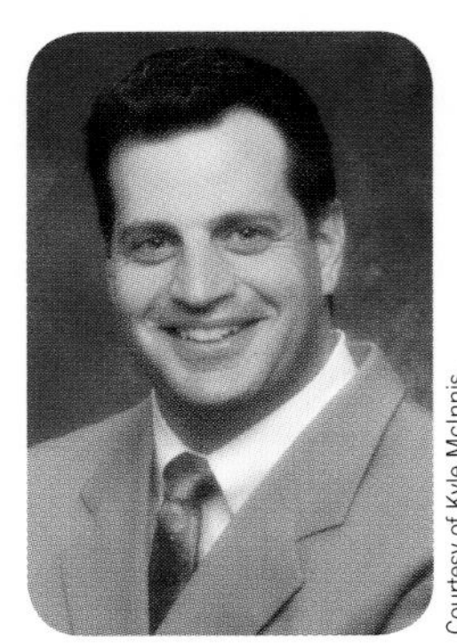
Courtesy of Kyle McInnis.

Michael Shipe, MS, RCEP, is an assistant professor of exercise science in the health, physical education and sport science department at Carson Newman College in Jefferson City, Tennessee. He attained his registered clinical exercise physiologist certification in 1999. Mr. Shipe served as the fitness director for the Blount Memorial Wellness Center from 1997 to 2001. He was director of the medical fitness and cardiac rehabilitation programs at Blount Memorial Hospital from 2002 to 2004. He is currently enrolled as a doctoral student in exercise science at the University of Tennessee.

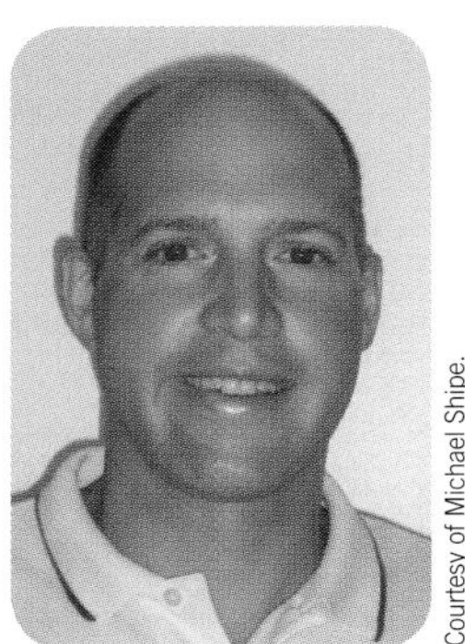
Courtesy of Michael Shipe.

Dixie L. Thompson, PhD, FACSM, is a professor in the department of exercise, sport, and leisure studies at the University of Tennessee at Knoxville. She focuses her research on body composition analysis and the effects of exercise on women's health. She is the director of the University of Tennessee's Center for Physical Activity and Health and associate editor in chief for *ACSM's Health and Fitness Journal,* and she has served as president of the Southeast chapter of ACSM. Dr. Thompson is a fellow of the American College of Sports Medicine.

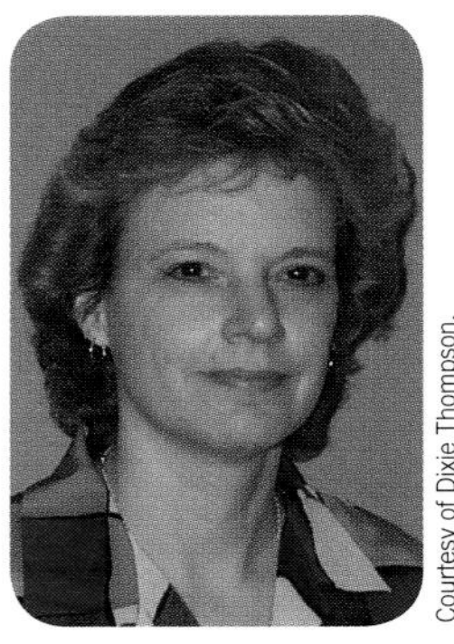
Courtesy of Dixie Thompson.